DICTIONARY
FOR
NURSES

Sphere Books Limited

Sphere Books Limited
27 Wrights Lane, London W8 5TZ

First published by Oxford University Press, 1984
with the title *Pocket Dictionary for Nurses*
Copyright © 1984 Market House Books Ltd
First published by Sphere Books Ltd 1987

TRADE

MARK

Set in Times

Printed and bound in Great Britain by
Cox & Wyman Ltd, Reading

PREFACE

THE *Pocket Dictionary for Nurses* is a new compilation which aims to reflect current clinical practice. It provides, in over 8000 entries, explanations of the terms and concepts likely to be encountered by nurses, therapists, radiographers, and those in similar professions during the course of their work. In addition to terms relating specifically to the nursing profession and the nursing process, there are many entries in the fields of medicine, surgery, anatomy and physiology, psychiatry, physiotherapy, and pharmacology (where trade names of commonly used drugs are listed at the end of entries for the appropriate official drug name).

Each entry contains a pronunciation guide, the part of speech, and a concisely written definition. The pronunciation guide, which is described in detail on page viii, follows that used in the *Oxford Paperback Dictionary* and provides an easy and accessible guide to correct pronunciation without the use of special symbols. Most definitions comprise a single sentence, but, where necessary, a second explanatory sentence is given. Many terms in medicine are used in combination with other phrases (for example *acute abscess*, *apical abscess*, etc.) and each of these phrases is treated as a separate definition within the main entry (*abscess* in this example). Derived terms (for example, adjectives derived from nouns) are not normally included as separate entries except where their meanings cannot be deduced from the words from which they are derived. Instead they are listed at the end of the definition of the parent word together with the part-of-speech and, where necessary, a pronunciation guide.

The Appendices include a comprehensive selection of tables of standard values for biochemical data, obtained from the *Oxford Textbook of Medicine*, together with tables of SI units and conversion tables to and from other systems of units.

In the preparation of this dictionary a range of entries has been adapted from the *Concise Medical Dictionary* published by the Oxford University Press in 1980 and by Corgi Books in 1982.

Consultant Editor
PAUL WAINWRIGHT M.Sc. SRN, RNT

General Editors
ROSALIND FERGUSSON BA
ELIZABETH MARTIN MA

PRONUNCIATION GUIDE

A pronunciation guide is given in brackets after the entry word and before the part of speech. Words of two or more syllables are broken up into small units, usually of one syllable, separated by hyphens. The stressed syllable in a word of two or more syllables is shown in **bold type**.

The sounds represented are as follows:

a *as in* back (bak), active (**ak**-tiv)
ă *as in* abduct (ăb-**dukt**), gamma (**gam**-ă)
ah *as in* after (**ahf**-ter), palm (pahm)
air *as in* aerosol (**air**-ŏ-sol), care (kair)
ar *as in* tar (tar), heart (hart)
aw *as in* jaw (jaw), gall (gawl)
ay *as in* mania (**may**-niă), grey (gray)
b *as in* bed (bed)
ch *as in* chin (chin)
d *as in* day (day)
e *as in* red (red)
ě *as in* bowel (**bow**-ěl)
ee *as in* see (see), haem (heem), caffeine (**kaf**-een)
eer *as in* fear (feer), serum (**seer**-ŭm)
er *as in* dermal (**der**-măl), labour (**lay**-ber)
ew *as in* dew (dew), nucleus (**new**-kli-ŭs)
ewr *as in* pure (pewr), dura (**dewr**-ă)
f *as in* fat (fat), phobia (**foh**-biă), cough (kof)
g *as in* gag (gag)
h *as in* hip (hip)
i *as in* fit (fit), acne (akni), reduction (ri-**duk**shŏn)
I *as in* eye (I), angiitis (an-ji-**I**-tis)
j *as in* jaw (jaw), gene (jeen), ridge (rij)
k *as in* kidney (**kid**-ni), chlorine (**klor**-een)

ks *as in* toxic (**toks**-ik)
kw *as in* quadrate (**kwod**-rayt)
l *as in* liver (**liv**-er)
m *as in* milk (milk)
n *as in* nit (nit)
ng *as in* sing (sing)
nk *as in* rank (rank), bronchus (**bronk**-ŭs)
o *as in* pot (pot)
ŏ *as in* buttock (**but**-ŏk)
oh *as in* home (hohm), post (pohst)
oi *as in* boil (boil)
oo *as in* food (food), croup (kroop), fluke (flook)
oor *as in* pruritus (proor-**I**-tŭs)
or *as in* organ (**or**-găn), wart (wort)
ow *as in* powder (**pow**-der), pouch (powch)
p *as in* pill (pil)
r *as in* rib (rib)
s *as in* skin (skin), cell (sel)
sh *as in* shock (shok), action (**ak**-shŏn)
t *as in* tone (tohn)
th *as in* bath (bahth)
th as in then (*th*en)
u *as in* pulp (pulp), blood (blud)
ŭ *as in* typhus (**ty**-fŭs)
uu *as in* hook (huuk)
v *as in* vein (vayn)
w *as in* wind (wind)
y *as in* yeast (yeast)
   or, when preceded by a consonant, *as in* bite (byt)
yoo *as in* unit (**yoo**-nit), formula (**form**-yoo-lă)
yoor *as in* ureter (yoor-**ee**-ter)
yr *as in* fire (fyr)
z *as in* zinc (zink), glucose (**gloo**-kohz)
zh as in vision (**vi***zh*-ŏn)

A consonant is sometimes doubled to prevent accidental mispronunciation of a syllable resembling a familiar word;

for example, **ass**-id (acid), rather than **as**-id; ultră-**sonn**-iks (ultrasonics), rather than ultră-**son**-iks.

An apostrophe is used (i) between two consonants forming a syllable, as in den-t'l (dental), and (ii) between two letters when the syllable might otherwise be mispronounced through resembling a familiar word, as in **th'e**-ra-pi (therapy), th'y (thigh), and tal'k (talc).

A

a- (an-) *prefix denoting* absence of; lacking; not.

ab- *prefix denoting* away from.

abarticulation (ab-ar-tik-yoo-lay-shŏn) *n.* 1. the dislocation of a joint. 2. a synovial joint (*see* diarthrosis).

abdomen (ab-dŏm-ĕn) *n.* the part of the body cavity below the chest (*see* thorax), from which it is separated by the diaphragm. The abdomen contains the organs of digestion – stomach, liver, intestines, etc. – and excretion – kidneys, bladder, etc., and is lined by a membrane, the peritoneum. **—abdominal** (ăb-**dom**-i-năl) *adj.*

abdominoperineal excision (ăb-dom-in-oh-pe-ri-nee-ăl) *n.* an operation for excision of the rectum in which incisions are made in both the abdomen and the perineum.

abdominoscopy (ăb-dom-i-**noss**-kŏ-pi) *n. see* laparoscopy.

abducens nerve (ăb-**dew**-sĕnz) *n.* the sixth cranial nerve (VI), which supplies the lateral rectus muscle of each eyeball.

abduct (ăb-**dukt**) *vb.* to move a limb or any other part away from the midline of the body. **—abduction** *n.*

abductor (ăb-**duk**-ter) *n.* any muscle that, when it contracts, moves one part of the body away from another or from the midline of the body.

aberrant (a-**be**-rănt) *adj.* abnormal: usually applied to a blood vessel or nerve that does not follow its normal course.

aberration (ab-er-**ay**-shŏn) *n.* 1. deviation from the normal. 2. the failure of a lens to focus light rays accurately.

ablation (ăb-**lay**-shŏn) *n.* surgical removal of tissue, a part of the body, or an abnormal growth, usually by cutting.

abnormal (ab-nor-măl) *adj.* deviating from the normal in structure, position, occurrence, etc.: *an abnormal growth.*

abnormality (ab-nor-**mal**-iti) *n.* 1. deviation from the normal or expected. 2. a malformation of deformity: *a developmental abnormality.*

abort (ă-**bort**) *vb.* 1. to terminate a process or disease before its full course has been run. 2. to remove or expel an embryo or fe-

Regions of the abdomen

tus from the womb before it is capable of independent existence. *See* abortion.

abortifacient (ă-bor-ti-**fay**-shĕnt) *n.* a drug that induces abortion or miscarriage.

abortion (ă-**bor**-shŏn) *n.* the expulsion or removal of an embryo or fetus from the womb at a stage of pregnancy when it is incapable of independent survival (i.e. at any time between conception and the 28th week of pregnancy). *complete a.* premature expulsion of the fetus and all its membranes. *criminal a.* (in Britain) abortion not carried out within the terms of the Abortion Act (1967). *habitual a.* abortion occurring in three or more successive pregnancies. *incomplete a.* retention by the womb of part of the fetus or its membranes during an abortion. *induced a.* the deliberate termination of a pregnancy before the 28th week. *inevitable a.* abortion that cannot be prevented as the fetus is dead. *missed a.* abortion in which the fetus is dead but not expelled from the womb. *spontaneous a.* miscarriage; naturally occurring abortion. *therapeutic a.* abortion induced to protect the life or health of the mother. *threatened a.* abdominal pain and bleeding from the womb while the fetus is still alive. —**abortionist** *n.* —**abortive** *adj.*

abortus (ă-**bor**-tŭs) *n.* a fetus, weighing less than 500 g, that is expelled from the mother's body either dead or incapable of surviving.

ABO system *n. see* blood group.

abrasion (ă-**bray**-zhŏn) *n.* a minor wound in which the surface of the skin or a mucous membrane is worn away by rubbing or scraping.

abreaction (ab-ree-**ak**-shŏn) *n.* the release of strong emotion associated with a buried memory. Abreaction may be induced as a treatment for hysteria, anxiety state, and other neurotic conditions.

abscess (**ab**-sis) *n.* a collection of pus enclosed by damaged and inflamed tissues. *acute a.* an abscess associated with pain, inflammation, and some fever. *apical a.* an abscess in the bone around the tip of the root of a tooth. *Brodie's a.* an abscess of bone due to chronic bacterial osteomyelitis. *cold* or *chronic a.* an abscess, usually due to tuberculosis organisms, in which there is little pain or inflammation. *psoas a.* a cold abscess in the psoas muscle (in the groin), which has spread from diseased vertebrae in the lower part of the spine. *subphrenic a.* an abscess in the space below the diaphragm, usually resulting from a spread of infection from the abdomen.

absorption (ăb-**sorp**-shŏn) *n.* the uptake of digested food from the intestine into the blood and lymphatic systems. *See also* assimilation, digestion.

abulia (ă-**boo**-liă) *n.* absence or impairment of will power, commonly a symptom of schizophrenia.

acanthosis (ak-ăn-**thoh**-sis) *n.* generalized thickening of the innermost (prickle-cell) layer of the epidermis, with abnormal multiplication and increase in the number of cells. *a. nigricans* dark warty growths, especially in skin folds such as the groin, armpits, and mouth, that are usually a sign of internal cancer.

acapnia (ă-**kap**-niă) *n.* a condition in which there is an abnormally low concentration of carbon dioxide in the blood.

acariasis (akă-ry-ă-sis) *n.* an infestation of mites and ticks.

acaricide (ă-**ka**-ri-syd) *n.* any chemical agent used for destroying mites and ticks.

acatalasia (ă-kat-ă-**lay**-ziă) *n.* an inborn lack of the enzyme catalase, leading to recurrent infections of the gums (gingivitis) and mouth.

accessory nerve (spinal accessory nerve) (ăk-**sess**-er-i) *n.* the eleventh cranial nerve (XI), which arises from two roots, cranial and spinal. Fibres from the cranial root form the recurrent laryngeal nerve, which supplies the internal laryngeal muscles; fibres from the spinal root supply the sternomastoid and trapezius muscles, in the neck region.

accommodation (ă-kom-ŏ-**day**-shŏn) *n.* adjustment of the shape of the lens to change the focus of the eye. When the ciliary muscle (*see* ciliary body) is relaxed, the lens is flattened and the eye is then able to focus on distant objects. To focus the eye on near objects the ciliary muscles contract and the lens becomes more spherical.

accouchement (ă-**koosh**-mahnt) *n.* delivery of a baby.

accountability (ă-kownt-ă-**bil**-iti) *n.* the obligation to disclose to others information about one's actions or the performance of tasks for which one is responsible.

accreditation (ă-kred-i-**tay**-shŏn) *n.* **1.** formal recognition by an organization of an individual as an approved and acknowledged representative, e.g. of a union or staff organization. **2.** (in the USA) the licensing of a hospital by government agencies, subject to its meeting certain prerequisite conditions.

accretion (ă-**kree**-shŏn) *n.* the accumulation of deposits in an organ or cavity. Calculi may be formed by accretion.

acephalus (ă-**sef**-ă-lŭs) *n.* a fetus without a head. —**acephalous** *adj.*

acetabuloplasty (ass-i-**tab**-yoo-loh-plas-ti) *n.* an operation in which the shape of the acetabulum is modified to correct congenital dislocation of the hip or to treat osteoarthritis.

acetabulum (cotyloid cavity) (ass-i-**tab**-yoo-lŭm) *n.* (*pl.* **acetabula**) either of the two deep sockets, one on each side of the hip bone, into which the head of the thigh bone (femur) fits.

acetarsol (ass-i-**tar**-sŏl) *n.* an arsenic-containing|drug|administered by mouth for the treatment of amoebic dysentery, yaws, and Vincent's angina; as vaginal tablets for vaginitis; and as a rectal suppository for proctitis.

acetate (**ass**-it-ayt) *n.* any salt or ester of acetic acid.

acetazolamide (ass-ee-tă-**zol**-ă-myd) *n.* a diuretic used in the treatment of glaucoma to reduce the pressure inside the eyeball. Trade names: **Acetazide**, **Diamox**.

acetic acid (ă-**see**-tik) *n.* the acid that is present in vinegar. It is used in the preparation of astringent and antiseptic medicines and in urine testing. Formula: CH_3COOH.

acetoacetic acid (ass-i-toh-ă-**see**-tik) *n.* an organic acid produced in large amounts by the liver in such conditions as starvation. Formula: CH_3COCH_2COOH. *See also* ketone.

acetohexamide (ass-i-toh-**heks**-ă-myd) *n.* a drug that reduces the level of blood sugar, administered by mouth in the treatment of diabetes mellitus.

acetonaemia (ass-i-toh-**nee**-miă) *n.* the presence of acetone bodies in the blood. *See* ketone.

acetone (**ass**-i-tohn) *n.* an organic compound that is produced by the liver in such conditions as starvation. Acetone is of great value as a solvent. Formula: CH_3COCH_3. *See also* ketone.

acetone body (ketone body) *n. see* ketone.

acetonuria (ass-i-toh-**newr**-iă) *n. see* ketonuria.

acetylcholine (ass-i-tyl-**koh**-leen) *n.* the acetic acid ester of the organic base choline: the neurotransmitter released at the synapses of parasympathetic nerves and at neuromuscular junctions. *See also* cholinesterase.

acetylcoenzyme A (ass-i-tyl-koh-en-zym) *n.* a compound formed by the combination of an acetate molecule with coenzyme A. Acetylcoenzyme A has an important role in the Krebs cycle.

acetylcysteine (ass-i-tyl-**siss**-ti-een) *n.* a drug that is administered as an aerosol for the treatment of respiratory diseases, such as bronchitis, and cystic fibrosis.

acetylsalicylic acid (ass-i-tyl-sa-li-sil-ik) *n. see* aspirin.

achalasia (cardiospasm) (ak-ă-**lay**-ziă) *n.* a condition in which the normal muscular activity of the oesophagus (gullet) is disturbed, which delays the passage of swallowed material.

Achilles tendon (ă-**kil**-eez) *n.* the tendon of the muscles of the calf of the leg (the gastrocnemius and soleus muscles), situated at the back of the ankle and attached to the calcaneus (heel bone).

achillorrhaphy (ak-i-lo-**răfi**) *n.* surgical repair of the Achilles tendon.

achillotomy (ak-i-**lot**-ŏmi) *n.* surgical division of the Achilles tendon.

achlorhydria (ay-klor-**hy**-driă) *n.* absence of hydrochloric acid in the stomach. It is sometimes associated with pernicious anaemia.

acholia (ă-**koh**-liă) *n.* absence or deficiency of bile secretion or failure of the bile to enter the alimentary canal.

acholuria (ak-oh-**lewr**-iă) *n.* absence of the bile pigments from the urine, which occurs in some forms of jaundice (*acholuric jaundice*). —**acholuric** *adj.*

achondroplasia (ă-kon-droh-**play**-ziă) *n.* an inherited disorder in which the bones of the arms and legs fail to grow to normal size. It results in a type of dwarfism characterized by short limbs, a normal-sized head and body, and normal intelligence. —**achondroplastic** (ă-kon-droh-**plas**-tik) *adj.*

achromatic (ak-roh-**mat**-ik) *adj.* without colour. —**achromasia** (ak-roh-**may**-ziă) *n.*

achromatopsia (ă-kroh-mă-**top**-siă) *n.* the inability to perceive colour. Such complete colour blindness is very rare and is usually determined by hereditary factors.

achylia (ă-**ky**-liă) *n.* absence of secretion. *a. gastrica* a nonsecreting stomach whose lining (mucosa) is atrophied.

acid (**ass**-id) *n.* a substance that releases hydrogen ions when dissolved in water, has a pH below 7 and turns litmus paper red, and reacts with a base to form a salt and water only. *Compare* base.

acidaemia (asid-ee-miă) *n.* a condition of abnormally high blood acidity. *See also* acidosis. *Compare* alkalaemia.

acid-base balance *n.* the balance between the amount of carbonic acid and bicarbonate in the blood, which must be maintained at a constant ratio of 1:20 in order to keep the hydrogen ion concentration of the plasma at a constant value (pH 7.4).

acid-fast *adj.* 1. describing bacteria that have been stained and continue to hold the stain after treatment with an acidic solution. 2. describing a stain that is not removed from a specimen by washing with an acidic solution.

acidity (ă-sid-iti) *n.* the state of being acid. The degree of acidity of a solution is measured on the pH scale (*see* pH).

acidosis (asid-oh-sis) *n.* a condition in which the acidity of body fluids and tissues is abnormally high. This arises because of a failure of the mechanisms responsible for maintaining a balance between acids and alkalis in the blood (*see* acid-base balance). —**acidotic** (asid-ot-ik) *adj.*

acid phosphatase *n.* an enzyme secreted in the seminal fluid by the prostate gland.

acinus (ass-in-ŭs) *n.* (*pl.* acini) 1. a small sac or cavity surrounded by the secretory cells of a gland. 2. (in the lung) the tissue supplied with air by one terminal bronchiole. —**acinous** *adj.*

acne (ak-ni) *n.* a skin disorder in which the sebaceous glands become inflamed. *a. vulgaris* the commonest variety of acne, generally starting in adolescence. It is caused by overactivity of the sebaceous glands and results in pustules and blackheads, mainly on the face, chest, and back. *See also* rosacea.

acoustic (ă-koo-stik) *adj.* of or relating to sound or the sense of hearing. *a. holography* a technique of building up a three-dimensional picture of structures within the body using ultrasound waves. *a. nerve see* vestibulocochlear nerve.

acquired (ă-kwyrd) *adj.* describing a condition or disorder contracted after birth and not attributable to hereditary causes. *Compare* congenital.

acquired immune deficiency syndrome *n. see* AIDS.

acriflavine (ak-ri-flay-vin) *n.* a dye used as an antiseptic on skin and mucous membranes and to disinfect contaminated wounds.

acro- *prefix denoting* 1. extremity; tip. 2. height; promontory. 3. extreme; intense.

acrocentric (ak-roh-sen-trik) *n.* a chromosome in which the centromere is situated at or very near one end. —**acrocentric** *adj.*

acrocyanosis (ak-roh-sy-ă-noh-sis) *n.* bluish-purple discoloration of the hands and feet due to slow circulation of the blood through the small vessels in the skin.

acrodynia (ak-roh-din-iă) *n. see* pink disease.

acromegaly (ak-roh-meg-ăli) *n.* increase in size of the hands, feet, and the face due to excessive production of growth hormone by a tumour of the anterior pituitary gland. *See also* gigantism.

acromion (ă-kroh-mi-ŏn) *n.* an oblong process at the top of the spine of the scapula, part of which articulates with the clavicle (collar bone) to form the

acromioclavicular joint. —**acromial**
adj.

acronyx (ak-rŏ-niks) *n.* an ingrowing toenail or fingernail. *See* ingrowing toenail.

acroparaesthesiae (ak-roh-pa-ristheez-i-ee) *n.* a tingling sensation in the hands and feet.

acrophobia (ak-rŏ-foh-biă) *n.* a morbid dread of heights.

acrosclerosis (ak-roh-skleer-oh-sis) *n.* a skin disease thought to be a type of generalized scleroderma, mainly affecting the hands, face, and feet.

acrosome (ak-rŏ-sohm) *n.* the caplike structure on the front end of a spermatozoon.

ACTH (**adrenocorticotrophic hormone, adrenocorticotrophin, corticotrophin**) *n.* a hormone synthesized and stored in the anterior pituitary gland, controlling the secretion of corticosteroid hormones from the adrenal gland. It is administered by injection to treat conditions such as rheumatic diseases (especially in children) and asthma.

actin (ak-tin) *n.* a protein, found in muscle, that plays an important role in the process of contraction. *See* striated muscle.

Actinomyces (ak-ti-noh-my-seez) *n.* a genus of Gram-positive nonmotile fungus-like bacteria that cause disease in animals and man. *A. israeli* the causative organism of human actinomycosis.

actinomycin (ak-ti-noh-my-sin) *n.* a cytotoxic drug that inhibits the growth of cancer cells. There are two forms, actinomycin C and actinomycin D, both of which are administered by injection.

actinomycosis (ak-ti-noh-my-koh-sis) *n.* a noncontagious disease caused by the bacterium *Actinomyces israeli* and resulting in the formation of multiple sinuses that open onto the skin. Actinomycosis most commonly affects the jaw but may also affect the lungs, brain, or intestines.

actinotherapy (ak-ti-noh-th'e-ră-pi) *n.* the treatment of disorders with infrared or ultraviolet radiation.

action potential (ak-shŏn) *n.* the change in voltage that occurs across the membrane of a nerve or muscle cell when a nerve impulse is triggered.

activator (ak-ti-vay-ter) *n.* a substance that stimulates a chemical change or reaction.

active movement (ak-tiv) *n.* movement brought about by a patient's own efforts. *Compare* passive movement.

active principle *n.* an ingredient of a drug that is actively involved in its therapeutic effect.

activity of daily living (**activity of living, ADL, AL**) (ak-tiv-iti) *n.* any of the routine activities that a healthy individual does for himself during the course of the day, such as eating, drinking, or washing.

actomyosin (ak-toh-my-oh-sin) *n.* a protein complex formed in muscle between actin and myosin during the process of contraction. *See* striated muscle.

acupuncture (ak-yoo-punk-cher) *n.* a traditional Chinese system of healing in which thin metal needles are inserted into selected points beneath the skin to relieve pain or induce anaesthesia.

acute (ă-kewt) *adj.* **1.** describing a disease of rapid onset, severe symptoms, and brief duration. *Compare* chronic. **2.** describing any intense symptom, such as severe pain.

acute abdomen *n.* an emergency surgical condition caused by damage to one or more abdominal organs following injury or disease.

acute rheumatism *n.* *see* rheumatic fever.

acystia (ă-sis-tiă) *n.* congenital absence of the bladder.

ad- *prefix denoting* towards or near.

adamantinoma (ad-ă-man-ti-noh-mă) *n.* *see* ameloblastoma.

Adam's apple (laryngeal prominence) (ad-ămz) *n.* a projection, lying just under the skin, of the thyroid cartilage of the larynx.

adaptation (ad-ăp-tay-shŏn) *n.* the phenomenon in which a sense organ shows a gradually diminishing response to continuous or repetitive stimulation.

addiction (ă-dik-shŏn) *n.* a state of dependence produced by the habitual taking of any of certain drugs. *See also* alcoholism, tolerance.

Addison's disease (ad-i-sŏnz) *n.* a syndrome due to inadequate secretion of corticosteroid hormones by the adrenal glands. Symptoms include weakness, loss of energy, low blood pressure, and dark pigmentation of the skin. [T. Addison (1793–1860), British physician]

adduct (ă-dukt) *vb.* to move a limb or any other part towards the midline of the body. —**adduction** *n.*

adductor (ă-duk-ter) *n.* any muscle that moves one part of the body towards another or towards the midline of the body.

aden- (adeno-) *prefix denoting* a gland or glands.

adenine (ad-ĕ-neen) *n.* one of the nitrogen-containing bases (*see* purine) that occurs in the nucleic

acids DNA and RNA. *See also* ATP.

adenitis (ad-ĕ-ny-tis) *n.* inflammation of one or more glands or lymph nodes.

adenocarcinoma (ad-in-oh-kar-si-noh-mă) *n.* (*pl.* **adenocarcinomata**) a malignant epithelial tumour arising from glandular tissue. The term is also applied to tumours showing a glandular growth pattern.

adenohypophysis (ad-in-oh-hy-pof-i-sis) *n.* *see* pituitary gland.

adenoidectomy (ad-in-oid-ek-tŏmi) *n.* surgical removal of the adenoids.

adenoids (pharyngeal tonsils) (ad-in-oidz) *pl.* *n.* the collection of lymphatic tissue at the rear of the nose. Enlargement of the adenoids may cause obstruction to breathing through the nose.

adenoma (ad-in-oh-mă) *n.* (*pl.* **adenomata**) a benign tumour of epithelial origin that is derived from glandular tissue or exhibits clearly defined glandular structures. Adenomas may become malignant (*see* adenocarcinoma).

adenomyoma (ad-in-oh-my-oh-mă) *n.* a benign tumour derived from glandular and muscular tissue. Adenomyomas frequently occur in the uterus.

adenopathy (ad-in-op-ăthi) *n.* disease of a gland, especially a lymphatic gland.

adenosclerosis (ad-in-oh-skleer-oh-sis) *n.* hardening of a gland, usually due to calcification.

adenosine (ă-den-ŏ-seen) *n.* a compound containing adenine and the sugar ribose: it occurs in ATP. *See also* nucleoside.

adenosine diphosphate *n.* *see* ADP.

adenosine monophosphate *n.* *see* AMP.

adenosine triphosphate *n. see* ATP.

adenosis (ad-in-**oh**-sis) *n.* (*pl.* **adenoses**) **1.** excessive growth or development of glands. **2.** any disease of a gland, especially of a lymph gland (node).

adenovirus (ad-in-oh-vy-rŭs) *n.* one of a group of DNA-containing viruses causing latent infections of the upper respiratory tract that produce symptoms resembling those of the common cold.

adhesion (ăd-**hee**-*zh*ŏn) *n.* **1.** the union of two normally separate surfaces by fibrous connective tissue developing in an inflamed or damaged region. (The fibrous tissue itself is also called an adhesion.) Adhesion between loops of intestine may occur following abdominal surgery. **2.** a healing process in which the edges of a wound fit together.

adiadochokinesis (ă-dy-ă-doh-koh-ki-**nee**-sis) *n. see* dysdiadochokinesis.

adiaphoresis (ă-dy-ă-fŏ-**ree**-sis) *n.* deficient or reduced secretion of sweat. —**adiaphoretic** (ă-dy-ă-fŏ-ret-ik) *adj.*

adipose tissue (ad-i-pohs) *n.* fibrous connective tissue packed with masses of fat cells. It forms a thick layer under the skin and occurs around the kidneys and in the buttocks.

adiposis (liposis) (ad-i-**poh**-sis) *n.* the presence of abnormally large accumulations of fat in the body. The condition may arise from overeating, hormone irregularities, or a metabolic disorder. *See also* obesity.

adiposuria (ad-i-poh-**sewr**-iă) *n. see* lipuria.

aditus (**ad**-i-tŭs) *n.* an anatomical opening or passage; for example, the opening of the tympanic cavity (middle ear) to the air spaces of the mastoid process.

adjuvant (**aj**-oo-vănt) *n.* any substance used in conjunction with another to enhance its activity.

adnexa (ad-**neks**-ă) *pl. n.* adjoining parts. *uterine a.* the Fallopian tubes and ovaries.

adolescence (ad-ŏ-**less**-ĕns) *n.* the period of development between puberty and adulthood. —**adolescent** *n., adj.*

ADP (adenosine diphosphate) *n.* a compound containing adenine, ribose, and two phosphate groups. ADP occurs in cells and is involved in processes requiring the transfer of energy (*see* ATP).

adrenalectomy (ă-dree-năl-ek-tŏmi) *n.* surgical removal of one or both adrenal glands.

adrenal glands (suprarenal glands) (ă-**dree**-năl) *pl. n.* two triangular endocrine glands, each of which covers the superior surface of a kidney. The *medulla* forms the grey core of the gland and produces adrenaline and noradrenaline. The *cortex* is a yellowish tissue surrounding the medulla; it produces corticosteroid hormones.

adrenaline (epinephrine) (ă-**dren**-ă-lin) *n.* an important hormone secreted by the medulla of the adrenal gland. It has widespread effects on circulation, the muscles, and sugar metabolism. The action of the heart is increased, the rate and depth of breathing are increased, and the metabolic rate is raised; the force of muscular contraction improves and the onset of muscular fatigue is delayed. At the same time the blood supply to the bladder and intestines is reduced, their muscular walls relax, and the sphincters contract. Adrenaline is administered by injection for the relief of bronchial asthma; it is also used during surgery to reduce blood loss by constricting vessels in the skin.

adrenergic (ad-rĕ-ner-jik) *adj.* describing nerve fibres that release noradrenaline as a neurotransmitter. *Compare* cholinergic.

adrenocorticotrophic hormone (adrenocorticotrophin) (ă-dree-noh-kor-ti-koh-trof-ik) *n. see* ACTH.

adrenogenital syndrome (ă-dree-noh-jen-it-ăl) *n.* precocious sexual development and apparent masculinization in girls, caused by overproduction of hormones by the adrenal cortex in infancy.

adrenolytic (ă-dree-noh-lit-ik) *adj.* inhibiting the activity of adrenergic nerves. Adrenolytic activity is opposite to that of adrenaline.

adsorbent (ăd-sor-bĕnt) *n.* a substance that attracts other substances to its surface to form a film. Charcoal and kaolin are adsorbents.

adsorption (ăd-sorp-shŏn) *n.* the formation of a layer of atoms or molecules of one substance on the surface of a solid or liquid of different substance. *See* absorbent.

advancement (ăd-vahns-mĕnt) *n.* the detachment by surgery of a muscle or tendon and its reattachment at a more advanced (anterior) point. The technique is used, for example, in the treatment of squint.

adventitia (tunica adventitia) (ad-ven-ti-shă) *n.* 1. the outer coat of the wall of a vein or artery. 2. the outer covering of various other organs or parts.

adventitious (ad-ven-ti-shŭs) *adj.* 1. occurring in a place other than the usual one. 2. relating to the adventitia.

Aëdes (ay-ee-deez) *n.* a genus of widely distributed mosquitoes occurring throughout the tropics and subtropics. *A. aegypti* the principal vector of dengue and yellow fever.

aegophony (e-gof-ŏni) *n. see* vocal resonance.

-aemia *suffix denoting* a specified condition of the blood.

aer- (aero-) *prefix denoting* air or gas.

aerobe (air-ohb) *n.* any organism, especially a microbe, that requires the presence of free oxygen for life and growth. *Compare* anaerobe. —**aerobic** (air-oh-bik) *adj.*

aerobic respiration *n.* a type of cellular respiration in which foodstuffs (carbohydrates) are completely oxidized by atmospheric oxygen, with the production of maximum chemical energy from the foodstuffs.

aerogenous (air-oj-ĕnŭs) *adj.* producing gas. The term is applied to bacteria such as *Clostridium welchii*, which causes gas gangrene.

aerophagy (air-off-ăji) *n.* the swallowing of air. Voluntary aerophagy is used to permit oesophageal speech after surgical removal of the larynx (usually for cancer).

aerosol (air-ŏ-sol) *n.* a suspension of extremely small liquid or solid particles in the air. Drugs in aerosol form may be administered by inhalation.

aetiology (etiology) (ee-ti-ol-ŏji) *n.* 1. the study or science of the causes of disease. 2. the cause of a specific disease.

afebrile (ay-feb-ryl) *adj.* without, or not showing any signs of, a fever.

affect (af-ekt) *n.* (in psychiatry) a wave of emotion or the emotion associated with a particular idea. —**affective** *adj.*

afferent (af-er-ĕnt) *adj.* 1. designating nerves or neurones that convey impulses to the brain or spinal cord. 2. designating blood vessels that feed a capillary network in an organ or part. 3. designating lymphatic vessels that enter a lymph node. *Compare* efferent.

affinity (ă-fin-iti) *n.* the chemical attraction of one substance to another or others.

aflatoxin (af-lă-toks-in) *n.* a poisonous substance produced in the spores of the fungus *Aspergillus flavus*, which infects peanuts. It is known to produce cancer in certain animals.

afterbirth (ahf-ter-berth) *n.* the placenta, umbilical cord, and ruptured membranes associated with the fetus, which normally become detached from the womb and expelled within a few hours of birth.

after-care (ahf-ter-kair) *n.* 1. long-term surveillance as an adjunct or supplement to formal medical treatment of those who are chronically sick or handicapped. After-care includes the provision of special aids and the adaptation of homes to improve daily living. 2. surveillance of convalescents.

after-image (ahf-ter-im-ij) *n.* an impression of an image that is registered by the brain for a brief moment after an object is removed from in front of the eye, or after the eye is closed.

after-pains (ahf-ter-paynz) *pl. n.* pains in the womb during the first few days after childbirth, caused by contraction of the womb muscles.

agalactia (ag-al-ak-tiă) *n.* absence or abnormally low production of milk in a woman who has just given birth.

agammaglobulinaemia (ă-gam-ă-glob-yoo-lin-ee-miă) *n.* a total deficiency of the plasma protein gamma globulin. *Compare* hypogammaglobulinaemia.

agar (ay-ger) *n.* an extract of certain seaweeds that forms a gel suitable for the solidification of liquid bacteriological culture media. Agar may also be used as a laxative.

agenesis (ă-jen-ĕsis) *n.* absence of an organ, usually due to total failure of its development in the embryo.

agglutination (clumping) (ă-gloo-tin-ay-shŏn) *n.* the sticking together of such microscopic antigenic particles as red blood cells or bacteria so that they form visible clumps. —**agglutinative** *adj.*

agglutinin (ă-gloo-tin-in) *n.* an antibody that brings about the agglutination of bacteria, blood cells, or other antigenic particles.

agglutinogen (ă-gloo-tin-oh-jĕn) *n.* any antigen that provokes formation of an agglutinin in the serum and is therefore likely to be involved in agglutination.

aglossia (ă-gloss-iă) *n.* congenital absence of the tongue.

aglutition (a-gloo-ti-shŏn) *n.* inability to swallow. *See also* dysphagia.

agnosia (ag-noh-ziă) *n.* a disorder of the brain whereby the patient cannot interpret sensations correctly although the sense organs and nerves conducting sensation to the brain are functioning normally.

agonist (prime mover) (ag-ŏ-nist) *n.* a muscle whose active contraction causes movement of a part of the body. Contraction of an agonist is associated with relaxation of its antagonist.

agoraphobia (ag-er-ă-foh-biă) *n.* a morbid fear of public places and/or of open spaces. *See also* phobia.

agranulocytosis (ă-gran-yoo-loh-sy-toh-sis) *n.* a disorder in which there is a severe acute deficiency of certain blood cells (neutrophils) as a result of damage to the bone marrow by toxic drugs or chemicals. It is characterized by fever, with ulceration of the mouth and throat, and rapidly leads to prostration and death.

agraphia (dysgraphia) (ă-graf-iă) *n.* an acquired inability to write, although the strength and coordination of the hand remain normal.

ague (ay-gew) *n. see* malaria.

AID *n. see* artificial insemination.

AIDS (acquired immune deficiency syndrome) (aydz) *n.* a syndrome, caused by a virus, in which the body's natural resistance to disease is destroyed, leaving it vulnerable to fatal infections and cancers (*see* Kaposi's sarcoma). It is the most prevalent among male homosexuals.

AIH *n. see* artificial insemination.

air bed (air) *n.* a bed with a mattress whose upper surface is perforated with thousands of holes through which air is forced under pressure, so that the patient is supported on a cushion of air. Air beds are invaluable for the treatment of patients with large areas of burns.

air embolism *n.* an air lock that obstructs the outflow of blood from the right ventricle of the heart. Tipping the patient head down, lying on the left side, may move the air lock.

air hunger *n.* difficulty in breathing characterized by sighing and gasping. It is caused by anoxia.

air sickness *n. see* travel sickness.

akinesia (ak-in-ee-ziă) *n.* a loss of normal muscular tonicity or responsiveness. **akinetic epilepsy** a form of epilepsy in which there is a sudden loss of muscular tonicity, making the patient fall with momentary loss of consciousness. **akinetic mutism** a state of complete physical unresponsiveness although the patient's eyes remain open and appear to follow movements. It is a consequence of damage to the base of the brain. —**akinetic** (a-kin-et-ik) *adj.*

ala (al-ă) *n.* (*pl.* **alae**) (in anatomy) a winglike structure.

alanine (al-ă-neen) *n. see* amino acid.

alastrim (ă-las-trim) *n.* a mild form of smallpox, causing only a sparse rash and low-grade fever. Medical name: **variola minor.**

Albee's operation (awl-beez) *n.* **1.** an operation to produce ankylosis of the hip. The upper surface of the femur and the corresponding part of the acetabulum are removed and the two exposed surfaces allowed to remain in contact. **2.** an operation to immobilize part of the spinal column, using a bone graft from the tibia. [F. H. Albee (1876–1945), US surgeon]

Albers-Schönberg disease (al-bers shern-berg) *n. see* osteopetrosis. [H. E. Albers-Schönberg (1865–1921), German radiologist]

albinism (al-bin-izm) *n.* the inherited absence of pigmentation in the skin, hair, and eyes (*see* albino).

albino (al-**bee**-noh) *n.* an individual lacking the normal body pigment (melanin). Albinos have white hair and pink skin and eyes.

albumin (**al**-bew-min) *n.* a protein that is soluble in water and coagulated by heat. *serum a.* a protein found in blood plasma that is important for the maintenance of plasma volume.

albuminuria (proteinuria) (al-bew-min-**yoor**-iă) *n.* the presence of serum albumin, serum globulin, or other serum proteins in the urine, which may be associated with kidney or heart disease. *orthostatic a.* albuminuria not associated with disease, occurring after strenuous exercise or after a long period of standing.

albumose (**al**-bew-mohz) *n.* a substance, intermediate between albumin and peptones, produced during the digestion of proteins by pepsin and other endopeptidases (*see* peptidase).

alcaptonuria (alkaptonuria) (al-kap-tŏn-**yoor**-iă) *n.* accumulation in the tissues and excretion in the urine of homogentisic acid due to congenital absence of homogentisic acid oxidase, an enzyme essential for the normal breakdown of the amino acids tyrosine and phenylalanine.

alcohol (**al**-kŏ-hol) *n.* any of a class of organic compounds formed when a hydroxyl group (–OH) is substituted for a hydrogen atom in a hydrocarbon. *ethyl a.* (*ethanol*) the alcohol in alcoholic drinks, produced by the fermentation of sugar by yeast. Formula: C_2H_5OH. 'Pure' alcohol contains not less than 94.9% by volume of ethyl alcohol. A solution of 70% alcohol can be used as a preservative or antiseptic. *See also* alcoholism. —**alcoholic** (al-kŏ-**hol**-ik) *adj., n.*

alcohol-fast *adj.* describing bacteria that have been stained and continue to hold the stain after treatment with alcohol.

Alcoholics Anonymous *n.* a voluntary agency of self help that is organized and operated locally among those with alcoholic dependency.

alcoholism (**al**-kŏ-hol-izm) *n.* the syndrome due to physical dependence on alcohol, such that sudden deprivation may cause withdrawal symptoms – tremor, anxiety, hallucinations, and delusions (*see* delirium (tremens)). Alcoholism impairs intellectual function, physical skills, memory, and judgment. Heavy consumption of alcohol also causes cardiomyopathy, peripheral neuritis, cirrhosis of the liver, and enteritis.

alcoholuria (al-kŏ-hol-**yoor**-iă) *n.* the presence of alcohol in the urine.

Aldomet (**al**-dŏ-met) *n. see* methyldopa.

aldosterone (al-**dos**-ter-ohn) *n.* a steroid hormone (*see* corticosteroid) that is synthesized and released by the adrenal cortex and acts on the kidney to regulate salt (potassium and sodium) and water balance.

aldosteronism (al-**dos**-tĕ-rŏ-nizm) *n.* overproduction of aldosterone, causing electrolyte imbalance and raised blood pressure (hypertension).

Aleppo boil (ă-**lep**-oh) *n. see* oriental sore.

aleukaemic (al-yoo-**kee**-mik) *adj.* describing a stage of leukaemia in which there is no increase in

salivary gland

soft palate (uvula)

buccal cavity

tongue

hard palate

epiglottis

mouth

salivary glands

larynx

oesophagus

diaphragm

gall bladder

bile duct

liver

duodenum

stomach

pancreas

ileum

colon

rectum

caecum

appendix

anus

The alimentary canal

the number of white cells in the blood.

alexia (ă-leks-iă) *n.* an acquired inability to read due to disease in the left hemisphere of the brain in a right-handed person. *agnostic a.* (*word blindness*) inability to identify letters and words not affecting the patient's ability to write.

algesimeter (al-jĕ-sim-it-er) *n.* a piece of equipment for determining the sensitivity of the skin to various touch stimuli, especially those causing pain.

-algia *suffix denoting* pain.

algid (al-jid) *adj.* cold: usually describing the cold clammy skin

associated with certain forms of malaria.

alienation (ay-li-ĕn-ay-shŏn) *n.* (in psychiatry) 1. the experience that one's thoughts are under the control of somebody else, or that other people participate in one's thinking. 2. insanity.

alimentary canal (ali-**ment**-er-i) *n.* the long passage, extending from the mouth to the anus, through which food passes to be digested and absorbed.

aliquot (al-i-kwot) *n.* one of a known number of equal parts of a compound or solution.

alkalaemia (al-kă-lee-miă) *n.* abnormally high blood alkalinity.

See also alkalosis. *Compare* acidaemia.

alkali (al-kă-ly) *n.* a base that is soluble in water. Alkaline solutions turn litmus paper blue. *See* base.

alkaloid (al-kă-loid) *n.* one of a diverse group of nitrogen-containing substances that are produced by plants and have potent effects on body function. Many alkaloids are important drugs, including morphine, quinine, atropine, and codeine.

alkalosis (al-kă-loh-sis) *n.* a condition in which the alkalinity of body fluids and tissues is abnormally high. This arises because of a failure of the mechanisms that usually maintain a balance between alkalis and acids in the arterial blood (*see* acid-base balance).

alkaptonuria *n. see* alcaptonuria.

alkylating agent (al-ki-lay-ting) *n.* a drug, such as mustine (nitrogen mustard), that disrupts the growth of a malignant tumour by damaging the DNA in the tumour cell nuclei.

allantois (al-ăn-toh-iss) *n.* the membranous sac that develops as an outgrowth of the embryonic hindgut. Its outer (mesodermal) layer carries blood vessels to the placenta and so forms part of the umbilical cord. —**allantoic** *adj.*

allele (**allelomorph**) (ă-leel) *n.* one of two or more alternative forms of a gene, only one of which can be present in a chromosome. —**allelic** *adj.*

allelomorph (ă-leel-oh-morf) *n. see* allele.

allergen (al-er-jĕn) *n.* any antigen that causes allergy in a hypersensitive person. —**allergenic** *adj.*

allergy (al-er-ji) *n.* a disorder in which the body becomes hypersensitive to particular antigens (called allergens), which provoke characteristic symptoms whenever they are subsequently encountered. Different allergies afflict different tissues and may have either local or general effects, varying from asthma and hay fever to severe dermatitis or gastroenteritis or extremely serious shock (*see* anaphylaxis). —**allergic** *adj.*

allocheiria (al-oh-keer-iă) *n.* a condition in which the sensation aroused by a stimulus applied to one side of the body is referred to the opposite side.

allograft (al-oh-grahft) *n. see* homograft.

allopathy (ă-lop-ă-thi) *n.* (in homeopathic medicine) the orthodox system of medicine, in which the use of drugs is directed to producing effects in the body that will directly oppose and so alleviate the symptoms of a disease. *Compare* homeopathy.

allopurinol (al-oh-pewr-i-nol) *n.* a drug administered by mouth in the treatment of chronic gout. It acts by reducing the level of uric acid in tissues and blood.

all-or-none law *n.* the principle that tissue, such as nerve fibres, can produce only one of two reactions to a stimulus. Regardless of the intensity of the stimulus, such tissue will show either a total response or no response at all.

allylestrenol (**allyloestrenol**) (al-il-eess-trĕ-nol) *n.* a synthetic female sex hormone (*see* progestogen) administered by mouth in the treatment of abnormal bleeding from the womb and threatened abortion. Trade name: **Gestanin.**

alopecia (baldness) (al-ŏ-**pee**-shiă) *n.* absence of hair from areas where it normally grows. *a. areata* a condition of unknown origin in which hair falls out in patches.

aloxiprin (ă-**loks**-i-prin) *n.* a compound made from aluminium oxide and aspirin.

alpha cells (al-fă) *pl. n.* the cells in the islets of Langerhans that produce glucagon. *Compare* beta cells.

alpha-fetoprotein (afp) (al-fă-fee-toh-**proh**-teen) *n.* a protein formed in the liver of the fetus and present in the amniotic fluid in small amounts. In anencephaly and spina bifida the amount of afp in the fluid is greatly increased in the first six months of pregnancy, and this can be detected by amniocentesis.

alprenolol (al-**pren**-ŏ-lol) *n.* a drug used to treat arrhythmia and angina of the heart and to reduce high blood pressure (*see* beta blocker).

ALS *n. see* antilymphocytic serum.

altitude sickness (mountain sickness) (**al**-ti-tewd) *n.* the condition that results from unaccustomed exposure to a high altitude (4500 m or more above sea level). Reduced atmospheric pressure and shortage of oxygen cause deep rapid breathing, which lowers the concentration of carbon dioxide in the blood.

aluminium hydroxide (al-yoo-min-iŭm) *n.* a safe slow-acting antacid and laxative. It is administered by mouth as a gel in the treatment of indigestion, gastric and duodenal ulcers, and reflux oesophagitis.

alveolitis (al-vee-oh-**ly**-tis) *n.* inflammation of an alveolus or alveoli. Chronic inflammation of the walls of the lung alveoli is usually caused by inhaled inorganic dusts (*see* pneumoconiosis) or organic dusts (*see* farmer's lung).

alveolus (al-vee-oh-lŭs) *n.* (*pl.* **alveoli**) **1.** (in the lung) a blind-ended air sac of microscopic size. **2.** the part of the upper or lower jawbone that supports the roots of the teeth (*see also* mandible, maxilla). **3.** the sac of a racemose gland (*see also* acinus). **4.** any other small cavity, depression, or sac. —**alveolar** *adj.*

Alzheimer's disease (**alts**-hy-merz) *n.* a progressive form of dementia occurring in middle age, for which there is no treatment. It is associated with diffuse degeneration of the brain. *Compare* Pick's disease. [A. Alzheimer (1864–1915), German physician]

amalgam (ă-**mal**-găm) *n.* any of a group of alloys containing mercury. In dentistry fillings are made by mixing a silver-tin alloy with mercury.

amantadine (ă-**man**-tă-deen) *n.* an antiviral drug used in the treatment of influenza infections and parkinsonism. Trade name: **Symmetrel.**

amaurosis (am-aw-**roh**-sis) *n.* partial or complete blindness. *a. fugax* a condition in which loss of vision is transient. —**amaurotic** (am-aw-**rot**-ik) *adj.*

amaurotic familial idiocy *n. see* Tay-Sachs disease.

ambivalence (am-**biv**-ălĕns) *n.* (in psychology) the condition of holding opposite feelings (such as love and hate) for the same person or object.

amblyopia (am-blee-oh-piă) *n.* poor sight, not due to any detectable disease of the eyeball or visual system. *a. ex anopsia* a condition in which factors such as squint (*see* strabismus), cataract, and other abnormalities of the optics of the eye (*see* refraction) impair its normal use in early childhood by preventing the formation of a clear image on the retina.

amblyoscope (orthoptoscope, synoptophore) (am-blee-ŏ-skohp) *n.* an instrument for measuring the angle of a squint and assessing the degree to which a person uses both eyes together.

ambulant (am-bew-lănt) *adj.* able to walk.

ambulatory (am-bew-layt-er-i) *adj.* relating to walking. *a. treatment* treatment that enables or encourages a patient to remain on his feet.

ambutonium (am-bew-toh-niŭm) *n.* a drug given by mouth to treat indigestion and peptic ulcer.

amelia (ă-mee-liă) *n.* congenital total absence of the arms or legs due to a developmental defect. It is one of the fetal abnormalities induced by the drug thalidomide taken early in pregnancy. *See also* phocomelia.

amelioration (ă-mee-li-er-ay-shŏn) *n.* general improvement in the condition of a patient; reduction in severity of the symptoms of a disease.

ameloblastoma (ă-mee-loh-blas-toh-mă) *n.* a locally malignant tumour of the jaw, formerly known as an *adamantinoma*.

amenorrhoea (am-en-ŏ-ree-ă) *n.* the absence or stopping of the menstrual periods. *primary a.* the nonappearance of menstrual periods at puberty, often because of a congenital defect (e.g. Turner's syndrome). *secondary a.* the stopping of menstrual periods after establishment at puberty, for reasons such as pituitary or thyroid gland deficiency, diabetes, mental disturbance, anorexia nervosa, or pregnancy.

amentia (ă-men-shă) *n.* failure of development of the intellectual faculties. *See* subnormality.

amethocaine (ă-meth-ŏ-kayn) *n.* a potent local anaesthetic. It is applied to skin or mucous membranes for eye, ear, nose and throat surgery, but it has also been employed for spinal anaesthesia.

ametropia (am-ě-troh-piă) *n.* any abnormality of refraction of the eye, resulting in blurring of the image formed on the retina. *See* astigmatism, hypermetropia, myopia. *Compare* emmetropia.

amiloride (ă-mil-ŏ-ryd) *n.* a diuretic that causes the increased excretion of sodium and chloride. Trade name: **Midamor**.

amino acid (ă-mee-noh) *n.* an organic compound containing an amino group ($-NH_2$) and a carboxyl group ($-COOH$). Amino acids are fundamental constituents of all proteins (see table). Some can be synthesized by the body; others (*see* essential amino acid) must be obtained from protein in the diet.

aminobenzoic acid (ă-mee-noh-ben-zoh-ik) *n. see* para-aminobenzoic acid.

aminophylline (ă-mee-noh-fil-een) *n.* a drug that relaxes smooth muscle and stimulates respiration. Administered by mouth or in suppositories, it is used in the treatment of asthma and emphysema, to dilate the coronary ar-

Amino acid	Abbreviation	Amino acid	Abbreviation
alanine	ala	*leucine	leu
arginine	arg	*lysine	lys
asparagine	asn	*methionine	met
aspartic acid	asp	*phenylalanine	phe
cysteine	cys	proline	pro
glutamic acid	glu	serine	ser
glutamine	gln	*threonine	thr
glycine	gly	*tryptophan	trp
histidine	his	tyrosine	tyr
*isoleucine	ile	*valine	val

*an essential amino acid

The amino acids occurring in proteins

teries in angina pectoris, and as a diuretic. *See also* theophylline.

aminosalicylic acid (ă-mee-noh-sali-sil-ik) *n. see* para-aminosalicylic acid.

amitosis (ami-**toh**-sis) *n.* division of the nucleus of a cell by a process, not involving mitosis, in which the nucleus is constricted into two.

amitriptyline (ami-**trip**-til-een) *n.* a tricyclic antidepressant drug that has a mild tranquillizing action. Trade names: **Elatrol, Tryptizol**.

ammonia (ă-**moh**-niă) *n.* a colourless gas with a pungent odour that can be cooled and compressed to form a liquid. Ammonium salts are used as astringents, diuretics, and expectorants and ammonia itself (in very dilute form) is used as a reflex stimulant. Formula: NH_3.

amnesia (am-**nee**-ziă) *n.* total or partial loss of memory following

physical injury, disease, drugs, or psychological trauma. *anterograde a.* loss of memory for events following the trauma. *retrograde a.* loss of memory for events preceding the trauma.

amniocentesis (am-ni-oh-sen-**tee**-sis) *n.* withdrawal of a sample of amniotic fluid surrounding an embryo in the womb, by means of a syringe inserted through the abdominal wall, to enable prenatal diagnosis of chromosomal abnormalities (such as Down's syndrome) and metabolic and other congenital disorders (such as spina bifida).

amniography (am-ni-**og**-răfi) *n.* the making of X-ray pictures (*amniograms*) of the amniotic sac, which enables the placenta and umbilical cord to be visualized.

amnion (**am**-ni-ŏn) *n.* the membrane that forms initially over the dorsal part of the embryo but soon expands to enclose it completely within the amniotic cavity. —**amniotic** (am-ni-ot-ik) *adj.*

amnioscopy (am-ni-**oss**-kŏ-pi) *n.* examination of the inside of the amniotic sac by means of an instrument (*amnioscope*) that is passed through the abdominal wall. *cervical a.* examination of the amniotic sac through the neck of the womb.

amniotic cavity *n.* the fluid-filled cavity between the embryo and the amnion. *See also* amniotic fluid.

amniotic fluid *n.* the fluid contained within the amniotic cavity. It surrounds the growing fetus, protecting it from external pressure. *See also* amniocentesis.

amniotomy (am-ni-**ot**-ŏmi) *n.* the artificial puncturing of the membranes surrounding the baby in the womb by means of a special instrument (*amniotome*). Labour generally follows naturally, but in some cases it must be started artificially by additional measures.

amodiaquine (am-oh-**dy**-ă-kwin) *n.* an antimalarial drug with effects and uses similar to those of chloroquine.

amoeba (ă-**mee**-bă) *n.* (*pl.* **amoebae**) any single-celled microscopic animal of jelly-like consistency and irregular and constantly changing shape. Some amoebae cause disease in man (*see* Entamoeba). *See also* Protozoa. —**amoebic** *adj.* —**amoeboid** *adj.*

amoebiasis (ami-by-ă-sis) *n. see* dysentery.

amoebicide (ă-**mee**-bi-syd) *n.* an agent that kills amoebae.

AMP (adenosine monophosphate) *n.* a compound containing ade-

nine, ribose, and one phosphate group. AMP occurs in cells and is involved in processes requiring the transfer of energy (*see* ATP).

ampere (**am**-pair) *n.* the basic SI unit of electric current. It is equal to the current flowing through a conductor of resistance 1 ohm when a potential difference of 1 volt is applied between its ends. Symbol: A.

amphetamine (am-**fet**-ămin) *n.* a sympathomimetic drug that has a marked stimulant action on the central nervous system. Administered by mouth, it has been used in the treatment of narcolepsy, mild depressive neuroses, and obesity. Tolerance of amphetamine develops rapidly, and prolonged use may lead to dependence.

amphiarthrosis (am-fi-arth-**roh**-sis) *n.* a slightly movable joint in which the bony surfaces are separated by fibrocartilage (*see* symphysis) or hyaline cartilage (*see* synchondrosis).

amphoric breath sounds (am-**fo**-rik) *pl. n. see* cavernous breath sounds.

amphotericin (am-foh-te-ri-sin) *n.* an antibiotic used to treat deep-seated fungal infections. It can be administered by mouth, but is usually given by intravenous injection.

ampicillin (am-pi-sil-in) *n.* an antibiotic administered by mouth or injection in the treatment of a variety of infections, including those of the urinary, respiratory, biliary, and intestinal tracts. Trade names: **Amcill, Penbritin, Polycillin, Principen.**

ampoule (ampule) (am-pool) *n.* a sealed glass or plastic capsule containing one dose of a drug in the form of a sterile solution for injection.

ampulla (am-**puul**-ă) *n.* (*pl.* **ampullae**) an enlarged or dilated ending of a tube or canal. *a. of Vater* the dilated part of the common bile duct where it is joined by the pancreatic duct. [A. Vater (1684–1751), German anatomist]

amputation (am-pew-**tay**-shŏn) *n.* the removal of a limb, part of a limb, or any other portion of the body (such as a breast).

amylase (**am**-i-layz) *n.* an enzyme that occurs in saliva and pancreatic juice and aids the digestion of starch, which it breaks down into glucose, maltose, and dextrins.

amyl nitrite (**am**-il) *n.* a drug that relaxes smooth muscle, especially that of blood vessels. Given by inhalation, amyl nitrite is used mainly in the treatment of angina pectoris.

amylobarbitone (ami-loh-**bar**-bi-tohn) *n.* an intermediate-acting barbiturate, administered by mouth as a hypnotic or injected intravenously to produce mental relaxation before psychoanalysis. Prolonged use may lead to dependence and overdosage has serious toxic effects (*see* barbiturism). Trade names: **Amytal, Amobarbital.**

amyloid (**am**-i-loid) *n.* a glycoprotein, resembling starch, that is deposited in the internal organs in amyloidosis.

amyloidosis (ami-loid-**oh**-sis) *n.* infiltration of the liver, kidneys, spleen, and other tissues with amyloid. *primary a.* amyloidosis without any apparent cause. *secondary a.* a late complication of such chronic infections as tuberculosis or leprosy.

amylopectin (ami-loh-**pek**-tin) *n.* *see* starch.

amylopsin (ami-**lop**-sin) *n.* an amylase found in the pancreatic juice.

amylose (**am**-i-lohz) *n.* *see* starch.

amyotonia congenita (floppy baby syndrome) (ay-my-ŏ-**toh**-niă kon-jen-**it**ă) *n.* a disorder, present at birth, in which the child's muscles are weak and floppy.

amyotrophy (ami-**ot**-rŏfi) *n.* a progressive loss of muscle bulk associated with weakness, caused by disease of the nerve that supplies the affected muscle.

an- *prefix. see* a-.

anabolic (ană-**bol**-ik) *adj.* promoting tissue growth by increasing the metabolic processes involved in protein synthesis. Anabolic agents are usually synthetic male sex hormones (*see* androgen).

anabolism (ă-**nab**-ŏl-izm) *n.* the synthesis of complex molecules, such as proteins and fats, from simpler ones by living things. *See also* anabolic, metabolism.

anacidity (ană-**sid**-iti) *n.* a deficiency or abnormal absence of acid in the body fluids.

anacrotism (ăn-**ak**-rŏt-izm) *n.* the condition in which there is an abnormal curve in the ascending line of a pulse tracing. It may be seen in cases of aortic stenosis. —**anacrotic** *adj.*

anaemia (ă-**nee**-miă) *n.* a reduction in the quantity of the oxygen-carrying pigment haemoglobin in the blood. The main symptoms are excessive tiredness and fatiguability, breathlessness on exertion, pallor, and poor resistance to infection. The many causes of anaemia include loss of blood (*haemorrhagic a.*); lack of iron (*iron-deficiency a.*); the increased destruction of red blood cells (*haemolytic a.*); and the impaired production of red blood cells (*see* aplastic anaemia; leukaemia; pernicious (anaemia)). Anaemias can be classified on the basis of the size of the red cells, which may be large (*macrocytic a.*), small (*microcytic a.*), or normal-sized (*normocytic a.*). —**anaemic** *adj.*

anaerobe (an-air-rohb) *n.* any organism, especially a microbe, that is able to live and grow in the absence of free oxygen. *Compare* aerobe. —**anaerobic** (an-air-**roh**-bik) *adj.*

anaerobic respiration *n.* a type of cellular respiration in which foodstuffs (usually carbohydrates) are never completely oxidized because molecular oxygen is not used.

anaesthesia (anis-**theez**-iă) *n.* loss of feeling or sensation in a part or all of the body, especially when induced by drugs. *general a.* total unconsciousness, usually achieved by administering a combination of injections and gases. It is induced for such major operations as removal of the stomach or a lung. *local a.* loss of feeling in a limited area of the body, induced for minor operations, particularly many dental procedures. It may be achieved by injections of substances such as lignocaine close to a local nerve, which deadens the tissues supplied by that nerve. *See also* spinal anaesthesia.

anaesthetic (anis-**thet**-ik) 1. *n.* an agent that reduces or abolishes sensation. *general a.* an anaesthetic, such as halothane, that affects the whole body. *local a.* an anaesthetic, such as lignocaine, that affects a particular region of

the body. 2. *adj.* reducing or abolishing sensation.

anaesthetist (ăn-**ees**-thĕt-ist) *n.* a medically qualified doctor who administers an anaesthetic to induce unconsciousness in a patient before a surgical operation.

anal (ay-năl) *adj.* of, relating to, or affecting the anus.

analeptic (ană-**lep**-tik) *n.* a drug that restores consciousness to a patient in a coma or faint. Analeptics stimulate the central nervous system to counteract the effects of large doses of narcotic drugs.

analgesia (an-ăl-**jeez**-iă) *n.* reduced sensibility to pain, without loss of consciousness and without the sense of touch necessarily being affected.

analgesic (an-ăl-**jee**-sik) 1. *n.* a drug that relieves pain. Aspirin and paracetamol are mild analgesics; morphine and pethidine are more potent. *See also* narcotic. 2. *adj.* relieving pain.

analogous (ă-**nal**-ŏgŭs) *adj.* describing organs or parts that have similar functions in different organisms although they do not have the same evolutionary origin or development. *Compare* homologous.

analysis (ă-**nal**-isis) *n.* (in psychology) any means of understanding complex mental processes or experiences. *See also* psychoanalysis.

analyst (an-ă-list) *n.* a person who performs analysis.

anaphase (an-ă-fayz) *n.* the third stage of mitosis and of each division of meiosis.

anaphylaxis (ană-fil-**aks**-is) *n.* an abnormal reaction to a particular antigen, e.g. a localized allergic attack. *anaphylactic shock* an ex-

treme and generalized allergic reaction in which widespread histamine release causes swelling (oedema), constriction of the bronchioles, heart failure, circulatory
collapse, and sometimes death.
—**anaphylactic** *adj*.

anaplasia (ană-**play**-ziă) *n.* a loss
of normal cell characteristics or
differentiation. Anaplasia is typical of malignant tumours.

anasarca (ană-**sar**-kă) *n.* massive
swelling of the legs, trunk, and
genitalia due to retention of
fluid (oedema): found in congestive heart failure and some forms
of renal failure.

anastomosis (ă-nass-tŏ-**moh**-sis) *n.*
1. (in anatomy) a communication
between two blood vessels without any intervening capillary network. *arteriovenous a.* a thick-
walled blood vessel that connects
an arteriole directly with a venule, found in the skin of the
lips, nose, ears, hands, and feet.
2. (in surgery) an artificial connection between two tubular organs or parts, especially between
two normally separate parts of
the intestine (a *short circuit*). *See
also* shunt.

anatomy (ă-**nat**-ŏmi) *n.* the study
of the structure of living organisms. In medicine it refers to the
study of the form and gross
structure of the various parts of
the human body. *See also* cytology, histology, physiology. —**anatomical** (ană-tom-i-k'l) *adj.* —**anatomist** *n.*

anconeus (an-koh-niŭs) *n.* a muscle behind the elbow that assists
in extending the forearm.

Ancylostoma (Ankylostoma) (an-si-
loh-**stoh**-ma) *n.* a genus of small
parasitic nematodes that inhabit
the small intestine (*see* hook-

worm). *A. duodenale* the species
that most commonly infests man.

ancylostomiasis (an-si-loh-stoh-
my-ăsis) *n.* an infestation of the
small intestine by the parasitic
hookworm *Ancylostoma
duodenale*. *See* hookworm (disease).

andr- (andro-) *prefix denoting* man
or the male sex.

androgen (**an**-drŏ-jĕn) *n.* one of a
group of steroid hormones, including testosterone and androsterone, that stimulate the development of male sex organs and
male secondary sexual characteristics. The principal source of
these hormones is the testis but
they are also secreted by the adrenal cortex and ovaries in small
amounts. In women excessive
production of androgens gives
rise to masculinization. Naturally
occurring and synthetic androgens are used in replacement
therapy, as anabolic agents, and
in the treatment of breast cancer. —**androgenic** *adj*.

androsterone (an-**drost**-er-ohn) *n.* a
steroid hormone (*see* androgen)
that is synthesized and released
by the testes and is responsible
for controlling male sexual development.

anencephaly (an-en-**sef**-ăli) *n.* partial or complete absence of the
bones of the rear of the skull
and of the cerebral hemispheres
of the brain. It occurs as a developmental defect and is not
compatible with life for more
than a few hours. *See also* alpha-
fetoprotein. —**anencephalous** *adj*.

anergy (**an**-er-ji) *n.* **1.** lack of response to a specific antigen or
allergen. **2.** lack of energy. —**an-
ergic** *adj*.

aneurin (vitamin B₁) (**an**-yoor-in)
n. see vitamin B.

aneurysm (an-yoor-izm) *n.* a balloon-like swelling in the wall of an artery, due to disease or congenital deficiency. *arteriovenous a.* a direct communication between an artery and vein, without an intervening capillary bed. *Charcot-Bouchard a.* a small aneurysm found within the brain of elderly and hypertensive subjects. Such aneurysms may rupture, causing cerebral haemorrhage. [J. M. Charcot (1825–93), French neurologist; C. J. Bouchard (1837–1915), French physician] *dissecting a.* a condition in which a tear occurs in the lining of the aorta, which allows blood to enter the wall and track along (dissect) the muscular coat. A dissecting aneurysm may rupture or it may compress the blood vessels arising from the aorta and produce infarction (localized necrosis) in the organs they supply. *ventricular a.* a condition that may develop in the wall of the left ventricle after myocardial infarction. Heart failure may result or thrombosis within the aneurysm may act as a source of embolism. —**aneurysmal** *adj.*

angi- (angio-) *prefix denoting* blood or lymph vessels.

angiectasis (an-ji-ek-tă-sis) *n.* abnormal dilation of blood vessels.

angiitis (vasculitis) (an-ji-I-tis) *n.* a patchy inflammation of the walls of small blood vessels.

angina (an-jy-nă) *n.* a sense of suffocation or suffocating pain. *a. pectoris* pain in the centre of the chest, which is induced by exercise and relieved by rest and may spread to the jaws and arms. Angina pectoris occurs when the demand for blood by the heart exceeds the supply of

the coronary arteries and it usually results from coronary artery atheroma. It may be prevented or relieved by such drugs as glyceryl trinitrate and propranolol. *See also* Ludwig's angina.

angiocardiography (an-ji-oh-kar-di-og-răfi) *n.* X-ray examination of the chambers of the heart after introducing a radio-opaque contrast medium into the blood in the heart. Its progress through the heart is followed by a rapid series of X-ray films or by the use of cine film (*see* cineangiocardiography). The X-ray is called an *angiocardiogram*.

angiography (an-ji-og-răfi) *n.* X-ray examination of blood vessels. A dye that is opaque to X-rays is injected into the artery and a rapid series of X-ray films (*angiograms*) is taken (*see* arteriography).

angiology (an-ji-ol-ŏji) *n.* the branch of medicine concerned with the structure, function, and diseases of blood vessels.

angioma (arteriovenous malformation) (an-ji-oh-mă) *n.* (*pl.* **angiomata**) a knot of distended blood vessels overlying and compressing the surface of the brain. *See also* haemangioma, lymphangioma.

angioneurotic oedema (an-ji-oh-newr-ot-ik) *n.* an allergic condition producing transient or persistent swelling of areas of skin accompanied by itching, which may be severe. *See also* urticaria.

angioplasty (an-ji-oh-plas-ti) *n.* surgical reshaping or reconstruction of blood vessels.

angiosarcoma (an-ji-oh-sar-koh-mă) *n.* a sarcoma arising in the blood vessels.

angiospasm (an-ji-oh-spazm) *n. see* Raynaud's disease.

angiotensin (an-ji-oh-fen-sin) *n.* a protein in the blood, derived from a plasma protein and released by the action of renin. Angiotensin causes constriction of blood vessels, thus raising blood pressure, and stimulates the secretion of aldosterone.

angstrom (ang-ström) *n.* a unit of length equal to one ten millionth of a millimetre (10^{-10} m), sometimes used to express wavelengths and interatomic distances. Symbol Å.

anhidrotic (an-hy-drot-ik) **1.** *n.* any drug that inhibits the secretion of sweat, such as parasympatholytic drugs. **2.** *adj.* inhibiting sweating.

anhydraemia (an-hy-dree-miă) *n.* a decrease in the proportion of water, and therefore plasma, in the blood.

anhydrous (an-hy-drŭs) *adj.* containing no water.

anidrosis (anhidrosis) (ani-droh-sis) *n.* the abnormal absence of sweating, accompanying disease or occurring as a congenital defect.

anileridine (ani-le-rid-een) *n.* a synthetic narcotic analgesic drug, given by mouth or by injection to relieve pain or support anaesthesia. Trade name: **Leritine**.

aniline (an-il-een) *n.* an oily compound obtained from coal tar and widely used in the preparation of dyes.

anion (anI-ŏn) *n.* a negatively charged ion, which moves towards the anode (positive electrode) when an electric current is passed through the solution containing it. *Compare* cation.

aniridia (ani-rid-iă) *n.* congenital absence of the iris (of the eye).

anisocytosis (an-I-soh-sy-toh-sis) *n.* an excessive variation in size between individual red blood cells.

anisomelia (an-I-soh-mee-liă) *n.* a difference in size or shape between the arms or the legs.

anisometropia (an-I-soh-mě-troh-piă) *n.* the condition in which the power of refraction in one eye differs markedly from that in the other.

ankle (an-k'l) *n.* **1.** the hinge joint between the leg and the foot. It consists of the talus (ankle bone), which projects into a socket formed by the lower ends of the tibia and fibula. **2.** the whole region of the ankle joint, including the tarsus and the lower parts of the tibia and fibula.

ankyloblepharon (anki-loh-blef-er-on) *n.* adhesion of the ciliary edges of the eyelids.

ankylosing spondylitis (anki-loh-zing) *n. see* spondylitis.

ankylosis (anki-loh-sis) *n.* fusion of the bones across a joint space, either by bony tissue (*bony a.*) or by shortening of connecting fibrous tissue (*fibrous a.*).

Ankylostoma (anki-loh-stoh-mă) *n. see* Ancylostoma.

annulus (an-yoo-lŭs) *n.* (in anatomy) a circular opening or ring-shaped structure. —**annular** *adj.*

anodyne (an-ŏ-dyn) *n.* any treatment or drug that soothes and eases pain.

anomaly (ă-nom-ăli) *n.* any deviation from the normal, especially a congenital or developmental defect. —**anomalous** *adj.*

anomia (ă-noh-miă) *n.* **1.** a form of aphasia in which the patient is unable to give the names of objects, but retains the ability to put words together into speech. **2.** absence of respect for laws and established customs, which is a feature of psychopathy.

anomie (an-oh-mi) *n.* a condition in which a person is no longer able to identify with or relate to others, resulting in apathy, loneliness, and distress.

anonychia (anŏ-nik-iă) *n.* congenital absence of one or more nails.

Anopheles (ă-nof-i-leez) *n.* a genus of widely distributed mosquitoes. The malarial parasite (*see* Plasmodium) is transmitted to man solely through the bite of female *Anopheles* mosquitoes.

anorchism (an-or-kizm) *n.* congenital absence of one or both testes.

anorexia (an-er-eks-iă) *n.* loss of appetite. *a. nervosa* a psychological illness, most common in female adolescents, in which the patients have an aversion to eating. The result is severe loss of weight and sometimes even death from starvation. The problem often starts with an obsessive desire to lose weight but the underlying cause of the illness is more complicated. Patients must usually be treated by psychotherapy.

anosmia (an-oz-miă) *n.* a loss of the sense of smell.

anovular (anovulatory) (an-ov-yooler) *adj.* not associated with the development and release of a female germ cell (ovum) in the ovary, as in *anovular menstruation.*

anoxaemia (an-oks-ee-miă) *n.* a condition in which there is less than the normal concentration of oxygen in the blood. *See also* hypoxaemia.

anoxia (an-oks-iă) *n.* a condition in which the tissues of the body receive inadequate amounts of oxygen. *See also* hypoxia. —**anoxic** *adj.*

ant- (anti-) *prefix denoting* opposed to; counteracting; relieving.

Antabuse (ant-ă-bews) *n. see* disulfiram.

antacid (ant-ass-id) *n.* a drug, such as sodium bicarbonate, that neutralizes the hydrochloric acid secreted in the digestive juices of the stomach. Antacids are used to relieve discomfort in disorders of the digestive system.

antagonist (an-tag-ŏn-ist) *n.* **1.** a muscle whose action (contraction) opposes that of another muscle (*see* agonist). **2.** a drug or other substance with opposite action to that of another drug or natural body chemical. —**antagonism** *n.*

antazoline (ant-az-ŏ-leen) *n.* a short-acting antihistamine drug, given by mouth to relieve the symptoms of allergic reactions.

ante- *prefix denoting* before.

anteflexion (anti-flek-shŏn) *n.* the abnormal bending forward of an organ, especially the bending of the body of the womb towards the front.

ante mortem (an-ti mor-těm) *adj.* before death. *Compare* post mortem.

antenatal (anti-nay-t'l) *adj.* of or relating to the period of pregnancy; before birth. *a. diagnosis see* prenatal diagnosis.

Antepar (an-ti-par) *n. see* piperazine.

antepartum (anti-par-tŭm) *adj.* occurring before the onset of labour.

anterior (an-teer-i-er) *adj.* **1.** describing or relating to the front (ventral) portion of the body or limbs. **2.** describing the front part of any organ.

anteversion (anti-**ver**-shŏn) *n.* the normal forward inclination of the womb.

anthelmintic (an-thel-**min**-tik) **1.** *n.* any drug, such as dichlorophen, or chemical agent used to destroy parasitic worms (helminths) and/or remove them from the body. **2.** *adj.* having the power to destroy or eliminate helminths.

anthracosis (an-thră-**koh**-sis) *n.* a lung disease – a form of pneumoconiosis – caused by coal dust. It affects mainly coal miners.

anthrax (**an**-thraks) *n.* an acute infectious disease of farm animals caused by the bacterium *Bacillus anthracis*. In man the disease attacks either the lungs, causing pneumonia (*woolsorter's disease*), or the skin, producing severe ulceration (*malignant pustule*). Anthrax can be treated with penicillin or tetracycline.

anthrop- (anthropo-) *prefix denoting* the human race.

antibiotic (anti-by-**ot**-ik) *n.* a substance, produced by or derived from a microorganism, that destroys or inhibits the growth of other microorganisms. Antibiotics are used to treat infections caused by organisms that are sensitive to them, usually bacteria or fungi. *See also* cephalosporin, chloramphenicol, penicillin, streptomycin, tetracycline.

antibody (**an**-ti-bodi) *n.* a special kind of blood protein that is synthesized in lymphoid tissue in response to the presence of a particular antigen and circulates in the plasma to attack the antigen and render it harmless. Antibody formation is the basis of both immunity and allergy; it is also responsible for tissue or organ rejection following transplantation.

anticholinergic (anti-koli-**ner**-jik) *adj.* inhibiting the action of acetylcholine. Parasympatholytic drugs are anticholinergic.

anticholinesterase (anti-koli-nes-ter-ayz) *n.* any substance that inhibits the action of cholinesterase and therefore allows acetylcholine to continue transmitting nerve impulses.

anticoagulant (anti-koh-**ag**-yoolǎnt) *n.* an agent, such as heparin or phenindione, that prevents the clotting of blood and is used in the treatment of such conditions as thrombosis and embolism. Incorrect dosage may result in haemorrhage.

anticonvulsant (anti-kŏn-**vul**-sǎnt) *n.* a drug, such as sodium valproate or phenytoin, that prevents or reduces the severity of fits (convulsions) in various types of epilepsy.

anti D *n.* the rhesus-factor antibody, formed by rhesus-negative individuals following exposure to rhesus-positive blood. *See* haemolytic disease of the newborn.

antidepressant (anti-di-**press**-ǎnt) *n.* a drug that alleviates the symptoms of depression. The most widely prescribed group are the *tricyclic antidepressants*, such as amitriptyline and imipramine. The other main group of antidepressants (*see* MAO inhibitor) have more severe sideeffects.

antidiuretic hormone (ADH) (anti-dy-yoor-et-ik) *n. see* vasopressin.

antidote (**an**-ti-doht) *n.* a drug that counteracts the effects of a poison.

antiemetic (anti-i-**met**-ik) *n.* a drug that prevents vomiting, used to treat such conditions as motion sickness and vertigo and to counteract nausea and vomiting caused by other drugs.

antigen (**an**-ti-jĕn) *n.* any substance that the body regards as foreign or potentially dangerous and against which it produces an antibody. —**antigenic** *adj.*

antihaemophilic factor (anti-heem-ŏ-fil-ik) *n. see* haemophilia.

antihistamine (anti-**hist**-ă-meen) *n.* a drug, such as mepyramine, that inhibits some of the effects of histamine in the body. Antihistamines are used mainly for the relief of hay fever, pruritus (itching), rhinitis, urticaria (nettle rash), and other allergic reactions. Many antihistamines, such as cyclizine, also have strong antiemetic activity and are used to prevent motion sickness. The most common side-effect of antihistamines is drowsiness and because of this they are sometimes used to promote sleep.

antilymphocytic serum (ALS) (anti-lim-foh-**sit**-ik) *n.* an antiserum containing antibodies that suppress lymphocytic activity. ALS may be given to prevent the immune reaction that causes tissue rejection following transplantation of such organs as kidneys.

antimetabolite (anti-mi-**tab**-ŏ-lyt) *n.* a drug that interferes with the normal metabolic processes within cells by combining with the enzymes responsible for them. Some drugs used in the treatment of cancer, e.g. fluorouracil, methotrexate, and mercaptopurine, are antimetabolites. Side-effects can be severe, involving blood cell disorders and digestive disturbances. *See also* cytotoxic drug.

antimitotic (anti-my-**tot**-ik) *n.* a drug that inhibits cell division and growth. The drugs used to treat cancer are mainly antimitotics. *See also* antimetabolite, cytotoxic drug.

antimony potassium tartrate (tartar emetic) (**an**-ti-mŏni) *n.* a toxic and irritating salt of antimony used for the treatment of schistosomiasis and leishmaniasis. It may produce severe side-effects, particularly vomiting, and should not be given to patients with heart, kidney, or liver disease.

antimycotic (anti-my-**kot**-ik) *n.* a drug active against fungi.

antiperistalsis (anti-pe-ri-**stal**-sis) *n.* a wave of contraction in the alimentary canal that passes in an oral (i.e. upward or backwards) direction. *Compare* peristalsis.

antipruritic (anti-**proor**-it-ik) *n.* an agent, such as calamine, that relieves itching (pruritus).

antipyretic (anti-py-**ret**-ik) *n.* a drug that reduces fever by lowering the body temperature.

antisepsis (anti-**sep**-sis) *n.* the elimination of bacteria, fungi, viruses, and other microorganisms that cause disease by the use of chemical or physical methods.

antiseptic (anti-**sep**-tik) *n.* a chemical, such as hexamine, that destroys or inhibits the growth of disease-causing bacteria and other microorganisms. Antiseptics are used externally to cleanse wounds and internally to treat infections of the intestine and bladder.

antiserum (anti-**seer**-ŭm) *n.* (*pl.* **antisera**) a serum that contains antibodies against antigens of a particular kind; it may be injected to treat, or give temporary protection against, specific diseases. Antisera are prepared in large quantities in such animals as horses.

antisocial (anti-**soh**-shăl) *adj.* contrary to the accepted standards of behaviour in society.

antispasmodic (anti-spaz-**mod**-ik) *n.* a drug that relieves spasm of smooth muscle. *See* spasmolytic.

antistatic (anti-**stat**-ik) *adj.* preventing the accumulation of static electricity.

antithrombin (anti-**throm**-bin) *n.* a substance or effect that inhibits the action of thrombin in the circulation, preventing unwanted clotting.

antitoxin (anti-**toks**-in) *n.* an antibody produced by the body to counteract a toxin formed by invading bacteria or from any other source.

antitragus (anti-**tray**-gŭs) *n.* a small projection of cartilage above the lobe of the ear, opposite the tragus. *See* pinna.

antitussive (anti-**tuss**-iv) *n.* a drug, such as pholcodine, that suppresses coughing.

antivenene (antivenin) (anti-ven-een) *n.* an antiserum containing antibodies against specific poisons in the venom of such an animal as a snake, spider, or scorpion.

antrectomy (an-trek-tŏmi) *n.* **1.** surgical removal of the bony walls of an antrum. *See* antrostomy. **2.** a surgical operation in which a part of the stomach (the antrum) is removed, used in the treatment of peptic ulcers.

antrostomy (an-**trost**-ŏmi) *n.* a surgical operation to produce an artificial opening to an antrum in a bone, so providing drainage for any fluid. The operation is sometimes carried out to treat infection of the paranasal sinuses.

antrum (an-**trŭm**) *n.* **1.** a cavity, especially a cavity in a bone. *a. of Highmore* the maxillary sinus (*see* paranasal sinuses). [N. Highmore (1613–85), English physician] *mastoid* (or *tympanic*) *a.* the space connecting the air cells of the mastoid process with the chamber of the inner ear. **2.** the part of the stomach adjoining the pylorus.

anuria (ă-**newr**-iă) *n.* failure of the kidneys to produce urine.

anus (ay-nŭs) *n.* the opening at the lower end of the alimentary canal, through which the faeces are discharged. It opens out from the rectum and is guarded by two sphincters. —**anal** *adj.*

anvil (an-vil) *n.* (in anatomy) *see* incus.

anxiety (ang-zy-iti) *n.* generalized pervasive fear. *a. state* a form of neurosis in which anxiety dominates the patient's life. It can be treated with psychotherapy, behaviour therapy, and tranquillizing drugs.

aorta (ay-or-tă) *n.* (*pl.* **aortae** or **aortas**) the main artery of the body, from which all others derive. *abdominal a.* the part of the descending aorta below the diaphragm. *arch of the a.* the part of the aorta that arches over the heart. *ascending a.* the part of the aorta that arises from the left ventricle. *descending a.* the part of the aorta that descends in front of the backbone. *thoracic a.* the part of the descending aorta from the arch of the aorta to the diaphragm. —**aortic** (ay-**or**-tik) *adj.*

aortic regurgitation *n.* reflux of blood from the aorta into the left ventricle during diastole.

Aortic regurgitation most commonly follows scarring of the aortic valve as a result of previous acute rheumatic fever, but it may also result from other conditions, such as syphilis or dissecting aneurysm.

aortic stenosis *n.* narrowing of the opening of the aortic valve due to fusion of the cusps that comprise the valve. It may result from previous rheumatic fever, or from calcification and scarring in a valve that has two cusps instead of the normal three, or it may be congenital.

aortic valve *n. see* semilunar valve.

aortitis (ay-or-ty-tis) *n.* inflammation of the aorta, which most commonly occurs as a late complication of syphilis.

aortography (ay-or-**tog**-răfi) *n.* X-ray examination of the aorta, which involves the injection into it of a radio-opaque contrast medium, after which a series of X-rays is taken (*see* angiocardiography).

aperient (ă-**peer**-iĕnt) *n.* a mild laxative.

aperistalsis (ay-pe-ri-**stal**-sis) *n.* the absence of peristaltic movement in the intestines.

apex (**ay**-peks) *n.* the tip or summit of an organ; for example the heart or lung. The apex of a tooth is the tip of the root. *See also* apical.

apex beat *n.* the impact of the heart against the chest wall during systole. It can be felt or heard to the left of the breastbone, in the space between the fifth and sixth ribs.

apgar score (**ap**-gar) *n.* a method of rapidly assessing the general state of a baby immediately after birth. A maximum of 2 points is given for each of the following signs: type of breathing, heart rate, colour, muscle tone, and response to stimuli. [V. Apgar (1909–), US anaesthetist]

aphagia (ă-**fay**-jiă) *n.* loss of the ability to swallow.

aphakia (ă-**fay**-kiă) *n.* absence of the lens of the eye: the state of the eye after a cataract has been removed.

aphasia (dysphasia) (ă-**fay**-ziă) *n.* a disorder of language affecting the generation of speech and its understanding. It is caused by disease in the left half of the brain (the dominant hemisphere) in a right-handed person. —**aphasic** *adj.*

aphonia (ă-**foh**-niă) *n.* absence of or loss of the voice through disease of the larynx or mouth.

aphrodisiac (afrŏ-**diz**-iak) *n.* an agent that stimulates sexual excitement.

aphtha (**af**-thă) *n.* (*pl.* **aphthae**) a small ulcer, occurring singly or in groups in the mouth as white or red spots. —**aphthous** *adj.*

apical (**ay**-pi-k'l) *adj.* of or relating to the apex of an organ or tooth. *a. abscess see* abscess.

apicectomy (ay-pi-**sek**-tŏmi) *n.* (in dentistry) surgical removal of the apex of the root of a tooth.

aplasia (ă-**play**-ziă) *n.* total or partial failure of development of an organ or tissue. *See also* agenesis. —**aplastic** (ay-**plas**-tik) *adj.*

aplastic anaemia *n.* a severe form of anaemia, resistant to therapy, in which the bone marrow fails to produce new blood cells. There are several causes, including a reaction to toxic drugs.

apnoea (ap-**nee**-ă) *n.* temporary cessation of breathing from any cause. —**apnoeic** *adj.*

apocrine (ap-ŏ-kryn) *adj.* **1.** describing sweat glands that occur only in hairy parts of the body, especially the armpit and groin. These glands develop in the hair follicles and appear after puberty has been reached. *Compare* eccrine. **2.** describing a type of gland that loses part of its protoplasm when secreting. *See* secretion.

apomorphine (apŏ-mor-feen) *n.* an emetic that produces its effect by direct action on the vomiting centre in the brain. It is administered by subcutaneous injection in the treatment of poisoning by noncorrosive substances that have been taken by mouth.

aponeurosis (apŏ-newr-oh-sis) *n.* a thin but strong fibrous sheet of tissue that replaces a tendon in muscles that are flat and sheetlike and have a wide area of attachment (e.g. to bones). —**aponeurotic** (apŏ-newr-ot-ik) *adj.*

apophysis (ă-pof-i-sis) *n.* a projection from a bone or any other part. *a. cerebri* the pineal body. —**apophyseal** *adj.*

apophysitis (ă-pof-i-sy-tis) *n.* inflammation of one or more of the synovial joints between the posterior arches of the vertebrae (*apophyseal joints*).

apoplexy (ap-ŏ-plek-si) *n. see* stroke.

appendectomy (ap-ĕn-dek-tŏmi) *n. US* appendicectomy.

appendicectomy (ă-pen-di-sek-tŏmi) *n.* surgical removal of the vermiform appendix. *See also* appendicitis.

appendicitis (ă-pen-di-sy-tis) *n.* inflammation of the vermiform appendix. *acute a.* the most common form of the condition, usually affecting young people. The chief symptom is abdominal pain, first central and later in the right lower abdomen, over the appendix. If not treated by surgical removal (appendicectomy) the condition usually progresses to cause an abscess or generalized peritonitis. *chronic a.* a popular diagnosis 20–50 years ago to explain recurrent pains in the lower abdomen. It is rare, and appendicectomy will not usually cure such pains.

appendicular (ap-ĕn-dik-yoo-ler) *adj.* **1.** relating to or affecting the vermiform appendix. **2.** relating to the limbs.

appendix (vermiform appendix) (ă-pen-diks) *n.* the short thin blind-ended tube, 7–10 cm long, that is attached to the end of the caecum. It has no known function in man and is liable to become infected and inflamed (*see* appendicitis).

apperception (ap-er-sep-shŏn) *n.* (in psychology) the process by which the qualities of an object, situation, etc., perceived by an individual are correlated with his/her preexisting knowledge.

applicator (ap-li-kay-ter) *n.* any device used to apply medication or treatment to a particular part of the body.

apposition (apŏ-zish-ŏn) *n.* the state of two structures, such as parts of the body, being in close contact. For example, the fingers are brought into apposition when the fist is clenched.

appraisal (ă-pray-z'l) *n.* a report on the progress or performance of an employee or learner (such as a student nurse), produced by a manager or tutor (such as a nursing officer or ward sister).

apraxia (dyspraxia) (ă-praks-iă) *n.* an inability to make skilled movements with accuracy. This is a disorder of the cerebral cortex most often caused by disease of the parietal lobes of the brain.

APT *n.* alum precipitated toxoid: a preparation used for immunization against diphtheria.

apyrexia (ap-I-**reks**-iă) *n.* the absence of fever.

aqua (**ak**-wă) *n.* water. *a. destillata* distilled water. *a. fortis* nitric acid.

aqueduct (**ak**-wi-dukt) *n.* (in anatomy) a canal containing fluid. *a. of the midbrain* (*cerebral a., a. of Sylvius*) a canal connecting the third and fourth ventricles. [F. Sylvius de la Boe (1614 – 72), French anatomist]

aqueous humour (**ay**-kwi-ŭs) *n.* the watery fluid that fills the chamber of the eye immediately behind the cornea and in front of the lens.

arachidonic acid (ă-rak-i-**don**-ik) *n.* *see* essential fatty acid.

arachnodactyly (ă-rak-noh-**dak**-tili) *n.* *see* Marfan's syndrome.

arachnoid (arachnoid mater) (ă-**rak**-noid) *n.* the middle of the three membranes covering the brain and spinal cord (*see* meninges), which has a fine, almost cobweb-like, texture. *a. villi* thin-walled projections of the arachnoid into the blood-filled sinuses of the dura, through which cerebrospinal fluid flows from the subarachnoid space into the bloodstream. Large villi (*Pacchionian bodies*) are found in the region of the superior sagittal sinus.

arbor (**ar**-ber) *n.* (in anatomy) a treelike structure. *a. vitae* **1.** the treelike outline of white matter seen in sections of the cerebellum. **2.** the treelike appearance

of the inner folds of the neck of the womb.

arborization (ar-ber-I-**zay**-shŏn) *n.* the branching termination of certain neurone processes.

arbovirus (ar-boh-vy-**rŭs**) *n.* one of a group of RNA-containing viruses that are transmitted by arthropods (hence *arthropod-borne* viruses) and cause diseases resulting in encephalitis or serious fever, such as dengue and yellow fever.

arch- (arche-, archi-, archo-) *prefix denoting* first; beginning; primitive; ancestral.

arcus (**ar**-kŭs) *n.* (in anatomy) an arch. *a. senilis* a greyish line in the periphery of the cornea, common in the elderly. It begins above and below the cornea but may become a continuous ring.

areola (ă-**ree**-ŏlă) *n.* **1.** the brownish or pink ring of tissue surrounding the nipple of the breast. **2.** the part of the iris that surrounds the pupil of the eye. **3.** a small space in a tissue. —**areolar** (ă-**ree**-ŏler) *adj.*

areolar tissue *n.* loose connective tissue consisting of a meshwork of collagen, elastic tissue, and reticular fibres interspersed with numerous connective tissue cells.

argentaffin cells (ar-**jen**-tă-fin) *pl. n.* cells that stain readily with silver salts. Such cells occur, for example, in the crypts of Lieberkühn in the intestine.

argentaffinoma (carcinoid) (ar-jen-tafi-**noh**-mă) *n.* a tumour of the argentaffin cells in the glands of the intestine. Argentaffinomas typically occur in the tip of the appendix and are among the commonest tumours of the small intestine.

arginine (**ar**-ji-neen) *n.* an amino acid that plays an important role in the formation of urea by the liver.

Argyll Robertson pupil (ar-**gyl** rob-ert-sŏn) *n.* a disorder of the eyes, common to several diseases of the central nervous system, in which the pupillary (light) reflex is absent. Although the pupils contract normally for near vision, they fail to contract in bright light. [D. Argyll Robertson (1837–1909), Scottish ophthalmologist]

ariboflavinosis (ă-ry-boh-flay-vin-**oh**-sis) *n.* the group of symptoms caused by deficiency of riboflavin (vitamin B_2). These symptoms include inflammation of the tongue and lips and sores in the corners of the mouth.

Arnold-Chiari malformation (ar-n'ld ki-**ar**-i) *n.* a congenital disorder in which there is distortion of the base of the skull with protrusion of the lower brainstem and parts of the cerebellum. [J. Arnold (1835–1915) and H. Chiari (1851–1916), German pathologists]

arrector pili (ă-**rek**-tor **pyly**) *n.* (*pl.* **arrectores pilorum**) a small erector muscle attached to the hair follicle. Contraction of the arrectores pilorum causes goose flesh.

arrhythmia (ă-**rith**-miă) *n.* any deviation from the normal rhythm (sinus rhythm) of the heart. Arrhythmias include ectopic beats, ectopic tachycardias, fibrillation, and heart block. *sinus a.* a normal variation in the heart rate, which accelerates slightly on inspiration and slows on expiration.

arsenic (ar-**sĕn**-ik) *n.* a poisonous greyish metallic element producing the symptoms of nausea, vomiting, diarrhoea, cramps, convulsions, and coma when ingested in large doses. Arsenic was formerly used in medicine, the most important arsenical drugs being *arsphenamine* (*Salvarsan*) and *neoarsphenamine*, used in the treatment of syphilis and dangerous parasitic diseases. Symbol: As.

arter- (arteri-, arterio-) *prefix denoting* an artery.

arteriectomy (ar-teer-i-**ek**-tŏmi) *n.* surgical excision of an artery or part of an artery.

arteriogram (ar-**teer**-i-oh-gram) *n.* a tracing of the wave form of an arterial pulse.

arteriography (ar-teer-i-**og**-răfi) *n.* X-ray examination of an artery that has been outlined by the injection of a radio-opaque contrast medium.

arteriole (ar-**teer**-i-ohl) *n.* a small branch of an artery, leading into many smaller vessels – the capillaries. By their constriction and dilation, under the regulation of the sympathetic nervous system, arterioles are the principal controllers of blood flow and pressure.

arteriopathy (ar-teer-i-**op**-ăthi) *n.* disease of an artery.

arterioplasty (ar-**teer**-i-oh-plas-ti) *n.* surgical reconstruction of an artery; for example, in the treatment of aneurysms.

arteriorrhaphy (ar-teer-i-**o**-răfi) *n.* suture of an artery.

arteriosclerosis (ar-teer-i-oh-skleer-**oh**-sis) *n.* any of several conditions affecting the arteries, such as atherosclerosis; *Mönckeberg's degeneration*, in which calcium is deposited in the arteries as part of the ageing process; and *arteriolarsclerosis*, in which the walls of small arteries become thickened due to ageing or hypertension.

arteriotomy (ar-teer-i-**ot**-ŏmi) *n.* an incision into, or a needle puncture of, the wall of an artery.

arteriovenous (ar-teer-i-oh-**vee**-nŭs) *adj.* relating to or affecting an artery and a vein. *a. malformation see* angioma.

arteritis (ar-ter-**I**-tis) *n.* an inflammatory disease affecting the muscular walls of the arteries. The affected vessels are swollen and tender and may become blocked. *temporal* or *giant-cell a.* a condition that occurs in the elderly. It most commonly affects the arteries of the scalp and blindness may result from thrombosis of the arteries to the eyes.

artery (**ar**-ter-i) *n.* a blood vessel carrying blood away from the heart. The walls of arteries contain smooth muscle fibres, which contract or relax under the control of the sympathetic nervous system. *See also* aorta, arteriole. —**arterial** (ar-teer-iăl) *adj.*

arthr- (**arthro-**) *prefix denoting* a joint.

arthralgia (arth-**ral**-jă) *n.* pain in a joint, without swelling or other signs of arthritis. *Compare* arthritis.

arthrectomy (arth-**rek**-tŏmi) *n.* surgical excision of a joint.

arthritis (arth-**ry**-tis) *n.* inflammation of one or more joints, characterized by swelling, warmth, redness of the overlying skin, pain, and restriction of motion. Any disease involving the synovial membranes or causing degeneration of cartilage may cause arthritis. Treatment of arthritis depends on the cause, but aspirin and similar analgesics are often used to suppress inflammation, and hence reduce pain and swelling. *See also* osteoarthritis, psoriasis, rheumatoid arthritis, haemarthrosis, pyarthrosis, hydrarthrosis. —**arthritic** (arth-**rit**-ik) *adj.*

arthroclasia (arth-roh-**klay**-ziă) *n.* the surgical breaking down of ankylosis in a joint to permit freer movement.

arthrodesis (arth-roh-**dee**-sis) *n.* fusion of bones across a joint space by surgical means, which eliminates movement.

arthrodynia (arth-roh-**din**-iă) *n.* pain in a joint.

arthrography (arth-**rog**-răfi) *n.* an X-ray technique for examining joints. A contrast medium (either air or a liquid opaque to X-rays) is injected into the joint space, allowing its outline and contents to be traced accurately.

arthropathy (arth-**rop**-ăthi) *n.* any disease or disorder involving a joint.

arthroplasty (**arth**-roh-plas-ti) *n.* surgical remodelling of a diseased joint. To prevent the ends of the bones fusing after the operation, a large gap may be created between them (*gap a.*), a barrier of artificial material may be inserted (*interposition a.*), or one or both bone ends may be replaced by a prosthesis of metal or plastic (*replacement a.*). *Mc-Kee-Farrar a.* replacement arthroplasty of the hip joint. Both the head of the femur and the acetabulum are replaced by metal prostheses; the replacement acetabulum is cemented into the bone.

arthroscope (**arth**-roh-skohp) *n.* an instrument for insertion into the cavity of a joint in order to inspect the contents.

vertebral

long thoracic

axillary

circumflex

superior mesenteric

renal

testicular (ovarian)

deep palmar arch

superficial palmar arch

descending branch of lateral femoral circumflex

anterior tibial

dorsalis pedis

common carotid

subclavian

aorta

heart

coeliac trunk

abdominal aorta

ulnar

inferior mesenteric

radial

common iliac

internal iliac

femoral

profunda femoris

The principal arteries of the body.

arthrotomy (arth-**rot**-ŏmi) *n.* surgical incision of a joint capsule in order to inspect the contents and drain pus (if it is present).

articulation (ar-tik-yoo-**lay**-shŏn) *n.* (in anatomy) the point or type of contact between two bones. *See* joint.

artificial insemination (ar-ti-**fish**-ăl) *n.* instrumental introduction of semen into the vagina in order that the woman may conceive. The semen specimen may be provided by the husband (*AIH – artificial insemination husband*) in cases of impotence or by an anonymous donor (*AID – artificial insemination donor*) in cases where the husband is sterile.

artificial kidney (dialyser) *n. see* haemodialysis.

artificial lung *n. see* respirator.

artificial respiration *n.* an emergency procedure for maintaining a flow of air into and out of a patient's lungs when the natural breathing reflexes are absent or insufficient. The simplest and most efficient method is the mouth-to-mouth technique (*see* kiss of life).

arytenoid cartilage (a-ri-**tee**-noid) *n.* either of the two pyramid-shaped cartilages that lie at the back of the larynx next to the upper edges of the cricoid cartilage.

asbestos (ass-**best**-os) *n.* a fibrous mineral that is incombustible and does not conduct heat. It is used in the form of fabric or boards for its heat-resistant properties.

asbestosis (ass-best-**oh**-sis) *n.* a lung disease – a form of pneumoconiosis – caused by fibres of asbestos inhaled by those who are exposed to large amounts of the mineral. *See also* mesothelioma.

ascariasis (askă-ry-ăsis) *n.* a disease caused by an infestation with the parasitic worm *Ascaris lumbricoides*. Adult worms in the intestine can cause abdominal pain, vomiting, constipation, diarrhoea, appendicitis, and peritonitis; migrating larvae in the lungs can provoke pneumonia.

Ascaris (**ass**-kă-ris) *n.* a genus of parasitic nematode worms. *A. lumbricoides* the largest of the human intestinal nematodes. Larvae hatch out in the intestine and then migrate via the hepatic portal vein, liver, heart, lungs, windpipe, and pharynx, before returning to the intestine where they later develop into adult worms (*see also* ascariasis).

Aschoff nodules (**ash**-off) *pl. n.* nodules that occur in the muscular and connective tissue of the heart in rheumatic myocarditis. [K. A. L. Aschoff (1866–1942), German pathologist]

ascites (hydroperitoneum) (ă-sy-teez) *n.* the accumulation of fluid in the peritoneal cavity, causing abdominal swelling. *See also* oedema.

ascorbic acid (ă-**skor**-bik) *n. see* vitamin C.

-ase *suffix denoting* an enzyme.

asepsis (ay-**sep**-sis) *n.* the complete absence of bacteria, fungi, viruses, or other microorganisms that could cause disease. Asepsis is the ideal state for the performance of surgical operations and is achieved by using sterilization techniques. —**aseptic** *adj.*

asparagine (ă-**spa**-ră-jeen) *n. see* amino acid.

aspartic acid (aspartate) (ă-**spar**-tik) *n. see* amino acid.

aspergillosis (ass-per-jil-**oh**-sis) *n.* a rare disease in which the fungus *Aspergillus fumigatus* grows freely in pre-existing lesions in the lungs and bronchioles. Occasionally the fungus attacks the mucous membranes of the eyes, nose, or urethra or such internal organs as the lungs, liver, and kidneys.

Aspergillus (ass-per-**jil**-ŭs) *n.* a genus of fungi, including many common moulds, some of which cause infections of the respiratory system in man. *A. fumigatus* the cause of aspergillosis.

aspermia (ă-**sperm**-iă) *n.* strictly, a lack or failure of formation of semen. More usually, however, the term is used to mean the total absence of sperm from the semen (*see* azoospermia).

asphyxia (ă-**sfiks**-iă) *n.* suffocation: a life-threatening condition in which oxygen is prevented from reaching the tissues by obstruction of or damage to any part of the respiratory system.

aspiration (ass-per-**ay**-shŏn) *n.* the withdrawal of fluid from the body by means of suction.

aspirator (**ass**-per-ay-ter) *n.* any of various instruments used for aspiration. Some employ hollow needles for removing fluid from cysts, inflamed joint cavities, etc., another kind is used to suck debris and water from the patient's mouth during dental treatment.

aspirin (acetylsalicylic acid) (**ass**-prin) *n.* a widely used drug that relieves pain and also reduces inflammation and fever. It is taken by mouth for the relief of headache, toothache, neuralgias, etc. It is also taken to reduce fever in influenza and the common cold. Aspirin may irritate the lining of the stomach, causing nausea, vomiting, pain, and bleeding.

assessment (ă-**ses**-měnt) *n.* **1.** the first stage of the nursing process, in which data about the patient's health status are collected and from which nursing diagnoses may be made. **2.** an examination set by an examining body to test a candidate's nursing skills.

assimilation (ă-simi-**lay**-shŏn) *n.* the process by which food substances are taken into the cells of the body after they have been digested and absorbed.

associate nurse (ă-**soh**-si-ăt) *n.* a nurse who provides care for a patient on the instructions of the patient's primary nurse or in her absence. *See* primary nursing.

association area (ă-soh-si-**ay**-shŏn) *n.* an area of cerebral cortex that lies away from the main areas that are concerned with the reception of sensory impulses and the start of motor impulses but is linked to them by many neurones (*association fibres*).

association of ideas *n.* (in psychology) linkage of one idea to another in a regular way according to their meaning. *See also* free association.

astereognosis (ă-ste-ri-ŏg-**noh**-sis) *n. see* agnosia.

asthenia (ass-**theen**-iă) *n.* weakness or loss of strength.

asthenic (ass-**th'en**-ik) *adj.* describing a personality disorder characterized by low energy, susceptibility to physical and emotional stress, and a diminished capacity for pleasure.

asthenopia (ass-thi-**noh**-piă) *n. see* eyestrain.

asthma (**ass**-mă) *n.* a condition characterized by paroxysmal attacks of bronchospasm, causing difficulty in breathing. *bronchial a.* asthma precipitated by exposure to one or more of a large range of stimuli, including allergens, exertion, emotions, and infections. Powerful drugs, including corticosteroids, are now available to control asthmatic attacks, which may be very serious and prolonged (*see* status asthmaticus). *cardiac a.* asthma that occurs in left ventricular heart failure and must be distinguished from bronchial asthma, for which the treatment is different. —**asthmatic** (ass-**mat**-ik) *adj.*

astigmatism (ă-**stig**-mă-tizm) *n.* a defect of vision in which the image of an object is distorted because not all the light from it comes to a focus on the retina. This is usually due to abnormal curvature of the cornea and/or lens, whose surface resembles part of the surface of an egg (rather than a sphere). —**astigmatic** (ass-tig-**mat**-ik) *adj.*

astragalus (ass-**trag**-ălŭs) *n. see* talus.

astringent (ă-**strin**-jěnt) *n.* a drug that causes cells to shrink by precipitating proteins from their surfaces. Astringents are used in lotions to harden and protect the skin and to reduce bleeding from minor abrasions.

astrocytoma (ass-troh-sy-**toh**-mă) *n.* any brain tumour derived from non-nervous supporting cells (glia), which may be benign or malignant. In adults astrocytomas are usually found in the cerebral hemispheres but in children they also occur in the cerebellum.

asymmetry (ay-**sim**-it-ri) *n.* (in anatomy) the state in which opposite parts of an organ or parts at opposite sides of the body do not correspond with each other. —**asymmetric** (ay-si-**met**-rik) *adj.*

asymptomatic (ay-simp-tŏm-**at**-ik) *adj.* not showing any symptoms of disease, whether disease is present or not.

asynclitism (ă-**sin**-klit-izm) *n.* the entry of the head of the baby at birth into the vagina at an oblique angle. *See also* Naegele's obliquity.

asynergia (a-sin-**er**-jiă) *n. see* dyssynergia.

asystole (ă-**sis**-tohl) *n.* a condition in which the heart no longer beats, accompanied by the absence of complexes in the electrocardiogram.

ataraxia (at-ă-**raks**-iă) *n.* a state of calmness and freedom from anxiety, especially the state produced by tranquillizing drugs.

atavism (at-ă-**vizm**) *n.* the phenomenon in which an individual has a character or disease known to have occurred in a remote ancestor but not in his parents.

ataxia (ă-**taks**-iă) *n.* the shaky movements and unsteady gait that result from the brain's failure to regulate the body's posture and the strength and direction of limb movements. *cerebellar a.* a condition in which the patient staggers when walking, cannot pronounce words properly, and has nystagmus. *Friedreich's a.* an inherited disorder appearing first in adolescence. It has the features of cerebellar ataxia, together with spasticity of the limbs. *sensory a.* ataxia that is exaggerated when the patient closes his eyes (*see* Romberg's sign). *See also* tabes dorsalis (locomotor ataxia). —**ataxic** *adj.*

Atebrin (at-eb-rin) *n. see* mepacrine.

atel- (atelo-) *prefix denoting* imperfect or incomplete development.

atalectasis (at-ĕ-lek-tă-sis) *n.* failure of part of the lung to expand. This occurs when the cells lining the alveoli are immature, as in premature babies, or damaged by inhaled substances or secretions.

atherogenic (ath-er-oh-jen-ik) *adj.* denoting a factor that may cause atheroma. Such factors include cigarette smoking, excessive consumption of animal fats and refined sugar, obesity, and inactivity.

atheroma (ath-er-oh-ma) *n.* degeneration of the walls of the arteries due to the formation in them of fatty plaques and scar tissue. This limits blood circulation and predisposes to thrombosis.

atherosclerosis (ath-er-oh-skleer-oh-sis) *n.* a disease of the arteries in which fatty plaques develop on their inner walls, with eventual obstruction of blood flow. *See* atheroma.

athetosis (ath-ĕ-toh-sis) *n.* a writhing involuntary movement especially affecting the hands, face, and tongue. It is usually a form of cerebral palsy.

athlete's foot (ath-leets) *n.* a fungus infection of the skin between the toes: a type of ringworm. Medical name: **tinea pedis**.

atlas (at-lăs) *n.* the first cervical vertebra, by means of which the skull is articulated to the backbone.

atom (at-ŏm) *n.* the smallest constituent of an element that can take part in a chemical reaction. An atom consists of a positively charged nucleus with negatively charged electrons orbiting around it.

atomizer (at-ŏ-my-zer) *n.* an instrument that reduces liquids to a fine spray of minute droplets.

atony (at-ŏni) *n.* a state in which muscles are floppy, lacking their normal elasticity. —**atonic** (ă-ton-ik) *adj.*

atopen (at-oh-pĕn) *n. see* atopy.

atopy (at-oh-pi) *n.* a form of allergy in which the hypersensitivity reaction may be distant from the region of contact with the substance (*atopen*) responsible. —**atopic** (ă-top-ik) *adj.*

ATP (adenosine triphosphate) *n.* a compound that contains adenine, ribose, and three phosphate groups and occurs in cells. The chemical bonds of the phosphate groups store energy needed by the cell, for muscle contraction; this energy is released when ATP is split into ADP or AMP. ATP is formed from ADP or AMP using energy produced by the breakdown of carbohydrates or other food substances. *See also* mitochondrion.

atresia (ă-tree-ziă) *n.* **1.** congenital absence or abnormal narrowing of a body opening. **2.** the degenerative process that affects the majority of ovarian follicles. Usually only one Graafian follicle will ovulate in each menstrual cycle. —**atretic** (ă-tret-ik) *adj.*

atri- (atrio-) *prefix denoting* an atrium, especially the atrium of the heart.

atrial (ay-tri-ăl) *adj.* of or relating to the atrium or atria. *a. fibrillation see* fibrillation. *a. septal defect see* septal defect.

atrioventricular (ay-tri-oh-ven-trik-yoo-ler) *adj.* relating to the atria and ventricles of the heart.

atrioventricular bundle (AV bundle, bundle of His) *n.* a bundle of modified heart muscle fibres (*Purkinje fibres*) passing from the atrioventricular (AV) node forward to the septum between the ventricles, where it divides into right and left bundles, one for each ventricle. The fibres transmit contraction waves from the atria, via the AV node, to the ventricles.

atrioventricular node (AV node) *n.* a mass of modified heart muscle situated in the lower middle part of the right atrium. It receives the impulse to contract from the sinoatrial node, via the atria, and transmits it through the atrioventricular bundle to the ventricles.

atrium (ay-tri-ŭm) *n.* (*pl.* **atria**) 1. either of the two upper chambers of the heart. The left atrium receives arterial blood from the lungs via the pulmonary artery; the right atrium receives venous blood from the venae cavae. *See also* auricle. 2. any of various anatomical chambers into which one or more cavities open. —**atrial** *adj.*

Atromid-S (at-roh-mid-ess) *n. see* clofibrate.

atrophy (at-rŏ-fi) *n.* the wasting away of a normally developed organ or tissue due to degeneration of cells. This may occur through undernourishment, disuse, or ageing. *muscular a.* atrophy of muscular tissue associated with various diseases, such as poliomyelitis.

atropine (at-rŏ-peen) *n.* a drug extracted from belladonna that inhibits the action of certain nerves of the autonomic nervous system (*see* parasympatholytic). Atropine relaxes smooth muscle and is used to treat biliary colic and renal colic. It also reduces secretions of the bronchial tubes, salivary glands, stomach, and intestines and is used before general anaesthesia and to relieve peptic ulcers. It is also used to dilate the pupil of the eye.

attenuation (ă-ten-yoo-ay-shŏn) *n.* reduction of the disease-producing ability (virulence) of a bacterium or virus so that it may be used for immunization.

atypical (ay-tip-ik-ăl) *adj.* not conforming to type.

audi- (audio-) *prefix denoting* hearing or sound.

audiogram (aw-di-oh-gram) *n.* the graphic record of a test of hearing carried out on an audiometer.

audiometer (awdi-om-it-er) *n.* an apparatus for measuring hearing at different sound frequencies, so helping in the diagnosis of deafness. —**audiometry** *n.*

audit (aw-dit) *n.* a means of measuring or analysing the structure, process, or outcomes of healthcare delivery, as a means of quality control.

auditory (aw-dit-er-i) *adj.* relating to the ear or to the sense of hearing. *a. nerve see* vestibulocochlear nerve.

Auerbach's plexus (myenteric plexus) (ow-er-bahks) *n.* a collection of nerve fibres – fine branches of the vagus nerve – within the walls of the intestine. It supplies the muscle layers and controls the movements of peristalsis. [L. Auerbach (1828–97), German anatomist]

aura (or-ă) *n.* the forewarning of an attack, as occurs in epilepsy and migraine.

aural (or-ăl) *adj.* relating to the ear.

An auriscope

Aureomycin (or-i-oh-**my**-sin) *n. see* chlortetracycline.

auricle (or-i-k'l) *n.* **1.** a small pouch in the wall of each atrium of the heart: the term is also used incorrectly as a synonym for atrium. **2.** *see* pinna.

auriscope (otoscope) (or-i-skohp) *n.* an apparatus for examining the eardrum and the external meatus.

auscultation (aw-skŭl-**tay**-shŏn) *n.* the process of listening, usually with a stethoscope, to sounds produced by movement of gas or liquid within the body, as an aid to diagnosis. —**auscultatory** *adj.*

Australia antigen (oss-**tray**-liă) *n.* an antigen that has been detected by serological tests in the serum of patients suffering from serum hepatitis.

aut- (auto-) *prefix denoting* self.

autism (aw-tizm) *n.* **1.** (**Kanner's syndrome, infantile autism**) a rare and severe psychiatric disorder of childhood marked by an inability to communicate by speech or to form normal personal relationships, repetitive and limited patterns of behaviour, and obsessive resistance to tiny changes in familiar surroundings. Most autistic children are intellectually subnormal. **2.** the condition of retreating from realistic thinking to self-centred fantasy thinking: a symptom of personality disorder and schizophrenia. —**autistic** *adj.*

autoantibody (aw-toh-**an**-ti-bodi) *n.* an antibody formed against one of the body's own components in an autoimmune disease.

autoclave (aw-tŏ-klayv) **1.** *n.* a piece of sterilizing equipment in which surgical instruments, dressings, etc., are treated with steam at high pressure. **2.** *vb.* to sterilize in an autoclave.

autograft (aw-tŏ-grahft) *n.* a tissue graft taken from one part of the body and transferred to another part of the same individual. Unlike homografts, autografts are not rejected by the body's immunity defences. *See also* skin (graft).

autoimmune disease (aw-toh-i-**mewn**) *n.* one of a group of otherwise unrelated disorders suspected of being caused by inflammation and destruction of tissues by autoantibodies. These disorders include pernicious anaemia, rheumatic fever, rheumatoid arthritis, glomerulonephritis, and Hashimoto's disease.

autoimmunity (aw-toh-i-**mewn**-iti) *n.* a disorder of the body's defence mechanisms in which antibodies are produced against certain components or products of its own tissues, treating them as foreign material and attacking them. *See* autoimmune disease, immunity.

autoinfection (aw-toh-in-**fek**-shŏn) *n.* **1.** infection by an organism that is already present in the body. **2.** infection transferred from one part of the body to another via the fingers, towels, etc.

autointoxication (aw-toh-in-toks-i-**kay**-shŏn) *n.* poisoning by a toxin formed within the body.

autolysis (aw-**tol**-i-sis) *n.* the destruction of tissues or cells brought about by the actions of their own enzymes. *See* lysosome.

automatism (aw-**tom**-ă-tizm) *n.* one of the symptoms of temporal lobe epilepsy, in which the patient performs well-organized movements during an attack.

autonomic nervous system (aw-tŏ-**nom**-ik) *n.* the part of the nervous system responsible for the control of bodily functions that are not consciously directed, including regular beating of the heart, intestinal movements, sweating, salivation, etc. *See* parasympathetic nervous system, sympathetic nervous system.

autonomy (aw-**tonn**-ŏmi) *n.* the right of personal freedom of action, said to be one of the characteristics of a profession.

autopsy (necropsy, post mortem) (aw-**top**-si) *n.* dissection and examination of a body after death in order to determine the cause of death or the presence of disease processes.

autoradiography (radioautography) (aw-toh-ray-di-**og**-răfi) *n.* a technique for examining the distribution of a radioactive tracer in the tissues of an experimental animal.

autosome (aw-tŏ-sohm) *n.* any chromosome that is not a sex chromosome and that occurs in pairs in diploid cells. —**autosomal** *adj.*

autosuggestion (aw-toh-sŭ-**jes**-chŏn) *n.* self-suggestion or self-conditioning that involves repeating ideas to oneself in order to change psychological or physiological states. *See* suggestion.

autotransfusion (aw-toh-trans-**few**-zhŏn) *n.* reintroduction into a patient of blood that has been lost from the patient's circulation during surgical operation.

aux- (auxo-) *prefix denoting* increase; growth.

avascular (ă-**vas**-kew-ler) *adj.* lacking blood vessels or having a poor blood supply.

aversion therapy (ă-**ver**-shŏn) *n.* a form of behaviour therapy that is used to reduce the occurrence of undesirable behaviour. The patient is conditioned by repeated pairing of some unpleasant stimulus with a stimulus related to the undesirable behaviour. *See also* sensitization.

avitaminosis (avi-tami-**noh**-sis) *n.* the condition caused by lack of a vitamin. *See also* deficiency disease.

avulsion (evulsion) (ă-**vul**-shŏn) *n.* the tearing or forcible separation of part of a structure.

axilla (ak-**sil**-ă) *n.* (*pl.* **axillae**) the armpit. —**axillary** *adj.*

axis (**aks**-is) *n.* **1.** a real or imaginary line through the centre of the body or one of its parts or a line about which the body or a part rotates. **2.** the second cervical vertebra, which articulates with the atlas vertebra above and allows rotational movement of the head.

axon (**aks**-on) *n.* a nerve fibre: a single process extending from the cell body of a neurone and carrying nerve impulses away from it.

azathioprine (ază-**th'y**-ŏ-preen) *n.* an immunosuppressive drug, used mainly to aid the survival of organ or tissue transplants. Trade name: **Imuran**.

azo- (azoto-) *prefix denoting* a nitrogenous compound, such as urea.

azoospermia (aspermia) (ay-zoh-ŏ-**sperm**-iă) *n.* the complete absence of sperm from the seminal fluid.

azotaemia (azŏ-**tee**-miă) *n.* a former name for uraemia.

azoturia (azŏ-**tewr**-iă) *n.* the presence in the urine of an abnormally high concentration of nitrogen-containing compounds, especially urea.

azygos vein (**az**-i-gos) *n.* an unpaired vein that arises from the inferior vena cava and drains into the superior vena cava, returning blood from the thorax and abdominal cavities.

B

Babinski reflex (ba-**bin**-ski) *n.* an upward movement of the great toe that is an abnormal plantar reflex indicating disease in the brain or spinal cord. [J. F. F. Babinski (1857–1932), French neurologist]

bacillaemia (ba-si-**lee**-miă) *n.* the presence of bacilli in the blood, resulting from infection.

bacille Calmette-Guérin (ba-**seel** kal-**met** gay-**ran**) *n. see* BCG. [A. L. C. Calmette (1863–1933) and C. Guérin (1872–1961), French bacteriologists]

bacilluria (ba-sil-**yoor**-iă) *n.* the presence of bacilli in the urine, resulting from a bladder or kidney infection. *See* cystitis.

bacillus (bă-**sil**-ŭs) *n.* (*pl.* **bacilli**) any rod-shaped bacterium. *See also* Bacillus, Lactobacillus, Streptobacillus.

Bacillus *n.* a large genus of Gram-positive spore-bearing rodlike bacteria. They are widely distributed in soil and air (usually as spores). *B. anthracis* a nonmotile species that causes anthrax. *B. polymyxa* the source of the polymyxin group of antibiotics. *B. subtilis* a species that may cause conjunctivitis in man; it also produces the antibiotic bacitracin.

bacitracin (ba-si-**tray**-sin) *n.* an antibiotic produced by certain strains of bacteria and effective against a number of microorganisms. It is usually applied externally, to treat infections of the skin, eyes, or nose.

backbone (spinal column, spine, vertebral column) (**bak**-bohn) *n.* the flexible bony column, extending from the base of the skull to the small of the back, that encloses and protects the spinal cord. It is made up of individual bones (*see* vertebra) connected by discs of fibrocartilage (*see* intervertebral disc). The backbone of a newborn baby contains 33 vertebrae: seven cervical, 12 thoracic, five lumbar, five sacral, and four coccygeal. In the adult the sacral and coccygeal vertebrae become fused into two single bones (sacrum and coccyx, respectively). Anatomical name: **rachis**.

bacteraemia (bak-ter-**ee**-miă) *n.* the presence of bacteria in the blood: a sign of infection.

cervical
vertebrae
(7)

thoracic
vertebrae
(12)

lumbar
vertebrae
(5)

sacrum
(5 fused)

coccyx
(4 fused)

A

B

The backbone, seen from the back (A) and left side (B)

bacteri- (bacterio-) *prefix denoting* bacteria.

bacteria (bak-**teer**-iă) *pl. n.* (*sing.* **bacterium**) a group of microorganisms all of which lack a distinct nuclear membrane and have a cell wall of unique composition. Most bacteria are unicellular; the cells may be spherical (*see* coc-

cus), rodlike (*see* bacillus), spiral (*see* Spirillum), comma-shaped (*see* Vibrio) or corkscrew-shaped (*see* spirochaete). Generally, they range in size between 0.5 and 5 μm. Motile species bear one or more fine hairs (flagella) arising from their surface. Most bacteria reproduce asexually by simple division of cells; some may reproduce sexually by conjugation. Bacteria live in soil, water, or air or as parasites of man, animals, and plants. Some parasitic bacteria cause diseases by producing poisons (*see* endotoxin, exotoxin). —**bacterial** *adj*.

bactericidal (bak-teer-i-sy-dăl) *adj*. capable of killing bacteria. Substances with this property include antibiotics, antiseptics, and disinfectants. *Compare* bacteriostatic. —**bactericide** *n*.

bacteriology (bak-teer-i-ol-ŏji) *n*. the science of bacteria. *See also* microbiology. —**bacteriological** *adj*. —**bacteriologist** *n*.

bacteriolysin (bak-teer-i-ol-i-sin) *n*. *see* lysin.

bacteriolysis (bak-teer-i-ol-i-sis) *n*. the destruction of bacteria by lysis. —**bacteriolytic** *adj*.

bacteriophage (**phage**) (bak-teer-i-oh-fayj) *n*. a virus that attacks bacteria. The phage grows and replicates in the bacterial cell, which is eventually destroyed with the release of new phages. Each phage acts specifically against a particular species of bacterium. This is utilized in *phage-typing*, a technique of identifying bacteria by the action of known phages on them.

bacteriostatic (bak-teer-i-oh-stat-ik) *adj*. capable of inhibiting or retarding the growth and multiplication of bacteria. *Compare* bactericidal.

bacterium (bak-teer-iŭm) *n*. *see* bacteria.

bacteriuria (bak-teer-i-yoor-iă) *n*. the presence of bacteria in the urine.

Bactrim (bak-trim) *n*. *see* co-trimoxazole.

Baghdad boil (bag-dad) *n*. *see* oriental sore.

BAL (**British Anti-Lewisite**) *n*. *see* dimercaprol.

balanitis (bal-ă-ny-tis) *n*. inflammation of the glans penis, usually associated with tightness of the foreskin (phimosis).

balanoposthitis (bal-ă-noh-posth'y-tis) *n*. inflammation of the foreskin and the surface of the underlying glans penis. It usually occurs as a consequence of phimosis and represents a more extensive local reaction than simple balanitis.

balantidiasis (bal-ăn-ti-dy-ă-sis) *n*. an infestation of the large intestine of man with the parasitic protozoan *Balantidium coli*. The parasite invades and destroys the intestinal wall, causing ulceration and necrosis, and the patient may experience diarrhoea and dysentery.

baldness (bawld-nis) *n*. *see* alopecia.

Balkan beam (**Balkan frame**) (bawl-kăn) *n*. a rectangular frame attached over a bed, used for the support of splints, pulleys, or slings for an immobilized limb.

ball-and-socket joint (bawl-ănd-sok-it) *n*. *see* enarthrosis.

ballottement (bă-lot-mĕnt) *n*. the technique of examining a fluid-filled part of the body to detect a floating object. During pregnancy, a sharp tap with the fingers, applied to the womb through the abdominal wall or the vagina, causes the fetus to move away and then return, with an answering tap, to its original position.

balneotherapy (bal-ni-oh-th'e-ră-pi) *n*. the treatment of disease by bathing, originally in the mineral-containing waters of hot springs. Today, specialized remedial treatment in baths is used to alleviate pain and improve blood circulation and limb mobility in conditions such as arthritis.

balsam (bawl-săm) *n.* an aromatic resinous substance of plant origin. *b. of Peru* a South American balsam used in skin preparations as a mild antiseptic. *See* friar's balsam.

bandage (band-ij) *n.* a piece of material, in the form of a pad or strip, applied to a wound or used to bind around an injured or diseased part of the body.

Bandl's ring (ban-d'lz) *n. see* retraction (ring). [L. Bandl (1842–92), German obstetrician]

Bankart's operation (bank-arts) *n.* an operation to repair a defect in the glenoid cavity in cases of recurrent dislocation of the shoulder. [A. S. B. Bankart (1879–1951), British orthopaedic surgeon]

Banti's syndrome (ban-teez) *n.* a disorder in which enlargement and overactivity of the spleen occurs as a result of increased pressure within the splenic vein. The commonest cause is cirrhosis of the liver. [G. Banti (1852–1925), Italian pathologist]

barbitone (barbital) (bar-bi-tohn) *n.* a long-acting barbiturate, used as a hypnotic, as a sedative, for the suppression of convulsions, as an analgesic, and as an anaesthetic. Trade name: **Veronal**.

barbiturate (bar-bit-yoor-ăt) *n.* any of a group of drugs derived from barbituric acid, such as amylobarbitone, phenobarbitone, and thiopentone, that depress activity of the central nervous system. Most are taken as sleeping pills; some are used as sedatives or anaesthetics. Because they produce psychological and physical dependence and have serious toxic side-effects (*see* barbiturism), barbiturates have been largely replaced in clinical use by safer drugs. The use of barbiturates with alcohol should be avoided.

barbiturism (bar-bit-yoor-izm) *n.* addiction to drugs of the barbiturate group. Signs of intoxication include slurring of speech, sleepiness, and loss of balance. Withdrawal of the drugs must be undertaken slowly.

barbotage (bar-bŏ-tah*z*h) *n.* a method of spinal anaesthesia in which a small amount of anaesthetic is injected into the subarachnoid space followed by withdrawal of cerebrospinal fluid into the syringe. This process is repeated until all the anaesthetic has been injected.

barium sulphate (bair-iŭm) *n.* a barium salt, insoluble in water, that is opaque to X-rays and is used as a contrast medium in radiography of the stomach and intestines. *See also* enema.

Barlow's disease (bar-lohz) *n.* infantile scurvy: scurvy occurring in young children due to dietary deficiency of vitamin C. [Sir T. Barlow (1845–1945), British physician]

baroreceptor (baroceptor) (ba-roh-ri-sep-ter) *n.* a collection of sensory nerve endings specialized to monitor changes in blood pressure. The main receptors lie in the carotid sinuses and the aortic arch.

Barr body (bar) *n. see* sex chromatin. [M. L. Barr (1908–), Canadian anatomist]

barrier nursing (ba-ri-er) *n.* the nursing care of an infectious patient in isolation from other patients, to prevent the spread of infection.

bartholinitis (vulvovaginitis) (bar-thŏ-li-ny-tis) *n.* inflammation of Bartholin's glands. *acute b.* bartholinitis in which the glands are blocked and an abscess develops. *chronic b.* bartholinitis in which cysts may form in the glands.

Bartholin's glands (greater vestibular glands) (bar-thŏ-linz) *pl. n.* a pair of glands that open at the junction of the vagina and the vulva. Their secretions lubricate the vulva and so assist penetration by the penis during coitus. [C. Bartholin (1655–1748), Danish anatomist]

basal cell carcinoma (bay-săl) *n. see* rodent ulcer.

basal ganglia *pl. n.* several large masses of grey matter embedded deep within the white matter of the cerebrum. They include the *caudate* and *lenticular nuclei* (together known as the *corpus striatum*) and the *amygdaloid nucleus*. The lenticular nucleus consists of the *putamen* and *globus pallidus*. The basal ganglia are involved with the regulation of voluntary movements at a subconscious level.

basal metabolism *n.* the minimum amount of energy expended by the body to maintain vital processes, e.g. respiration, circulation, and digestion. It is expressed in terms of heat production per unit of body surface area per day (*basal metabolic rate – BMR*). BMR is normally determined indirectly, by measuring the respiratory quotient. Measurements are best taken during a period of least activity, i.e. during sleep and 12–18 hours after a meal, under controlled temperature conditions.

basal narcosis *n.* preliminary unconsciousness induced in a patient by administration of a narcotic drug prior to administration of a general anaesthetic by inhalation.

base (bayss) *n.* **1.** the main ingredient of an ointment or other medicinal preparation. **2.** a substance that releases hydroxyl ions when dissolved in water, has a pH greater than 7 and turns litmus paper blue, and reacts with an acid to form a salt and water only. *Compare* acid.

basement membrane (bayss-měnt) *n.* the thin delicate membrane that lies at the base of an epithelium.

basilar artery (ba-si-ler) *n.* an artery in the base of the brain, formed by the union of the two vertebral arteries.

basilic vein (bă-zil-ik) *n.* a large vein in the arm, extending from the hand along the back of the forearm, then passing forward to the inner side of the arm at the elbow.

basophil (bay-sŏ-fil) *n.* a variety of white blood cell distinguished by the presence in its cytoplasm of coarse granules that stain purple-black with Romanowsky stains. Basophils are capable of ingesting foreign particles and contain histamine and heparin.

basophilia (bay-sŏ-fil-iă) *n.* **1.** a property of a microscopic structure whereby it shows an affinity for basic dyes. **2.** an increase in the number of basophils in the blood. —**basophilic** *adj.*

Batchelor plaster (ba-chě-ler) *n.* a type of plaster that keeps both legs abducted and medially rotated, used to correct congenital dislocation of the hip. [J. S. Batchelor (1905–), British orthopaedic surgeon]

battered baby syndrome (bat-erd) *n.* injuries inflicted on babies or young children by their parents. Battering commonly takes the form of facial bruises, cigarette burns, bites, head injuries (often with brain damage), and fractured bones; it may be triggered by such crises as an unwanted pregnancy, unemployment, and debts.

battledore placenta (bat-t'l-dor) *n.* a placenta to which the umbilical cord is attached at the margin (rather than at the centre).

Bazin's disease (ba-zanz) *n.* a disease of young women in which tender nodules develop under the skin in the calves. The nodules may break down and ulcerate though they may clear up spontaneously. Medical name: **erythema induratum.** [A. P. E. Bazin (1807–78), French dermatologist]

BCG (bacille Calmette-Guérin) *n.* a strain of tubercle bacillus that has lost the power to cause tuberculosis but retains its antigenic activity; it is therefore used to prepare a vaccine against the disease.

bearing down (bair-ing down) *n.* **1.** the expulsive uterine contractions of a woman in the second stage of labour. **2.** a sensation of heaviness and descent in the pelvis associated with pelvic tumours and certain other disorders.

bed bug (bed bug) *n.* a bloodsucking insect of the genus *Cimex*, especially *C. lectularius*. They live and lay their eggs in the crevices of walls and furniture and emerge at night to suck blood; their bites leave a route for bacterial infection.

bed occupancy *n.* the number of hospital beds occupied by patients expressed as a percentage of the total beds available in the ward, specialty, hospital, area, or region. It is used to assess the demands for hospital beds and hence to gauge an appropriate balance between health needs and residential (hospital) resources.

bedsore (decubitus ulcer, pressure sore) (bed-sor) *n.* an ulcerated area of skin caused by irritation and continuous pressure on part of the body in a bedridden patient. Careful nursing is necessary to prevent local gangrene. The patient's position should be changed frequently, and the buttocks, heels, elbows, and other regions at risk kept dry and clean.

bedwetting (bed-wet-ing) *n. see* enuresis.

behavioural objective (bi-hayv-yer-ăl) *n.* the goal of a particular nursing intervention or a specific lesson, in terms of what a person is expected to be able to do as a result of it.

behaviourism (bi-hayv-yer-izm) *n.* an approach to psychology postulating that only observable behaviour need be studied, thus denying any importance to unconscious processes. **—behaviourist** *n.*

behaviour therapy (bi-hayv-yer) *n.* treatment based on the belief that psychological problems are the products of faulty learning and not the symptoms of an underlying disease. *See also* aversion therapy, conditioning, desensitization.

bejel (endemic syphilis) (bej-ĕl) *n.* a long-lasting nonvenereal form of syphilis, particularly prevalent where standards of personal hygiene are low. The disease is spread among children and adults by direct body contact.

belladonna (bel-ă-don-ă) *n.* **1.** deadly nightshade (*Atropa belladonna*). **2.** the poisonous alkaloid derived from deadly nightshade, from which atropine and hyoscyamine are extracted.

belle indifférence (bel an-di-fay-rahns) *n.* inappropriate calmness in the face of distressing physical symptoms, characteristic of patients with conversion hysteria.

Bellocq's cannula (Bellocq's sound) (bel-oks) *n.* a curved hollow tube used for inserting a plug into the nose to arrest nosebleeding. [J. J. Bellocq (1732–1807), French surgeon]

Bell's palsy (belz) *n.* paralysis of the facial nerve causing weakness of the muscles of one side of the face and an inability to close the eye. [Sir C. Bell (1774–1842), Scottish physiologist]

belly (bel-i) *n.* **1.** the abdomen or abdominal cavity. **2.** the central fleshy portion of a muscle.

Bence-Jones protein (Bence-Jones albumose) (benss-joh'nz) *n.* a protein of low molecular weight found in the urine of patients with multiple myeloma, lymphoma, leukaemia, and Hodgkin's disease. [H. Bence-Jones (1814–73), British physician]

bendrofluazide (bendroflumethazide) (ben-droh-floo-ă-zyd) *n.* a potent diuretic used in the treatment of conditions involving retention of fluid, such as hypertension and oedema.

bends (bendz) *n. see* compressed air illness.

Benedict's test (ben-i-dikts) *n.* a test for the presence of sugar in urine or other liquids, using a solution of sodium or potassium citrate, sodium carbonate, and copper sulphate (*Benedict's solution*). [S. R. Benedict (1884–1936), US chemist]

benethamine penicillin (ben-eth-ă-min) *n.* an antibiotic, derived from benzylpenicillin, effective against most Gram-positive bacteria.

benign (bi-nyn) *adj.* **1.** describing a tumour that is not cancerous. **2.** describing any disorder or condition that does not produce harmful effects. *Compare* malignant.

benorylate (ben-or-il-ayt) *n.* a drug, derived from paracetamol, that relieves pain, inflammation, and fever. It is an alternative to aspirin, particularly in the treatment of rheumatoid arthritis. Trade name: **Benoral.**

benzalkonium (ben-zăl-koh-niŭm) *n.* a detergent disinfectant with the same uses and effects as cetrimide.

benzathine penicillin (ben-ză-theen) *n.* a long-acting antibiotic, given by mouth or intramuscular injection, that is effective against most Gram-positive bacteria (streptococci, staphylococci, and pneumococci). Trade names: **Bicillin, Penidural.** *See also* penicillin.

benzene (ben-zeen) *n.* a toxic liquid hydrocarbon. Continued inhalation of benzene vapour may result in aplastic anaemia or a form of leukaemia. Formula: C_6H_6.

benzhexol (benz-heks-ol) *n.* a drug that acts in a similar way to atropine. Taken by mouth, it is used mainly to reduce muscle spasm in parkinsonism. Trade names: **Artane, Pipanol.**

benzocaine (ben-zoh-kayn) *n.* a local anaesthetic applied externally to relieve painful conditions of the skin and mucous membranes. Virtually nontoxic, it can also be administered orally to treat mouth lacerations or gastric ulcers.

benzodiazepines (ben-zoh-dy-az-ĕ-peenz) *pl. n.* a group of minor tranquillizers and hypnotics, including diazepam and oxazepam.

benzoic acid (ben-zoh-ik) *n.* an antiseptic used as a preservative and to treat fungal infections of the skin.

benzoin (ben-zoh-in) *n.* a fragrant gum resin used as a constituent of friar's balsam.

benzthiazide (benz-th'y-ă-zyd) *n.* a diuretic used in the treatment of conditions involving fluid retention. Trade name: **Exna.**

benztropine (benz-trŏ-peen) *n.* a drug similar to atropine, used mainly in the treatment of parkinsonism to reduce rigidity and muscle cramps.

benzyl benzoate (ben-zyl ben-zoh-ayt) *n.* an oily aromatic liquid that is applied externally for the treatment of scabies.

benzylpenicillin (ben-zyl-pen-i-sil-in) *n. see* penicillin.

beriberi (b'e-ri-b'e-ri) *n.* a nutritional disorder due to deficiency of vitamin B_1 (thiamin). It is widespread in communities in which the diet is based on polished rice. *dry b.* a form of beriberi in which there is extreme emaciation. *wet b.* a form of beriberi in which there is an accumulation of tissue fluid (oedema). There is nervous degeneration in both forms of the dis-

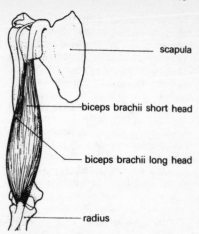

The biceps muscle of the arm

ease and death from heart failure is often the outcome.

berylliosis (b'e-ri-li-oh-sis) *n.* poisoning by inhalation of beryllium or its compounds. This may be acute and sometimes fatal, but is more often chronic with the development of fibrosis affecting all parts of the lungs.

beta blocker (bee-tă) *n.* a drug, such as oxprenolol or propranolol, that prevents stimulation of the beta-adrenergic receptors of the nerves of the sympathetic nervous system and therefore decreases the activity of the heart.

beta cells *pl. n.* the cells of the islets of Langerhans that produce insulin. *Compare* alpha cells.

betamethasone (bee-tă-meth-ă-sohn) *n.* a synthetic corticosteroid drug with effects and uses similar to those of prednisolone. The side-effects are those of cortisone. Trade names: **Betnelan, Betnesol, Betnovate.**

betatron (bee-tă-tron) *n.* a device used to accelerate a stream of electrons (*beta particles*) into a beam of radiation that can be used in radiotherapy.

bethanidine (beth-**an**-i-deen) *n.* a drug that is administered orally to lower blood pressure. Trade names: **Bethamid, Esbatal**.

bezoar (**bee**-zor) *n.* a mass of swallowed foreign material within the stomach.

bi- *prefix denoting* two; double.

bicarbonate (by-**kar**-bŏ-nit) *n.* a salt containing the ion HCO_3^-. *b. of soda see* sodium bicarbonate.

biceps (**by**-seps) *n.* a muscle with two heads. *b. brachii* a muscle that extends from the shoulder to the elbow and is responsible for flexing the arm and forearm. *b. femoris* a muscle at the back of the thigh, responsible for flexing the knee.

biconcave (by-**kon**-kayv) *adj.* having a hollowed surface on both sides. Biconcave lenses are used to correct short-sightedness. *Compare* biconvex.

biconvex (by-**kon**-veks) *adj.* having a surface on each side that curves outwards. Biconcave lenses are used to correct long-sightedness. *Compare* biconcave.

bicornuate (by-**kor**-new-it) *adj.* having two hornlike processes or projections. The term is applied to an abnormal uterus that is divided into two separate halves at the upper end.

bicuspid (by-**kus**-pid) *adj.* having two cusps, as in the premolar teeth and the mitral valve of the heart. *b. valve see* mitral valve.

bifid (**by**-fid) *adj.* split or cleft into two parts.

bifocal lenses (by-**foh**-kăl) *pl. n.* glasses in which the upper part of the lens is shaped to give a sharp image of distant objects and the lower part is for use in near vision, such as reading. *See also* multifocal lenses.

bifurcation (by-fer-**kay**-shŏn) *n.* (in anatomy) the point at which division into two branches occurs; for example in blood vessels or in the trachea.

bigeminy (by-**jem**-ini) *n.* the condition in which alternate ectopic beats of the heart are transmitted to the pulse and felt as a double pulse beat (*pulsus bigeminus*).

bilateral (by-**lat**-er-ăl) *adj.* (in anatomy) relating to or affecting both sides of the body or of a tissue or organ or both of a pair of organs.

bile (byl) *n.* a thick alkaline fluid that is secreted by the liver and stored in the gall bladder. It is ejected intermittently into the duodenum, where it helps to emulsify fats so that they can be more easily digested. Bile may be yellow, green, or brown; its constituents include bile pigments and salts, lecithin, and cholesterol.

bile acids *pl. n.* the organic acids in bile; mostly occurring as bile salts. They are cholic acid, deoxycholic acid, glycocholic acid, and taurocholic acid.

bile duct *n.* any of the ducts that convey bile from the liver. Many small ducts unite to form the main bile duct, the *hepatic duct*. This joins the *cystic duct*, which leads from the gall bladder, to form the *common bile duct*, which drains into the duodenum.

bile pigments *pl. n.* coloured compounds – breakdown products of the blood pigment haemoglobin – that are excreted in bile. The two most important bile pigments are *bilirubin*, which is orange or yellow, and its oxidized form *biliverdin*, which is green. Mixed with the intestinal contents, they give the brown colour to the faeces (*see* urobilinogen).

bile salts *pl. n.* sodium glycocholate and sodium taurocholate – the alkaline salts of bile – necessary for the emulsification of fats.

Bilharzia (bil-**harts**-iă) *n. see* Schistosoma.

bilharziasis (bil-harts-I-ă-sis) *n. see* schistosomiasis.

bili- *prefix denoting* bile.

biliary (**bil**-yer-i) *adj.* relating to or affecting the bile duct or bile. *b. colic* severe steady pain in the upper abdomen (in the mid-line or to the right) resulting from obstruction of the gall bladder or common bile duct, usually by a stone. Vomiting often occurs simultaneously. *b. fistula see* fistula.

bilious (**bil**-yŭs) *adj.* **1.** containing bile. **2.** a lay term used to describe attacks of nausea or vomiting.

bilirubin (bili-**roo**-bin) *n. see* bile pigments.

biliuria (**choluria**) (bili-**yoor**-iă) *n.* the presence of bile in the urine: a feature of certain forms of jaundice.

biliverdin (bili-**ver**-din) *n. see* bile pigments.

Billroth's operation (**bil**-rohts) *n.* an operation in which the lower part of the stomach is removed and the remaining portion joined to the duodenum (*B. o. I*) or the lower stomach and duodenum are removed, with attachment of the remaining stomach to the jejunum (*B. o. II*). *See* gastrectomy. [C. A. T. Billroth (1829–94), Austrian surgeon]

bimanual (by-**man**-yoo-ăl) *adj.* us-

ing two hands to perform an activity, such as a gynaecological examination.

binaural (byn-**or**-ăl) *adj.* relating to or involving the use of both ears.

binder (**byn**-der) *n.* a bandage that is wound around a part of the body, usually the abdomen, to apply pressure or to give support or protection.

binocular (bin-**ok**-yoo-ler) *adj.* relating to or involving the use of both eyes. *b. vision* the acquired ability to focus both eyes on an object at the same time, so that only one image is seen.

binovular (bin-**ov**-yoo-ler) *adj.* derived from two separate ova, as are fraternal twins. *Compare* uniovular.

bio- *prefix denoting* life or living organisms.

bioassay (by-oh-**ass**-ay) *n.* estimation of the activity or potency of a drug or other substance by comparing its effects on living organisms with effects of a preparation of known strength.

biochemistry (by-oh-**kem**-istri) *n.* the study of the chemical processes and substances occurring in living things. —**biochemical** *adj.* —**biochemist** *n.*

biogenesis (by-oh-**jen**-i-sis) *n.* the theory that living organisms can arise only from other living organisms and not from nonliving matter.

biology (by-**ol**-ŏji) *n.* the study of living organisms including their structure and working and their relationships with one another and with the inanimate world. —**biological** (by-ŏ-**loj**-ik-ăl) *adj.* —**biologist** *n.*

bionics (by-**on**-iks) *n.* the science of mechanical or electronic systems that function in the same way as, or have characteristics of, living systems. *Compare* cybernetics. −**bionic** *adj.*

bionomics (by-ŏ-**nom**-iks) *n. see* ecology.

biopsy (**by**-op-si) *n.* the removal of a small piece of living tissue from an organ or part of the body for microscopic examination.

biostatistics (by-oh-stă-**tist**-iks) *n.* statistical information and techniques used with special reference to studies of health and social problems. *See also* demography, vital statistics.

biotin (**by**-ŏ-tin) *n.* a vitamin of the B complex that is essential for the metabolism of fat, being involved in fatty acid synthesis and gluconeogenesis. Rich sources of the vitamin are egg yolk, yeast, and liver.

bipara (**bip**-er-ă) *n.* a woman who has been pregnant twice and has given birth to a living child at the end of each pregnancy.

biparous (**bip**-er-ŭs) *adj.* giving birth to two children at the end of a pregnancy.

bipolar (by-**poh**-ler) *adj.* (in neurology) describing a neurone (nerve cell) that has two processes extending in different directions from its cell body.

birth (berth) *n.* (in obstetrics) *see* labour.

birth control *n.* the use of contraception or sterilization (male or female) to prevent unwanted pregnancies.

birthmark (**berth**-mark) *n.* a skin blemish or mark present at birth.

birth rate *n. see* fertility rate.

bisacodyl (bis-ak-oh-dil) *n.* a laxative that acts on the large intestine to cause reflex movement and bowel evacuation. It is administered by mouth or in a

Types of bistoury

suppository. Trade name: **Dulcolax**.

bisexual (by-**seks**-yoo-ăl) *adj.* **1.** describing an individual who is sexually attracted to both men and women. **2.** describing an individual who possesses the qualities of both sexes.

bismuth salts (**biz**-mŭth) *pl. n.* salts of bismuth used in some antacid mixtures and as protective agents in skin powders and pastes. They were formerly widely used in the treatment of syphilis.

bistoury (**bis**-ter-i) *n.* a narrow surgical knife, with a straight or curved blade.

bite-wing (**byt**-wing) *n.* a dental X-ray film that provides a view of the crowns of the teeth in part of both upper and lower jaws.

bivalve (**by**-valv) *adj.* consisting of or possessing two valves or sections. *b. cast* a plaster cast that is cut into anterior and posterior sections to monitor pressure beneath the cast. *b. speculum* a vaginal speculum that has two blades.

black eye (blak) *n.* bruising of the eyelids.

blackhead (**blak**-hed) *n.* a plug formed of fatty material (sebum and keratin) in the outlet of a sebaceous gland in the skin. Oxidation of the keratin in the blackhead is the cause of the black coloration. *See also* acne. Medical name: **comedo**.

blackwater fever (blak-waw-ter) *n.* a rare and serious complication of malignant tertian (falciparum) malaria in which there is massive destruction of the red blood cells, leading to the presence of the blood pigment haemoglobin in the urine.

bladder (blad-er) *n.* **1.** (**urinary bladder**) a sac-shaped organ that has a wall of smooth muscle and stores the urine produced by the kidneys. **2.** any of several other hollow organs containing fluid, such as the gail bladder.

bladderworm (blad-er-werm) *n. see* cysticercus.

Blalock-Taussig operation (blay-lok taw-sig) *n.* an operation in which the pulmonary artery is anastomosed to the subclavian artery, performed on patients with tetralogy of Fallot. [A. Blalock (1899–1964), US surgeon; H. B. Taussig (1898–   ), US paediatrician]

bland (bland) *adj.* nonirritating; mild; soothing: applied to foods and diets.

-blast *suffix denoting* a formative cell.

blasto- *prefix denoting* a germ cell or embryo.

blastocyst (blast-oh-sist) *n.* an early stage of embryonic development that consists of a hollow ball of cells with a localized thickening (the *inner cell mass*) that will develop into the actual embryo. *See also* implantation.

blastomycosis (blast-oh-my-koh-sis) *n.* any disease caused by parasitic fungi of the genus *Blastomyces*, which may affect the skin (forming wartlike ulcers and tumours) or involve various internal tissues.

blastula (blast-yoo-lă) *n.* an early stage of the embryonic development of many animals. The equivalent stage in mammals (including man) is the blastocyst.

bleeding (bleed-ing) *n. see* haemorrhage.

bleeding time *n.* the time taken for bleeding to cease from a small wound, such as a puncture in a finger or ear lobe. It is used as a test of platelet function.

blenn- (blenno-) *prefix denoting* mucus.

blennorrhagia (blen-ŏ-ray-jiă) *n.* a copious discharge of mucus, particularly from the urethra.

blennorrhoea (blen-ŏ-ree-ă) *n.* a profuse watery discharge from the urethra.

bleomycin (bli-oh-my-sin) *n.* an antibiotic with action against cancer cells, administered by injection in the treatment of Hodgkin's disease and other lymphomas and in squamous-cell carcinoma.

blephar- (blepharo-) *prefix denoting* the eyelid.

blepharitis (blef-ă-ry-tis) *n.* inflammation of the eyelids.

blepharon (blef-er-ŏn) *n. see* eyelid.

blepharospasm (blef-er-oh-spazm) *n.* involuntary tight contraction of the eyelids, usually in response to painful conditions of the eye.

blindness (blynd-nis) *n.* the inability to see. For administrative purposes, the term also covers cases of partial blindness (*see* blind register). The commonest causes of blindness worldwide are trachoma, onchocerciasis, and vitamin A deficiency, and in Great Britain diabetes mellitus, myopic degeneration, and glaucoma. *See also* colour blindness, day blindness, night blindness, snow blindness.

blind register (blynd) *n.* (in Britain) a list of persons who are technically blind due to reduced visual acuity or who have severely restricted fields of vision.

blind spot *n.* the small area of the retina of the eye where the nerve fibres from the light-sensitive cells lead into the optic nerve. There are no rods or cones in this area and hence it does not register light. Anatomical name: **punctum caecum**.

blister (blis-ter) *n.* a swelling containing watery fluid (serum) and sometimes also blood (*blood b.*) or pus, within or just beneath the skin.

block (blok) *n.* any interruption of physiological or mental function, brought about intentionally (as part of a therapeutic procedure) or by disease. *See also* heart block, nerve block.

blood (blud) *n.* a fluid tissue that circulates throughout the body, via the arteries and veins, providing a vehicle by which an immense variety of different substances are transported between the various organs and tissues. It is composed of cells (*see* blood cell), which are suspended in a liquid medium (*see* plasma).

blood bank *n.* a department within a hospital or blood transfusion centre in which blood collected from donors is stored prior to transfusion.

blood-brain barrier *n.* the mechanism whereby the circulating blood is kept separate from the tissue fluids surrounding the brain cells. It is a semipermeable membrane allowing solutions to pass through it but excluding solid particles and large molecules.

blood casts *pl. n.* fragments of cel-

small lymphocyte

erythrocyte

large lymphocyte

neutrophil

monocyte

eosinophil

platelets

basophil

granulocytes

Types of blood cells

lular material (*see* cast) to which blood cells are attached, which are derived from the kidney tubules and are excreted in the urine in certain kidney diseases.

blood cell (blood corpuscle) *n.* any of the cells that are present in the blood in health or disease. The cells may be subclassified into two major categories: red cells (*see* erythrocyte) and white cells (*see* leucocyte).

blood clot *n.* a solid mass formed as the result of blood coagulation, either within the blood vessels and heart or elsewhere. *See also* thrombosis.

Donor's blood group	Blood group of people donor can receive blood from	Blood group of people donor can give blood to
A	A,O	A,AB
B	B,O	B,AB
AB	A,B,AB,O	AB
O	O	A,B,AB,O

blood clotting *n. see* blood coagulation.

blood coagulation (blood clotting) *n.* the process whereby blood is converted from a liquid to a solid state. The process involves the interaction of a variety of substances (*see* coagulation factors) and leads to the production of the enzyme thromboplastin, which converts the soluble blood protein fibrinogen to the insoluble protein fibrin. Blood coagulation is an essential mechanism for the arrest of bleeding.

blood corpuscle *n. see* blood cell.

blood count *n.* the numbers of different blood cells in a known volume of blood, usually expressed as the number of cells per litre. *See also* differential leucocyte count.

blood donor *n.* a person who gives blood for storage in a blood bank.

blood group *n.* any one of the many types into which a person's blood may be classified, based on the presence or absence of certain inherited antigens on the surface of the red blood cells. Blood of one group contains antibodies in the serum that react against the cells of other groups. One of the most important blood group systems is the *ABO system*. It is based on the presence or absence of antigens A and B: blood of groups A and B contains antigens A and B, respectively; group AB contains both antigens and group O neither. Blood of group A contains antibodies to antigen B; group B blood contains anti-A antibodies; group AB has neither antibody and group O has both. The table illustrates which blood groups can be used in transfusion for each of the four groups. *See also* rhesus factor.

blood plasma *n. see* plasma.

blood poisoning *n.* the presence of either bacterial toxins or large numbers of bacteria in the bloodstream causing serious illness. *See* pyaemia, septicaemia, toxaemia.

blood pressure *n.* the pressure of blood against the walls of the main arteries. Pressure is highest during systole, when the ventricles are contracting (*systolic pressure*), and lowest during diastole, when the ventricles are relaxing and refilling (*diastolic pressure*). Blood pressure is measured – in millimetres of mercury – by means of a sphygmomanometer at the brachial artery of the arm. A young adult would be expected to have a systolic pressure of around 120 mm and a diastolic pressure of 80 mm. These are recorded as 120/80. *See also* hypertension, hypotension.

blood serum *n. see* serum.

blood sugar *n*. the concentration of glucose in the blood, normally expressed in millimoles per litre. The normal range is 3.5 – 5.5 mmol/l. Blood-sugar estimation is an important investigation in a variety of diseases, most notably in diabetes mellitus. *See also* hyperglycaemia, hypoglycaemia.

blood test *n*. any test designed to discover abnormalities in a sample of a person's blood or to determine the blood group.

blood transfusion *n*. *see* transfusion.

blood vessel *n*. a tube carrying blood away from or towards the heart. *See* artery, arteriole, vein, venule, capillary.

blue baby (bloo) *n*. an infant suffering from congenital malformation of the heart as a result of which some or all of the blue (deoxygenated) blood is pumped around the body instead of passing through the lungs to be oxygenated.

body (**bod**-i) *n*. **1.** an entire animal organism. **2.** the trunk of an individual, excluding the limbs. **3.** the main or largest part of an organ. **4.** a solid discrete mass of tissue; e.g. the carotid body. *See also* corpus.

body image (**body schema**) *n*. the individual's concept of the disposition of his limbs and the identity of the different parts of his body.

body temperature *n*. the intensity of heat of the body, as measured by a thermometer. In most normal individuals body temperature is maintained at about 37°C (98.4°F). A rise in body temperature occurs in fever.

Boeck's disease (beks) *n*. a form of sarcoidosis. [C. P. M. Boeck

Section of the shaft of a long bone (above) with detail of a single Haversian system (below)

(1845 – 1913), Norwegian dermatologist]

boil (boil) *n*. a tender inflamed area of the skin containing pus.

The infection is usually caused by the bacterium *Staphylococcus aureus* entering through a hair follicle or a break in the skin. Boils usually heal when the pus is released or with antibiotic treatment, though occasionally they may cause more widespread infection. Medical name: **furuncle**.

bolus (boh-lŭs) *n.* a soft mass of chewed food that is ready to be swallowed.

bone (bohn) *n.* the hard extremely dense connective tissue that forms the skeleton of the body. It is composed of a matrix of collagen fibres impregnated with bone salts (chiefly calcium carbonate and calcium phosphate). *compact b.* the outer shell of bones, consisting of a hard virtually solid mass made up of bony tissue arranged in concentric layers (*Haversian systems*). *spongy b.* bone found beneath the outer shell; it consists of a meshwork of bony bars (*trabeculae*) with many interconnecting spaces containing marrow.

bone marrow (marrow) *n.* the tissue contained within the internal cavities of the bones. At birth, these cavities are filled entirely with blood-forming *myeloid tissue* (*red marrow*) but in later life the marrow in the limb bones is replaced by fat (*yellow marrow*).

Bonney's blue (bon-iz) *n.* a dye consisting of a mixture of crystal violet and brilliant green. It is used as a skin disinfectant and to demonstrate the presence of a fistula, by instilling it via a cannula and tracing its path. [W. F. V. Bonney (1872–1953), British gynaecologist]

bony labyrinth (boh-ni) *n. see* labyrinth.

borax (bor-aks) *n.* a mild astringent with a weak antiseptic action, applied externally to skin and mucous membranes. Borax and boric acid are used in mouth and nasal washes, gargles, eye lotions and contact-lens solutions, and in dusting powder.

borborygmus (bor-ber-ig-mŭs) *n.* (*pl.* **borborygmi**) an abdominal gurgle due to movement of fluid and gas in the intestine.

Bordetella (bor-dĕ-tel-ă) *n.* a genus of tiny Gram-negative aerobic bacteria. *B. pertussis* the cause of whooping cough.

boric acid (bor-ik) *n. see* borax.

Bornholm disease (devil's grip, epidemic myalgia, epidemic pleurodynia) (born-holm) *n.* a disease caused by Coxsackie viruses. It is spread by contact; symptoms include fever, headache, and attacks of severe pain in the lower chest. The illness lasts about a week and is rarely fatal.

botulism (bot-yoo-lizm) *n.* a serious form of food poisoning from foods containing the toxin produced by the bacterium *Clostridium botulinum*, which thrives in improperly preserved foods. The toxin selectively affects the central nervous system; some cases are fatal.

bougie (boo-zhee) *n.* a hollow or solid cylindrical instrument, usually flexible, that is inserted into tubular passages, such as the oesophagus (gullet), rectum, or urethra. Bougies are used in diagnosis and treatment, particularly by enlarging strictures.

bowel (bow-ĕl) *n. see* intestine.

bow-legs (boh-legz) *pl. n.* abnormal out-curving of the legs, resulting in a gap between the knees on standing. Medical name: **genu varum**.

central sulcus

choroid plexus of third ventricle

corpus callosum

pineal body

thalamus

cerebral aqueduct

hypothalamus

optic chiasma

fourth ventricle

infundibulum

vermis

pituitary body

mamillary body

white matter of cerebellum

pons Varolii

medulla oblongata

The brain (midsagittal section)

Bowman's capsule (boh-mănz) *n.* *see* glomerulus. [Sir W. P. Bowman (1816–92), British physician]

brachi- (brachio-) *prefix denoting* the arm.

brachial (brayk-iăl) *adj.* relating to or affecting the arm.

brachial artery *n.* an artery that extends from the axillary artery at the armpit, down the side and inner surface of the upper arm to the elbow, where it divides into the radial and ulnar arteries.

brachial plexus *n.* a network of nerves, arising from the spine at the base of the neck, from which arise the nerves supplying the arm, forearm and hand, and parts of the shoulder girdle. *See also* radial (nerve).

brachium (brayk-iŭm) *n.* (*pl.* **brachia**) the arm, especially the part of the arm between the shoulder and the elbow.

brachy- *prefix denoting* shortness.

brachycephaly (brak-i-sef-ăli) *n.*

shortness of the skull, with a cephalic index of about 80. —**brachycephalic** *adj.*

Bradford's frame (brad-ferdz) *n.* a rectangular metal frame with canvas slings attached, used to support and immobilize a patient in a prone or supine position. [E. H. Bradford (1848–1926), US orthopaedic surgeon]

brady- *prefix denoting* slowness.

bradycardia (brad-i-kar-diă) *n.* slowing of the heart rate to less than 50 beats per minute.

bradykinin (brad-i-ky-nin) *n.* a naturally occurring polypeptide consisting of nine amino acids; it is a very powerful vasodilator and causes contraction of smooth muscle.

brain (brayn) *n.* the enlarged and highly developed mass of nervous tissue that forms the upper end of the central nervous system. It is invested by three connective tissue membranes (*see* meninges) and floats in cerebrospinal fluid within the rigid casing formed by the bones of the skull. *See also* forebrain, hindbrain, midbrain. Anatomical name: **encephalon**.

brain death *n. see* death.

brainstem (**brayn**-stem) *n.* the enlarged extension upwards within the skull of the spinal cord, consisting of the medulla oblongata, the pons, and the midbrain.

branchial cyst (**brank**-iăl) *n.* a cyst that arises at the site of one of the embryonic pharyngeal pouches due to a developmental anomaly.

branchial pouch *n. see* pharyngeal pouch.

Longitudinal section through a breast

Braun's splint

Braun's splint (brawnz) *n.* a metal splint with attachments for pulleys, used to support or apply traction to a fractured lower limb. [H. F. W. Braun (1862–1934), German surgeon]

breakbone fever (**brayk**-bohn) *n. see* dengue.

breast (brest) *n.* **1.** the mammary gland of a woman: one of two compound glands that produce milk. Each breast consists of glandular lobules – the milk-secreting areas – embedded in fatty tissue. The milk passes from the lobules into *lactiferous ducts*, each of which discharges through a separate orifice in the nipple. *See also* lactation. Anatomical name: **mamma**. **2.** the front part of the chest (thorax).

breastbone (**brest**-bohn) *n. see* sternum.

breast cancer *n.* a malignant tumour of the breast, usually a carcinoma but sometimes a sarcoma. It is rare in men but is the commonest form of cancer in women, in some cases involving both breasts.

breathing (**breeth**-ing) *n.* the alternation of active inhalation of air into the lungs through the mouth or nose with the passive exhalation of the air. Breathing is part

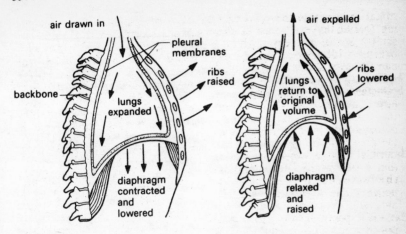

Position of the diaphragm (from the side) during breathing

of respiration and is sometimes called *external respiration*.

breathlessness (breth-lis-nis) *n. see* dyspnoea.

breath sounds (breth) *pl. n.* the sounds heard through a stethoscope placed over the lungs during breathing. *See* bronchial breath sounds, cavernous breath sounds, vesicular breath sounds.

breech presentation (breech) *n.* the position of a baby in the womb such that it would be delivered buttocks first (instead of the normal head-first position).

bregma (breg-mǎ) *n.* the point on the top of the skull at which the coronal and sagittal sutures meet. In a young infant this is an opening, the anterior fontanelle.

Bright's disease (bryts) *n. see* nephritis. [R. Bright (1789–1858), British physician]

brilliant green (bril-yǎnt) *n.* an aniline dye used as an antiseptic.

British Anti-Lewisite (BAL) (brit-ish anti-loo-i-syt) *n. see* dimercaprol.

Broadbent's sign (brawd-bents) *n.* retraction of the left side and back near the 11th and 12th ribs with every heartbeat, indicating adhesions between the pericardium and the diaphragm. [Sir W. H. Broadbent (1835–1907), British physician]

broad ligaments (brawd) *pl. n.* folds of peritoneum extending from each side of the uterus to the lateral walls of the pelvis, supporting the uterus, and Fallopian tubes, and forming a partition across the pelvic cavity.

Broca's area (broh-kǎz) *n.* the area of cerebral motor cortex responsible for the initiation of speech. It is situated in the left frontal lobe in most (but not all) right-handed people. [P. P. Broca (1824–80), French surgeon]

Brodie's abscess (broh-diz) *n. see* abscess. [Sir B. C. Brodie (1783–1862), British surgeon]

bromhexine (brom-heks-een) *n.* an expectorant that acts by increasing the volume and reducing the viscosity of bronchial secretions.

It is used in the treatment of bronchitis and may cause nausea. Trade name: **Bisolvon**.

bromides (broh-mydz) *pl. n.* salts of bromine, including potassium bromide, once widely used as sedatives because of their depressant action on the central nervous system. *See also* bromism.

bromidrosis (broh-mi-**droh**-sis) *n.* bacterial breakdown of sweat, usually in the armpit or on the feet, which causes an unpleasant smell.

bromism (broh-mizm) *n.* a group of symptoms, including drowsiness, loss of sensation, and slurred speech, caused by excessive intake of bromides.

bromsulphthalein (brom-**sulf**-thǎ-lin) *n.* a blue dye used in tests of liver function.

bronch- (**broncho-**) *prefix denoting* the bronchial tree.

bronchial breath sounds (bronk-iǎl) *pl. n.* breath sounds transmitted through consolidated lungs in pneumonia; they are similar to the sounds heard normally over the larger bronchi and are louder and harsher than vesicular breath sounds.

bronchial tree *n.* a branching system of tubes conducting air from the trachea to the lungs: includes the bronchi and their subdivisions and the bronchioles.

bronchiectasis (bronk-i-ek-tǎ-sis) *n.* widening of the bronchi or their branches. It may be congenital or it may result from infection or obstruction. Pus may form in the widened bronchus so that the patient coughs up purulent sputum, which may contain blood. Treatment consists of antibiotic drugs to control the infection and physiotherapy to drain the sputum. Surgery may be used if only a few segments of the bronchi are affected.

bronchiole (bronk-i-ohl) *n.* a subdivision of the bronchial tree that does not contain cartilage or mucous glands in its wall. The smallest bronchioles open into the alveoli. —**bronchiolar** *adj.*

bronchiolitis (bronk-i-oh-ly-tis) *n.* inflammation of the bronchioles, due to infection by bacteria or viruses.

bronchitis (brong-ky-tis) *n.* inflammation of the bronchi. *acute b.* bronchitis caused by viruses or bacteria. It is characterized by coughing, the production of mucopurulent sputum, and bronchospasm. *chronic b.* bronchitis in which the patient coughs up excessive mucus secreted by enlarged bronchial mucous glands; the bronchospasm cannot be relieved by bronchodilator drugs. The disease is particularly prevalent in Britain in association with cigarette smoking, air pollution, and emphysema.

bronchoconstrictor (brong-koh-kŏn-strik-ter) *n.* a drug that causes narrowing of the air passages by producing spasm of bronchial smooth muscle.

bronchodilator (brong-koh-dy-lay-ter) *n.* an agent, such as ephedrine or salbutamol, that causes widening of the air passages by relaxing bronchial smooth muscle.

broncography (brong-**kog**-rǎfi) *n.* X-ray examination of the bronchial tree after it has been made visible by the injection of radio-opaque dye or the inhalation of radio-opaque particles.

bronchomycosis (brong-koh-my-**koh**-sis) *n.* any of various fungal infections of the bronchi, such as candidiasis of the lungs.

bronchophony (brong-kof-ŏni) *n.* *see* vocal resonance.

bronchopleural (brong-koh-**ploor**-ăl) *adj.* relating to a bronchus and the pleura. **b. fistula** an abnormal communication (*see* fistula) between a bronchus and the pleural cavity.

bronchopneumonia (brong-koh-new-**moh**-niă) *n.* *see* pneumonia.

bronchopulmonary (brong-koh-**pul**-mŏn-er-i) *adj.* relating to the lungs and the bronchial tree.

bronchoscope (**bronk**-ŏ-skohp) *n.* an instrument used to look into the trachea and bronchi. With the aid of a bronchoscope the bronchial tree can be washed out and samples of tissue and foreign bodies can be removed with long forceps. —**bronchoscopy** (brong-**kos**-kŏ-pi) *n.*

bronchospasm (**brong**-koh-spazm) *n.* narrowing of bronchi by muscular contraction in response to some stimulus, as in asthma and bronchitis. Some types of bronchospasm can be relieved by bronchodilator drugs; others, such as chronic bronchitis, cannot.

bronchospirometry (brong-koh-spy-rom-itri) *n.* a technique used to assess the efficiency of ventilation of a lung or of a segment of the lung.

bronchus (**bronk**-ŭs) *n.* (*pl.* **bronchi**) any of the air passages beyond the trachea that has cartilage and mucous glands in its wall. *See also* bronchiole. —**bronchial** *adj.*

brown fat (brown) *n.* a type of fat occurring in the adipose tissue of many animal species that can be rapidly metabolized to produce heat energy.

Brown-Séquard syndrome (brown say-kar) *n.* the neurological condition resulting when the spinal cord has been partly cut through. Below the lesion there is a spastic paralysis on the same side and a loss of pain and temperature sensation on the opposite side. [C. E. Brown-Séquard (1818 – 94), French physiologist]

Brucella (broo-**sel**-ă) *n.* a genus of Gram-negative aerobic spherical or rodlike parasitic bacteria responsible for brucellosis (undulant fever) in man and contagious abortion in cattle, pigs, sheep, and goats. The principal species are *B. abortus* and *B. melitensis.*

brucellosis (Malta fever, Mediterranean fever, undulant fever) (broo-si-**loh**-sis) *n.* a chronic disease of farm animals caused by bacteria of the genus *Brucella*, which can be transmitted to man either by contact with an infected animal or by drinking nonpasteurized contaminated milk. Symptoms include headache and sickness, progressing to chronic fever and the swelling of lymph nodes.

Brufen (broo-fĕn) *n.* *see* ibuprofen.

bruise (contusion) (brooz) *n.* an area of skin discoloration caused by the escape of blood from ruptured underlying vessels following injury.

bruit (broot) *n.* *see* murmur.

Brunner's glands (brun-erz) *pl. n.* compound glands of the small intestine, found in the duodenum and the upper part of the jejunum. They are embedded in the submucosa and secrete mucus. [J. C. Brunner (1653 – 1727), Swiss anatomist]

bubo (bew-boh) *n.* a swollen inflamed lymph node in the armpit or groin, commonly developing in venereal disease, bubonic plague, and leishmaniasis.

bubonic plague (bew-**bon**-ik) *n. see* plague.

buccal (buk-ăl) *adj.* relating to the mouth or the hollow part of the cheek.

buccinator (buks-i-nay-ter) *n.* a muscle of the cheek that has its origin in the maxilla and mandible. It is responsible for compressing the cheek and is important in mastication.

Buerger's disease (ber-gerz) *n.* an inflammatory condition affecting the arteries, especially the arteries of the legs. The condition may lead to gangrene of the limbs and venous or coronary thrombosis. Medical name: **thromboangiitis obliterans**. [L. Buerger (1879–1943), US physician]

buffer (buf-er) *n.* a solution whose hydrogen ion concentration (pH) remains virtually unchanged by dilution or by the addition of acid or alkali. *See also* acid-base balance.

bulb (bulb) *n.* (in anatomy) any rounded structure or a rounded expansion at the end of an organ or part.

bulbar (bul-ber) *adj.* **1.** relating to or affecting the medulla oblongata. **2.** relating to a bulb.

bulbourethral glands (bul-bo-yoor-ee-thrăl) *n. see* Cowper's glands.

bulimia (bew-**lim**-iă) *n.* insatiable over-eating. This symptom may be psychogenic, as in anorexia nervosa; or it may be due to neurological causes, such as a lesion of the hypothalamus.

bulla (buul-ă) *n.* (*pl.* **bullae**) **1.** a large blister, containing serous fluid. **2.** (in anatomy) a rounded bony prominence. **3.** a thin-walled air-filled space within the lung, arising congenitally or in emphysema. —**bullous** *adj.*

Buller's shield (buul-erz) *n.* a protective shield placed over one eye when the other is infected. It consists of a watch glass fixed in position with adhesive tape. [F. Buller (1844–1905), Canadian ophthalmologist]

bundle (bun-d'l) *n.* a group of nerve fibres situated close together and running in the same direction.

bundle branch block *n.* a defect in the specialized conducting tissue of the heart that is recognised as an electrocardiographic abnormality.

bundle of His (hiss) *n. see* atrioventricular bundle. [L. His (1863–1934), German physiologist]

bunion (bun-yŏn) *n.* a swelling of the joint between the great toe and the first metatarsal bone. A bursa often develops over the site and the great toe becomes displaced towards the others. Bunions are usually caused by ill-fitting shoes and may require surgical treatment.

buphthalmos (hydrophthalmos) (buf-**thal**-mŏs) *n.* infantile or congenital glaucoma: increased pressure within the eye due to a defect in the development of the tissues through which fluid drains from the eye.

bupivacaine (bew-piv-ă-kayn) *n.* a potent local anaesthetic, used mainly for regional nerve block. Trade name: **Marcain**.

Burkitt's tumour (Burkitt's lymphoma) (ber-kits) *n.* a malignant tumour of the lymphatic system, most commonly affecting children and largely confined to tropical Africa. It can arise at various sites, most commonly the facial structures, such as the jaw, and in the abdomen. [D. P. Burkitt (1911–), Irish surgeon]

burn (bern) *n.* tissue damage caused by such agents as heat, chemicals, electricity, sunlight, or nuclear radiation. Burns cause swelling and blistering; loss of plasma from damaged blood vessels may lead to severe shock. There is also a risk of bacterial infection. *first-degree b.* a burn affecting only the outer layer (epidermis) of the skin. *second-degree b.* a burn in which both the epidermis and the underlying dermis are damaged. *third-degree b.* a burn that involves damage or destruction of the skin to its full depth and damage to the tissues beneath.

burr (ber) *n.* a bit for a surgical drill that is used for cutting into tooth or bone.

bursa (ber-să) *n.* (*pl.* **bursae**) a small sac of fibrous tissue that is lined with synovial membrane and filled with fluid. Bursae help to reduce friction; they are normally formed round joints and in places where ligaments and tendons pass over bones.

bursa of Fabricius (fă-brish-ŭs) *n.* a mass of lymphoid tissue occurring as an outgrowth of the cloaca of young birds. It is an important source of B-lymphocytes. [H. Fabricius (1537–1619), Italian anatomist]

bursitis (ber-sy-tis) *n.* inflammation of a bursa, resulting from injury, infection, or rheumatoid synovitis. It produces pain and sometimes restricts movement at a nearby joint. *See also* housemaid's knee.

busulphan (bew-sul-fan) *n.* a drug that destroys cancer cells by acting on the bone marrow. It is administered by mouth, mainly in the treatment of chronic myeloid leukaemia. Trade name: **Myleran.**

butacaine (bew-tă-kayn) *n.* a local anaesthetic used mainly in eye, ear, nose, and throat surgery. Trade name: **Butyn.**

butobarbitone (**butobarbital**) (bew-toh-bar-bi-tohn) *n.* an intermediate-acting barbiturate, used for the treatment of insomnia and for sedation. Trade name: **Soneryl.**

buttock (but-ŏk) *n.* either of the two fleshy protuberances at the lower posterior section of the trunk, consisting of muscles (*see* gluteus) and fat. Anatomical name: **natis.**

byssinosis (bis-i-noh-sis) *n.* an industrial disease of the lungs caused by inhalation of dusts of cotton, flax, or hemp.

C

C 1. *symbol for* carbon. **2.** *abbreviation of* Celsius *or* centigrade.

Ca *symbol for* calcium.

cac- (**caco-**) *prefix denoting* disease or deformity.

cachet (kash-ay) *n.* a flat capsule containing a drug that has an unpleasant taste. The cachet is swallowed intact by the patient.

cachexia (kă-keks-iă) *n.* a condition of abnormally low weight, weakness, and general bodily decline associated with chronic disease, such as cancer.

cadaver (kă-dav-er) *n.* a dead body, especially one preserved and used for dissection and anatomical study.

caecosigmoidostomy (see-koh-sigmoid-**ost**-ŏmi) *n.* an operation in which the caecum is joined to the sigmoid colon.

caecostomy (see-**kost**-ŏmi) *n.* an operation in which the caecum is brought through the abdominal wall and opened in order to drain or decompress the intestine.

caecum (see-kŭm) *n.* a blind-ended pouch at the junction of the small and large intestines, to which the vermiform appendix is attached. —**caecal** *adj.*

Caesarean section (siz-**air**-iăn) *n.* a surgical operation for delivering a baby through the abdominal wall. It is carried out when there are risks to the baby or to the mother from normal childbirth.

caesium-137 (seez-iŭm) *n.* an artificial radioactive isotope of the metallic element caesium, used in radiotherapy. Symbol: Cs¹³⁷. *See also* telecurietherapy.

caffeine (**kaf**-een) *n.* an alkaloid drug, present in coffee and tea, that has a stimulant action on the central nervous system and is a weak diuretic. It is used in analgesic preparations.

caisson disease (**kay**-sŏn) *n. see* compressed air illness.

calamine (**kal**-ă-myn) *n.* a preparation of zinc carbonate used as a mild astringent on the skin in the form of a lotion, cream, or ointment.

calc- (**calci-**, **calco-**) *prefix denoting* calcium or calcium salts.

calcaneus (**heel bone**) (kal-**kay**-niŭs) *n.* the large bone in the tarsus of the foot that forms the projection of the heel behind the foot.

calcareous (kal-**kair**-iŭs) *adj.* containing calcium, especially calcium carbonate; chalky.

calciferol (kal-**sif**-er-ol) *n. see* vitamin D.

calcification (kal-si-fi-**kay**-shŏn) *n.* the deposition of calcium salts in tissue. This occurs as part of the normal process of bone formation (*see* ossification).

calcinosis (kal-si-**noh**-sis) *n.* the abnormal deposition of calcium salts in the tissues.

calcitonin (kal-si-**toh**-nin) *n. see* thyrocalcitonin.

calcium (**kal**-siŭm) *n.* a metallic element that is an important constituent of bones, teeth, and blood. It is also essential for many metabolic processes, including nerve function, muscle contraction, and blood clotting. Symbol: Ca.

calcium carbonate (kar-bŏ-nayt) *n.* a salt of calcium that neutralizes acids and is used in many antacid preparations. Formula: $CaCO_3$.

calcium gluconate and **lactate** (**gloo**-kŏ-nayt, **lak**-tayt) *n.* salts of calcium used to treat and prevent calcium-deficiency disorders, such as tetany and rickets. Formulae: $(CH_2OH(CHOH)_4COO)_2Ca.H_2O$; $(CH_3CHOHCOO)_2Ca.5H_2O$.

calculosis (kal-kew-**loh**-sis) *n.* the presence of multiple calculi in an organ.

calculus (**kal**-kew-lŭs) *n.* (*pl.* **calculi**) **1.** a stone: a hard pebble-like mass formed within the body, particularly in the gall bladder (*see* gallstone) or anywhere in the urinary tract. **2.** a calcified deposit that forms on the surfaces of teeth.

Caldwell-Luc operation (**kawld**-wel look) *n.* an operation in which the maxillary sinus is drained through an incision above the upper canine tooth. [G. W. Caldwell (1834–1918), US otolaryngologist; H. Luc (1855–1925), French laryngologist]

calibrator (kal-i-bray-ter) *n*. **1.** an instrument used for measuring the size of a tube or opening. **2.** an instrument used for dilating a tubular part, such as the gullet.

calliper (caliper) (kal-i-per) *n*. **1.** an instrument with two prongs or jaws, used for measuring diameters, particularly of the pelvis in obstetrics. **2.** (also called **calliper splint**) a leg splint consisting of two metal rods that are attached to a padded ring at the top of the leg and end in spurs that fit into the heel of the patient's shoe. It is used to support paralysed, fractured, or deformed limbs by taking the weight of the body at the pelvis.

callosity (callus) (kă-los-iti) *n*. a hard thick area of skin occurring in parts of the body subject to pressure or friction, particularly the soles of the feet and palms of the hands.

callus (kal-ŭs) *n*. **1.** a mass of blood, connective tissue, and bone-forming cells that forms around the bone ends following a fracture. It eventually develops into new bone that unites the fracture. **2.** *see* callosity.

calor (kal-er) *n*. heat: one of the four classical signs of inflammation in a tissue. *See also* dolor, rubor, tumor.

calorie (kal-er-i) *n*. a unit of heat equal to the amount of heat required to raise the temperature of 1 gram of water from 14.5°C to 15.5°C (the 15° calorie). One *Calorie* (*kilocalorie* or *kilogram calorie*) is equal to 1000 calories; this unit is used to indicate the energy value of foods. Both these units have now largely been replaced by the joule and kilojoule respectively (1 calorie = 4.1855 joules).

calorific (kal-er-if-ik) *adj*. producing heat.

calorimeter (kal-er-im-it-er) *n*. any apparatus used to measure the heat lost or gained during various chemical and physical changes. Calorimeters are used to determine the energy value of different foods. —**calorimetry** *n*.

calvaria (kal-vair-iă) *n*. the vault of the skull.

calyx (kay-liks) *n*. (*pl*. **calyces**) a cup-shaped part, especially any of the divisions of the pelvis of the kidney.

camphor (kam-fer) *n*. a crystalline substance obtained from the tree *Cinnamomum camphora* that has been used to treat flatulence. *Camphorated oil* (camphor in cottonseed oil) is used in liniments as a counterirritant.

canal (kă-nal) *n*. a tubular channel or passage; e.g. the alimentary canal.

canaliculus (ka-nă-lik-yoo-lŭs) *n*. (*pl*. **canaliculi**) a small channel or canal. Canaliculi occur, for example, in compact bone, linking lacunae containing bone cells, and in the liver, transporting bile to the bile duct.

cancellous (kan-si-lŭs) *adj*. latticelike: applied to spongy bone, which contains many spaces.

cancer (kan-ser) *n*. any malignant tumour, including carcinoma and sarcoma. It arises from the abnormal and uncontrolled division of cells that then invade and destroy the surrounding tissues. The cancer cells spread (*see* metastasis), setting up secondary tumours at sites distant from the original tumour. There are probably many causative factors, some of which are known; for example, cigarette smoking is associated with lung cancer, radiation with some bone sarcomas and leukaemia. Treatment of cancer depends on the type of tumour, the site of the primary tumour, and the extent of spread.

cancrum (canker) (kank-rŭm) *n.* ulceration, mainly of the lips and mouth (*c. oris*). *See* noma.

Candida (kan-di-dă) *n.* a genus of yeastlike fungi (formerly called *Monilia*) that inhabit the vagina and alimentary tract. *C. albicans* a small oval budding species primarily responsible for candidiasis.

candidiasis (kan-di-dy-ă-sis) *n.* infection with a yeastlike fungus of the genus *Candida*, usually the species *C. albicans*. The infection – formerly called *moniliasis* – is usually superficial, occurring in moist areas of the body, such as the skin folds, mouth, respiratory tract, and vagina (candidiasis of the mouth and vagina is popularly known as *thrush*). It is treated with antibiotics – especially nystatin – applied locally, inhaled, or taken by mouth.

canine (eye tooth) (kay-nyn) *n.* the third tooth from the midline of each jaw. There are thus four canines, two in each jaw.

canker (kank-er) *n. see* cancrum.

cannabis (kan-ă-bis) *n.* a drug prepared from the Indian hemp plant (*Cannabis sativa*), also known as *pot*, *marihuana*, *hashish*, and *bhang*. It produces euphoria and hallucinations and has no therapeutic value; its use is illegal. *See also* dependence.

cannula (kan-yoo-lă) *n.* a hollow tube designed for insertion into a body cavity. The tube contains a sharp pointed solid core (*trocar*), which facilitates its insertion and is withdrawn when the cannula is in place.

cantharidin (kan-tha-ri-din) *n.* the active principle of *cantharides* (*see* Spanish fly). A toxic and irritant chemical, cantharidin causes blistering of the skin and was formerly used in veterinary medicine as a counterirritant and vesicant.

canthus (kan-thŭs) *n.* either corner of the eye; the angle at which the upper and lower eyelids meet. —**canthal** *adj.*

cap (kap) *n.* a covering or a cover-like part.

capillary (kă-pil-er-i) *n.* an extremely narrow blood vessel. Capillaries form networks in most tissues; they are supplied with blood by arterioles and drained by venules. The vessel wall is only one cell thick, which enables exchange of oxygen, carbon dioxide, water, salts, etc., between the blood and the tissues.

capitate (kap-i-tayt) *adj.* head-shaped; having a rounded extremity. *c. bone* a bone of the wrist (*see* carpus). It articulates with the scaphoid and lunate bones behind and with the third metacarpal bone in front.

capitellum (kap-i-tel-ŭm) *n. see* capitulum.

capitulum (kă-pit-yoo-lŭm) *n.* the small rounded end of a bone that articulates with another bone. *c. humeri* (or *capitellum*) the round prominence at the elbow end of the humerus that articulates with the radius.

capreomycin (kap-ri-oh-**my**-sin) *n.* an antibiotic drug, derived from the bacterium *Streptomyces capreolus*, that is administered by intramuscular injection in the treatment of tuberculosis.

capsule (**kaps**-yool) *n.* **1.** a membrane, sheath, or other structure that encloses a tissue or organ. *joint c.* the fibrous tissue, including the synovial membrane, that surrounds a freely movable joint. **2.** a soluble case, usually made of gelatin, in which certain drugs are administered. **3.** the slimy substance that forms a protective layer around certain bacteria.

capsulitis (kaps-yoo-**ly**-tis) *n.* inflammation of a joint capsule.

capsulotomy (kaps-yoo-**lot**-ŏmi) *n.* an incision into the capsule of the lens, made after some operations for cataract in which the capsule is not removed.

caput succedaneum (**kap**-ŭt suk-si-**day**-niŭm) *n.* a temporary swelling of the soft parts of the head of a newly born infant that occurs during birth, due to compression by the muscles of the neck of the womb.

carbachol (**kar**-bă-kol) *n.* a parasympathomimetic drug used to relieve pressure within the eye in glaucoma. It is also used after surgical operations to restore the function of inactive bowels or bladder. Trade name: **Carcholin.**

carbamazepine (kar-bă-**maz**-ĕ-peen) *n.* an anticonvulsant drug used in the treatment of epilepsy and to relieve the pain of trigeminal neuralgia. Trade name: **Tegretol.**

carbenicillin (kar-ben-i-sil-in) *n.* a synthetic penicillin. Administered by intramuscular injection, it is effective against a wide range of bacterial infections. Trade name: **Pyopen.**

carbenoxolone (kar-bĕ-**noks**-ŏ-lohn) *n.* a drug that reduces inflammation, administered by mouth in the treatment of gastric ulcers or ulcers of the mouth. Trade names: **Biogastrone, Bioral.**

carbimazole (kar-**bim**-ă-zohl) *n.* a drug used to reduce the production of thyroid hormone in cases of overactivity of the gland (thyrotoxicosis). Trade names: **Bimazol, Neo-Mercazole.**

carbohydrate (kar-boh-**hy**-drayt) *n.* any one of a large group of compounds, including the sugars and starch, that contain carbon, hydrogen, and oxygen and have the general formula $C_x(H_2O)_y$. Carbohydrates are important as a source of energy: they are manufactured by plants and obtained by animals and man from the diet, being one of the three main constituents of food. *See also* disaccharide, monosaccharide, polysaccharide.

carbol fuchsin (kar-bol **fuuk**-sin) *n.* a red stain for bacteria and fungi, consisting of carbolic acid and fuchsin dissolved in alcohol and water.

carbolic acid (kar-**bol**-ik) *n. see* phenol.

carbon dioxide (**kar**-bŏn dy-ok-syd) *n.* a colourless gas formed in the tissues during metabolism and carried in the blood to the lungs, where it is exhaled (an increase in the concentration of this gas in the blood stimulates respiration). It forms a solid (dry ice) at −75°C (at atmospheric pressure) and in this form is used as a refrigerant. Formula: CO_2.

carbonic anhydrase (kar-**bon**-ik an-**hy**-drayz) *n.* an enzyme that catalyses the breakdown of carbonic acid into carbon dioxide and water or the combination of carbon dioxide and water to form carbonic acid. It therefore facilitates the transport of carbon dioxide from the tissues to the lungs.

carbon monoxide (mŏn-**ok**-syd) *n.* a colourless almost odourless gas that is very poisonous. When breathed in it combines with haemoglobin in the red blood cells (*see* carboxyhaemoglobin). Carbon monoxide is present in coal gas and motor exhaust fumes. Formula: CO.

carbon tetrachloride (tet-ră-**klor**-ryd) *n.* a pungent volatile fluid used as a dry-cleaner. When inhaled or swallowed it may severely damage the heart, liver, and kidneys. Treatment is by administration of oxygen.

carboxyhaemoglobin (kar-boks-i-heem-ŏ-**gloh**-bin) *n.* a substance formed when carbon monoxide combines with the pigment haemoglobin in the blood. Carboxyhaemoglobin is incapable of transporting oxygen to the tissues and this is the cause of death in carbon monoxide poisoning.

carboxyhaemoglobinaemia (kar-boks-i-heem-ŏ-gloh-bi-**nee**-miă) *n.* the presence of carboxyhaemoglobin in the blood.

carbromal (kar-**broh**-măl) *n.* a weak sedative and hypnotic, given by mouth and used in the treatment of mild insomnia. Its action lasts for a few hours but prolonged use may lead to dependence.

carbuncle (kar-bung-kŭl) *n.* a collection of boils with multiple drainage channels. The infection is usually caused by *Staphylococ-*

cus aureus and normally results in an extensive slough of skin.

carcin- (**carcino-**) *prefix denoting* cancer or carcinoma.

carcinogen (kar-**sin**-ŏ-jin) *n.* any substance that, when exposed to living tissue, may cause the production of a carcinoma. —**carcinogenic** (kar-sin-ŏ-**jen**-ik) *adj.*

carcinoid (**kar**-sin-oid) *n. see* argentaffinoma.

carcinoma (kar-sin-**oh**-mă) *n.* any cancer that arises in epithelium, the tissue that lines the skin and internal organs of the body. It may occur in any tissue containing epithelial cells. Organs may exhibit more than one type of carcinoma; for example, an adenocarcinoma and a squamous carcinoma may be found in the cervix (but not usually concurrently). —**carcinomatous** *adj.*

carcinomatosis (kar-sin-oh-mă-**toh**-sis) *n.* carcinoma that has spread widely throughout the body.

cardi- (**cardio-**) *prefix denoting* the heart.

cardia (**kar**-diă) *n.* **1.** the opening at the upper end of the stomach that connects with the oesophagus (gullet). **2.** the heart.

cardiac (**kar**-di-ak) *adj.* **1.** of, relating to, or affecting the heart. **2.** of or relating to the upper part of the stomach (*see* cardia).

cardiac arrest *n.* the cessation of effective pumping action of the heart, which most commonly occurs when the muscle fibres of the ventricles start to beat rapidly without pumping any blood (ventricular fibrillation) or when the heart stops beating completely (asystole). There is abrupt loss of consciousness, absence of the pulse, and breathing stops. Unless treated promptly, irreversible brain damage and death follow within minutes. Some patients may be resuscitated by massage of the heart, artificial respiration, and defibrillation.

cardiac cycle *n.* the sequence of events between one heart beat and the next, normally occupying less than a second. *See* diastole, systole.

cardiac muscle *n.* the specialized muscle of which the walls of the heart are composed. It consists of a network of branching elongated cells (fibres).

cardiac reflex *n.* reflex control of the heart rate.

cardinal ligaments (Mackenrodt's ligaments) (kar-din-ăl) *pl. n.* fan-shaped sheets of fascia that extend from the vagina and the cervix of the womb to the walls of the pelvis.

cardiology (kar-di-ol-ŏji) *n.* the science concerned with the study of the structure, function, and diseases of the heart. —**cardiologist** *n.*

cardiomyopathy (kar-di-oh-my-op-ă-thi) *n.* any chronic disorder affecting the muscle of the heart. It may result in enlargement of the heart, heart failure, arrhythmias, and embolism.

cardiomyotomy (Heller's operation) (kar-di-oh-my-ot-ŏmi) *n.* surgical splitting of the muscular ring at the junction of the stomach and oesophagus to relieve achalasia.

cardiopathy (kar-di-op-ă-thi) *n.* any disease of the heart. —**cardiopathic** (kar-di-oh-path-ik) *adj.*

cardiopulmonary bypass (kar-di-oh-pul-mŏn-er-i) *n.* a method by which the circulation to the body is maintained while the heart is deliberately stopped during heart surgery. The function of the heart and lungs is carried out by a pump-oxygenator (heart-lung machine) until the natural circulation is restored.

cardiospasm (kar-di-oh-spazm) *n.* see achalasia.

cardiotocography (kar-di-oh-tŏ-kog-răfi) *n.* the automatic recording in graphic form of fetal heart rate and the amplitude, duration, and frequency of the muscular contractions of the womb during labour.

cardiotomy syndrome (postcardiotomy syndrome) (kar-di-ot-ŏmi) *n.* a condition that may develop after surgery to the heart and the pericardium and is characterized by fever and pericarditis. Pneumonia and pleurisy may form part of the syndrome.

cardiovascular system (circulatory system) (kar-di-oh-vas-kew-ler) *n.* the heart together with two networks of blood vessels – the systemic circulation and the pulmonary circulation. The cardiovascular system effects the circulation of blood around the body, which brings about transport of nutrients and oxygen to the tissues and the removal of waste products.

cardioversion (countershock) (kar-di-oh-ver-shŏn) *n.* a method of restoring the normal rhythm of the heart in patients with increased heart rate due to arrhythmia. A controlled direct-current shock is given through electrodes placed on the chest wall of the anaesthetized patient. The apparatus is called a *cardiovertor*.

care plan (kair) *n.* see planning.

caries (kair-eez) *n.* decay and crumbling of the substance of a tooth (*dental c.*) or a bone. —**carious** *adj.*

The origin and main branches
of the carotid arteries

carina (kă-**ree**-nă) *n.* a keel-like
structure, such as the keel-shaped
cartilage at the bifurcation of the
trachea into the two main
bronchi.

cariogenic (kair-i-oh-**jen**-ik) *adj.*
causing caries, particularly dental
caries.

carminative (kar-**min**-ă-tiv) *n.* a
drug that relieves flatulence, used
to treat gastric discomfort and
colic.

carneous mole (**kar**-niŭs) *n.* a
fleshy mass that develops from
blood clots, membranes, or
pieces of placenta left in the
womb after abortion.

carotenaemia (ka-rŏ-ti-**nee**-miă) *n.*
see xanthaemia.

carotene (**ka**-rŏ-teen) *n.* a yellow,
orange, red, or brown plant pig-
ment; one of the carotenoids.
The most important form,
β-carotene, can be converted in
the body to retinol (vitamin A).

carotenoid (kă-**rot**-in-oid) *n.* any
one of a group of about 100
naturally occurring yellow to red
pigments found mostly in plants.

carotid artery (kă-**rot**-id) *n.* either
of the two main arteries in the

neck whose branches supply the
head and neck.

carotid body *n.* a small mass of
tissue in the carotid sinus containing chemoreceptors that monitor levels of oxygen, carbon dioxide, and hydrogen ions in the
blood.

carotid sinus *n.* a pocket in the
wall of the carotid artery, at its
division in the neck, containing
receptors that monitor blood
pressure (baroreceptors).

carp- (carpo-) *prefix denoting* the
wrist (carpus).

carpal (**kar**-păl) **1.** *adj.* relating to
the wrist. **2.** *n.* any of the bones
forming the carpus.

carpal tunnel syndrome *n.* compression of the median nerve as
it enters the palm of the hand.
This causes pain and numbness
in the index and middle fingers
and weakness of the abductor
muscle of the thumb.

carphology (floccillation) (kar-
fol-ŏji) *n.* plucking at the bed-
clothes by a delirious patient.
This is often a sign of extreme

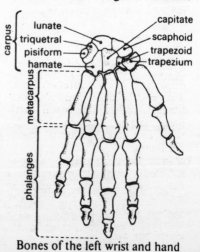

Bones of the left wrist and hand

exhaustion and may be the prelude to death.

carpopedal spasm (kar-poh-**pee**-d'l) *n. see* spasm.

carpus (**kar**-pŭs) *n.* the eight bones of the wrist (see illustration). The carpus articulates with the metacarpals distally and with the humerus and radius proximally.

carrier (**ka**-ri-er) *n.* **1.** a person who harbours the microorganisms causing a particular disease without experiencing signs or symptoms of infection and who can transmit the disease to others. **2.** (in genetics) a person who bears a gene for an abnormal trait without showing signs of the disorder. **3.** an animal, usually an insect, that passively transmits infectious organisms from one animal to another or from an animal to man. *See also* vector.

cartilage (**kar**-til-ij) *n.* a dense connective tissue, consisting chiefly of chondroitin sulphate, that is capable of withstanding considerable pressure. In the fetus and infant cartilage occurs in many parts of the body, but most of this cartilage disappears during development. *elastic c.* cartilage occurring in the external ear. *fibrocartilage* cartilage occurring in the intervertebral discs and tendons. *hyaline c.* cartilage found in the costal cartilages, larynx, trachea, bronchi, nose, and at the joints of movable bones.

caruncle (**ka**-rŭng-kŭl) *n.* a small red fleshy swelling. *hymenal c.* a caruncle occurring around the mucous membrane lining the vaginal opening. *lacrimal c.* the red prominence at the inner angle of the eye.

Hyaline cartilage

Elastic cartilage

Fibrocartilage
Types of cartilage

cascara (cascara sagrada) (kaskar-ă) *n.* the dried bark of an American buckthorn, *Rhamnus purshiana*, used as a laxative.

caseation (kay-si-**ay**-shŏn) *n.* the breakdown of diseased tissue into a dry cheeselike mass: a type of degeneration associated with tubercular lesions.

casein (kay-si-in) *n.* a milk protein. Casein is precipitated out of milk in acid conditions or by the action of rennin. It is very easily prepared and is useful as a protein supplement, particularly in the treatment of malnutrition.

caseinogen (kay-si-**in**-ŏ-jin) *n.* a protein, present in milk, that is converted into casein by the action of rennin.

cast (kahst) *n.* **1.** a rigid casing designed to immobilize part of the body, usually a fractured limb, until healing has progressed sufficiently. It is made with open-woven bandage impregnated with plaster of Paris and applied while wet. **2.** a mass of dead cellular, fatty, and other material that forms within a body cavity and takes its shape. It may then be released and appear elsewhere.

castor oil (**kahst**-er) *n.* an irritant laxative administered by mouth to relieve constipation. It is also used with zinc as an ointment to treat skin irritations, such as napkin rash and bedsores.

castration (kas-**tray**-shŏn) *n.* removal of the sex glands (the testes or the ovaries).

cata- *prefix denoting* downward or against.

catabolism (kă-**tab**-ŏl-izm) *n.* the chemical decomposition of complex substances by the body to form simpler ones, accompanied by the release of energy. *See also* metabolism. —**catabolic** (kat-ă-**bol**-ik) *adj.*

catalase (**kat**-ă-layz) *n.* an enzyme, present in many cells (including red blood cells and liver cells), that catalyses the breakdown of hydrogen peroxide.

catalepsy (**kat**-ă-lep-si) *n.* the abnormal maintenance of postures or physical attitudes, occurring in catatonia.

catalyst (**kat**-ă-list) *n.* a substance that alters the rate of a chemical reaction but is itself unchanged at the end of the reaction. The catalysts of biochemical reactions are the enzymes.

catamenia (kat-ă-**mee**-niă) *n. see* menstruation.

cataphoresis (kat-ă-fŏ-**ree**-sis) *n.* the introduction into the tissues of positively charged ionized substances (cations) by the use of a direct electric current. *See* iontophoresis.

cataplexy (**kat**-ă-pleks-i) *n.* a recurrent condition in which the patient suddenly collapses to the ground without loss of consciousness. Any strong emotion can provoke an attack.

cataract (**kat**-ă-rakt) *n.* any opacity in the lens of the eye, resulting in blurred vision. Cataracts most commonly occur in the elderly (*senile c.*), but some are congenital or due to metabolic disease, such as diabetes. Cataract is treated by surgical removal of the affected lens (*c. extraction*).

catarrh (kă-**tar**) *n.* the excessive secretion of thick phlegm or mucus by the mucous membrane of the nose, nasal sinuses, nasopharynx, or air passages.

catatonia (kat-ă-**toh**-niă) *n.* a syndrome of motor abnormalities associated with an abnormal mental state. The symptoms may be *excited*: stereotypy and purposeless violence; or *inhibited*, including stupor, catalepsy, and negativism. Commonly they are features of catatonic schizophrenia but they are also seen in other conditions, including encephalitis and hysteria. —**catatonic** *adj.*

catchment area (kach-měnt) *n.* the geographic area from which a hospital can expect to receive patients and on which in Britain the designated population of the hospital is based.

catecholamines (kat-ě-kol-ă-meenz) *pl. n.* a group of physiologically important substances, including adrenaline, noradrenaline, and dopamine, with different roles (mainly as neurotransmitters) in the functioning of the sympathetic and central nervous systems.

catgut (kat-gut) *n.* a fibrous material prepared from the tissues of animals, usually from sheep intestines, used to sew up wounds and tie off blood vessels during surgery. The catgut gradually dissolves and is absorbed by the tissues, so that the stitches do not have to be removed later.

catharsis (kă-thar-sis) *n.* purging or cleansing out of the bowels by giving the patient a laxative (cathartic) to stimulate intestinal activity.

cathartic (kă-thar-tik) *n. see* laxative.

catheter (kath-it-er) *n.* a tube for insertion into a narrow opening so that fluids may be introduced or removed. *urinary c.* a catheter passed into the bladder through the urethra to allow drainage of urine in certain disorders and to empty the bladder before abdominal operations.

catheterization (kath-it-er-I-zay-shŏn) *n.* the introduction of a catheter into a hollow organ.

cardiac c. the introduction of special catheters into the various chambers of the heart via the arteries and veins of the arms or legs. It provides data on pressures and blood flow within the various chambers of the heart. *urethral c.* the introduction of a catheter into the bladder to relieve obstruction to the outflow of urine.

cation (katI-ŏn) *n.* a positively charged ion, which moves towards the cathode (negative electrode) when an electric current is passed through the solution containing it. *Compare* anion.

cat-scratch fever (kat-skrach) *n.* an infectious virus disease transmitted to man following injury to the skin by a cat scratch, splinter, or thorn. Mild fever and glandular swelling develop about a week after infection.

cauda (kaw-dă) *n.* a tail-like structure. *c. equina* a bundle of nerve roots from the lumbar, sacral, and coccygeal spinal nerves that descend from the spinal cord to their respective openings in the vertebral column.

caudal (kaw-d'l) *adj.* relating to the lower part or tail end of the body.

caul (kawl) *n.* **1.** (in obstetrics) a membrane, part of the amnion, that may cover an infant's head at birth. **2.** (in anatomy) *see* omentum.

causalgia (kaw-zal-jiă) *n.* an intensely unpleasant burning pain felt in a limb where there has been partial damage to the sympathetic and somatic sensory nerves.

caustic (kaw-stik) *n.* an agent, such as silver nitrate, that causes irritation and burning and destroys tissue. Caustic agents may

plasma membrane

cytoplasm

centrosome

nucleus

nucleolus

fibrils

nucleoplasm

pores in nuclear membrane

rough endoplasmic reticulum

ribosomes

glycogen granules

Golgi apparatus

centrioles

lysosomes

nuclear membrane

chromatin

smooth endoplasmic reticulum

fat droplets

mitochondria

An animal cell (microscopical structure)

be used to remove dead skin, warts, etc.

cauterize (kaw-tĕ-ryz) *vb.* to destroy tissues by direct application of a heated instrument (known as a *cautery*): used for the removal of small warts or other growths. —**cautery** *n.*

cavernous breath sounds (amphoric breath sounds) (kav-er-nŭs) *pl. n.* hollow breath sounds heard over cavities in the lung.

cavernous sinus *n.* one of the paired cavities within the sphenoid bone, at the base of the skull behind the eye sockets, into which blood drains from the brain, eye, nose, and upper cheek before leaving the skull through connections with the internal jugular and facial veins.

cavity (kav-iti) *n.* **1.** (in anatomy) a hollow enclosed area; for example, the abdominal cavity or the buccal cavity (mouth). **2.** (in dentistry) the hole in a tooth

caused by caries or abrasion or formed by a dentist to retain a filling.

-cele (-coele) *suffix denoting* swelling, hernia, or tumour.

cell (sel) *n.* the basic unit of all living organisms, which can reproduce itself exactly (*see* mitosis). Cells contain cytoplasm, in which are suspended a nucleus and other structures (organelles) specialized to carry out particular activities in the cell. Complex organisms such as man are built up of millions of cells that are specially adapted to carry out particular functions.

cell division *n.* reproduction of cells by division first of the chromosomes (karyokinesis) and then of the cytoplasm (cytokinesis). Cell division to produce more body (somatic) cells is by mitosis; cell division during the formation of gametes is by meiosis.

cellulitis (sel-yoo-ly-tis) *n.* inflammation of the connective tissue between adjacent tissues and organs. This is commonly due to bacterial infection and usually requires antibiotic treatment to prevent its spread to the bloodstream.

cellulose (sel-yoo-lohz) *n.* a carbohydrate consisting of linked glucose units. It is an important constituent of plant cell walls. Cellulose cannot be digested by man and is a component of dietary fibre (roughage).

Celsius temperature (centigrade temperature) (sel-si-ŭs) *n.* temperature expressed on a scale in which the melting point of ice is assigned a temperature of 0° and the boiling point of water a temperature of 100°. The formula for converting from Celsius (C) to Fahrenheit (F) is: $F = \frac{9}{5}(C + 32)$. *See also* Fahrenheit temperature. [A. Celsius (1701–44), Swedish astronomer]

cement (si-ment) *n.* 1. a substance used in dentistry to fix into place an inlay or crown or to form a filling. 2. *see* cementum.

cementum (cement) (si-men-tŭm) *n.* a thin layer of hard tissue on the surface of the root of a tooth. It anchors the fibres of the periodontal membrane to the tooth.

censor (sen-ser) *n.* (in psychology) the mechanism, postulated by Freud, that suppresses or modifies desires that are inappropriate or feared.

-centesis *suffix denoting* puncture or perforation.

centi- *prefix denoting* one hundredth or a hundred.

centigrade temperature (sent-i-grayd) *n. see* Celsius temperature.

central nervous system (CNS) (sen-trăl) *n.* the brain and the spinal cord, as opposed to the peripheral nervous system. The CNS is responsible for the integration of all nervous activities.

central venous pressure *n.* blood pressure in the right atrium, recorded by means of a catheter inserted into the vena cava and attached to a manometer. It is monitored particularly after heart surgery.

centri- *prefix denoting* centre.

centrifugal (sen-tri-few-găl) *adj.* moving away from a centre, as from the brain to the peripheral tissues.

centrifuge (sen-tri-fewj) *n.* a device for separating components of different densities in a liquid, using centrifugal force. The liquid is placed in special containers that are spun at high speed around a central axis.

centriole (sen-tri-ohl) *n.* a small particle found in the cytoplasm of cells, near the nucleus. Centrioles are involved in the formation of the spindle and aster during cell division.

centripetal (sen-trip-it'l) *adj.* moving towards a centre, as from the peripheral tissues to the brain.

centromere (kinetochore) (sen-trŏ-meer) *n.* the part of a chromosome that joins the two chromatids to each other and becomes attached to the spindle during mitosis and meiosis. When chromosome division takes place the centromeres split longitudinally.

centrosome (centrosphere) (sen-trŏ-sohm) *n.* an area of clear cytoplasm, found next to the nucleus in nondividing cells, that contains the centrioles.

centrosphere (sen-trŏ-sfeer) *n.* **1.** an area of clear cytoplasm seen in dividing cells around the poles of the spindle. **2.** *see* centrosome.

cephal- (cephalo-) *prefix denoting* the head.

cephalalgia (sef-ă-lal-jiă) *n.* pain in the head; headache.

cephalexin (sef-ă-leks-in) *n.* a semisynthetic antibiotic, administered by mouth, used in the treatment of a variety of infections. *See* cephalosporin. Trade names: **Ceporex, Keflex.**

cephalhaematoma (sef-ăl-heem-ă-toh-mă) *n.* an egg-sized swelling on the head caused by a collection of bloody fluid between one of the skull bones and its covering membrane (periosteum). It is most commonly seen in newborn infants delivered with the aid of forceps or subjected to pressures during passage through the birth canal. No treatment is necessary and the swelling disappears in a few weeks.

cephalic (si-fal-ik) *adj.* of or relating to the head.

cephalic index *n.* a measure of the shape of a skull, commonly used in craniometry.

cephalic version *n.* a procedure for turning a fetus that is lying in a breech or transverse position so that its head will enter the birth passage first.

cephalocele (si-fal-ŏ-seel) *n.* protrusion of the contents of the skull through a defect in the bones of the skull. *See* neural tube defect.

cephalogram (sef-ă-loh-gram) *n.* a special standardized X-ray picture that can be used to measure alterations in the growth of skull bones.

cephalometry (sef-ă-lom-itri) *n.*

measurement of the head, particularly measurement of the head of a fetus by radiography.

cephaloridine (sef-ă-lo-rid-een) *n.* a semisynthetic antibiotic, given by intravenous or intramuscular injection. It is used in the treatment of a variety of severe infections, including those of bones, joints, the bloodstream, and the urinary and respiratory tracts. *See* cephalosporin. Trade name: **Loridine.**

cephalosporin (sef-ă-loh-spor-in) *n.* any one of a group of semisynthetic antibiotics, derived from the mould *Cephalosporium*, which are effective against a wide range of microorganisms and are therefore used in a variety of infections (*see* cephalexin, cephaloridine, cephalothin sodium). Cross-sensitivity with penicillin may occur and the principal side-effects are allergic reactions and irritation of the digestive tract.

cephalothin sodium (sef-ă-loh-thin) *n.* a semisynthetic antibiotic, given by intramuscular or intravenous injection in the treatment of a number of infections. *See* cephalosporin. Trade name: **Keflin.**

cerebellum (se-ri-bel-ŭm) *n.* the largest part of the hindbrain, bulging back behind the pons and the medulla oblongata and overhung by the occipital lobes of the cerebrum. The cerebellum is essential for the maintenance of muscle tone, balance, and the synchronization of activity in groups of muscles under voluntary control, converting muscular contractions into smooth coordinated movement. —**cerebellar** *adj.*

cerebr- (cerebri-, cerebro-) *prefix denoting* the cerebrum or brain.

cerebral aqueduct (se-ri-brăl) *n.* *see* aqueduct.

cerebral cortex *n.* the intricately folded outer layer of the cerebrum, making up some 40% of the brain by weight. It is directly responsible for consciousness, with essential roles in perception, memory, thought, mental ability, and intellect, and it is responsible for initiating voluntary activity.

cerebral haemorrhage *n.* bleeding from a cerebral artery into the tissue of the brain. It is usually caused by degenerative disease of the blood vessels and high blood pressure. The symptoms vary from a transient weakness or numbness to profound coma and death. *See also* atheroma, hypertension, stroke.

cerebral hemisphere *n.* one of the two paired halves of the cerebrum.

cerebral palsy *n.* a developmental abnormality of the brain resulting in weakness and incoordination of the limbs and often caused by injury during birth. The most common disability is a spastic paralysis (an affected child is called a *spastic*), which may slowly increase from contractures to cause fixed deformities of the limbs.

cerebration (se-ri-**bray**-shŏn) *n.* **1.** the functioning of the brain as a whole. **2.** the unconscious activities of the brain.

cerebrospinal fever (spotted fever) (se-ri-broh-**spy**-năl) *n.* a type of meningitis caused by the bacterium *Neisseria meningitidis*. Symptoms include severe headache, fever, stiffness of the neck muscles, and a rash of small red spots on the trunk. Without treatment death can occur within a week, but administration of penicillin or sulphonamide drugs is usually effective.

cerebrospinal fluid (CSF) *n.* the clear watery fluid that surrounds and protects the brain and spinal cord. It is contained in the subarachnoid space and circulates in the ventricles of the brain and in the central canal of the spinal cord.

cerebrovascular accident (se-ri-broh-vas-kew-ler) *n.* the clinical syndrome accompanying a sudden and severe attack of cerebrovascular disease, which leads to a stroke.

cerebrovascular disease *n.* any disorder of the blood vessels of the brain and its covering membranes (meninges). Most cases are due to atheroma and/or hypertension, clinical effects being caused by rupture of diseased blood vessels or inadequacy of the blood supply to the brain, due to cerebral thrombosis or embolism.

- parieto-occipital fissure
- parietal lobe
- central sulcus
- frontal lobe
- lateral sulcus
- temporal lobe
- occipital lobe

Lobes of cerebrum (from right side)

cerebrum (telencephalon) (se-ri-brŭm) *n.* the largest and most highly developed part of the brain, composed of the two cerebral hemispheres, separated from each other by the longitudinal fissure in the midline and connected at the base by the corpus callosum. The cerebrum is responsible for the initiation and coordination of all voluntary activity in the body and for governing the functioning of lower parts of the nervous system. —**cerebral** *adj.*

cerumen (earwax) (si-roo-men) *n.* the waxy material that is secreted by the sebaceous glands in the external auditory meatus of the outer ear.

cervic- (cervico-) *prefix denoting* **1.** the neck. **2.** the cervix, especially of the uterus.

cervical (ser-vy-kăl) *adj.* **1.** of or relating to the neck. *c. vertebrae* the seven bones making up the neck region of the backbone. *See also* vertebra. **2.** of, relating to, or affecting the cervix of an organ, especially the cervix of the womb. *c. smear* a specimen of cellular material scraped from the cervix of the womb and examined under a microscope in order to determine whether cancer is present.

cervicitis (ser-vi-sy-tis) *n.* inflammation of the cervix of the womb.

cervix (ser-viks) *n.* a necklike part. *c. uteri* the narrow passage at the lower end of the uterus (womb), which connects with the vagina.

cestode (ses-tohd) *n. see* tapeworm.

cetrimide (set-ri-myd) *n.* a detergent disinfectant, used for cleansing skin surfaces and wounds, sterilizing surgical instruments and babies' napkins, and in shampoos. Trade name: **Cetavlon.**

chalazion (meibomian cyst) (kă-lay-zi-ŏn) *n.* a swollen sebaceous gland in the eyelid, caused by chronic inflammation following blockage of the gland's duct.

chancre (shang-ker) *n.* a painless ulcer that develops on the lips, penis, urethra, or eyelid as the primary symptom of such infections as sleeping sickness and syphilis.

chancroid (shank-roid) *n. see* soft sore.

charcoal (char-kohl) *n.* a fine black powder, a form of carbon that is the residue from the partial burning of wood and other organic materials. *activated c.* charcoal that has been treated to increase its properties as an adsorbent, used as an emergency antidote to various poisons.

Charcot-Marie-Tooth disease (peroneal muscular atrophy) (shar-koh mă-ree tooth) *n.* an inherited disease of the peripheral nerves causing a gradually progressive weakness and wasting of the muscles of the legs and the lower part of the thighs. The hands and arms are eventually affected. [J. M. Charcot (1825–93), French neurologist; P. Marie (1853–1940), French physician; H. H. Tooth (1856–1925), British physician]

Charcot's joint *n.* a damaged, swollen, and deformed joint, often the knee, resulting from repeated minor injuries of which the patient is unaware because the nerves that normally register pain are not functioning. The condition may occur in syphilis, diabetes mellitus, and syringomyelia.

Charnley clamps (**charn**-li) *pl. n.* parallel metal rods driven through the ends of two bones that are to be joined to form an arthrodesis. The rods are connected on each side of the joint by bolts bearing wing nuts; tightening of the screw arrangements forces the surfaces of the bones together. [Sir J. Charnley (1911–   ), British orthopaedic surgeon]

cheil- (**cheilo-**) *prefix denoting* the lip(s).

cheilitis (ky-**ly**-tis) *n.* inflammation of the lips.

cheiloplasty (ky-loh-plasti) *n. see* labioplasty.

cheiloschisis (ky-**losk**-i-sis) *n. see* harelip.

cheilosis (ky-**loh**-sis) *n.* swollen cracked bright-red lips. This is a common symptom of many nutritional disorders, including ariboflavinosis (vitamin B_2 deficiency).

cheir- (**cheiro-**) *prefix denoting* the hand(s).

cheiropompholyx (ky-roh-**pom**-fŏ-liks) *n.* a type of eczema affecting the sides and fronts of the palms and fingers, with a similar distribution on the feet.

chelating agent (kee-**layt**-ing) *n.* a chemical compound that forms complexes by binding metal ions. Some chelating agents, including desferrioxamine and penicillamine, are drugs used to treat metal poisoning: the metal is bound to the drug and excreted safely.

cheloid (kee-loid) *n. see* keloid.

chem- (**chemo-**) *prefix denoting* chemical or chemistry.

chemoreceptor (kee-moh-ri-**sep**-ter) *n.* a cell or group of cells that responds to the presence of specific chemical compounds by initiating an impulse in a sensory nerve. Chemoreceptors are found in the taste buds and in the mucous membranes of the nose. *See also* receptor.

chemosis (ki-**moh**-sis) *n.* swelling (oedema) of the conjunctiva.

chemotaxis (kee-moh-**taks**-iss) *n.* movement of a cell or organism in response to the stimulus of a gradient of chemical concentration.

chemotherapy (kee-moh-**th'e**-ră-pi) *n.* the prevention or treatment of disease by the use of chemical substances. The term is sometimes restricted to the treatment of infectious diseases with antibiotics and other drugs or to the control of cancer with antimetabolites and similar drugs (in contrast to radiotherapy).

chest (chest) *n. see* thorax.

Cheyne-Stokes respiration (chayn stohks) *n.* a striking form of breathing in which there is a cyclical variation in the rate, which becomes slower until breathing stops for several seconds before speeding up to a peak and then slowing again. It occurs particularly in states of coma. [J. Cheyne (1777–1836), Scottish physician; W. Stokes (1804–78), Irish physician]

chiasma (ky-**az**-mă) *n.* (*pl.* **chiasmata**) *see* optic (chiasma).

chickenpox (**chik**-in-poks) *n.* a mild highly infectious disease caused by a herpesvirus that is transmitted by airborne droplets. Symptoms are mild fever followed by an itchy rash of dark red pimples that spread from the trunk to the face, scalp, and limbs. These develop into blisters and then scabs, which drop off after about 12 days. The patient is infectious from the onset of symptoms until all the spots have gone. Medical name: **varicella**.

Chief Administrative Medical Officer *n.* a physician at Area level under the NHS (Scotland) Act.

chilblain (chil-blayn) *n.* a red round itchy swelling of the skin, occurring generally on the fingers or toes in cold weather. *See also* perniosis. Medical name: **pernio**.

childbed (chyld-bed) *n. see* puerperium.

childbirth (chyld-berth) *n. see* labour.

child health clinic (CHC) (chyld) *n.* (in Britain) a special clinic for the routine care of infants and preschool children. The service provides screening tests for congenital dislocation of hips, suppressed squint, and impaired speech and/or hearing, education for mothers (especially those having their first child) in feeding techniques and hygiene, and immunizations against infectious diseases.

chir- (chiro-) *prefix denoting* the hand(s). *See also* cheir-.

chiropody (podiatry) (ki-rop-ŏdi) *n.* the study and care of the foot, including its normal structure, its diseases, and their treatment. **—chiropodist** *n.*

chiropractic (ky-rŏ-prak-tik) *n.* a system of treating diseases by manipulation, mainly of the vertebrae of the backbone. It is based on the theory that nearly all disorders can be traced to the incorrect alignment of bones, with consequent malfunctioning of nerves and muscle throughout the body. **—chiropractor** (ky-rŏ-prak-ter) *n.*

chloasma (melasma) (kloh-az-mă)

n. the appearance of brown patches, mainly on the forehead, temples, and cheeks. It is due to a localized increase in the dark pigment melanin and may occur in pregnancy, during the menopause, or as a side-effect of the contraceptive pill.

chlor- (chloro-) *prefix denoting* 1. chlorine or chlorides. 2. green.

chloracne (klor-ak-ni) *n.* an occupational acne-like skin disorder that occurs after regular contact with chlorinated hydrocarbons.

chloral hydrate (klor-ăl hy-drayt) *n.* a sedative and hypnotic drug used, mainly in children and the elderly, to induce sleep or as a daytime sedative. It is usually given by mouth as a syrup, although it can be administered rectally. Trade names: **Noctec, Somnos**.

chlorambucil (klor-am-bew-sil) *n.* a drug that destroys cancer cells. It is given by mouth and used mainly in the treatment of chronic leukaemias. Prolonged large doses may cause damage to the bone marrow. Trade name: **Leukeran**.

chloramphenicol (klor-am-fen-i-kol) *n.* an antibiotic that is effective against a wide variety of microorganisms. However, due to its serious side-effects, especially damage to the bone marrow, it is usually reserved for serious infections (such as typhoid fever) when less toxic drugs are ineffective. Trade names: **Chloromycetin, Mycinol**, etc.

chlorbutol (klor-bew-tol) *n.* an antibacterial and antifungal agent used in injection solutions, in eye and nose drops, in powder form for irritational skin conditions, and occasionally by mouth as a mild sedative in travel sickness.

chlorcyclizine (klor-sy-kliz-een) *n.* an antihistamine drug that is slow-acting but produces longlasting effects. Given by mouth, it is used mainly to relieve the symptoms of allergic reactions and to prevent travel sickness. Trade names: **Di-paralene, Histantine**.

chlordiazepoxide (klor-dy-az-i-**pok**-syd) *n.* a sedative and tranquillizing drug with muscle relaxant properties, administered by mouth or injection. Trade names: **Librium, Diapox, Elenium**. *See also* tranquillizer.

chlorhexidine (klor-**heks**-i-deen) *n.* an antiseptic used in solutions, creams, gels, and lozenges as a general disinfectant for skin and mucous membranes, as a preservative (for example, in eye drops), or as a mouthwash to control mouth infections. Trade name: **Hibitane**.

chlorine (**klor**-een) *n.* an extremely pungent gaseous element with antiseptic and bleaching properties. It is widely used to sterilize drinking water and purify swimming baths. In high concentrations it is toxic. Symbol: Cl.

chlormethiazole (klor-mi-**th'y**-ă-zohl) *n.* a sedative and hypnotic drug administered by mouth or injection to treat insomnia in the elderly (when associated with confusion, agitation, and restlessness) and drug withdrawal symptoms (especially in alcoholism). Trade name: **Heminevrin**.

chlorocresol (klo-roh-**kree**-sol) *n.* an antiseptic derived from phenol, used as a general disinfectant and, at low concentrations, as a preservative in injections,

creams, and lotions and also in eye drops.

chloroform (**klo**-rŏ-form) *n.* a volatile liquid formerly widely used as a general anaesthetic. Chloroform is now used only in low concentrations as a flavouring agent and preservative, in the treatment of flatulence, and in liniments as a rubefacient.

chloroma (klo-roh-mă) *n.* a tumour that arises in association with myeloid leukaemia and consists essentially of a mass of leukaemic cells. A freshly cut specimen of the tumour appears green, but the colour rapidly disappears on exposure to air.

chlorophenothane (klo-roh-**feen**-ŏ-thayn) *n. see* DDT.

chlorophyll (**klo**-rŏ-fil) *n.* one of a group of green pigments, found in all green plants and some bacteria, that absorb light to provide energy for the synthesis of carbohydrates from carbon dioxide and water (photosynthesis).

chloroquine (**klo**-roh-kween) *n.* a drug used principally in the treatment and prevention of malaria but also used in rheumatoid arthritis, certain liver infections and skin conditions, and lupus erythematosus. It is administered by mouth or injection; a side-effect of prolonged use in large doses is eye damage. Trade names: **Avloclor, Nivaquine**.

chlorothiazide (klo-roh-**th'y**-ă-zyd) *n.* a diuretic administered by mouth to treat fluid retention (oedema) and high blood pressure (hypertension). Trade name: **Saluric**.

chlorotrianisene (klo-roh-try-**an**-i-seen) *n.* a synthetic oestrogen administered by mouth to treat symptoms of the menopause, to suppress lactation in mothers not breast feeding, and to relieve symptoms in cancer of the prostate gland. Trade name: **Tace**.

chloroxylenol (klo-roh-zy-li-nol) *n*. an antiseptic, derived from phenol but less toxic and more selective in bactericidal activity, used mainly in solution as a skin disinfectant. Trade name: **Dettol**.

chlorpheniramine (klor-fen-I-rămeen) *n*. a potent antihistamine used to treat such allergies as hay fever, rhinitis, and urticaria. It is administered by mouth or, to relieve severe conditions, by injection. Trade name: **Piriton**.

chlorpromazine (klor-**prom**-ă-zeen) *n*. a major tranquillizer and sedative used to treat anxiety, tension, and agitation, to control nausea and vomiting, to enhance the effects of analgesics, and in preparation for or induction of anaesthesia. Chlorpromazine is administered by mouth or injection or as a rectal suppository. Trade names: **Chloractil**, **Largactil**.

chlorpropamide (klor-**proh**-pă-myd) *n*. a drug that reduces blood sugar levels and is administered by mouth to treat diabetes in adults. Trade names: **Diabinese**, **Melitase**. *See also* sulphonylurea.

chlorprothixene (klor-prŏ-**thiks**-een) *n*. a major tranquillizer and sedative that is administered by mouth to treat agitation, anxiety, insomnia, delusions, and hallucinations. Trade name: **Taractan**.

chlortetracycline (klor-tet-răsy-kleen) *n*. an antibiotic active against many bacteria and fungi. It is administered by mouth or injection or as ointment or cream (for skin and eye infections). Trade names: **Aureomycin**, **Chlortetrin**, **Deteclo**.

chlorthalidone (klor-**thal**-i-dohn) *n*. a diuretic administered by mouth to treat fluid retention (oedema) and high blood pressure (hypertension). Trade name: **Hygroton**.

choana (koh-ă-nă) *n*. (*pl.* **choanae**) a funnel-shaped opening, particularly either of the two openings between the nasal cavity and the pharynx.

chocolate cyst (**chok**-ŏ-lit) *n*. a cyst filled with dark fluid, occurring in the ovary in endometriosis.

chol- (chole-, cholo-) *prefix denoting* bile.

cholaemia (kol-**eem**-iă) *n*. the presence of bile or bile pigments in the blood. *See* jaundice.

cholagogue (**kol**-ă-gog) *n*. a drug that stimulates the flow of bile from the gall bladder and bile ducts into the duodenum.

cholangiography (kol-anji-**og**-răfi) *n*. X-ray examination of the bile ducts, used to demonstrate the site and nature of any obstruction to the ducts or to show the presence of stones within them. A medium that is opaque to X-rays is introduced into the ducts by injection into the bloodstream, the liver, the bile ducts themselves, or the duodenal opening of the ducts.

cholangiolitis (kol-anji-ŏ-**ly**-tis) *n*. inflammation of the smallest bile ducts (*cholangioles*). *See* cholangitis.

cholangitis (kol-an-**jy**-tis) *n*. inflammation of the bile ducts, often caused by an obstruction in the ducts. Initial treatment is by antibiotics, but removal of the obstruction is essential for permanent cure.

cholecalciferol (koli-kal-**sif**-er-ol) *n*. *see* vitamin D.

cholecyst- *prefix denoting* the gall bladder.

cholecystectomy (koli-sis-**tek**-tŏmi) *n.* surgical removal of the gall bladder, usually for cholecystitis or gallstones.

cholecystenterostomy (koli-sist-en-ter-**ost**-ŏmi) *n.* a surgical procedure in which the gall bladder is joined to the small intestine. It is performed in order to allow bile to pass from the liver to the intestine when the common bile duct is obstructed by an irremovable cause.

cholecystitis (koli-sis-**ty**-tis) *n.* inflammation of the gall bladder.

cholecystoduodenostomy (koli-sis-toh-dew-oh-di-**nost**-ŏmi) *n.* a form of cholecystenterostomy in which the gall bladder is joined to the duodenum.

cholecystogastrostomy (koli-sis-toh-gas-**trost**-ŏmi) *n.* a form of cholecystenterostomy in which the gall bladder is joined to the stomach. It is rarely performed.

cholecystography (koli-sis-**tog**-răfi) *n.* X-ray examination of the gall bladder. A compound opaque to X-rays is administered by mouth and an X-ray photograph (*cholecystogram*) is taken.

cholecystojejunostomy (koli-sis-toh-jĕ-joo-**nost**-ŏmi) *n.* a form of cholecystoenterostomy in which the gall bladder is joined to the jejunum.

cholecystokinin-pancreozymin (koli-sis-toh-**ky**-nin pank-ri-oh-**zy**-min) *n.* a hormone from the small intestine (duodenum) that causes contraction of the gall bladder and expulsion of bile into the intestine and stimulates the production of digestive enzymes by the pancreas.

cholecystolithiasis (koli-sis-toh-lith-**I**-ă-sis) *n. see* cholelithiasis.

cholecystotomy (koli-sis-**tot**-ŏmi) *n.* a surgical operation in which the gall bladder is opened, usually to remove gallstones.

choledoch- (choledocho-) *prefix denoting* the common bile duct.

choledocholithiasis (koli-dok-oh-lith-**I**-ă-sis) *n.* stones within the common bile duct. The stones usually form in the gall bladder and pass into the bile duct, but they may develop within the duct after cholecystectomy.

choledochotomy (koli-dŏ-**kot**-ŏmi) *n.* a surgical operation in which the common bile duct is opened, to search for or to remove stones within it.

cholelithiasis (cholecystolithiasis) (koli-lith-**I**-ă-sis) *n.* the formation of stones in the gall bladder or bile duct (*see* gallstone).

cholelithotomy (koli-lith-**ot**-ŏmi) *n.* removal of gallstones by cholecystotomy.

cholera (**kol**-er-ă) *n.* an acute infection of the small intestine by the bacterium *Vibrio cholerae*, which causes severe vomiting and diarrhoea (known as *ricewater stools*) leading to dehydration. The disease is contracted from contaminated food or drinking water and often occurs in epidemics. The patient is treated by intravenous infusion of salt solution; antibiotics only hasten recovery. The mortality rate in untreated cases is over 50%. Vaccination against cholera is effective for only 6–9 months.

choleresis (kol-er-**ee**-sis) *n.* the production of bile by the liver.

choleretic (kol-er-et-ik) *n.* an agent that stimulates the secretion of bile by the liver thereby increasing the flow of bile.

cholestasis (koli-**stay**-sis) *n.* failure of normal amounts of bile to reach the intestine, resulting in obstructive jaundice. The symptoms are jaundice with dark urine, pale faeces, and usually itching (pruritus).

cholesteatoma (koli-sti-ă-**toh**-mă) *n.* a mass consisting mainly of cellular debris in which cholesterol crystals may be demonstrated. Cholesteatomas occur mainly in the middle ear.

cholesterol (kŏl-**est**-er-ol) *n.* a fat-like material (a sterol) present in the blood and most tissues, especially nervous tissue. Elevated blood concentration of cholesterol is often associated with atheroma, of which cholesterol is a major component. Cholesterol is also a constituent of gallstones.

cholesterosis (kŏl-est-er-**oh**-sis) *n.* a form of chronic cholecystitis in which small crystals of cholesterol are deposited on the internal wall of the gall bladder. The crystals may enlarge to become gallstones.

cholestyramine (koli-**sty**-ră-meen) *n.* a drug that binds with bile salts so that they are excreted. It is administered by mouth to relieve conditions due to irritant effects of bile salts – such as the itching that occurs in obstructive jaundice – and also to lower the blood levels of cholesterol and other fats. Trade names: **Cuemid, Questran.**

cholic acid (**cholalic acid**) (**kol**-ik) *n. see* bile acids.

choline (**koh**-leen) *n.* a basic compound important in the synthesis of phosphatidylcholine (lecithin) and other phospholipids and of acetylcholine. It is also involved in the transport of fat in the body. Choline is sometimes classed as a vitamin but, although it is essential for life, it can be synthesized in the body.

cholinergic (koh-lin-**er**-jik) *adj.* describing nerve fibres that release acetylcholine as a neurotransmitter. *Compare* adrenergic.

choline salicylate (să-**lis**-i-layt) *n.* an analgesic, related to aspirin, that is applied locally to relieve earache, mouth ulcers, and other painful conditions. Trade names: **Audax, Bonjela, Teejel.**

cholinesterase (koh-lin-**est**-er-ayz) *n.* an enzyme that breaks down a choline ester into its choline and acid components. The term usually refers to *acetylcholinesterase*, which breaks down the neurotransmitter acetylcholine into choline and acetic acid.

choline theophyllinate (thi-ŏ-**fil**-i-nayt) *n.* a drug used to dilate the air passages in asthma and chronic bronchitis. It is administered by mouth and can cause digestive upsets and nausea. Trade name: **Choledyl.**

choluria (kol-**yoor**-iă) *n.* bile in the urine, which occurs when the level of bile in the blood is raised, especially in obstructive jaundice.

chondr- (chondro-) *prefix denoting* cartilage.

chondritis (kon-**dry**-tis) *n.* any inflammatory condition affecting cartilage.

chondroblast (kon-droh-blast) *n.* a cell that produces the matrix of cartilage.

chondroblastoma (kon-droh-blas-**toh**-mă) *n.* a tumour derived from chondroblasts, having the appearance of a mass of well-differentiated cartilage.

chondroclast (kon-droh-klast) *n.* a cell that is concerned with the absorption of cartilage.

85 **choroidocyclitis**

chondrocyte (kon-droh-syt) *n.* a cartilage cell, found embedded in the matrix.

chondroma (kon-**droh**-mă) *n.* a benign tumour of cartilage-forming cells, which may occur at the growing end of any bone but is found most commonly in the bones of the feet and hands. *See also* dyschondroplasia, enchondroma, ecchondroma.

chondromalacia (kon-droh-mă-lay-shiă) *n.* degeneration of cartilage at a joint. *c. patellae* a roughening of the inner surface of the kneecap, resulting in pain, a grating sensation, and a feeling of instability on movement.

chondrosarcoma (kon-droh-sar-koh-ma) *n.* (*pl.* **chondrosarcomata**) a malignant tumour of cartilage cells, occurring in a bone.

chord- (chordo-) *prefix denoting* 1. a cord. 2. the notochord.

chorda (kor-da) *n.* (*pl.* **chordae**) a cord, tendon, or nerve fibre. *chordae tendineae* stringlike processes in the heart that attach the margins of the mitral and tricuspid valve leaflets to projections of the wall of the ventricle (*papillary muscles*).

chordee (kor-dee) *n.* acute angulation of the penis. It may result from Peyronie's disease or, in a child, from hypospadias.

chorditis (kor-dy-tis) *n.* inflammation of a vocal cord. *See* laryngitis.

chordotomy (kor-dot-ŏmi) *n. see* cordotomy.

chorea (ko-ree-ă) *n.* a jerky involuntary movement particularly affecting the shoulders, hips, and face. The symptoms are due to disease of the basal ganglia. *Huntington's c.* an inherited form in which the involuntary movements are accompanied by a progressive dementia: there is widespread neuronal degeneration throughout the brain. *Sydenham's c.* chorea that affects children and is associated with rheumatic fever. It responds to mild sedatives.

chorion (kor-iŏn) *n.* the embryonic membrane that totally surrounds the embryo from the time of implantation. —**chorionic** *adj.*

chorionepithelioma (choriocarcinoma) (kor-i-ŏn-ep-i-theel-i-oh-mă) *n.* a rare form of cancer originating in the chorion and affecting the womb or the site of a pregnancy outside the womb. Chorionepithelioma is highly malignant; it may occur after hydatidiform mole, pregnancy, or abortion.

chorionic gonadotrophin (human chorionic gonadotrophin, HCG) (kor-i-on-ik) *n.* a hormone, similar to the pituitary gonadotrophins, produced by the placenta during pregnancy. Large amounts are excreted in the urine, and this is used as the basis for most pregnancy tests. HCG is given by injection to treat such conditions as delayed puberty, undescended testes, and premenstrual tension.

chorionic villi *pl. n. see* villus.

choroid (ko-roid) *n.* the layer of the eyeball between the retina and the sclera. It contains blood vessels and a pigment that absorbs excess light and so prevents blurring of vision. *See* eye.

choroiditis (ko-roid-I-tis) *n.* inflammation of the choroid layer of the eye. Vision becomes blurred but the eye is usually painless. *See* uveitis.

choroidocyclitis (ko-roid-oh-sy-kly-tis) *n.* inflammation of the choroid layer and the ciliary body of the eye.

choroid plexus *n.* a rich network of blood vessels, derived from those of the pia mater, in each of the brain's ventricles. It is responsible for the production of cerebrospinal fluid.

Christmas disease (kris-măs) *n.* a disorder that is identical in its effects to haemophilia, but is due to a deficiency of a different blood coagulation factor, the *Christmas factor* (Factor IX).

chrom- (chromo-) *prefix denoting* colour or pigment.

-chromasia *suffix denoting* staining or pigmentation.

chromat- (chromato-) *prefix denoting* colour or pigmentation.

chromatid (kroh-mă-tid) *n.* one of the two threadlike strands formed by longitudinal division of a chromosome during mitosis and meiosis. They remain attached at the centromere.

chromatin (kroh-mă-tin) *n.* the material of a cell nucleus that stains with basic dyes and consists of DNA and protein: the substance of which the chromosomes are made.

chromatography (kroh-mă-**tog**-răfi) *n.* any of several techniques for separating the components of a mixture by selective absorption. In two such techniques, widely used in medicine, a sample of the mixture is placed at the edge of a sheet of filter paper (*paper c.*) or a column of a powdered absorbent (*column c.*). The components of the mixture are absorbed to different extents and thus move along the paper or column at different rates.

chromatolysis (kroh-mă-**tol**-i-sis) *n.* the dispersal or disintegration of the microscopic structures within

the nerve cells that normally produce proteins. It is part of the cell's response to injury.

chromatophore (kroh-mă-tŏ-for) *n.* a cell containing pigment. In man chromatophores containing melanin are found in the skin, hair, and eyes.

chromatosis (kroh-mă-**toh**-sis) *n.* abnormal pigmentation of the skin, as occurs in Addison's disease.

chromic acid (kroh-mik) *n.* a compound of chromium used in solution as a caustic for the removal of warts. Formula: CrO_3.

chromosome (kroh-mŏ-sohm) *n.* one of the threadlike structures in a cell nucleus that carry the genetic information in the form of genes. It is composed of a long double filament of DNA coiled into a helix together with associated proteins. The nucleus of each human somatic cell contains 46 chromosomes, 23 being of maternal and 23 of paternal origin. *See also* chromatid, centromere, sex chromosome. —**chromosomal** *adj.*

chronic (kron-ik) *adj.* describing a disease of long duration involving very slow changes. Such disease is often of gradual onset. *Compare* acute.

Chronic Sick and Disabled Persons Act (1970) (in Britain) an Act providing for the identification and care of those suffering from a chronic or degenerative disease for which there is no cure and which can be only partially alleviated by treatment.

Chvostek's sign (vos-teks) *n.* a spasm of the facial muscles elicited by lightly tapping the facial nerve. It is a sign of tetany. [F. Chvostek (1835–84), Austrian surgeon]

chyle (kyl) *n.* an alkaline milky liquid found within the lacteals after a period of absorption. It consists of lymph with a suspension of minute droplets of digested fats, which have been absorbed from the small intestine.

chyluria (kyl-**yoor**-iă) *n.* the presence of chyle in the urine.

chyme (kym) *n.* the semiliquid acid mass that is the form in which food passes from the stomach to the small intestine. It is produced by the action of gastric juice and the churning movements of the stomach.

chymotrypsin (ky-moh-**trip**-sin) *n.* a protein-digesting enzyme (*see* peptidase). It is secreted by the pancreas in an inactive form, *chymotrypsinogen*, that is converted into chymotrypsin in the duodenum by the action of trypsin.

chymotrypsinogen (ky-moh-trip-sin-ŏ-jin) *n. see* chymotrypsin.

cicatrix (**sik**-ă-triks) *n.* a scar: any mark left after the healing of a wound, where the damaged tissues fail to repair themselves completely and are replaced by connective tissue.

-cide *suffix denoting* killer or killing.

ciliary body (**sil**-i-er-i) *n.* the part of the eye that connects the choroid with the iris. It consists of three zones: the *ciliary ring*, which adjoins the choroid; the *ciliary processes*, a series of about 70 radial ridges behind the iris to which the suspensory ligament of the lens is attached; and the *ciliary muscle*, contraction of which alters the curvature of the lens (*see* accommodation).

cilium (**sil**-iŭm) *n.* (*pl.* **cilia**) 1. a hairlike process, large numbers of which are found on certain epithelial cells, particularly the epithelium that lines the upper respiratory tract, and on certain protozoa. 2. an eyelash or eyelid. —**ciliary** *adj.*

cimetidine (si-**met**-i-deen) *n.* a drug that reduces secretion of acid in the stomach and is administered by mouth or injection to treat digestive disorders such as stomach and duodenal ulcers. Trade name: **Tagamet**.

Cimex (**sy**-meks) *n. see* bed bug.

cinchocaine (**sink**-ŏ-kayn) *n.* a local anaesthetic used in dental and other operations and to relieve pain. It is applied directly to the skin or mucous membranes or injected at the site where anaesthesia is required or into the spine.

cinchona (sing-**koh**-nă) *n.* the dried bark of *Cinchona* trees, formerly used in medicine to stimulate the appetite and to prevent haemorrhage and diarrhoea. Cinchona is the source of quinine.

cinchonism (**sink**-ŏ-nizm) *n.* poisoning caused by an overdose of cinchona or the alkaloids quinine, quinidine, or cinchonine derived from it. The symptoms include ringing noises in the ears, dizziness, and blurring of vision.

cineangiocardiography (sini-an-ji-oh-kar-di-**og**-răfi) *n.* a form of angiocardiography in which the X-ray pictures are recorded on cine film. This allows the dynamic movements of the heart to be studied when the film is projected.

cineradiography (sini-ray-di-**og**-răfi) *n.* the technique of taking a rapid succession of X-ray photographs, to capture on film events that occur rapidly during a particular radiographic investigation.

cingulum (sing-yoo-lŭm) *n.* (*pl.* **cingula**) a curved bundle of nerve fibres in each cerebral hemisphere, nearly encircling its connection with the corpus callosum. *See* cerebrum.

circadian rhythm (ser-kay-diăn) *n.* the periodic rhythm, synchronized approximately to the 24-hour day/night cycle, seen in various metabolic activities of most living organisms (e.g. sleeping, hormone secretion).

circle of Willis (ser-kŭl ŏv wil-iss) *n.* a circle on the undersurface of the brain formed by linked branches of the arteries that supply the brain. This helps to maintain the blood supply in the event of a feeding vessel being blocked. [T. Willis (1621–75), English anatomist]

circulation (ser-kew-lay-shŏn) *n.* **1.** the movement of a fluid in a circular course, especially the passage of blood through the cardiovascular system. **2.** the system of vessels effecting this passage. *pulmonary c.* circulation of blood between the heart and lungs. Deoxygenated blood passes to the lungs from the right ventricle via the pulmonary artery; oxygenated blood returns to the left atrium via the pulmonary vein. *systemic c.* circulation of blood between the heart and all parts of the body except the lungs. Oxygenated blood leaves the aorta and deoxygenated blood returns into the vena cava. *See also* collateral circulation. —**circulatory** *adj.*

circum- *prefix denoting* around; surrounding.

circumcision (ser-kŭm-sizh-ŏn) *n.* surgical removal of the foreskin of the penis. This operation is usually performed for religious and ethnic reasons but is sometimes required for medical conditions, mainly phimosis and paraphimosis.

circumduction (ser-kŭm-duk-shŏn) *n.* a circular movement, such as that made by a limb.

circumflex nerve (ser-kŭm-fleks) *n.* a mixed sensory and motor nerve of the upper arm. It arises from the fifth and sixth cervical segments of the spinal cord and is distributed to the deltoid muscle of the shoulder and the overlying skin.

circumoral (ser-kŭm-or-ăl) *adj.* situated around the mouth.

cirrhosis (si-roh-sis) *n.* a condition in which the liver responds to injury or death of some of its cells by producing interlacing strands of fibrous tissue between which are nodules of regenerating cells. Causes include alcoholism (*alcoholic c.*), viral hepatitis (*postnecrotic c.*), chronic obstruction of the common bile duct (*secondary biliary c.*), autoimmune diseases (*primary biliary c.*), and chronic heart failure (*cardiac c.*). Complications include portal hypertension, ascites, hepatic encephalopathy, and hepatoma. —**cirrhotic** *adj.*

cirs- (**cirso-**) *prefix denoting* a varicose vein.

cirsoid (ser-soid) *adj.* describing the distended knotted appearance of a varicose vein.

cisterna (sis-ter-nă) *n.* (*pl.* **cisternae**) **1.** one of the enlarged spaces beneath the arachnoid that act as reservoirs for cerebrospinal fluid. *c. magna* the largest of the cisternae, lying beneath the cerebellum and behind the medulla oblongata. **2.** a dilatation at the lower end of the thoracic duct, into which the

noncrushing clamp

twin gastrointestinal clamp

Intestinal clamps

great lymph ducts of the lower limbs drain.

citric acid (sit-rik) *n.* an organic acid found naturally in citrus fruits. Citric acid is formed in the first stage of the Krebs cycle. Formula: $CH_2(COOH)C(OH)(COOH)CH_2COOH$.

citric acid cycle *n.* see Krebs cycle.

citrulline (sit-rŭ-leen) *n.* an amino acid produced by the liver as a by-product during the conversion of ammonia to urea.

clamp (klamp) *n.* a surgical instrument designed to compress a structure, such as a blood vessel or a cut end of the intestine.

clasmocyte (klaz-mŏ-syt) *n.* see macrophage.

claudication (klaw-di-kay-shŏn) *n.* limping. *intermittent c.* a cramping pain in the calf and leg muscles, induced by exercise and relieved by rest, that is caused by an inadequate supply of blood to the affected muscles.

claustrophobia (klaw-strŏ-**foh**-biă) *n.* a morbid fear of enclosed places. *See also* phobia.

clavicle (klav-i-kŭl) *n.* the collar bone: a long slender curved bone, a pair of which form the front part of the shoulder girdle. —**clavicular** (klă-vik-yoo-ler) *adj.*

clavus (klay-vŭs) *n.* **1.** *see* corn. **2.** a sharp pain in the head, as if a nail were being driven in.

claw-foot (klaw-fuut) *n.* an excessively arched foot, giving an unnaturally high instep. In most cases the cause is unknown, but the deformity may sometimes be due to an imbalance between the muscles flexing the toes and the shorter muscles that extend them. Medical name: **pes cavus**.

claw-hand (klaw-hand) *n.* flexion and contraction of the fingers with extension at the joints between the fingers and the hand, giving a claw-like appearance. Causes of claw-hand include injuries, syringomyelia, and leprosy. *See also* Dupuytren's contracture.

cleavage (kleev-ij) *n.* (in embryology) the process of repeated cell division of the fertilized egg to form a ball of cells that becomes the blastocyst.

cleft palate (kleft) *n.* a fissure in the midline of the palate due to failure of the two sides to fuse in embryonic development. Only part of the palate may be affected, or the cleft may extend the full length and be associated with a cleft in the upper lip (*see* harelip).

cleid- (**cleido-, clid-, clido-**) *prefix denoting* the clavicle (collar bone).

cleidocranial dysostosis (kly-doh-kray-niăl dis-os-toh-sis) *n.* a congenital defect of bone formation in which the skull bones ossify imperfectly and the collar bones (clavicles) are absent.

climacteric (kly-mak-ter-ik) *n.* **1.** *see* menopause. **2.** declining sexual drive and fertility in men, usually occurring in middle age.

clindamycin (klin-dă-my-sin) *n.* an antibiotic administered by mouth to treat serious bacterial infections.

clinic (klin-ik) *n.* **1.** an establishment or department of a hospital devoted to the treatment of particular diseases or the medical care of out-patients. **2.** a gathering of instructors, students, and patients, usually in a hospital ward, for the examination and treatment of the patients.

clinical medicine (klin-i-kăl) *n.* the branch of medicine dealing with the study of patients in bed and the diagnosis and treatment of disease at the bedside, as opposed to the study of disease by pathology or other laboratory work.

clitoridectomy (klit-er-id-ek-tŏmi) *n.* surgical removal of the clitoris.

clitoris (klit-er-iss) *n.* the female counterpart of the penis, which contains erectile tissue (*see* corpus (cavernosum)) but is unconnected with the urethra. It becomes erect under conditions of sexual stimulation.

cloaca (kloh-ay-kă) *n.* the most posterior part of the embryonic hindgut. It becomes divided into the rectum and the urinogenital sinus.

clofibrate (kloh-fy-brayt) *n.* a drug that reduces the levels of blood lipids, including cholesterol, and is administered by mouth to treat atherosclerosis and angina. Trade names: **Atromid-S**, **Liprinal**.

clomipramine (kloh-mip-ră-meen) *n.* a drug administered by mouth or injection to treat various depressive states (*see* antidepressant). Trade name: **Anafranil**.

clomocycline (kloh-moh-sy-kleen) *n.* an antibiotic administered by mouth to treat infections caused by a variety of microorganisms and also used for long-term treatment of acne. Trade name: **Megaclor**.

clonazepam (kloh-naz-ĕ-pam) *n.* a drug with anticonvulsant properties, administered by mouth or injection to treat epilepsy and other conditions involving seizures. Trade name: **Rivotril**.

clone (klohn) **1.** *n.* a group of cells (usually bacteria) descended from a single cell by asexual reproduction and therefore genetically identical to each other and to the parent cell. **2.** *vb.* to form a clone.

clonic (klon-ik) *adj.* of, relating to, or resembling clonus. The term is most commonly used to describe the rhythmical limb movements in convulsive epilepsy (*see* grand mal).

clonidine (kloh-ni-deen) *n.* a drug administered by mouth or injection to treat high blood pressure (hypertension) and migraine. Trade name: **Catapres**.

clonus (kloh-nŭs) *n.* rhythmical contraction of a muscle in response to a suddenly applied and then sustained stretch stimulus. It is most readily obtained at the ankle and is usually a sign of disease in the brain or spinal cord.

clopamide (kloh-pă-myd) *n.* a diuretic administered by mouth to treat fluid retention (oedema) and high blood pressure (hypertension). Trade name: **Brinaldix**.

clorexolone (klor-eks-ŏ-lohn) *n.* a diuretic with prolonged action, administered by mouth to treat fluid retention (oedema) and high blood pressure (hypertension). Trade name: **Nefrolan**.

Clostridium (klo-**strid**-iŭm) *n.* a genus of mostly Gram-positive anaerobic spore-forming rodlike
bacteria commonly found in soil
and in the intestinal tract of
man and animals. *C. botulinum*
a species that grows freely in
badly preserved canned foods,
producing a toxin causing serious
food poisoning (*see* botulism).
C. tetani a species that causes
tetanus on contamination of
wounds. *C. welchii* (*C. perfr-
ingens*, *Welch's bacillus*) a species
that causes blood poisoning,
food poisoning, and gas gangrene.

clotrimazole (kloh-**trim**-ă-zohl) *n.*
an antiseptic used to treat all
types of fungal skin infections,
including ringworm and infections of the genital organs. It is
applied to the infected part as
cream or solution or as vaginal
pessaries. Trade name: **Canesten**.

clotting factors (**klot**-ing) *pl. n. see*
coagulation factors.

clotting time *n. see* coagulation
time.

cloxacillin sodium (kloks-ă-sil-in)
n. an antibiotic, derived from
penicillin, administered by mouth
or injection to treat many bacterial infections. Trade name:
Orbenin.

clubbing (**klub**-ing) *n.* thickening
of the tissues at the bases of the
finger and toe nails so that the
normal angle between the nail
and the digit is filled in. In extreme cases the digit end becomes bulbous like a club or
drumstick. Clubbing is seen in
some diseases of the heart and
respiratory system and as a
harmless congenital abnormality.

club-foot (**klub**-fuut) *n. see* talipes.

clumping (**klump**-ing) *n. see* agglutination.

Clutton's joint (klu-t'nz,) *n.* a swollen joint, usually the knee,
caused by inflammation of the
synovial membranes due to congenital syphilis. [H. H. Clutton
(1850 – 1909), British surgeon]

CMV *n. see* cytomegalovirus.

CNS *n. see* central nervous system.

coagulant (koh-**ag**-yoo-lănt) *n.* any
substance capable of converting
blood from a liquid to a solid
state. *See* blood coagulation.

coagulase (koh-**ag**-yoo-layz) *n.* an
enzyme, formed by disease-producing varieties of certain bacteria of the genus *Staphylococcus*,
that causes blood plasma to coagulate. Staphylococci that are
positive when tested for coagulase production are classified as
belonging to the species *Staphylococcus aureus*.

coagulation (koh-ag-yoo-**lay**-shŏn)
n. the process by which a colloidal liquid changes to a jellylike
mass. *See* blood coagulation.

coagulation factors (clotting factors) *pl. n.* a group of substances
present in blood plasma that are
responsible for the conversion of
blood from a liquid to a solid
state (*see* blood coagulation). Although they have specific names,
most coagulation factors are referred to by an agreed set of
Roman numerals.

coagulation time (clotting time) *n.*
the time taken for blood or
blood plasma to coagulate (*see*
blood coagulation).

coagulum (koh-**ag**-yoo-lŭm) *n.* a
mass of coagulated matter, such
as that formed when blood clots.

coalesce (koh-ă-less) *vb.* to grow
together or unite. —**coalescence**
n.

coarctation (koh-ark-**tay**-shŏn) *n.* (of the aorta) a congenital narrowing of a short segment of the aorta, resulting in high blood pressure in the upper part of the body and arms and low blood pressure in the legs. The defect is corrected surgically.

cobalt (**koh**-bawlt) *n.* a metallic element that forms part of the vitamin B_{12} molecule. Symbol: Co. *cobalt-60* (*radiocobalt*) a powerful emitter of gamma radiation, used in the radiation treatment of cancer (*see* radiotherapy, telecurietherapy).

cocaine (kŏ-**kayn**) *n.* an alkaloid, derived from the leaves of the coca plant (*Erythroxylon coca*) or prepared synthetically, sometimes used as a local anaesthetic in eye, ear, nose, and throat surgery. Since it may lead to psychological dependence, cocaine has largely been replaced by safer anaesthetics.

cocainism (koh-**kayn**-izm) *n.* **1.** the habitual use of, or addiction to, cocaine in order to experience its intoxicating effects. **2.** the mental and physical deterioration resulting from addiction to cocaine.

coccus (**kok**-ŭs) *n.* (*pl.* **cocci**) any spherical bacterium. *See also* gonococcus, meningococcus, Micrococcus, pneumococcus, Staphylococcus, Streptococcus.

coccy- (coccyg-, coccygo-) *prefix denoting* the coccyx.

coccydynia (kok-si-**din**-iă) *n.* pain in the coccyx and the neighbouring area.

coccyx (**kok**-siks) *n.* (*pl.* **coccyges** or **coccyxes**) the lowermost element of the backbone: the vestigial human tail. It consists of four rudimentary *coccygeal vertebrae* fused to form a triangular bone that articulates with the sa-crum. *See also* vertebra. —**coccygeal** (kok-**sij**-iăl) *adj.*

cochlea (**kok**-liă) *n.* the spiral organ of the labyrinth of the ear, which is concerned with the reception and analysis of sound. —**cochlear** (kok-li-er) *adj.*

cochlear duct (**scala media**) *n. see* scala.

cochlear nerve *n.* the nerve connecting the cochlea to the brain and therefore responsible for the nerve impulses relating to hearing. It forms part of the vestibulocochlear nerve.

codeine (koh-**deen**) *n.* an analgesic derived from morphine but less potent as a pain killer and sedative and less toxic. It is administered by mouth or injection to relieve pain and also to suppress coughs.

cod liver oil (kod) *n.* a pale yellow oil, extracted from the livers of cod and related fish, that is rich in vitamins A and D and used in the treatment and prevention of deficiencies of these vitamins (e.g. rickets).

-coele *suffix denoting* **1.** a body cavity. **2.** *see* -cele.

coeli- (coelio-) *prefix denoting* the abdomen or belly.

coeliac (**seel**-i-ak) *adj.* of or relating to the abdominal region. *c. trunk* a branch of the abdominal aorta supplying the stomach, spleen, liver, and gall bladder.

coeliac disease *n.* a condition in which the small intestine fails to digest and absorb food. It is due to sensitivity of the intestinal lining to the protein gliadin, which is contained in gluten in the germ of wheat and rye and causes atrophy of the digestive and absorptive cells of the intestine. Symptoms include stunted growth, distended abdomen, and pale frothy foul-smelling stools. Medical name: **gluten enteropathy**.

coelioscopy (see-li-**os**-kŏpi) *n.* the technique of introducing an endoscope through an incision in the abdominal wall to examine the intestines and other organs within the abdominal cavity.

coenzyme (koh-**en**-zym) *n.* a nonprotein organic compound that, in the presence of an enzyme, plays an essential role in the reaction that is catalysed by the enzyme.

coffee-ground vomit (kof-ee-grownd) *n.* vomit containing gastric juices and small dark fragments of partly digested blood, indicating slow bleeding in the upper gastrointestinal tract.

cognition (kog-**nish**-ŏn) *n.* a group of mental activities (including perception, recognition, and judgment) that leads to awareness of an object or situation. *Compare* conation.

coitus (**sexual intercourse, copulation**) (koh-it-ŭs) *n.* sexual contact between a man and a woman during which the erect penis enters the vagina and is moved within it by pelvic thrusts until ejaculation occurs. *c. interruptus* an unreliable contraceptive method in which the penis is removed from the vagina before ejaculation of semen. *See also* orgasm. —**coital** *adj.*

col- (coli-, colo-) *prefix denoting* the colon.

colchicine (kol-chi-seen) *n.* a drug obtained from the meadow saffron (*Colchicum autumnale*), administered by mouth to relieve pain in attacks of gout.

cold (common cold) (kohld) *n.* a widespread infectious virus disease causing inflammation of the mucous membranes of the nose, throat, and bronchial tubes. Symptoms include a sore throat, stuffy or runny nose, headache, cough, and general malaise.

cold sore *n. see* herpes (simplex).

colectomy (kŏ-**lek**-tŏmi) *n.* surgical removal of the colon (*total c.*) or a segment of the colon (*partial c.*). *See also* hemicolectomy, proctocolectomy.

colic (**kol**-ik) *n.* severe abdominal pain, usually of fluctuating severity, with waves of pain seconds or a few minutes apart. *infantile c.* colic that is common among babies, due to wind in the intestine associated with feeding difficulties. *intestinal c.* colic due to partial or complete obstruction of the intestine or to constipation. Medical names: **enteralgia**, **tormina**. *See also* biliary (colic).

coliform bacteria (kol-i-form) *pl. n.* a group of Gram-negative rodlike bacteria that are normally found in the gastrointestinal tract and have the ability to ferment the sugar lactose. It includes the genera *Enterobacter*, *Escherichia*, and *Klebsiella*.

colistin (kŏ-**list**-in) *n.* an antibiotic administered by mouth to treat gastroenteritis and other bacterial infections. Trade name: **Colomycin**.

colitis (kŏ-**ly**-tis) *n.* inflammation of the colon. The usual symptoms are diarrhoea, sometimes with blood and mucus, and lower abdominal pain. *mucous c. see* irritable bowel syndrome. *ulcerative c.* (*idiopathic proctocolitis*) colitis of varying severity in which the rectum (*see* proctitis) as well as a varying amount of the colon become inflamed and ulcerated; its cause is unknown.

collagen (kol-ă-jin) *n.* a protein that is the principal constituent of white fibrous connective tissue (as occurs in tendons). Collagen is also found in skin, bone, cartilage, and ligaments.

collagen disease (connective-tissue disease) *n.* any one of a group of diseases that are characterized by degenerative changes in collagen. They include dermatomyositis, lupus erythematosus, and polyarteritis nodosa.

collar bone (kol-er) *n. see* clavicle.

collateral (kŏ-lat-er-ăl) **1.** *adj.* accessory or secondary. **2.** *n.* a branch (e.g. of a nerve fibre) that is at right angles to the main part.

collateral circulation *n.* **1.** an alternative route provided for the blood by secondary vessels when a primary vessel becomes blocked. **2.** the channels of communication between the blood vessels supplying the heart.

Colles' fracture (kol-iss) *n. see* fracture. [A. Colles (1773–1843), Irish surgeon]

collodion (kŏ-loh-diŏn) *n.* a syrupy solution of nitrocellulose in a mixture of alcohol and ether. When applied to minor wounds it evaporates to leave a thin clear transparent skin. Flexible collodion also contains camphor and castor oil, which allow the skin to stretch a little more.

colloid (kol-oid) *n.* a mixture in which particles of one component (diameter 10^{-6}–10^{-4} mm) are dispersed in a continuous phase of another component. —**colloidal** *adj.*

collyrium (ko-leer-iŭm) *n.* a medicated solution used to bathe the eyes.

coloboma (kolŏ-boh-mă) *n.* (*pl.* **colobomata**) a defect in the de-

splenic flexure
descending colon
transverse colon
ileum
hepatic flexure
haustra
sigmoid colon
rectum
appendix
ascending colon
caecum

The colon

velopment of the eye causing abnormalities ranging in severity from a notch in the lower part of the iris, making it pear-shaped, to defects in the lower part of the retina and choroid.

colon (koh-lŏn) *n.* the main part of the large intestine, which consists of four sections – the *ascending, transverse, descending,* and *sigmoid colons* (see illustration). The colon absorbs large amounts of water and electrolytes from the undigested food passed on from the small intestine. At intervals strong peristaltic movements move the dehydrated contents (faeces) towards the rectum. —**colonic** (koh-lon-ik) *adj.*

colonic irrigation *n.* washing out the contents of the large bowel by means of copious enemas, using either water, with or without soap, or other medication.

colonoscopy (koh-lŏn-**os**-kŏpi) *n*. a procedure for examining the interior of the entire colon and rectum using a flexible illuminated fibreoptic instrument (*colonoscope*) introduced through the anus.

colony (**kol**-ŏni) *n*. a discrete population or mass of microorganisms, usually bacteria, all of which are considered to have developed from a single parent cell. *See also* culture.

colorimeter (kul-ŏ-**rim**-it-er) *n*. an instrument for determining the concentration of a particular compound in a preparation by comparing the intensity of colour in it with that in a standard preparation of known concentration.

colostomy (kŏ-**lost**-ŏmi) *n*. a surgical operation in which a part of the colon is brought through the abdominal wall and opened in order to drain or decompress the intestine. The colostomy may be temporary, eventually being closed to restore continuity; or permanent, usually when the rectum or lower colon has been removed.

colostrum (kŏ-**los**-trŭm) *n*. the first secretion from the breast, occurring shortly after, or sometimes before, birth. It contains serum, white blood cells, and protective antibodies.

colour blindness (**kul**-er) *n*. any of various conditions in which certain colours are confused with one another. True lack of colour appreciation is extremely rare (*see* monochromat); the most common type of colour blindness is red-blindness (*see* Daltonism). *See also* deuteranopia, tritanopia.

colp- (colpo-) *prefix denoting* the vagina.

colpitis (kol-**py**-tis) *n*. inflammation of the vagina. *See* vaginitis.

colpocele (vaginocele) (**kol**-poh-seel) *n*. **1.** a hernia protruding into the vagina. **2.** *see* colpoptosis.

colpohysterectomy (kol-poh-hiss-ter-ek-**tŏmi**) *n*. surgical removal of the womb through the vagina. *See* hysterectomy.

colpoperineorrhaphy (colpoperineoplasty) (kol-poh-pe-ri-ni-o-**răfi**) *n*. a tissue grafting operation for repairing tears in the vagina and the perineum.

colpopexy (**kol**-poh-peks-i) *n*. the stitching of a displaced vagina to the abdominal wall.

colpoptosis (colpocele) (kol-poh-**toh**-sis) *n*. the dropping of the vagina from its normal position, which may happen under the action of gravity if the supporting tissues are weak.

colporrhaphy (kol-**po**-răfi) *n*. stitching of the vagina in order to reduce its laxity in cases of prolapse of the bladder (*anterior c.*) or rectum (*posterior c.*).

colposcope (vaginoscope) (**kol**-poh-skohp) *n*. an instrument that is inserted into the vagina and permits visual examination of the neck of the womb and the upper part of the vagina in which it lies. —**colposcopy** (kol-**pos**-kŏpi) *n*.

colpotomy (kol-**pot**-ŏmi) *n*. an incision made into the wall of the vagina.

column (**kol**-ŭm) *n*. (in anatomy) any pillar-shaped structure, especially any of the tracts of grey matter found in the spinal cord.

coma (**koh**-mă) *n*. a state of unrousable unconsciousness. Its severity is sometimes graded according to the presence or absence of withdrawal responses to painful stimuli and pupillary and corneal reflexes.

comatose (koh-mă-tohs) *adj.* in a state of coma; unconscious.

comedo (kom-i-doh) *n.* (*pl.* **comedones**) *see* blackhead.

commensal (kŏ-men-săl) *n.* an organism that lives in close association with another of a different species without either harming or benefiting it. *Compare* symbiosis. —**commensalism** *n.*

comminuted fracture (kom-i-newtid) *n. see* fracture.

commissure (kom-iss-yoor) *n.* **1.** a bundle of nerve fibres that crosses the midline of the central nervous system, often connecting similar structures on each side. **2.** any other tissue connecting two similar structures.

communicable disease (contagious disease, infectious disease) (kŏ-mew-nik-ăbŭl) *n.* any disease that can be transmitted from one person to another. This may occur by direct physical contact, by common handling of a contaminated object (*see* fomes), through a disease carrier, or by spread of infected droplets exhaled into the air.

Community Health Council (CHC) (kŏ-mew-niti) *n.* (in Britain) a group of local residents appointed to voice the views of patients in relation to the National Health Service.

community medicine *n.* the branch of medicine concerned with assessing needs and trends in health and disease of populations as distinct from individuals. It includes epidemiology, public health, preventive medicine, health care planning, and evaluation of services.

community nurses *pl. n.* (in Britain) a generic term for health visitors, domiciliary midwives, and home nurses. *See also* domiciliary services.

community physician *n.* (in Britain) a doctor of consultant status with special postgraduate training in community medicine.

compatibility (kŏm-pati-bil-iti) *n.* the degree to which the body's defence systems will tolerate the presence of intruding foreign material, such as blood when transfused or a kidney when transplanted. *Compare* incompatibility. *See also* histocompatibility, immunity. —**compatible** *adj.*

compensation (kom-pen-say-shŏn) *n.* **1.** the act of making up for a functional or structural deficiency. For example, compensation for the loss of a diseased kidney is brought about by an increase in size of the remaining kidney, so restoring the urine-producing capacity. **2.** (in psychoanalysis) the act of exaggerating an approved character trait to make up for a weakness in an opposite trait.

complement (kom-pli-měnt) *n.* a substance in the blood, consisting of a group of nine different fractions, that aids the body's defences when antibodies combine with invading antigens. *See also* immunity.

complement fixation *n.* the binding of complement to the complex that is formed when an antibody reacts with a specific antigen. Because complement is taken up from the serum only when such a reaction has occurred, testing for the presence of complement after mixing a suspension of a known organism with a patient's serum can give confirmation of infection with a suspected organism.

complex (**kom**-pleks) *n.* (in psychoanalysis) an emotionally charged and repressed group of ideas and beliefs that is capable of influencing an individual's behaviour.

complication (kom-pli-**kay**-shŏn) *n.* a disease or condition arising during the course of or as a consequence of another disease.

compos mentis (kom-pŏs **men**-tis) *adj.* of sound mind; sane.

compress (**kom**-press) *n.* a pad of material soaked in hot or cold water and applied to an injured part of the body to relieve the pain of inflammation.

compressed air illness (caisson disease) (kŏm-**prest**) *n.* a syndrome occurring in people working under high pressure in diving bells or at great depths with breathing apparatus. On return to normal atmospheric pressure nitrogen dissolved in the bloodstream expands to form bubbles, causing pain (the *bends*) and blocking the circulation in small blood vessels in the brain and elsewhere (*decompression sickness*). Symptoms may be eliminated by returning the victim to a higher atmospheric pressure and reducing this gradually.

compression (kŏm-**presh**-ŏn) *n.* the state in which an organ, tissue, or part is subject to pressure. *cerebral c.* pressure on brain tissue from a cerebral tumour, intracranial haematoma, etc.

compulsion (kŏm-**pul**-shŏn) *n.* an obsession that takes the form of a motor act, such as repetitive washing based on a fear of contamination.

compulsory admission (kŏm-**pul**-ser-i) *n.* (in Britain) the entry and detention of a person within an institution (hospital or Part III Accommodation) without his consent, either because of mental illness (*see* Mental Health Act) or severe social deprivation. *Compare* voluntary admission.

conation (koh-**nay**-shŏn) *n.* the group of mental activities (including drives, will, and instincts) that leads to purposeful action. *Compare* cognition.

conception (kŏn-**sep**-shŏn) *n.* **1.** (in gynaecology) the start of pregnancy, when a male germ cell (sperm) fertilizes a female germ cell (ovum) in the Fallopian tube. **2.** (in psychology) an idea or mental impression.

conceptus (kŏn-**sep**-tŭs) *n.* the products of conception: the developing infant and its enclosing membrane at all stages in the womb.

concha (konk-ă) *n.* (*pl.* **conchae**) (in anatomy) any part resembling a shell. *c. auriculae* a depression on the outer surface of the pinna (auricle), which leads to the external auditory meatus of the outer ear. *See also* nasal (concha).

concordance (kŏn-**kor**-dănss) *n.* similarity of any physical characteristic that is found in both of a pair of twins.

concretion (kŏn-**kree**-shŏn) *n.* a stony mass formed within such an organ as the kidney, especially the coating of an internal organ or a foreign body with calcium salts. *See also* calculus.

concussion (kŏn-**kush**-ŏn) *n.* a limited period of unconsciousness caused by injury to the head. It may last for a few seconds or a few hours. *See also* punchdrunk syndrome.

condenser (kŏn-**den**-ser) *n.* (in microscopy) an arrangement of lenses beneath the stage of a microscope. It can be adjusted to provide correct focusing of light on the microscope slide.

conditioned reflex (kŏn-**dish**-ŏnd) *n.* a reflex in which the response occurs not to the sensory stimulus that normally causes it but to a separate stimulus, which has been learnt to be associated with it.

conditioning (kŏn-**dish**-ŏn-ing) *n.* the establishment of new behaviour by modifying the stimulus/response associations.

condom (**French letter, rubber**) (kon-**dŏm**) *n.* a sheath made of latex rubber, plastic, or silk that is fitted over the penis during sexual intercourse. A condom is a reasonably reliable contraceptive; it also protects both partners against the transmission of venereal diseases.

conduction (kŏn-**duk**-shŏn) *n.* **1.** (in physics) the process in which heat is transferred through a substance from regions of higher to regions of lower temperature. **2.** (in physiology) the passage of a nerve impulse.

conductor (kŏn-**duk**-ter) *n.* **1.** (in physics) a substance capable of transmitting heat (e.g. copper, silver) or electricity. **2.** (in surgery) a grooved surgical director.

condyle (kon-dil) *n.* a rounded protuberance that occurs at the ends of some bones, e.g. the occipital bone, and forms an articulation with another bone.

condyloma (kon-di-**loh**-mă) *n.* a raised wartlike growth. *c. acuminatum* the commonest type of condyloma, found on the vulva, under the foreskin, or on the skin of the anal region. Condylomas are infectious and are probably transmitted during sexual contact. *c. latum* an infectious warty lesion of the secondary stage of syphilis, occurring around the vulva or anus.

cone (kohn) *n.* one of the two types of light-sensitive cells in the retina of the eye (*compare* rod). Cones are essential for acute vision and can also distinguish colours.

confabulation (kŏn-fab-yoo-lay-shŏn) *n.* the invention of circumstantial but fictitious detail about events supposed to have occurred in the past. Usually this is to disguise a loss of memory; it typically occurs in Korsakoff's syndrome.

confection (kŏn-**fek**-shŏn) *n.* (in pharmacy) a sweet substance that is combined with a medicinal preparation to make it suitable for administration.

conflict (kon-flikt) *n.* (in psychology) the state produced when a stimulus produces two opposing reactions. Conflict has been used to explain the development of neurotic disorders, and the resolution of conflict remains an important part of psychoanalysis. *See also* conversion.

congenital (kŏn-**jen**-it'l) *adj.* describing a condition that is recognized at birth or that is believed to have been present since birth. Congenital malformations include all disorders present at birth whether they are inherited or caused by an environmental factor.

congenital dislocation of the hip *n.* an abnormality of the hip joint, present at birth, in which the head of the femur fails to articulate with the acetabulum because the latter is too shallow.

congenital heart disease *n. see* blue baby.

congestion (kŏn-**jes**-chŏn) *n.* an accumulation of blood within an organ, which is the result of back pressure within its veins (for example congestion of the lungs and liver occurs in heart failure).

Congo red (kon-goh) *n.* a dark-red or reddish-brown pigment that becomes blue in acidic conditions. It is used as a histological stain.

conization (ko-ny-**zay**-shŏn) *n.* surgical removal of a cone of tissue. The technique is commonly used in excising a portion of the cervix (neck) of the womb.

conjugate (conjugate diameter, true conjugate) (kon-**jŭg**-it) *n.* the distance between the front and rear of the pelvis measured from the most prominent part of the sacrum to the back of the pubic symphysis. It is estimated by subtracting 1.3–1.9 cm from the distance between the lower edge of the symphysis and the sacrum (the *diagonal c.*). If the true conjugate is less than about 10.2 cm, delivery of an infant through the natural passages may be difficult or impossible.

conjunctiva (kon-junk-**ty**-vă) *n.* the delicate mucous membrane that covers the front of the eye and lines the inside of the eyelids. —**conjunctival** *adj.*

conjunctivitis (pink eye) (kŏn-junk-ti-**vy**-tis) *n.* inflammation of the conjunctiva, which becomes red and swollen and produces a watery or pus-containing discharge. Conjunctivitis is caused by infection, allergy, or physical or chemical irritation. *See also* trachoma, ophthalmia (neonatorum).

connective tissue (kŏ-**nek**-tiv) *n.* the tissue that supports, binds, or separates more specialized tissues and organs or functions as a packing tissue of the body. It consists of an amorphous matrix of mucopolysaccharides (*ground substance*) in which may be embedded white (collagenous), yellow (elastic), and reticular fibres, fat cells, fibroblasts, mast cells, and macrophages. Forms of connective tissue include bone, cartilage, tendons, ligaments, and adipose, areolar, and elastic tissues.

connective-tissue disease *n. see* collagen disease.

Conn's syndrome (konz) *n.* a condition resulting from overproduction of the hormone aldosterone due to disease of the adrenal cortex. *See* aldosteronism. [W. J. Conn (1907–), US physician]

consanguinity (kon-sang-**win**-iti) *n.* relationship by blood; the sharing of a common ancestor within a few generations.

consensus management (kŏn-sen-sŭs) *n.* a style of management practised in the National Health Service, in which multidisciplinary management teams make decisions based on discussion and mutual agreement.

conservative treatment (kŏn-**ser**-vă-tiv) *n.* treatment aimed at preventing a condition from becoming worse, in the expectation that either natural healing will occur or progress of the disease will be so slow that no drastic treatment will be justified. *Compare* radical treatment.

consolidation (kŏn-soli-**day**-shŏn) *n.* **1.** the state of the lung in which the alveoli (air sacs) are filled with fluid produced by inflamed tissue, as in pneumonia. **2.** the stage of repair of a broken bone following callus formation, during which the callus is transformed by osteoblasts into mature bone.

constipation (kon-sti-**pay**-shŏn) *n.* a condition in which bowel evacuations occur infrequently, or in which the faeces are hard and small, or where passage of faeces causes difficulty or pain. Recurrent or longstanding constipation is treated by increasing dietary fibre (roughage), laxatives, or enemas.

constrictor (kŏn-**strik**-ter) *n.* any muscle that compresses an organ or causes a hollow organ or part to contract.

consultant (kŏn-**sul**-t'nt) *n.* a fully trained specialist in a branch of medicine who accepts total responsibility for patient care.

consumption (kŏn-**sump**-shŏn) *n.* any disease causing wasting of tissues, especially (formerly) pulmonary tuberculosis. —**consumptive** *adj.*

contact (**kon**-takt) *n.* transmission of an infectious disease by touching or handling an infected person or animal (*direct c.*) or by inhaling airborne droplets, etc., containing the infective microorganism (*indirect c.*).

contact lenses *pl. n.* glass or plastic lenses worn directly against the eye, separated from it only by a film of tear fluid. Contact lenses are used mainly in place of glasses to correct errors of refraction, but they may be used for protection in some types of corneal disease.

contagious disease (kŏn-**tay**-jŭs) *n.* originally, a disease transmitted only by direct physical contact: now usually taken to mean any communicable disease.

contra- *prefix denoting* against or opposite.

contraception (kon-tră-**sep**-shŏn) *n.* the prevention of unwanted pregnancy. *See* coitus (interruptus), condom, diaphragm, IUD, oral contraceptive, rhythm method, sterilization.

contraction (kŏn-**trak**-shŏn) *n.* the shortening of a muscle in response to a motor nerve impulse. This generates tension in the muscle, usually causing movement.

contracture (kŏn-**trak**-cher) *n.* fibrosis of muscle tissue producing shrinkage and shortening of the muscle without generating any strength. *See also* Dupuytren's contracture, Volkmann's contracture.

contraindication (kon-tră-in-di-**kay**-shŏn) *n.* any factor in a patient's condition that makes it unwise to pursue a certain line of treatment.

contralateral (kon-tră-**lat**-er-ăl) *adj.* on or affecting the opposite side of the body.

contrast medium (**kon**-trahst) *n.* any substance, such as barium sulphate, that is used to improve visibility of structures during radiography. *See also* radio-opaque.

contrecoup (kon-tră-**koo**) *n.* injury of a part resulting from a blow on its opposite side. This may happen, for example, if a blow on the back of the head causes the front of the brain to be pushed against the inner surface of the skull.

contusion (kŏn-**tew**-*zh*ŏn) *n. see* bruise.

convection (kŏn-**vek**-shŏn) *n.* the transfer of heat through a liquid or gas by movement of the heated portions of the liquid or gas.

conversion (kŏn-**ver**-shŏn) *n.* (in psychiatry) the expression of conflict as physical symptoms.

convolution (kon-vŏ-**loo**-shŏn) *n.* a folding or twisting, such as one of the many that cause the fissures, sulci, and gyri of the surface of the cerebrum.

convulsion (kŏn-**vul**-shŏn) *n.* an involuntary contraction of the muscles producing contortion of the body and limbs. Rhythmic convulsions of the limbs are part of grand mal epilepsy.

Cooley's anaemia (**koo**-liz) *n. see* thalassaemia. [T. B. Cooley (1871–1945), US paediatrician]

Coomb's test (koomz) *n.* a means of detecting antibodies on the surface of red blood cells that can precipitate simple proteins (globulins) in the blood serum. The test is used in the diagnosis of haemolytic anaemia. [R. R. A. Coombs (1921–), British immunologist]

copper sulphate (**kop**-er) *n.* a salt of copper that, in solution, has been used as a fungicide and is a constituent of Fehling's and Benedict's solutions, used to test for the presence of glucose in the urine. Formula: $CuSO_4$.

copr- (copro-) *prefix denoting* faeces.

coprolalia (kop-rŏ-**lay**-liă) *n.* the repetitive speaking of obscene words. It can be involuntary, as part of the Gilles de la Tourette syndrome.

coprolith (**kop**-rŏ-lith) *n.* a mass of hard faeces within the colon or rectum, due to chronic constipation. It may become calcified.

coproporphyrin (kop-rŏ-**por**-fi-rin) *n.* a porphyrin compound that is formed during the synthesis of protoporphyrin IX. Coproporphyrin is excreted in the faeces during the process of red blood cell formation.

copulation (kop-yoo-**lay**-shŏn) *n. see* coitus.

cor (kor) *n.* the heart. *c. pulmonale* enlargement of the right ventricle of the heart resulting from disease of the lungs or pulmonary arteries.

coracoid process (ko-ră-koid) *n.* a beaklike process that curves upwards and forwards from the top of the scápula, over the shoulder-joint.

cord (kord) *n.* any long flexible structure, which may be solid or tubular. Examples include the spermatic cord, spinal cord, umbilical cord, and vocal cord.

cordectomy (kor-**dek**-tŏmi) *n.* surgical removal of a vocal cord.

cordotomy (chordotomy) (kor-**dot**-ŏmi) *n.* a surgical procedure for the relief of severe and persistent pain in the pelvis or lower limbs, in which the tracts of the spinal cord transmitting the sensation of pain to consciousness are severed in the cervical (neck) region.

corium (**kor**-iŭm) *n. see* dermis.

corn (korn) *n.* an area of hard thickened skin on or between the toes: a type of callosity produced by ill-fitting shoes. Medical name: **clavus**.

cornea (**korn**-iă) *n.* the transparent circular part of the front of the eyeball. It refracts the light entering the eye onto the lens, which then focuses it onto the retina. —**corneal** (**korn**-iăl) *adj.*

corneal graft *n. see* keratoplasty.

cornification (kor-ni-fi-**kay**-shŏn) *n. see* keratinization.

cornu (**kor**-new) *n.* (*pl.* **cornua**) (in anatomy) a horn-shaped structure. *See also* horn.

corona (kŏ-**roh**-nă) *n.* a crown or crownlike structure. *c. capitis* the crown of the head.

coronal (ko-**rŏ**-năl) *adj.* relating to the crown of the head or of a tooth. *c. plane* the plane that divides the body into dorsal and ventral parts. *c. suture* the immovable joint between the frontal and parietal bones (*see* skull).

coronary arteries (ko-rŏn-er-i) *pl. n.* the arteries supplying blood to the heart. They arise from the aorta, just above the aortic valve, and form branches that encircle the heart.

coronary thrombosis *n.* the formation of a blood clot (thrombus) in the coronary artery, which obstructs the flow of blood to the heart. *See* myocardial infarction.

coroner (ko-rŏn-er) *n.* the official who presides at an inquest. He must be either a medical practitioner or a lawyer of at least five years standing.

coronoid process (ko-rŏn-oid) *n.* **1.** a process on the upper end of the ulna. It forms part of the notch that articulates with the humerus. **2.** the process on the ramus of the mandible to which the temporalis muscle is attached.

corpus (kor-pŭs) *n.* (*pl.* **corpora**) any mass of tissue that can be distinguished from its surroundings. *c. callosum* the broad band of nervous tissue that connects the two cerebral hemispheres. *c. cavernosum* either of a pair of cylindrical blood sinuses that form the erectile tissue of the penis and clitoris. *c. luteum* the glandular tissue in the ovary that forms at the site of a ruptured Graafian follicle after ovulation. It secretes the hormone progesterone, which prepares the womb

for implantation. If implantation fails the corpus luteum degenerates. If an embryo becomes implanted the corpus luteum continues to secrete progesterone until the fourth month of pregnancy. *c. spongiosum* the blood sinus that surrounds the urethra of the male. Together with the corpora cavernosa, it forms the erectile tissue of the penis. *c. striatum* the part of the basal ganglia in the cerebral hemispheres of the brain consisting of the caudate nucleus and the lentiform nucleus.

corpuscle (kor-pŭs-ŭl) *n.* any small particle, cell, or mass of tissue.

corrective (kŏ-rek-tiv) *n.* any drug or agent that modifies the action of another substance.

Corrigan's pulse (water-hammer pulse) (ko-ri-gănz) *n.* a pulse characterized by an initial surge followed by a sudden collapse, usually due to aortic regurgitation. [Sir D. J. Corrigan (1802–80), Irish physician]

cortex (kor-teks) *n.* (*pl.* **cortices**) the outer part of an organ, situated immediately beneath its capsule or outer membrane. —**cortical** (kor-ti-kăl) *adj.*

corticosteroid (corticoid) (kor-ti-koh-steer-oid) *n.* any steroid hormone synthesized by the adrenal cortex. *See* glucocorticoid, mineralocorticoid.

corticotrophin (kor-ti-koh-**troh**-fin) *n. see* ACTH.

cortisol (kor-ti-sol) *n. see* hydrocortisone.

cortisone (kor-tiz-ohn) *n.* a naturally occurring corticosteroid that is used mainly to treat deficiency of corticosteroid hormones in Addison's disease and following surgical removal of the adrenal glands. It is administered by mouth or injection and may cause serious side-effects such as stomach ulcers, muscle and bone damage, and eye changes.

Corynebacterium (kŏ-ry-ni-bak-teer-iŭm) *n.* a genus of Gram-positive, mostly aerobic, non-motile rodlike bacteria. *C. diphtheriae* (*Klebs-Loeffler bacillus*) the causative organism of diphtheria. It occurs in one of three forms: *gravis*, *intermedius*, and *mitis*.

coryza (cold in the head) (kŏ-ry-ză) *n.* a catarrhal inflammation of the mucous membrane in the nose due to either a cold or hay fever. *See also* catarrh.

cost- (costo-) *prefix denoting* the rib(s).

costal (kos-t'l) *adj.* of or relating to the ribs. *c. cartilage* a cartilage that connects a rib to the breastbone (sternum).

costive (kost-iv) *adj.* constipated.

cot death (kot) *n.* the death of a baby, usually occurring overnight while it is in its cot, from an unidentifiable cause.

co-trimoxazole (koh-tri-**moks**-ă-zohl) *n.* an antibacterial drug consisting of sulphamethoxazole and trimethoprim. Co-trimoxazole is taken by mouth and is particularly useful for treating urinary-tract infections (such as cystitis). Trade names: **Bactrim**, **Septrin**.

cotyledon (kot-i-**lee**-dŏn) *n.* any of the major convex subdivisions of the mature placenta. Each cotyledon contains a major branch of the umbilical blood vessels.

cotyloid cavity (kot-i-loid) *n. see* acetabulum.

coughing (kof-ing) *n.* a form of violent exhalation by which irritant particles in the airways can be expelled. Medical name: **tussis**.

coulomb (koo-lom) *n.* the SI unit of electric charge, equal to the quantity of electricity transferred by 1 ampere in 1 second. Symbol: C.

counselling (kown-sĕl-ing) *n.* a method of approaching psychological difficulties in adjustment that aims to help the client work out his own problems.

counterextension (kownt-er-eks-ten-shŏn) *n.* an orthopaedic procedure consisting of traction on one part of a limb, while the remainder of the limb is held steady: used particularly in the treatment of a fractured femur.

counterirritant (kownt-er-i-ri-t'nt) *n.* an agent, such as methyl salicylate, that causes irritation when applied to the skin and is used in order to relieve more deep-seated pain or discomfort. —**counterirritation** *n.*

countertraction (kownt-er-trak-shŏn) *n.* the use of a balancing opposing force during traction. To arrange that traction on a limb does not pull the patient out of bed, countertraction is often produced by applying tension to metal pins temporarily inserted into the opposite end of the bone.

Cowper's glands (bulbourethral glands) (kow-perz) *pl. n.* a pair of small glands that open into the urethra at the base of the penis. Their secretion contributes to the seminal fluid. [W. Cowper (1666–1709), English surgeon]

cowpox (kow-poks) *n.* a virus infection of cows' udders, transmitted to man by direct contact, causing very mild symptoms similar to smallpox. An attack confers immunity to smallpox. Medical name: **vaccinia**.

cox- **(coxo-)** *prefix denoting* the hip.

coxa (koks-ă) *n.* (*pl.* **coxae**) 1. the hip bone. 2. the hip joint. *c. valga* a deformity of the hip joint in which the angle between the neck and shaft of the femur is abnormally increased. *c. vara* a deformity of the hip joint in which the angle between the neck and shaft of the femur is abnormally decreased.

coxalgia (koks-al-jiă) *n.* 1. pain in the hip joint. 2. disease of the hip joint.

Coxsackie virus (kok-sak-i) *n.* one of a group of RNA-containing viruses that are able to multiply in the gastrointestinal tract (*see* enterovirus). Type A viruses generally cause less severe diseases, although some cause meningitis and severe throat infections. Type B viruses cause inflammation or degeneration of brain, skeletal muscle, or heart tissue (*see* Bornholm disease).

crab louse (krab) *n. see* Phthirus.

cradle (kray-d'l) *n.* a framework of metal strips or other material that forms a cage over an injured part of the body of a patient lying in bed, to protect it from the pressure of the bedclothes.

cramp (kramp) *n.* prolonged painful contraction of a muscle. It is sometimes caused by an imbalance of the salts in the body, but is more often a result of fatigue, imperfect posture, or stress. *occupational c.* spasm in the muscles making it impossible to perform a specific task but allowing the use of these muscles for any other movement.

crani- **(cranio-)** *prefix denoting* the skull.

cranial nerves (kray-niăl) *pl. n.* the 12 pairs of nerves that arise directly from the brain and leave the skull through separate apertures. *Compare* spinal nerves.

craniometry (kray-ni-om-itri) *n.* the science of measuring the differences in size and shape of skulls.

craniopagus (**dicephalus**) (kray-ni-op-ăgŭs) *n.* Siamese twins united by their heads.

craniopharyngioma (kray-ni-oh-fă-rinj-i-oh-mă) *n.* a brain tumour derived from remnants of *Rathke's pouch*, an embryologic structure from which the pituitary gland is partly formed.

craniostenosis (kray-ni-oh-sti-noh-sis) *n.* premature closing of the sutures between the cranial bones during development, resulting in deformities of the skull.

craniotabes (kray-ni-oh-tay-beez) *n.* abnormal thinness and brittleness of the bones of the vault of the skull, occurring in children with rickets.

craniotomy (kray-ni-ot-ŏmi) *n.* 1. surgical removal of a portion of the skull, performed to expose the brain and meninges for inspection or biopsy or to relieve excessive intracranial pressure (as in a subdural haematoma). 2. surgical perforation of the skull of a dead fetus during difficult labour, so that delivery may continue.

cranium (kray-niŭm) *n.* the part of the skeleton that encloses the brain. It consists of eight bones connected together by immovable joints (*see* skull). —**cranial** *adj.*

creatine (kree-ă-teen) *n.* a product of protein metabolism found in muscle. *c. phosphate* (*phosphocrea-*

tine, phosphagen) the phosphate of creatine, which acts as a store of high-energy phosphate in muscle and serves to maintain adequate amounts of ATP.

creatinine (kree-**at**-i-neen) *n.* a substance derived from creatine and creatine phosphate in muscle. Creatinine is excreted in the urine.

creatinuria (kree-at-in-**yoor**-iă) *n.* an excess of the nitrogenous compound creatine in the urine.

creatorrhoea (kree-at-ŏ-**ree**-ă) *n.* the passage of excessive nitrogen in the faeces due to failure of digestion or absorption in the small intestine. It is found particularly in pancreatic failure. *See* cystic fibrosis, pancreatitis.

Credé's method (kray**dayz**) *n.* 1. a technique for expelling the placenta from the womb. Downward pressure is applied to the womb through the abdominal wall in the direction of the birth canal. 2. the application of 1% silver nitrate solution to the eyes of a newborn baby whose mother has gonorrhoea, to prevent the development of ophthalmia neonatorum. [K. S. F. Credé (1819–92), German gynaecologist]

creeping eruption (larva migrans) (**kreep**-ing) *n.* a skin disease caused either by larvae of nematode worms (e.g. *Ancylostoma braziliense*) or by the maggots of certain flies. The larvae burrow within the skin tissues, their movements marked by long thin red lines that cause the patient intense irritation.

crepitation (rale) (krep-i-**tay**-shŏn) *n.* a soft fine crackling sound heard in the lungs through the stethoscope. Crepitations are not normally heard in healthy lungs.

crepitus (**krep**-itŭs) *n.* 1. a crackling sound or grating feeling produced by bone rubbing on bone or roughened cartilage, detected on movement of an arthritic joint. 2. a similar sound heard with a stethoscope over an inflamed lung when the patient breathes in.

cresol (**kree**-sol) *n.* a strong antiseptic effective against many microorganisms and used mostly in soap solutions as a general disinfectant. Cresol solutions irritate the skin and if taken by mouth are corrosive and cause pain, nausea, and vomiting.

crest (krest) *n.* a ridge or linear protuberance, particularly on a bone.

cretinism (**kret**-in-izm) *n.* a syndrome of dwarfism, mental retardation, and coarseness of the skin and facial features due to congenital hypothyroidism.

cribriform plate (**krib**-ri-form) *n.* *see* ethmoid bone.

cricoid cartilage (**kry**-koid) *n.* the cartilage, shaped like a signet ring, that forms part of the anterior and lateral walls and most of the posterior wall of the larynx.

crisis (**kry**-sis) *n.* (*pl.* crises) 1. the turning point of a disease, after which the patient either improves or deteriorates. Since the advent of antibiotics, infections seldom reach the point of crisis. 2. the occurrence of sudden severe pain in certain diseases. *See also* Dietl's crisis.

crista (**krist**-ă) *n.* (*pl.* cristae) 1. the sensory structure within the ampulla of a semicircular canal within the inner ear. 2. one of the infoldings of the inner membrane of a mitochondrion. **3.** any anatomical structure resembling a crest.

Crohn's disease (krohnz) *n.* a condition in which segments of the alimentary tract become inflamed, thickened, and ulcerated. It usually affects the terminal part of the ileum; its acute form (*acute ileitis*) may mimic appendicitis. Chronic disease often causes partial obstruction of the intestine, leading to pain, diarrhoea, and malabsorption. Alternative names: **regional enteritis**, **regional ileitis**. [B. B. Crohn (1884–), US physician]

cromolyn sodium (kroh-mŏ-lin) *n.* a drug used to prevent and treat asthma and allergic bronchitis. It is administered by inhalation and may cause throat irritation. Trade name: **Intal**.

cross-infection (kros-in-fek-shŏn) *n.* the transfer of infection from one patient to another in hospital.

crotamiton (kroh-tă-my-tŏn) *n.* a drug that destroys mites and is used to treat scabies and similar skin infections and also to relieve itching. It is applied to the skin as a lotion or ointment. Trade name: **Eurax**.

croup (kroop) *n.* inflammation and obstruction of the larynx in young children, generally resulting from a viral infection of the respiratory tract (*see* laryngotracheobronchitis). The symptoms are those of laryngitis, accompanied by harsh difficult breathing (*see* stridor), a rising pulse rate, restlessness, and cyanosis.

crown (krown) *n.* **1.** the part of a tooth above the gum. **2.** a dental restoration that covers most or all of the natural crown. **3.** *see* corona.

crowning (krown-ing) *n.* the stage of labour when only the upper part of the infant's head is visible, tightly encircled by the margins of the vaginal opening.

crude rate (krood) *n.* the total number of events (e.g. cases of lung cancer) expressed as a percentage (or rate per 1000, etc.) of the whole population.

crural (kroor-ăl) *adj.* **1.** relating to the thigh or leg. **2.** relating to the crura cerebri (*see* crus).

crus (kruus) *n.* (*pl.* **crura**) an elongated process or part of a structure. *c. cerebri* one of two symmetrical nerve tracts situated between the medulla oblongata and the cerebral hemispheres.

crush syndrome (krush) *n.* the condition resulting from crushing accidents in which large areas of muscle are damaged, characterized by severe shock resulting from blood and fluid loss and oliguria leading to kidney failure.

cry- (cryo-) prefix denoting cold.

cryaesthesia (kry-iss-theez-iă) *n.* **1.** exceptional sensitivity to low temperature. **2.** a sensation of coldness.

cryoprecipitate (kry-oh-pri-sip-i-tăt) *n.* a precipitate produced by freezing and thawing under controlled conditions, such as the residue obtained from fresh frozen blood plasma that has been thawed at 4°C. This residue is used in the control of bleeding in haemophilia.

cryoprobe (kry-oh-prohb) *n.* an instrument used in cryosurgery, which has a fine tip cooled by allowing carbon dioxide or nitrous oxide gas to expand within it.

cryosurgery (kry-oh-ser-jer-i) *n.* the use of extreme cold in a localized part of the body to freeze and destroy unwanted tissues. Cryosurgery is commonly used for the removal of cataracts and the destruction of certain bone tumours. *See* cryoprobe.

cryotherapy (kry-oh-**th'e**-ră-pi) *n.* the use of cold in the treatment of disorders. *See* cryosurgery, hypothermia (def. 2). *Compare* thermotherapy.

crypt (kript) *n.* a small sac, follicle, or cavity; for example, the crypts of Lieberkühn (*see* Lieberkühn's glands).

crypt- (**crypto-**) *prefix denoting* concealed.

Cryptococcus (krip-toh-kok-ŭs) *n.* a genus of unicellular yeastlike fungi that cause disease in man. They are found in soil and pigeon droppings. *C. neoformans* a species that attacks the lungs and brain.

cryptogenic (krip-toh-jen-ik) *adj.* of obscure or unknown cause.

cryptomenorrhoea (krip-toh-men-ŏ-ree-ă) *n.* absence of blood flow when the internal symptoms of menstruation are present. The condition may arise because the hymen lacks an opening or because of some other obstruction.

cryptorchidism (**cryptorchism**) (krip-or-kid-izm) *n.* the condition in which the testes fail to descend into the scrotum and are retained within the abdomen or inguinal canal. —**cryptorchid** *adj.*, *n.*

crystal violet (**gentian violet**) (**kris**-t'l vy-ŏ-lit) *n.* an antiseptic dye used to treat some skin infections due to bacteria and fungi and also some worm infestations. Crystal violet is administered by mouth, as pessaries, or as ointments, paints, and solutions. The dye is also used to stain tissues and microorganisms for microscopical study.

CSF *n. see* cerebrospinal fluid.

CT scanner *n.* computerized tomography scanner: an X-ray scanner incorporating a computer, used to provide an integrated three-dimensional image of the soft structures of the body, particularly the brain. It can reveal the presence of tumours, fluid, etc.

cubital (**kew**-bit'l) *adj.* relating to the elbow or forearm. *c. fossa* the depression at the front of the elbow.

cuboid bone (**kew**-boid) *n.* the outer bone of the tarsus, which articulates with the fourth and fifth metatarsal bones in front and with the calcaneus (heel bone) behind.

cuirass (kwi-**ras**) *n. see* respirator.

culdoscope (kul-doh-skohp) *n.* a tubular instrument with lenses and a light source, used for direct observation of the womb, ovaries, and Fallopian tubes (*culdoscopy*). The instrument is passed through the wall of the vagina behind to the neck of the womb. *See also* endoscope.

culture (**kul**-cher) **1.** *n.* a population of microorganisms, usually bacteria, grown in a solid or liquid laboratory medium (*c. medium*), which is usually agar, broth, or gelatin. *stock c.* a permanent bacterial culture, from which subcultures are made. *See also* tissue culture. **2.** *vb.* to grow bacteria or other microorganisms in cultures.

cumulative action (kew-mew-lă-tiv) *n.* the toxic effects of a drug produced by repeated administration of small doses at intervals that are not long enough for it to be either broken down or excreted by the body.

cuneiform bones (kew-ni-form) *pl. n.* three bones in the tarsus that articulate with the first, second, and third metatarsal bones in front. All three bones articulate with the navicular bone behind.

cupola (kew-pŏ-lă) *n.* **1.** the small dome at the end of the cochlea. **2.** any of several dome-shaped anatomical structures.

curare (kew-rar-i) *n.* an extract from the bark of South American trees (*Strychnos* and *Chondodendron* species) that relaxes and paralyses voluntary muscle. Curare was formerly employed to control the muscle spasms of tetanus and, more recently, as a muscle relaxant in surgical operations. It has now been replaced in surgery by tubocurarine.

curettage (curettement) (kewr-i-tij) *n.* the scraping of the internal surface of an organ or body cavity by means of a spoon-shaped instrument (*curette*). Curettage is usually performed to remove diseased tissue or to obtain a specimen for diagnostic purposes. *See also* dilatation and curettage.

curette (kewr-et) *n.* *see* curettage.

curie (kewr-ee) *n.* a unit for expressing the activity of a radioactive substance, equal to 3.7×10^{10} disintegrations per second. Symbol: Ci.

Cushing's syndrome (kuush-ingz) *n.* the condition resulting from excess amounts of corticosteroid hormones in the body. Symptoms include weight gain, reddening of the face and neck, excess growth of body and facial hair, raised blood pressure, loss of mineral from the bones (osteoporosis), raised blood glucose levels, and sometimes mental disturbances. The syndrome may be due to overstimulation of the adrenal glands by excessive amounts of the hormone ACTH, secreted either by a tumour of the pituitary gland (*Cushing's disease*) or by a malignant tumour in the lung or elsewhere. [H. W. Cushing (1869–1939), US surgeon]

cusp (kusp) *n.* **1.** any of the cone-shaped prominences on the teeth, especially the premolars and molars. **2.** a pocket or fold of the membrane lining the heart or of the layer of the wall of a vein, several of which form a valve. When the blood flows backwards the cusps fill up and become distended, so closing the valve.

cutaneous (kew-tay-niŭs) *adj.* relating to the skin.

cuticle (kew-ti-kŭl) *n.* **1.** the epidermis of the skin. **2.** a layer of solid or semisolid material that is secreted by and covers an epithelium. **3.** a layer of cells, such as the outer layer of cells in a hair.

cutis (kew-tis) *n.* *see* skin.

cyan- (cyano-) *prefix denoting* blue.

cyanide (sy-ă-nyd) *n.* any of the notoriously poisonous salts of hydrocyanic acid. Cyanides combine with and render inactive the enzymes of the tissues responsible for cellular respiration, and therefore they kill extremely quickly.

cyanocobalamin (vitamin B$_{12}$) (sy-ă-noh-koh-bal-ă-min) *n.* *see* vitamin B.

cyanosis (sy-ă-noh-sis) *n.* a bluish discoloration of the skin and mucous membranes resulting from an inadequate amount of oxygen in the blood. Cyanosis is associated with heart failure, lung diseases, the breathing of oxygen-deficient atmospheres, and asphyxia. Cyanosis is also seen in blue babies, because of congenital heart defects. —**cyanotic** *adj.*

cybernetics (sy-ber-**net**-iks) *n.* the science of communication processes and automatic control systems in both machines and living things: a study linking the working of the brain and nervous system with the functioning of computers and automated feedback devices. *See also* bionics.

cycl- (cyclo-) *prefix denoting* 1. cycle or cyclic. 2. the ciliary body.

cyclandelate (sy-**klan**-di-layt) *n.* a vasodilator drug administered by mouth to improve circulation in cerebrovascular disease and other conditions in which blood flow is reduced. Trade name: **Cyclospasmol**.

cyclical vomiting (sy-klik-ăl) *n.* recurrent attacks of vomiting, often associated with acidosis, occurring in children but with no apparent cause.

cyclitis (sy-**kly**-tis) *n.* inflammation of the ciliary body of the eye (*see* uveitis).

cyclizine (sy-kliz-een) *n.* a drug with antihistamine properties, administered by mouth to prevent and relieve nausea and vomiting in travel sickness, vertigo, disorders of the inner ear, and postoperative sickness. Trade names: **Marzine, Valoid**.

cyclobarbitone (sy-kloh-**bar**-bi-tohn) *n.* a barbiturate drug administered by mouth as a hypnotic and sedative in cases of insomnia and anxiety. Trade name: **Phanodorm**.

cyclodialysis (sy-kloh-dy-**al**-i-sis) *n.* an operation for glaucoma in which part of the ciliary body is separated from its attachment to the sclera. The aim is to improve the drainage of fluid and thus reduce the pressure within the eye.

cyclopenthiazide (sy-kloh-pen-**th'y**-ă-zyd) *n.* a diuretic administered by mouth to treat oedema, high blood pressure, and heart failure. Trade name: **Navidrex**.

cyclopentolate (sy-kloh-**pen**-tŏ-layt) *n.* a drug, similar to atropine, that is used in eye drops to paralyse the ciliary muscles and dilate the pupil for eye examinations and to treat some types of eye inflammation. Trade names: **Mydrilate, Cyclopentolate Hydrochloride Minims**.

cyclophosphamide (sy-kloh-**fos**-fă-myd) *n.* a drug administered by mouth or injection to treat some cancers, often in combination with other cytotoxic drugs. It also has immunosuppressive properties and is used in prolonging the survival of tissue transplants and in other conditions requiring reduced immune response. Trade name: **Endoxana**.

cycloplegia (sy-kloh-**plee**-jiă) *n.* paralysis of the ciliary muscle of the eye (*see* ciliary body). This causes inability to alter the focus of the eye and is usually accompanied by paralysis of the muscles of the pupil, resulting in fixed dilation of the pupil (mydriasis).

cyclopropane (sy-kloh-**proh**-payn) *n.* a general anaesthetic, administered by inhalation for all types of surgical operation. It can cause postoperative nausea, vomiting, and headache.

cycloserine (sy-kloh-**seer**-een) *n.* an antibiotic, active against a wide range of bacteria, administered by mouth as supporting treatment in tuberculosis and in some infections of the urinary tract.

cyclothymia (sy-kloh-**th'y**-miă) *n.* the occurrence of marked swings of mood from cheerfulness to misery. These fluctuations usually represent a personality disorder, and are not as great as those of manic-depressive psychosis.

cyclotomy (sy-**klot**-ŏmi) *n.* surgical incision of the ciliary body of the eye.

cyesis (sy-**ee**-sis) *n.* pregnancy. *See also* pseudocyesis.

cyn- (cyno-) *prefix denoting* a dog or dogs.

cyproheptadine (sy-proh-**hep**-tă-deen) *n.* a potent antihistamine administered by mouth to treat allergies and itching skin conditions; it is also used to stimulate the appetite. Trade name: **Periactin**.

cyst (sist) *n.* **1.** an abnormal sac or closed cavity lined with epithelium and filled with liquid or semisolid matter. There are many varieties of cysts occurring in different parts of the body. *See* dermoid cyst, hydatid, ovarian cyst, retention cyst, sebaceous cyst. **2.** a dormant stage produced during the life cycle of certain protozoan parasites of the alimentary canal, including *Giardia* and *Entamoeba*. **3.** a structure formed by and surrounding the larvae of certain parasitic worms.

cyst- (cysto-) *prefix denoting* **1.** a bladder, especially the urinary bladder. **2.** a cyst.

cystadenoma (sis-tad-i-**noh**-mă) *n.* an adenoma showing a cystic structure.

cystalgia (sis-**tal**-jiă) *n.* pain in the urinary bladder. This is common in cystitis and when there are stones in the bladder and is occasionally present in bladder cancer.

cystectomy (sis-**tek**-tŏmi) *n.* surgical removal of the urinary bladder. The ureters draining the urine from the kidneys are reimplanted into the colon (*see* ureterosigmoidostomy) or into the ileus (*see* ileal conduit).

cysteine (sis-ti-een) *n.* a sulphur-containing amino acid that is an important constituent of many enzymes.

cystic (sis-tik) *adj.* **1.** of, relating to, or characterized by cysts. **2.** of or relating to the gall bladder or urinary bladder. *c. duct see* bile duct.

cysticercosis (sis-ti-ser-**koh**-sis) *n.* a disease caused by the presence of tapeworm larvae (*see* cysticercus) of the species *Taenia solium* in any of the body tissues. The presence of cysticerci in the muscles causes pain and weakness; in the brain the symptoms are more serious, including mental deterioration, paralysis, giddiness, epileptic attacks, and convulsions.

cysticercus (bladderworm) (sis-ti-ser-kŭs) *n.* a larval stage of some tapeworms in which the scolex and neck are invaginated into a large fluid-filled cyst. *See* cysticercosis.

cystic fibrosis (fibrocystic disease of the pancreas, mucoviscidosis) *n.* a hereditary disease affecting the exocrine glands. The abnormality results in the production of thick mucus, which obstructs the intestinal glands (causing meconium ileus in newborn babies), pancreas (causing deficiency of pancreatic enzymes), and bronchi (causing bronchiectasis). Respiratory infections, which may be severe, are a common complication.

cystine (sis-teen) *n. see* amino acid.

cystinosis (sis-ti-noh-sis) *n.* an inborn defect in the absorption and metabolism of amino acids, leading to abnormal accumulation of the amino acid cystine in the blood, kidneys, and lymphatic system. Excess excretion of cystine in the urine (*cystinuria*) leads to the formation of cystine stones in the kidneys. *See also* Fanconi syndrome.

cystinuria (sis-tin-yoor-iă) *n. see* cystinosis.

cystitis (sis-ty-tis) *n.* inflammation of the urinary bladder, often caused by infection. It is usually accompanied by the desire to pass urine frequently, with a degree of burning.

cystitome (sis-ti-tohm) *n.* a small knife with a tiny curved or hooked blade, used to cut the lens capsule in some operations for cataract.

cystocele (sis-tŏ-seel) *n.* prolapse of the base of the bladder in women. It is usually due to weakness of the pelvic floor after childbirth and causes bulging of the anterior wall of the vagina on straining.

cystography (sis-tog-răfi) *n.* X-ray examination of the urinary bladder after the injection of a contrast medium. The X-ray photographs or films thus obtained are known as *cystograms*.

cystolithiasis (sis-toh-lith-I-ă-sis) *n.* the presence of stones (calculi) in the urinary bladder. The stones cause pain, the passage of bloody urine, and interruption of the urinary stream and should be removed surgically. *See* calculus.

cystometer (sis-tom-it-er) *n.* an apparatus for measuring pressure within the bladder. —**cystometry** *n.*

cystopexy (vesicofixation) (sis-toh-peksi) *n.* a surgical operation to fix the urinary bladder (or a portion of it) in a different position. It may be performed as part of the repair or correction of a prolapsed bladder.

cystoscopy (sis-tos-kŏpi) *n.* examination of the bladder by means of an instrument (*cystoscope*) inserted via the urethra.

cystostomy (sis-tost-ŏmi) *n.* the operation of creating an artificial opening between the bladder and the anterior abdominal wall. This provides a temporary or permanent drainage route for urine.

cystotomy (sis-tot-ŏmi) *n.* surgical incision into the urinary bladder, usually by cutting through the abdominal wall above the pubic symphysis (*suprapubic c.*).

cyt- (cyto-) *prefix denoting* **1.** cell(s). **2.** cytoplasm.

cytarabine (sy-ta-ră-been) *n.* a cytotoxic drug used to suppress the symptoms of some types of leukaemia. It is administered by injection and can damage the bone marrow, leading to various blood cell disorders. Trade name: **Cytosar**.

-cyte *suffix denoting* a cell.

cytochemistry (sy-toh-kem-istri) *n.* the study of chemical compounds and their activities in living cells.

cytogenetics (sy-toh-ji-net-iks) *n.* a science that links the study of inheritance (genetics) with that of cells (cytology); it is concerned mainly with the study of the chromosomes, especially their origin, structure, and functions.

cytokinesis (sy-toh-ki-**nee**-sis) *n.* *see* karyokinesis.

cytology (sy-**tol**-ŏji) *n.* the study of the structure and function of cells. *exfoliative c.* the examination of cells under a microscope, used in the diagnosis of various diseases, e.g. cancer (*see* cervical (smear)). *See also* biopsy. —**cytological** *adj.*

cytolysis (sy-**tol**-i-sis) *n.* the breakdown of cells, particularly by destruction of their outer membranes.

cytomegalovirus (CMV) (sy-toh-meg-ă-loh-vy-rŭs) *n.* a virus belonging to the herpesvirus group. It normally causes only mild symptoms, but if contracted by a pregnant woman it may give rise to congenital mental handicap in her child.

cytometer (sy-**tom**-it-er) *n.* an instrument for determining the number of cells in a given quantity of fluid, such as blood, cerebrospinal fluid, or urine. *See* haemocytometer.

cytopenia (sy-toh-**pee**-niă) *n.* a deficiency of one or more of the various types of blood cells. *See* eosinopenia, erythropenia, lymphopenia, neutropenia, pancytopenia, thrombocytopenia.

cytoplasm (sy-toh-plazm) *n.* the jelly-like substance that surrounds the nucleus of a cell. *See also* protoplasm. —**cytoplasmic** *adj.*

cytosine (sy-toh-seen) *n.* one of the nitrogen-containing bases (*see* pyrimidine) that occurs in the nucleic acid DNA.

cytosome (sy-toh-sohm) *n.* the part of a cell that is outside the nucleus.

cytotoxic drug (sy-toh-**toks**-ik) *n.* a drug that damages or destroys cells and is used to treat various types of cancer. Examples are cyclophosphamide, cytarabine, and mustine; they destroy cancer cells by inhibiting cell division but they also affect normal cells, particularly in bone marrow, skin, stomach lining, and fetal tissue, and dosage must be carefully controlled. *See also* antimetabolite.

cytotoxin (sy-toh-**toks**-in) *n.* any substance that has a toxic action on specific cells.

D

dacry- (dacryo-) *prefix denoting* **1.** tears. **2.** the lacrimal apparatus.

dacryoadenitis (dak-ri-oh-ad-i-ny-tis) *n.* inflammation of the tear-producing gland. *See* lacrimal (apparatus).

dacryocystitis (dak-ri-oh-sis-ty-tis) *n.* inflammation of the lacrimal sac, usually occurring when the duct draining the tears into the nose is blocked. *See* lacrimal (apparatus).

dacryocystorhinostomy (dak-ri-oh-sis-toh-ry-**nost**-ŏmi) *n.* an operation to relieve blockage of the nasolacrimal duct (which drains tears into the nose), in which a communication is made between the lacrimal sac and the nose by removing the intervening bone. *See* dacryocystitis, lacrimal (apparatus).

dacryolith (**dak**-ri-oh-lith) *n.* a stone in the lacrimal canaliculus or lacrimal sac. *See* lacrimal (apparatus).

dacryoma (dak-ri-**oh**-mă) *n.* a harmless tumour-like swelling obstructing any of the ducts associated with the lacrimal apparatus.

dactyl- *prefix denoting* the digits (fingers or toes).

dactylion (dak-til-iŏn) *n. see* syndactyly.

dactylitis (dak-ti-ly-tis) *n.* inflammation of a finger .or toe caused by bone infection (as in tuberculous osteomyelitis) or rheumatic disease.

dactylology (dak-ti-lol-ŏji) *n.* the representation of speech by finger movements: deaf and dumb language.

Daltonism (protanopia) (dawl-tŏn-izm) *n.* red-blindness: a defect in colour vision in which a person cannot distinguish between reds and greens. The term has been used to refer to colour blindness in general. [J. Dalton (1766–1844), British chemist]

D and C *n. see* dilatation and curettage.

dandruff (scurf) (dan-druf) *n.* a common condition in which the scalp is covered with small flakes of dead skin, which come away when the hair is brushed or combed. The flakes are white if too little sebum is produced and yellow with excess secretion of sebum. Medical name: **pityriasis capitis.**

dangerous drugs (dayn-jer-ŭs) *pl. n. see* Misuse of Drugs Act (1971).

dapsone (dap-sohn) *n.* a drug (*see* sulphone) administered by mouth or injection to treat leprosy and some types of dermatitis.

dark adaptation (dark) *n.* the changes that take place in the retina and pupil of the eye enabling vision in very dim light. *See* rod. *Compare* light adaptation.

day blindness (day) *n.* comparatively good vision in poor light

but poor vision in good illumination. The condition is usually congenital and associated with poor visual acuity and defective colour vision. Medical name: **hemeralopia.** *Compare* night blindness.

day hospital *n. see* hospital.

DDT (chlorophenothane, dicophane) *n.* a powerful insecticide that has been in wide use for many years. The quantities now present in the environment – in the form of stores accumulated in animal tissues – raise the question of possible harmful effects on the body.

de- *prefix denoting* **1.** removal or loss. **2.** reversal.

dead space (ded) *n.* **1.** any part of the respiratory tract containing air that does not participate in the exchange of oxygen and carbon dioxide. **2.** a cavity that remains in an incompletely closed wound, in which blood may. accumulate and delay healing.

deafness (def-nis) *n.* partial or total loss of hearing in one or both ears. *conductive d.* deafness that is due to a defect in the conduction of sound from the external ear to the internal ear, often caused by middle-ear infection (*see* otitis (media)). *perceptive d.* deafness that is due to a lesion of the cochlea in the inner ear, the auditory nerve, or the auditory centres in the brain. *See also* hearing aid, Rinne's test, Weber's test.

deamination (dee-ami-**nay**-shŏn) *n.* a process that occurs in the liver during the metabolism of amino acids. The amino group $(-NH_2)$ is removed from an amino acid and converted to ammonia, which is ultimately converted to urea and excreted.

death (deth) *n.* absence of vital functions. *brain d.* permanent functional death of the centres in the brainstem that control respiration and other vital reflexes. Usually two independent medical opinions are required before brain death is agreed, but organs such as kidneys may then legally be removed for transplantation surgery before the heart has stopped.

death certificate *n.* a medical certificate stating the cause of a person's death, usually also stating the deceased's marital status, occupation, and age.

debility (di-**bil**-iti) *n.* physical weakness; loss of strength and power.

debridement (di-**breed**-měnt) *n.* the process of cleaning an open wound by removal of foreign material and dead tissue, so that healing may occur without hindrance.

debrisoquine (deb-**ris**-oh-kween) *n.* a potent drug administered by mouth to treat high blood pressure (hypertension). Trade name: **Declinax**.

dec- (**deca-**) *prefix denoting* ten.

Decadron (**dek**-ă-dron) *n. see* dexamethasone.

decalcification (dee-kal-sifi-**kay**-shŏn) *n.* loss or removal of calcium salts from a bone or tooth.

decapitation (di-kapi-**tay**-shŏn) *n.* removal of the head, usually the head of a dead fetus to enable delivery to take place. This procedure is now very rare.

decapsulation (dee-kaps-yoo-**lay**-shŏn) *n.* the surgical removal of a capsule from an organ; for example, the stripping of the membrane that envelops the kidney.

decay (di-**kay**) *n.* (in bacteriology) the decomposition of organic matter due to microbial action.

deci- *prefix denoting* a tenth.

decidua (di-**sid**-yoo-ă) *n.* the modified mucous membrane that lines the wall of the uterus during pregnancy and is shed with the afterbirth at parturition (*see* endometrium). *d. basalis* the region of the decidua where the embryo is attached. *d. capsularis* the thin layer of the decidua that covers the embryo. *d. parietalis* the region of the decidua that is not in contact with the embryo. —**decidual** *adj.*

deciduoma (di-sid-yoo-**oh**-mă) *n.* a mass of tissue within the womb derived from remnants of decidua. *See also* chorionepithelioma (malignant deciduoma).

decompensation (dee-kom-pen-**say**-shŏn) *n.* inability of the heart to maintain an adequate circulation in the face of an increased workload or some structural defect.

decomposition (dee-kom-pŏ-**zish**-ŏn) *n.* the gradual disintegration of dead organic matter, usually foodstuffs or tissues, by the chemical action of bacteria and/or fungi.

decompression (dee-kŏm-**presh**-ŏn) *n.* **1.** the reduction of pressure on an organ or part of the body by surgical intervention. Raised pressure in the fluid of the brain can be lowered by cutting into the dura mater; cardiac compression – the abnormal presence of blood or fluid round the heart – can be cured by cutting the pericardium. **2.** the gradual reduction of atmospheric pressure for deep-sea divers. *See* compressed air illness.

decompression sickness *n. see* compressed air illness.

decongestant (dee-kŏn-**jest**-ănt) *n.* an agent that reduces or relieves nasal congestion. Most nasal decongestants are sympathomimetic drugs, applied either locally, in the form of nasal sprays or drops, or taken by mouth.

decortication (dee-kor-ti-**kay**-shŏn) *n.* **1.** the removal of the outside layer (cortex) from an organ or structure, such as the kidney. **2.** an operation for removing the blood clot and scar tissue that forms after bleeding into the chest cavity.

decubitus (di-**kew**-bit-ŭs) *n.* the recumbent position.

decubitus ulcer *n. see* bedsore.

decussation (dee-kus-**ay**-shŏn) *n.* a point at which two or more structures of the body cross to the opposite side. The term is used particularly for the point at which nerve fibres cross over in the central nervous system.

defecation (def-i-**kay**-shŏn) *n.* the expulsion of faeces through the anus.

defence mechanism (di-**fenss**) *n.* the means whereby an undesirable impulse can be avoided or controlled (*see* censor). Defence mechanisms include repression, projection, and reaction formation.

deferent (**def**-er-ĕnt) *adj.* **1.** carrying away from or down from. **2.** relating to the vas deferens.

defervescence (def-er-ves-ĕns) *n.* the disappearance of a fever, a process that may occur rapidly or take several days.

defibrillation (dee-fib-ri-**lay**-shŏn) *n.* administration of a controlled electric shock to restore normal heart rhythm in cases of cardiac arrest due to ventricular fibrilla-

tion. The apparatus (*defibrillator*) administers the shock either through electrodes placed on the chest wall over the heart or directly to the heart after the chest has been opened surgically.

defibrination (dee-fib-ri-**nay**-shŏn) *n.* the removal of fibrin, one of the plasma proteins that causes coagulation, from a sample of blood.

deficiency disease (di-**fish**-ĕn-si) *n.* any disease caused by the lack of an essential nutrient in the diet. Such nutrients include vitamins, essential amino acids, and essential fatty acids.

degeneration (di-jen-er-**ay**-shŏn) *n.* the deterioration and loss of specialized function of the cells of a tissue or organ. The changes may be caused by a defective blood supply or by disease. Degeneration may involve the deposition of calcium salts, fat (*see* fatty degeneration), or fibrous tissue in the affected organ or tissue. *See also* infiltration.

deglutition (dee-gloo-**tish**-ŏn) *n. see* swallowing.

dehiscence (di-**hiss**-ĕns) *n.* a splitting open, as of a surgical wound.

dehydration (dee-hy-**dray**-shŏn) *n.* loss or deficiency of water in body tissues. The condition may result from inadequate water intake and/or from excessive removal of water from the body; for example, by sweating, vomiting, or diarrhoea.

dehydrogenase (dee-hy-**droj**-ĕ-nayz) *n. see* oxidoreductase.

déjà vu (day-*zha*-**vew**) *n.* a vivid psychic experience in which immediately contemporary events seem to be a repetition of previous happenings. It is a symptom

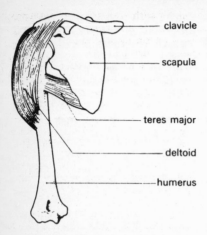

clavicle

scapula

teres major

deltoid

humerus

The deltoid muscle

of temporal lobe epilepsy. *See also* jamais vu.

Delhi boil (**del**-i) *n.* see oriental sore.

delirium (di-li-ri-ŭm) *n.* an acute disorder of the mental processes accompanying organic brain disease. It may be manifested by illusions, disorientation, hallucinations, or extreme excitement and occurs in metabolic disorders, intoxication, deficiency diseases, and infections. *d. tremens* a psychosis caused by alcoholism, usually seen as a withdrawal syndrome in chronic alcoholics. Features include anxiety, tremor, sweating, and vivid hallucinations.

deltoid (**del**-toid) *n.* a thick triangular muscle that covers the shoulder joint. It is responsible for raising the arm away from the side of the body.

delusion (di-**loo**-zhŏn) *n.* an irrationally held belief that cannot be altered by rational argument. It may be a symptom of schizophrenia, manic-depressive psy-

chosis, or an organic psychosis. *See also* paranoia.

demarcation (dee-mar-**kay**-shŏn) *n.* the marking of a limit or boundary. *line of d.* a red or black line marking the boundary between necrotic and healthy tissue in gangrene.

dementia (di-**men**-shă) *n.* a chronic or persistent disorder of the mental processes due to organic brain disease. It is marked by memory disorders, changes in personality, deterioration in personal care, impaired reasoning ability, and disorientation. *presenile d.* dementia that occurs in young or middle-aged people. *See* Alzheimer's disease, Pick's disease.

demethylchlortetracycline (dee-meth-yl-klor-tet-ră-sy-kleen) *n.* an antibiotic that is active against a wide range of bacteria and is administered by mouth to treat various infections. Trade name: **Ledermycin.**

demi- *prefix denoting* half.

demography (di-**mog**-răfi) *n.* the study of the populations of the world, their racial make-up, movements, birth rates, death rates, and other factors affecting the quality of life within them.

demulcent (di-**mul**-sĕnt) *n.* a soothing agent that protects the mucous membranes and relieves irritation.

demyelination (dee-my-ĕ-li-**nay**-shŏn) *n.* a disease process selectively damaging the myelin sheaths in the central or peripheral nervous system. Demyelination may be the primary disorder, as in multiple sclerosis, or it may occur after head injury or strokes.

dendrite (**den**-dryt) *n.* one of the shorter branching processes of the cell body of a neurone, which makes contact with other neurones at synapses and carries nerve impulses from them into the cell body.

dendritic ulcer (den-**drit**-ik) *n.* a branching ulcer of the surface of the cornea caused by herpes simplex virus.

denervation (de-ner-**vay**-shŏn) *n.* interruption of the nerve supply to the muscles and skin. A denervated area of skin loses all forms of sensation and its subsequent ability to heal and renew its tissues is impaired.

dengue (breakbone fever) (deng-i) *n.* a viral disease that occurs throughout the tropics and subtropics; it is transmitted to man principally by the mosquito *Aëdes aegypti*. Symptoms include severe pains in the joints and muscles, headache, fever, and an irritating rash.

denial (di-**ny**-ǎl) *n.* a psychological process in which an individual refuses to accept an aspect of reality. It is seen particularly in dying patients who refuse to accept their impending death.

Denis Browne splint (den-iss brown) *n.* a splint used for the correction of club-foot in early infancy. [Sir Denis J. W. Browne (1892–1967), British orthopaedic surgeon]

dens (denz) *n.* a tooth or tooth-shaped structure.

dent- (denti-, dento-) *prefix denoting* the teeth.

dental auxiliary (den-t'l) *n.* any of various assistants to a dentist.

dental caries *n. see* caries.

dentate (den-tayt) *adj.* serrated; having toothlike projections.

dentifrice (dent-i-fris) *n.* a powder or paste for cleaning the teeth. It consists of a fine abrasive com-bined with a soap or detergent, to which are added flavouring and colouring materials.

dentine (**den**-teen) *n.* the calcified part of a tooth, between the enamel and the pulp.

dentistry (**den**-tist-ri) *n.* the profession concerned with care and treatment of diseases of the teeth, gums, and jaws.

dentition (den-**tish**-ŏn) *n.* the number, type, and arrangement of the teeth as a whole in the mouth. *adult* (*permanent*) *d.* the 32 teeth usually present by the age of 21, made up of incisors, canines, premolars, and molars. *milk* (*deciduous*) *d.* the teeth of young children, which are progressively lost in preparation for the eruption of the adult teeth. It consists of 20 teeth, made up of incisors, canines, and molars only.

denture (**den**-cher) *n.* a removable prosthesis, made partially or wholly of plastic, bearing one or more false teeth.

deodorant (dee-**oh**-der-ǎnt) *n.* an agent that reduces or removes unpleasant body odours by destroying bacteria that live on the skin and break down sweat. Deodorant preparations often contain an antiseptic.

deoxycholic acid (dee-oks-i-**koh**-lik) *n. see* bile acids.

deoxycorticosterone (dee-oks-i-kor-ti-koh-**steer**-ohn) *n.* a hormone, synthesized and released by the adrenal cortex, that regulates salt and water balance. *See also* corticosteroid.

deoxyribonucleic acid (dee-oks-i-ry-boh-new-**klee**-ik) *n. see* DNA.

Department of Health and Social Security *n.* a department of central government that supports the Secretary of State for Health

molars | incisors | molars

canines | canines

Deciduous dentition

R | L

premolars | incisors | premolars
molars | | molars

canines | canines

Permanent dentition

and Social Services in meeting his obligations, which include the National Health Service and the prevention and control of infectious diseases. Information is collated, priorities assessed, and resources allocated to Regional and District Health Authorities.

dependence (drug dependence) (di-pen-dăns) *n.* **1.** the physical and/or psychological effects produced by the habitual taking of certain drugs, characterized by a compulsion to continue taking the drug. *physical d.* dependence in which withdrawal of the drug causes specific symptoms (*withdrawal symptoms*), such as sweating, vomiting, or tremors, that are reversed by further doses. It may be induced by alcohol, morphine, heroin, and cocaine. *psychological d.* dependence in which repeated use of a drug induces reliance on it for a state of well-being and contentment, but there are no physical withdrawal symptoms if use of the drug is stopped. It may be induced by nicotine in tobacco, cannabis, and such drugs as barbiturates and amphetamines. **2.** a state of reliance on others for aspects of self-care, sometimes used as a measure of nursing workload.

depersonalization (dee-per-sŏ-nă-ly-zay-shŏn) *n.* a state in which a person feels himself becoming unreal or strangely altered, or feels that his mind is becoming separated from his body. Severe feelings of depersonalization occur in conditions such as anxiety neurosis, schizophrenia, and epilepsy. *See also* derealization.

depilatory (di-**pil**-ă-ter-i) *n.* an agent applied to the skin to remove hair.

depolarization (dee-poh-lă-ry-zay-shŏn) *n.* the sudden surge of charged particles across the membrane of a nerve or muscle cell that accompanies a physicochemical change in the membrane and cancels out, or reverses, its resting potential to produce an action potential.

depressant (di-**pres**-ănt) *n.* an agent that reduces the normal activity of any body system or function. Drugs such as general anaesthetics, barbiturates, and opiates are depressants of the central nervous system and respiration.

depression (di-**presh**-ŏn) *n.* a mental state characterized by excessive sadness. Activity can be agitated or retarded and sleep, appetite, and concentration are disturbed. Depression may be caused by loss or frustration, or by conditions such as manic-depressive psychosis. Treatment is with antidepressant drugs and/or psychotherapy. *See also* endogenous, reactive.

depressor (di-**pres**-er) *n.* **1.** a muscle that causes lowering of part of the body. **2.** a nerve that lowers blood pressure.

dequalinium (dek-wă-**lin**-iŭm) *n.* an antiseptic, active against some bacteria and fungi, used as lozenges or paint to treat mouth and throat infections.

deradenitis (der-ad-i-ny-tis) *n.* inflammation of the lymph nodes in the neck.

Derbyshire neck (**dar**-bi-sher) *n.* endemic goitre, once common in Derbyshire due to lack of iodine in the soil and water.

derealization (dee-riă-ly-zay-shŏn) *n.* a feeling of unreality in which the environment is experienced as unreal and strange. It occurs in association with depersonalization or with the conditions that cause depersonalization.

dereism (**dee**-ri-izm) *n.* undirected fantasy thinking that fails to respect the realities of life. It may be a feature of schizophrenia.

derm- (derma-, dermo-, dermat(o)-) *prefix denoting* the skin.

-derm *suffix denoting* **1.** the skin. **2.** a germ layer.

dermal (**der**-măl) *adj.* relating to or affecting the skin, especially the dermis.

dermatitis (der-mă-**ty**-tis) *n.* inflammation of the skin caused by an outside agent. The skin is red and itchy and small blisters may develop. *eczematous d.* a condition associated wih eczema. It may result from direct irritation of the skin by a substance or it may be an allergic reaction to a particular substance that has been in contact with the skin, injected, or taken by mouth. *noneczematous d.* (*occupational d.*) dermatitis not associated with eczema and often caused by industrial substances.

dermatoglyphics (der-mă-**toh**-glif-iks) *n.* the study of the patterns of finger, palm, toe, and sole prints. These patterns, which are unique to each individual, are of interest to anthropologists and to doctors studying genetic disorders. They are also of value in criminology. *See also* fingerprint.

dermatology (der-mă-**tol**-ŏji) *n.* the medical specialty concerned with the diagnosis and treatment of skin disorders. —**dermatological** *adj.* —**dermatologist** *n.*

dermatome (der-mă-tohm) *n.* a surgical instrument used for cutting thin slices of skin in some skin grafting operations.

dermatomycosis (der-mă-toh-my-koh-sis) *n.* any infection of the skin caused by fungi.

dermatomyositis (der-mă-toh-my-oh-sy-tis) *n.* an inflammatory disorder of the skin and underlying tissues, including the muscles. A bluish-red skin eruption occurs on the face, scalp, neck, shoulders, and hands and is later accompanied by severe swelling. The condition is one of the collagen diseases; it is often associated with internal cancer.

dermatophyte (der-mă-toh-fyt) *n.* any microscopic fungus that grows on the skin and mucous membranes. There are three main genera: *Microsporum*, *Epidermophyton*, and *Trichophyton*.

dermatophytosis (der-mă-toh-fy-toh-sis) *n.* any fungus infection of the skin; more specifically, an infection caused by the parasitic fungus *Epidermophyton*.

dermatoplasty (der-mă-toh-plasti) *n.* replacement of damaged or destroyed skin by surgery. *See* plastic surgery, skin (graft).

dermatosis (der-mă-toh-sis) *n.* any disease of skin, particularly one without inflammation.

dermis (**corium**) (der-mis) *n.* the true skin: the thick layer of living tissue that lies beneath the epidermis. —**dermal** *adj.*

dermographia (der-moh-graf-iă) *n.* a local allergic reaction caused by pressure on the skin. People with such highly sensitive skin can 'write' on it with a finger or blunt instrument, the pressure producing lasting weals.

dermoid (der-moid) **1.** *adj.* resembling the skin. **2.** *n. see* dermoid cyst.

dermoid cyst (**dermoid**) *n.* a cyst containing hair, hair follicles, and sebaceous glands, usually found at sites marking the fusion of developing sections of the body in the embryo.

Descemet's membrane (dess-ě-mayz) *n.* the elastic membrane that lines the inner surface of the cornea of the eye, next to the aqueous humour. [J. Descemet (1732–1810), French anatomist]

desensitization (dee-sen-si-ty-zay-shŏn) *n.* **1.** (*or* **hyposensitization**) a method for reducing the effects of a known allergen by injecting, over a period, gradually increasing doses of the allergen, until resistance is built up. *See* allergy. **2.** a technique used in the behaviour therapy of phobic states. The thing that is feared is very gradually introduced to the patient, in conjunction with relaxation therapy, so that he is able to cope with progressively closer approximations to it.

deserpidine (dee-ser-pi-deen) *n.* a drug that reduces blood pressure and is administered by mouth to treat essential hypertension (*see* sympatholytic). Trade name: **Harmonyl**.

desferrioxamine (dess-ferri-oks-ă-meen) *n.* a drug that combines with iron in body tissues and fluids and is administered by mouth, injection, or as eye drops to treat iron poisoning or diseases involving iron storage in parts of the body (*see* haemochromatosis). Trade name: **Desferal**.

desipramine (dess-ip-ră-meen) *n.* a tricyclic antidepressant drug administered by mouth or injection. Trade name: **Pertofran**.

desquamation (des-kwă-may-shŏn) *n.* the process in which the outer layer of the epidermis of the skin is removed by scaling.

detached retina (di-tacht) *n.* separation of the retina from the choroid, causing loss of vision in the affected part of the retina. The condition can be treated surgically by creating patches of scar tissue between the retina and the choroid (*see* photocoagulation), which – combined with plombage – stick it back into place.

detergent (di-ter-jĕnt) *n.* a synthetic cleansing agent that removes all impurities from a surface by reacting with grease and suspended particles, including bacteria and other microorganisms.

detoxication (detoxification) (dee-toksi-kay-shŏn) *n.* the process whereby toxic substances are removed or toxic effects neutralized. It is one of the functions of the liver.

detrition (di-trish-ŏn) *n.* the process of wearing away solid bodies (e.g. bones) by friction or use.

detritus (di-try-tŭs) *n.* particles of matter produced by disintegration, tissue death, etc.

detrusor muscle (di-troo-ser) *n.* a band of smooth muscle fibres that form the outer muscular coat of the urinary bladder and are attached to the pubis.

Dettol (det-ol) *n. see* chloroxylenol.

detumescence (dee-tew-mes-ĕns) *n.* **1.** the reverse of erection, whereby the erect penis or clito-

ris becomes flaccid after orgasm. **2.** subsidence of a swelling.

deut- (deuto-, deuter(o)-) *prefix denoting* two, second, or secondary.

deuteranopia (dew-ter-ă-noh-piă) *n.* a defect in colour vision in which reds, yellows, and greens are confused. *Compare* tritanopia.

deviation (dee-vi-ay-shŏn) *n.* (in ophthalmology) any abnormal position of one or both eyes. Deviations of both eyes may occur in brain disease. Deviations of one eye come into the category of squint (*see* strabismus).

Devic's disease (dev-iks) *n. see* neuromyelitis optica. [E. Devic, French physician]

dexamethasone (deks-ă-meth-ă-zohn) *n.* a corticosteroid drug administered by mouth or injection principally to treat severe allergies, skin and eye diseases, rheumatic and other inflammatory conditions, and hormone and blood disorders. Trade names: **Decadron, Oradexon**.

dexamphetamine (deks-am-fet-ămin) *n.* a drug with actions and effects similar to those of amphetamine. Trade names: **Dexamed, Dexedrine**.

dextr- (dextro-) *prefix denoting* **1.** the right side. **2.** (in chemistry) dextrorotation.

dextran (deks-tran) *n.* a carbohydrate, consisting of branched chains of glucose units, that is a storage product of bacteria and yeasts. Preparations of dextran solution are used in transfusions, to increase the volume of plasma.

dextrin (deks-trin) *n.* a carbohydrate formed as an intermediate product in the digestion of starch by the enzyme amylase. Dextrin is used in the preparation of pharmaceutical products and surgical dressings.

dextrocardia (deks-troh-**kar**-diă) *n.* a congenital defect in which the position of the heart is a mirror image of its normal position, with the apex of the ventricles pointing to the right.

dextromoramide (deks-troh-**mor**-ă-myd) *n.* an analgesic administered by mouth, injection, or as suppositories to relieve moderate or severe pain. Dextromoramide is similar to morphine and can cause morphine-type dependence. Trade name: **Palfium**.

dextropropoxyphene (deks-troh-prŏ-**poks**-i-feen) *n.* an analgesic administered by mouth to relieve mild or moderate pain.

dextrose (**deks**-trohz) *n. see* glucose.

dhobie itch (**doh**-bi) *n.* a skin disease – a type of allergic dermatitis – caused by clothes laundry-marked with ink used in India by native laundrymen (or women).

di- *prefix denoting* two or double.

dia- *prefix denoting* **1.** through. **2.** throughout or completely. **3.** apart.

diabetes (dy-ă-**bee**-teez) *n.* any disorder of metabolism causing excessive thirst and the production of large volumes of urine. *d. insipidus* a rare form of diabetes that is due to deficiency of the pituitary hormone vasopressin. *d. mellitus* a disorder of carbohydrate metabolism in which sugars in the body are not oxidized to produce energy due to lack of the pancreatic hormone insulin. The accumulation of sugar leads to its appearance in the blood (hyperglycaemia), then in the urine; symptoms include thirst, loss of weight, and the excessive

production of urine. The use of fats as an alternative source of energy leads to disturbances of the acid-base balance, ketosis, and eventually to convulsions preceding *diabetic coma*. Treatment is based on a carefully controlled diet, with adequate carbohydrate for the body's needs, together with injections of insulin or drugs (such as tolbutamide) that are taken by mouth to lower blood-glucose levels. Lack of balance in the diet or in the amount of insulin taken leads to hypoglycaemia. *See also* haemochromatosis. —**diabetic** (dy-ă-**bet**-ik) *adj., n.*

diaclasia (dy-ă-**klay**-ziă) *n.* a fracture made deliberately by a surgeon to correct a deformity in a bone, which has usually resulted from a badly set or untreated fracture.

diagnosis (dy-ăg-**noh**-sis) *n.* the process of determining the nature of a disorder by considering the patient's signs and symptoms, medical background, and – when necessary – results of laboratory tests and X-ray examinations. *differential d.* diagnosis of a condition whose signs and/ or symptoms are shared by various other conditions. *See also* prenatal diagnosis. *Compare* prognosis. —**diagnostic** (dy-ăg-**noss**-tik) *adj.*

dialyser (**dy**-ă-ly-zer) *n.* a piece of apparatus for separating components of a liquid mixture by dialysis, especially an artificial kidney (*see* haemodialysis).

dialysis (dy-**al**-i-sis) *n.* a method of separating particles of different dimensions in a liquid mixture, using a thin semipermeable membrane. A solution of the mixture is separated from distilled water by the membrane; the solutes pass through the membrane into the water while the proteins, etc., are retained. The principle of dialysis is used in the artificial kidney (*see* haemodialysis).

diamorphine (dy-ă-**mor**-feen) *n. see* heroin.

diapedesis (dy-ă-pě-**dee**-sis) *n.* migration of cells through the walls of blood capillaries into the tissue spaces. Diapedesis is an important part of the reaction of tissues to injury (*see* inflammation).

diaphoresis (dy-ă-fer-**ee**-sis) *n.* the process of sweating, especially excessive sweating. *See* sweat.

diaphoretic (sudorific) (dy-ă-fer-et-ik) *n.* a drug, such as pilocarpine, that causes an increase in sweating. Antipyretic drugs also have diaphoretic activity.

diaphragm (dy-ă-fram) *n.* **1.** (in anatomy) a thin musculomembranous dome-shaped muscle that separates the thoracic and abdominal cavities. It plays an important role in breathing. There are openings in the diaphragm through which the oesophagus, blood vessels, and nerves pass. **2.** a hemispherical rubber cap fitted inside the vagina over the neck of the womb as a contraceptive. When combined with the use of a chemical spermicide the diaphragm provides reasonably reliable contraception.

diaphysis (dy-**af**-i-sis) *n.* the shaft (central part) of a long bone. *Compare* epiphysis.

diarrhoea (dy-ă-**ree**-ă) *n.* frequent bowel evacuation or the passage of abnormally soft or liquid faeces. Its causes include intestinal infections, other forms of intesti-

A synovial joint

nal inflammation, anxiety, and the irritable bowel syndrome. Severe or prolonged diarrhoea may lead to excess losses of fluid, salts, and nutrients in the faeces.

diarthrosis (synovial joint) (dy-arth-**roh**-sis) *n.* a freely movable joint. The ends of the adjoining bones are covered with a thin cartilaginous sheet, and the bones are linked by a ligament lined with synovial membrane, which secretes synovial fluid.

diastase (dy-ă-stayz) *n.* an enzyme that hydrolyses starch in barley grain to produce maltose during the malting process. It has been used to aid the digestion of starch in some digestive disorders.

diastasis (dy-**ast**-ă-sis) *n.* dislocation of bones at an immovable or slightly movable joint, as at the pubic symphysis.

diastole (dy-**ast**-ŏ-li) *n.* the period between two contractions of the heart, when the muscle of the heart relaxes and allows the chambers to fill with blood. *See also* blood pressure, systole. —**diastolic** (dy-ă-**stol**-ik) *adj.*

diastolic pressure *n. see* blood pressure.

diathermy (dy-ă-therm-i) *n.* the production of heat in a part of the body by means of a high-frequency electric current passed between two electrodes placed on the patient's skin. The heat generated can be used in the treatment of deep-seated pain in rheumatic and arthritic conditions. *d. knife* a knife generating heat that coagulates blood and is used to make bloodless surgical incisions. *d. snare* (or *needle*) an electrically heated snare (or needle) used to destroy unwanted tissue (*see* electrocautery).

diathesis (dy-ath-i-sis) *n.* a higher than average tendency to acquire certain diseases, such as allergies, rheumatic diseases, or gout. Such diseases may run in families, but they are not inherited.

diazepam (dy-az-ĕ-pam) *n.* a tranquillizer with muscle-relaxant and anticonvulsant properties, administered by mouth or injection to relieve anxiety and tension and in the treatment of epilepsy and muscular rheumatism. Trade name: **Valium.**

diazoxide (dy-ă-zok-syd) *n.* a drug used to lower blood pressure in patients with hypertension and also used to treat conditions in which the levels of blood sugar are low. It is administered by mouth or (for hypertension) injection.

dibenzepin (dy-benz-ĕ-pin) *n.* an antidepressant drug administered by mouth. Trade name: **Noveril.**

dicephalus (dy-sef-ă-lŭs) *n. see* craniopagus.

dichloralphenazone (dy-klor-ăl-fen-ă-zohn) *n.* a sedative administered by mouth to relieve pain, fever, and restlessness, mainly in children and elderly patients. It can cause dependence of the barbiturate-alcohol type. Trade names: **Paedo-Sed, Welldorm.**

dichlorophen (dy-klor-ŏ-fen) *n.* an anthelmintic drug administered by mouth to treat human tapeworm infestation. Trade name: **Anthiphen.**

dichlorphenamide (dy-klor-fen-ă-myd) *n.* a diuretic administered by mouth to reduce pressure within the eye in the treatment of glaucoma. Trade names: **Daranide, Oratrol.**

dichromatic (dy-kroh-mat-ik) *adj.* describing the state of colour vision of those who can appreciate only two of the three primary colours. *Compare* trichromatic.

Dick test (dik) *n.* a test for susceptibility to scarlet fever. [G. F. Dick (1881–1967) and G. R. H. Dick (1881–1963), US physicians]

dicophane (dy-koh-fayn) *n. see* DDT.

dicoumarol (dy-koo-mer-ol) *n.* an anticoagulant drug administered by mouth in the treatment of coronary and venous thrombosis. Dicoumarol has now largely been replaced in clinical use by phenindione or warfarin.

dicrotism (dy-krŏ-tizm) *n.* a condition in which the pulse is felt as a double beat for each contraction of the heart. It may be seen in typhoid fever. —**dicrotic** (dy-krot-ik) *adj.*

dicyclomine (dy-sy-klŏ-meen) *n.* a drug that reduces spasms of smooth muscle and is administered by mouth to relieve peptic ulcer, infantile colic, colitis, and related conditions. Trade name: **Merbentyl.**

didym- (**didymo-**) *prefix denoting* the testis.

dienoestrol (dy-in-ee-strol) *n.* a synthetic female sex hormone (*see* oestrogen) administered by mouth to treat symptoms of the menopause, to suppress lactation, and to relieve symptoms in cancer of the breast or prostate. It is also applied as a cream to relieve itching or inflammation of the vagina and in acne. Trade name: **Hormofemin**.

diet (**dy**-ĕt) *n.* the mixture of foods that a person eats. *balanced d.* a diet that contains adequate quantities of all the nutrients.

dietary fibre (**roughage**) (**dy**-it-er-i) *n.* the part of food that cannot be digested and absorbed to produce energy. Foods with a high fibre content include wholemeal cereals and flour, root vegetables, nuts, and fruit. Dietary fibre is considered by some to be helpful in the prevention of such diseases as diverticulosis, constipation, appendicitis, obesity, and diabetes mellitus.

dietetics (dy-i-tet-iks) *n.* the application of the principles of nutrition to the selection of food and the feeding of individuals and groups.

diethylcarbamazine (dy-eth-yl-kar-bam-ă-zeen) *n.* an anthelmintic drug that is administered by mouth in the treatment of filariasis, loiasis, and onchocerciasis.

diethylpropion (dy-eth-yl-**proh**-pi-on) *n.* a drug, similar to amphetamine, that suppresses the appetite and is administered by mouth in the treatment of obesity. Dependence of the amphetamine type can occur. Trade names: **Apesate, Tenuate**.

Dietl's crisis (dee-t'lz) *n.* acute ob-struction of a kidney causing severe pain in the loins. The obstruction usually occurs at the junction of the renal pelvis and the ureter, causing the kidney to become distended with accumulated urine (*see* hydronephrosis). [J. Dietl (1804–78), Polish physician]

differential diagnosis (dif-er-en-shăl) *n. see* diagnosis.

differential leucocyte count (**differential blood count**) *n.* a determination of the proportions of the different kinds of white cells (leucocytes) present in a sample of blood. The information often aids diagnosis of disease.

differentiation (dif-er-en-shi-ay-shŏn) *n.* the process in embryonic development during which unspecialized cells or tissues become specialized for particular functions.

diffusion (di-few-zhŏn) *n.* the mixing of one liquid or gas with another by the random movement of their particles.

digestion (dy-**jes**-chŏn) *n.* the process in which ingested food is broken down in the alimentary canal into a form that can be absorbed and assimilated by the tissues of the body.

digit (**dij**-it) *n.* a finger or toe. —**digital** *adj.*

digitalis (dij-i-tay-lis) *n.* an extract from the dried leaves of foxgloves (*Digitalis* species), which contains various substances, including digitoxin and digoxin, that stimulate heart muscle. Used to treat heart failure, it is administered by mouth or, in emergency, by injection. *See also* digitalization.

digitalization (dij-it-ă-ly-**zay**-shŏn) *n.* the administration of the drug digitalis or one of its purified derivatives to a patient with heart failure until the optimum level has been reached in the heart tissues.

digitoxin (dij-i-**toks**-in) *n.* a drug that increases heart muscle contraction and is administered by mouth or injection in heart failure. It is slow-acting but the effects are prolonged.

digoxin (dy-**goks**-in) *n.* a drug that increases heart muscle contraction and is administered by mouth or injection in heart failure. It is rapidly effective and the effects are short-lived.

dihydrocodeine (dy-hy-drŏ-**koh**-deen) *n.* a drug administered by mouth or injection to relieve pain and suppress coughs (*see* analgesic, antitussive).

diiodohydroxyquinoline (dy-I-ŏ-doh-hy-droks-i-**kwin**-ŏ-leen) *n.* an antiseptic administered by mouth or as pessaries to treat bowel infections and dysentery. Trade name: **Diodoquin.**

dilatation (dy-lă-**tay**-shŏn) *n.* the enlargement or expansion of a hollow organ (such as a blood vessel) or cavity.

dilatation and curettage (D and C) *n.* an operation in which the neck of the womb is expanded, using a dilator, and the lining of the womb is peeled off with a curette (*see* curettage). It is performed for a variety of reasons, including removal of cysts or tumours and examination of the womb lining in the diagnosis of gynaecological disorders.

dilator (dy-**lay**-ter) *n.* **1.** an instrument used to enlarge a body opening or cavity. **2.** a drug, applied either locally or systemically, that causes expansion of a structure. *See also* vasodilator. **3.** a muscle that, by its action,

opens an aperture or orifice in the body.

dill water (dil) *n.* a preparation containing a volatile oil extracted from the dill plant (*Anethum graveolens*), used to treat flatulence in infants.

diloxanide (dil-**oks**-ă-nyd) *n.* an antiseptic administered by mouth to treat bowel infections.

dimenhydrinate (dy-men-hy-dri-nayt) *n.* an antihistamine administered by mouth or injection to prevent and treat travel sickness, nausea and vomiting due to other causes, vertigo, and inner ear disturbances. Trade name: **Dramamine.**

dimercaprol (dy-mer-**kap**-rol) *n.* a drug that combines with metals in the body and is administered by injection to treat poisoning by antimony, arsenic, bismuth, gold, mercury, and thallium and in Wilson's disease. Trade name: **British Anti-Lewisite (BAL).**

dimethothiazine (dy-meth-oh-**th'y**-ă-zeen) *n.* an antihistamine administered by mouth to treat allergies such as hay fever. Trade name: **Banistyl.**

dimetria (uterus duplex, uterus didelphys) (dy-**mee**-triă) *n.* the condition of having a double womb.

dioctyl sodium sulphosuccinate (dy-**ok**-tyl soh-di-ŭm sul-foh-**suk**-si-nayt) *n.* a softening agent that is given by mouth or in suppositories, often together with a laxative, to relieve constipation. It is also used in solution to soften ear wax.

diodone (**dy**-ŏ-dohn) *n.* an iodine-containing compound that is radio-opaque and therefore useful in radiographic examination, especially pyelography.

dioptre (dy-**op**-ter) *n*. the unit of measurement of the power of refraction of a lens. One dioptre is the power of a lens that brings parallel light rays to a focus at a point one metre from the lens, after passing through it.

diphenhydramine (dy-fen-**hy**-dră-meen) *n*. an antihistamine administered by mouth or injection to treat allergic conditions, such as hay fever and rhinitis, and in cough mixtures. Trade name: **Benadryl**.

diphenoxylate (dy-fen-**oks**-i-layt) *n*. a drug administered by mouth, often in combination with atropine, to treat diarrhoea. It is also used after colostomy or ileostomy to reduce the frequency and fluidity of the stools.

diphtheria (dif-**theer**-iă) *n*. an acute highly contagious infection, caused by the bacterium *Corynebacterium diphtheriae*, generally affecting the throat but occasionally other mucous membranes and the skin. Early symptoms are a sore throat, weakness, and mild fever; later, a soft grey membrane forms across the throat, constricting the air passages and causing difficulty in breathing and swallowing. Bacteria multiply at the site of infection and release a toxin into the bloodstream, which damages heart and nerves. An effective immunization programme has now made diphtheria rare in most Western countries (*see also* Schick test).

diphtheroid (dif-ther-oid) *adj*. resembling diphtheria (especially the membrane formed in diphtheria) or the bacteria that cause it.

diphyllobothriasis (dy-fil-oh-bo-thry-ă-sis) *n*. an infestation of the intestine with the broad tapeworm, *Diphyllobothrium latum*, which sometimes causes nausea, malnutrition, diarrhoea, and anaemia resulting from impaired absorption of vitamin B_{12} through the gut.

dipipanone (dy-**pip**-ă-nohn) *n*. a potent analgesic drug administered by mouth or injection to relieve severe pain.

dipl- (diplo-) *prefix denoting* double.

diplacusis (dip-lă-**kew**-sis) *n*. perception of a single sound as double owing to a defect of the cochlea in the inner ear.

diplegia (dy-**plee**-jă) *n*. paralysis involving both sides of the body and affecting the legs more severely than the arms. *cerebral d.* a form of cerebral palsy in which there is widespread damage, in both cerebral hemispheres, of the brain cells that control the movements of the limbs. —**diplegic** *adj*.

diplococcus (dip-loh-**kok**-ŭs) *n*. any of a group of nonmotile parasitic spherical bacteria that occur in pairs. The group includes the pneumococcus.

diploë (**dip**-loh-ee) *n*. the latticelike tissue that lies between the inner and outer layers of the skull.

diploid (**dip**-loid) *adj*. describing cells, nuclei, or organisms in which each chromosome except the Y sex chromosome is represented twice. *Compare* haploid. —**diploid** *n*.

diplopia (di-**ploh**-piă) *n*. double vision: the simultaneous awareness of two images of the one object. It is usually due to a disturbance in the coordinated movements of the muscles that move the eyeball, and covering one eye will abolish it.

diprophylline (di-**prof**-i-leen) *n.* a drug that relaxes bronchial muscle and stimulates heart muscle. It is administered by mouth, injection, or in suppositories to relieve symptoms in asthma and bronchitis and to treat congestive heart failure. Trade. names: **Neutraphylline, Silbephylline.**

dipsomania (dip-sŏ-**may**-niă) *n.* morbid and insatiable craving for alcohol, occurring in paroxysms. Only a small proportion of alcoholics show this symptom. *See* alcoholism.

dipyridamole (dy-py-**rid**-ă-mohl) *n.* a drug that dilates the blood vessels of the heart. It is used to treat reduced heart activity and is given by mouth or injection.

director (di-**rek**-ter) *n.* an instrument used to guide the extent and direction of a surgical incision.

dis- *prefix denoting* separation.

Disabled Living Foundation (dis-ay-**bŭld**) *n.* (in Britain) a voluntary agency interested in all aspects of the care of those with handicaps and in improving their quality of life.

disabled person *n.* a person suffering from some handicap that prevents the performance of some activity.

Disablement Resettlement Officer (dis-**ay**-bŭl-měnt) *n.* a member of the Employment Service Division who assists handicapped people in finding and keeping suitable employment.

disaccharide (dy-**sak**-ă-ryd) *n.* a carbohydrate consisting of two linked monosaccharide units. The most common disaccharides are maltose, lactose, and sucrose.

disarticulation (dis-ar-tik-yoo-lay-shŏn) *n.* separation of two bones at a joint. This may be the result of an injury or it may be done by the surgeon at operation in the course of amputation.

disc (disk) *n.* (in anatomy) a rounded flattened structure, such as an intervertebral disc or the optic disc.

discharge rate (**dis**-charj) *n.* the number of cases of a specified disease discharged from hospitals related to the population of the catchment area: usually expressed regionally per 10,000.

discission (dis-si*z*h-ŏn) *n.* an operation for cataract in which the front of the lens capsule is cut extensively by a fine knife or needle inserted through the edge of the cornea. Subsequently the lens is absorbed naturally into the surrounding fluid of the eye.

discrete (dis-**kreet**) *adj.* composed of several parts: describing lesions that are separate and do not run into each other.

disease (di-**zeez**) *n.* a disorder with a specific cause and recognizable signs and symptoms; any bodily abnormality or failure to function properly, except that resulting directly from physical injury (the latter, however, may open the way for disease).

disimpaction (dis-im-**pak**-shŏn) *n.* the process of separating the broken ends of a bone when they have been forcibly driven together during a fracture.

disinfectant (dis-in-fek-tănt) *n.* an agent that destroys or removes bacteria and other microorganisms and is used to cleanse surgical instruments and other objects. Examples are cresol, hexachlorophane, and phenol.

disinfection (dis-in-**fek**-shŏn) *n.* the process of eliminating infective microorganisms from contaminated instruments, clothing, or surroundings by using physical means or chemicals (disinfectants).

disinfestation (dis-in-fes-**tay**-shŏn) *n.* the destruction of insect pests and other animal parasites. This generally involves the use of insecticides.

dislocation (luxation) (dis-lŏ-**kay**-shŏn) *n.* displacement from their normal position of bones meeting at a joint. The bones are restored to their normal positions by manipulation, which may require local or general anaesthesia (*see* reduction). *Compare* subluxation.

disopyramide (dy-soh-**py**-ră-myd) *n.* a parasympatholytic drug administered by mouth to treat various heart conditions involving abnormal heart rates. Trade names: **Norpace**, **Rythmodan**.

disorientation (dis-or-i-ĕn-**tay**-shŏn) *n.* the state produced by loss of awareness of space, time, or personality. It can be the result of drugs, anxiety, or organic disease (such as dementia or Korsakoff's syndrome).

dispensary (dis-**pen**-ser-i) *n.* a place where medicines are made up by a pharmacist according to the doctor's prescription and dispensed to patients.

dissection (dis-**sek**-shŏn) *n.* the cutting apart and separation of the body tissues along the natural divisions of the organs and different tissues in the course of an operation. Dissection of corpses is carried out for the study of anatomy.

disseminated (dis-**sem**-in-ayt-id) *adj.* widely distributed in an organ (or organs) or in the whole body. The term may refer to disease organisms or to pathological changes.

disseminated sclerosis *n. see* multiple sclerosis.

dissociation (dis-soh-si-**ay**-shŏn) *n.* (in psychiatry) the process whereby thoughts and ideas can be split off from consciousness and may function independently, allowing conflicting opinions to be held at the same time about the same object. Dissociation may be the main factor in cases of hysterical fugue and multiple personalities.

distal (**dis**-t'l) *adj.* (in anatomy) situated away from the origin or point of attachment or from the median line of the body. *Compare* proximal.

distichiasis (dis-ti-**ky**-ă-sis) *n.* a very rare condition in which there is an extra row of eyelashes behind the normal ones. They may rub on the cornea.

district nurse (**dis**-trikt) *see* home nurse.

disulfiram (dy-**sul**-fi-ram) *n.* a drug administered by mouth in the treatment of chronic alcoholism. It acts as a deterrent by producing unpleasant effects, such as headache, nausea, and vomiting, when taken with alcohol. Trade name: **Antabuse**.

dithranol (**dith**-ră-nol) *n.* a drug applied to the skin as an ointment or paste to treat ringworm infections, psoriasis, and other skin conditions. It may irritate the skin on application.

diuresis (dy-yoor-**ee**-sis) *n.* increased secretion of urine by the kidneys. This normally follows the drinking of more fluid than the body requires, but it can be stimulated by the administration of a diuretic.

diuretic (dy-yoor-et-ik) *n.* a drug, such as chlorothiazide, frusemide, or triamterene, that increases the volume of urine produced by promoting the excretion of salts and water from the kidney. Diuretics are used in the treatment of oedema, high blood pressure, and glaucoma.

diurnal (dy-**ern**-ăl) *adj.* occurring during the day.

divaricator (dy-va-ri-kay-ter) *n.* **1.** a hinged wooden splint used for correcting congenital dislocation of the hip. **2.** a scissor-like surgical instrument used to divide portions of tissue into two separate parts during an operation.

diverticular disease (dy-ver-tik-yoo-ler) *n.* a condition in which there are diverticula (*see* diverticulum) in the colon associated with lower abdominal pain and disturbed bowel habit. The pain is due to spasm of the muscles of the intestine and not to inflammation of the diverticula (*compare* diverticulitis).

diverticulitis (dy-ver-tik-yoo-ly-tis) *n.* inflammation of a diverticulum, most commonly of one or more colonic diverticula. This type of diverticulitis is caused by infection and causes lower abdominal pain with diarrhoea or constipation. A Meckel's diverticulum sometimes becomes inflamed due to infection, causing symptoms similar to appendicitis. *Compare* diverticular disease.

diverticulosis (dy-ver-tik-yoo-loh-sis) *n.* a condition in which diverticula exist in a segment of the intestine without evidence of inflammation (*compare* diverticulitis).

diverticulum (dy-ver-tik-yoo-lŭm)

n. (*pl.* **diverticula**) a sac or pouch formed at weak points in the walls of the alimentary tract. *colonic d.* a diverticulum that affects the colon. They are sometimes associated with abdominal pain or altered bowel habit (*see* diverticular disease, diverticulitis). *jejunal d.* a diverticulum that affects the small intestine. They are often multiple and may give rise to abdominal discomfort and malabsorption. *Meckel's d.* a diverticulum that occurs in the ileum as a congenital abnormality. It may become inflamed, mimicking appendicitis, or it may form a peptic ulcer, causing pain, bleeding, or perforation.

division (di-**vizh**-ŏn) *n.* the separation of an organ or tissue into parts by surgery.

divulsor (dy-**vul**-ser) *n.* a surgical instrument used to dilate forcibly any canal or cavity, usually the urethra.

dizygotic twins (dy-zy-**got**-ik) *pl.* *n.* *see* twins.

DNA (deoxyribonucleic acid) *n.* the genetic material of nearly all living organisms, which controls heredity and is located in the cell nucleus (*see* chromosome, gene). DNA is a nucleic acid composed of two strands made up of units called nucleotides, wound around each other into a double helix. The DNA molecule can make exact copies of itself by the process of replication, thereby passing on the genetic information to the daughter cells when the cell divides.

Doctor (**dok**-ter) *n.* **1.** the title given to a recipient of a higher university degree than a Master's degree. The degree *Medicinae Doctor* (MD) is awarded by some British universities as a research degree. **2.** a courtesy title given to a qualified medical practitioner, i.e. one who has been registered by the General Medical Council.

Döderlein's bacillus (ded-er-lynz) *n.* the bacterium *Lactobacillus acidophilus*, occurring normally in the vagina and its secretions. *See* Lactobacillus. [A. S. G. Döderlein (1860–1941), German obstetrician and gynaecologist]

dolich- (dolicho-) *prefix denoting* long.

dolichocephaly (doli-koh-sef-ăli) *n.* the condition of having a relatively long skull, with a cephalic index of 75 or less. —**dolichocephalic** *adj.*

dolor (dol-er) *n.* pain: one of the four classical signs of inflammation in a tissue. *See also* calor, rubor, tumor.

dolorimetry (dol-er-im-itri) *n.* the measurement of pain. *See* algesimeter.

domiciliary midwife (dom-i-sil-yer-i) *n.* (in Britain) a State Registered Nurse with special training in midwifery (both hospital and domiciliary practice).

domiciliary services *pl. n.* (in Britain) health and social services that are available in the home and are distinguished from hospital-based services.

dominant (dom-i-nănt) *adj.* (in genetics) describing a gene (or its corresponding characteristic) whose effect is shown in the individual whether its allele is the same or different. *Compare* recessive. —**dominant** *n.*

domiphen (doh-mi-fen) *n.* an antiseptic administered in the form of lozenges to treat bacterial and fungal infections of the mouth and throat. It is also used in so-lution for cleansing wounds, treating fungal infections of the skin, etc.

donor (doh-ner) *n.* a person who makes his own tissues or organs available for use by someone else. For example, a donor may provide blood for transfusion or a kidney for transplantation.

dopa (doh-pă) *n.* dihydroxyphenylalanine: a physiologically important compound that forms an intermediate stage in the synthesis of catecholamines from the essential amino acid tyrosine. The form L-dopa is administered for the treatment of parkinsonism.

dopamine (doh-pă-meen) *n.* a catecholamine derived from dopa that is an intermediate in the synthesis of noradrenaline. It is found in high concentrations in the adrenal medulla and is also in the caudate nucleus (*see* basal ganglia), where it may function as a neurotransmitter.

dors- (dorsi-, dorso-) *prefix denoting* **1.** the back. **2.** dorsal.

dorsal (dor-săl) *adj.* relating to or situated at or close to the back of the body or to the posterior part of an organ.

dorsiflexion (dor-si-flek-shŏn) *n.* backward flexion of the foot or hand or their digits; i.e. bending towards the upper surface.

dorsoventral (dor-soh-ven-trăl) *adj.* (in anatomy) extending from the back (dorsal) surface to the front (ventral) surface.

dorsum (dor-sŭm) *n.* **1.** the back. **2.** the upper or posterior surface of a part of the body.

dose (dohs) *n.* a carefully measured quantity of a drug that is prescribed by a doctor to be given to a patient at any one time.

dosimetry (doh-**sim**-itri) *n.* the calculation of appropriate doses for given conditions, usually the calculation of correct amounts of radiation for the treatment of cancer in different parts of the body. *See* radiotherapy.

double vision (**dub**-ŭl) *n. see* diplopia.

douche (doosh) *n.* a forceful jet of water used for cleaning any part of the body, most commonly the vagina.

Down's syndrome (downz) *n.* a form of mental subnormality due to a chromosome defect (there are three no. 21 chromosomes instead of the usual two). The main physical features include a slightly oblique slant to the eyes, as in the Mongolian races (hence the former name of this condition – *mongolism*); a round head; flat nasal bridge; and short stature. The ultimate mental attainment is about that of a five-year-old child, i.e. an IQ of 50 – 60. Medical name: **trisomy 21**. [J. L. H. Down (1828 – 96), British physician]

doxepin (**doks**-ĕ-pin) *n.* a drug administered by mouth to relieve depression, especially when associated with anxiety (*see* antidepressant, tranquillizer). Trade name: **Sinequan.**

doxorubicin (doks-oh-**roo**-bi-sin) *n.* an antibiotic isolated from *Streptomyces peucetius caesius* and used mainly in the treatment of leukaemia and various other forms of cancer. It is administered by injection or infusion; side-effects include bone marrow depression, baldness, gastrointestinal disturbances, and heart damage. Trade name: **Adriamycin.**

doxycycline (doks-i-sy-kleen) *n.* an antibiotic administered by mouth to treat infections caused by a wide range of bacteria and other microorganisms. Trade name: **Vibramycin.**

DPT vaccine *n.* a combined vaccine against diphtheria, whooping-cough, and tetanus organisms, prepared from their toxoids and other antigens.

dracontiasis (drak-on-ty-ă-sis) *n.* a tropical disease caused by the parasitic nematode *Dracunculus medinensis* (*see* guinea worm). The disease is transmitted to man via contaminated drinking water. The worm migrates to the skin surface and eventually forms a large blister, usually on the legs or arms, which bursts and may ulcerate and become infected.

Dracunculus (dra-**kunk**-yoo-lŭs) *n. see* guinea worm.

dragee (dra-**zhay**) *n.* a pill that has been coated with sugar.

drain (drayn) **1.** *n.* a device, usually a tube or wick, used to draw fluid from an internal body cavity to the surface. **2.** *vb. see* drainage.

drainage (**drayn**-ij) *n.* the drawing off of fluid from a cavity in the body, usually fluid that has accumulated abnormally. *See also* drain.

drastic (**dras**-tik) *n.* any agent causing a major change in a body function.

draw-sheet (**draw**-sheet) *n.* a sheet placed beneath a patient in bed that may be pulled under the patient when one portion has been soiled or become uncomfortably wrinkled.

drepanocyte (sickle cell) (drep-ă-noh-syt) *n. see* sickle-cell disease.

drepanocytosis (drep-ă-noh-sy-toh-sis) *n. see* sickle-cell disease.

dressing (dres-ing) *n.* material applied to a wound or diseased part of the body, with or without medication, to give protection and assist healing.

drill (dril) *n.* (in dentistry) the instrument most commonly used for the removal of caries and for the drilling and cutting of bone in dental surgery.

drip (intravenous drip) (drip) *n.* apparatus for the continuous injection (transfusion) of blood, plasma, saline, glucose solution, or other fluid into a vein. The fluid flows under gravity from a suspended bottle through a tube ending in a hollow needle inserted into the patient's vein.

dropsy (drop-si) *n. see* oedema.

drostanolone (dros-tan-ŏ-lohn) *n.* a synthetic male sex hormone (*see* androgen) administered by injection in the treatment of breast cancer, often in conjunction with other drug treatment or surgery. Trade name: **Masteril**.

drug (drug) *n.* any substance that affects the structure or functioning of a living organism. Drugs are widely used for the prevention, diagnosis, and treatment of disease and for the relief of symptoms.

drug dependence *n. see* dependence.

Duchenne dystrophy (dew-shen) *n. see* muscular dystrophy. [G. B. A. Duchenne (1806–75), French neurologist]

Ducrey's bacillus (doo-krayz) *n.* the bacterium *Haemophilus ducreyi. See* Haemophilus. [A. Ducrey (1860–1940), Italian dermatologist]

duct (dukt) *n.* a tubelike structure or channel, especially one for carrying glandular secretions.

ductless gland (dukt-lis) *n. see* endocrine gland.

ductule (duk-tewl) *n.* a small duct or channel.

ductus arteriosus (duk-tŭs ar-teer-i-oh-sŭs) *n.* a blood vessel in the fetus connecting the pulmonary artery directly to the ascending aorta, so bypassing the pulmonary circulation. It normally closes after birth. *patent d. a.* failure of the ductus to close, producing a continuous murmur and consequences similar to those of a septal defect.

dumbness (dum-nis) *n. see* mutism.

Dumdum fever (dum-dum) *n. see* kala-azar.

dumping syndrome (dump-ing) *n.* a group of symptoms that sometimes occur after stomach operations, particularly gastrectomy. After a meal, especially one rich in carbohydrate, the patient feels faint and weak and may sweat and become pale.

duo- *prefix denoting* two.

duoden- (duodeno-) *prefix denoting* the duodenum.

duodenal ulcer (dew-ŏ-deen-ăl) *n.* an ulcer in the duodenum, caused by the action of acid and pepsin on the duodenal lining (mucosa) of a susceptible individual. Symptoms include pain in the upper abdomen and vomiting; complications include bleeding, perforation, and obstruction due to scarring.

duodenostomy (dew-ŏ-di-nost-ŏmi) *n.* an operation in which the duodenum is brought through the abdominal wall and opened, usually in order to introduce food. *See also* gastroduodenostomy.

duodenum (dew-ŏ-deen-ŭm) *n.* the first of the three parts of the small intestine. It extends from the pylorus of the stomach to the jejunum. The duodenum receives bile from the gall bladder and pancreatic juice from the pancreas. —**duodenal** *adj.*

Dupuytren's contracture (dew-pwee-**trahnz**) *n.* forward curvature of one or more fingers (usually the third and/or fourth) due to fixation of the flexor tendon of the affected finger to the skin of the palm. [Baron G. Dupuytren (1777–1835), French surgeon]

dura (**dura mater, pachymeninx**) (**dewr**-ă) *n.* the thickest and outermost of the three meninges surrounding the brain and spinal cord. —**dural** *adj.*

dwarfism (**dworf**-izm) *n.* abnormally short stature. The most common cause is achondroplasia. Dwarfism may also be caused by a deficiency of growth hormone due to a defect in the pituitary gland; a genetic defect in the response to growth hormone; thyroid deficiency (*see* cretinism); chronic diseases such as rickets; renal failure; and intestinal malabsorption.

dydrogesterone (dy-droh-**jest**-er-ohn) *n.* a synthetic female sex hormone (*see* progestogen) administered by mouth to treat menstrual abnormalities (such as dysmenorrhoea) and infertility and to prevent miscarriage. Trade name: **Duphaston**.

dynamometer (dy-nă-**mom**-it-er) *n.* a device for recording the force of a muscular contraction. A small hand-held dynamometer may be used to record the strength of a patient's grip.

-dynia *suffix denoting* pain.

dys- *prefix denoting* difficult, abnormal, or impaired.

dysaesthesiae (dis-iss-**theez**-i-ee) *pl. n.* the abnormal and sometimes unpleasant sensations felt by a patient with partial damage to a peripheral nerve when his skin is touched. *Compare* paraesthesiae.

dysarthria (dis-**arth**-riă) *n.* a speech disorder in which the pronunciation is unclear although the linguistic content and meaning are normal.

dysbarism (dis-bar-izm) *n.* any clinical syndrome due to a difference between the atmospheric pressure outside the body and the pressure of air or gas within a body cavity. *See* compressed air illness.

dyschezia (dis-**kee**-ziă) *n.* a form of constipation resulting from a long period of voluntary suppression of the urge to defecate. The rectum becomes distended with faeces and bowel movements are difficult or painful.

dyschondroplasia (dis-kon-droh-**play**-ziă) *n.* a condition due to faulty ossification of cartilage, resulting in development of many benign cartilaginous tumours (*see* chondroma). The bones involved may become stunted and deformed.

dyscoria (dis-**kor**-iă) *n.* abnormality in the shape or form of the pupil of the eye.

dyscrasia (dis-**kray**-ziă) *n.* an abnormal state of the body or part of the body, especially one due to abnormal development or metabolism.

dysdiadochokinesis (**adia-dochokinesis**) (dis-dy-ad-ŏ-koh-ki-nee-sis) *n.* clumsiness in performing rapidly alternating movements. It is a sign of disease of the cerebellum.

dysentery (**dis**-ĕn-tri) *n.* an infection of the intestinal tract causing severe diarrhoea with blood and mucus. *amoebic d.* (*amoebiasis*) dysentery caused by the protozoan *Entamoeba histolytica*. It is mainly confined to tropical and subtropical countries. *bacillary d.* dysentery caused by bacteria of the genus *Shigella*. Epidemics are common in overcrowded insanitary conditions. *Compare* cholera.

dysfunction (dis-**funk**-shŏn) *n.* impairment or abnormality in the functioning of an organ.

dysgenesis (dis-**jen**-i-sis) *n.* faulty development.

dysgerminoma (germinoma, gonocytoma) (dis-jer-mi-**noh**-mă) *n.* a malignant tumour of the ovary, thought to arise from primitive germ cells; it is homologous to the seminoma of the testis. The tumours are very sensitive to radiotherapy. Dysgerminomas are also known as *large cell carcinomas* or *alveolar sarcomas of the ovary*.

dysgraphia (dis-**graf**-iă) *n. see* agraphia.

dysidrosis (dyshidrosis) (dis-i-**droh**-sis) *n.* any abnormality of sweating or the sweat glands other than hyperidrosis, hypoidrosis, or anidrosis; for example, changes in the colour or smell of sweat.

dyskinesia (dis-ki-**nee**-ziă) *n.* a group of involuntary movements, including chorea and dystonia, that appear to be a fragmentation of the normal smoothly controlled limb and facial movements.

dyslalia (dis-**lay**-liă) *n.* a speech disorder in which the patient uses a vocabulary or range of sounds that is peculiar to him.

dyslexia (dis-**leks**-ia) *n.* a developmental disorder selectively affecting a child's ability to learn to read and write. It is sometimes called *specific d.* or *developmental d.* to distinguish it from acquired difficulties with reading and writing. *Compare* alexia. —**dyslexic** *adj.*

dyslogia (dis-**loh**-jiă) *n.* disturbed and incoherent speech. This may be due to dementia, aphasia, subnormality, or mental illness.

dysmenorrhoea (dis-men-ŏ-**ree**-ă) *n.* painful or difficult menstruation. *primary* (*essential*) *d.* dysmenorrhoea that begins with the first period and has no apparent cause. *secondary d.* dysmenorrhoea that is experienced at some stage following the establishment of normal periods, for reasons including inflammation of the womb lining or blockage of the blood flow.

dyspareunia (dis-pă-**roo**-niă) *n.* painful or difficult sexual intercourse experienced by a woman. Psychological or physical factors may be responsible (*see* vaginismus).

dyspepsia (indigestion) (dis-**pep**-siă) *n.* disordered digestion: usually applied to pain or discomfort in the lower chest or abdomen after eating and sometimes accompanied by nausea or vomiting. —**dyspeptic** *adj.*

dysphagia (dis-**fay**-jiă) *n.* a condition in which the action of swallowing is either difficult to perform, painful (*see* odynophagia), or in which swallowed material seems to be held up in its passage to the stomach.

dysphasia (dis-**fay**-ziă) *n. see* aphasia.

dysphemia (dis-**fee**-miă) *n. see* stammering.

dysphonia (dis-**foh**-niă) *n.* difficulty in speaking due to a disorder of the larynx, vocal cords, tongue, or mouth. *Compare* dysarthria, aphasia.

dysplasia (**alloplasia, heteroplasia**) (dis-**play**-ziă) *n.* abnormal development of skin, bone, or other tissues.

dyspnoea (disp-**nee**-ă) *n.* laboured or difficult breathing. Dyspnoea can be due to obstruction to the flow of air into and out of the lungs (as in bronchitis and asthma), various diseases affecting the tissue of the lung, or heart disease.

dyspraxia (dis-**praks**-iă) *n. see* apraxia.

dysrhythmia (dis-**rith**-miă) *n.* abnormality in a rhythm, such as the rhythm of speech or of brain waves as recorded on an EEG.

dyssynergia (**asynergia**) (dis-sin-er-jiă) *n.* clumsily uncoordinated movements found in patients with disease of the cerebellum.

dystocia (dis-**toh**-siă) *n.* difficult birth. It may be caused by abnormalities in the fetus (*fetal d.*), such as excessive size or malpresentation, or by abnormalities in the mother (*maternal d.*), such as an abnormally small pelvis or failure of the womb muscles to contract.

dystonia (dis-**toh**-niă) *n.* a postural disorder caused by disease of the basal ganglia in the brain. There is spasm in the muscles of the shoulders, neck, and trunk. The arm is often held in a rotated position and the head is drawn back and to one side.

dystrophia adiposogenitalis (dis-**troh**-fiă adi-poh-soh-jen-i-**tahl**-iss) *n. see* Fröhlich's syndrome.

dystrophia myotonica (my-ŏ-**ton**-ikă) *n.* a type of muscular dystrophy in which the muscle weakness and wasting is accompanied by an unnatural prolongation of the muscular contraction after any voluntary effort (*see* myotonia). The disease can affect both sexes (it is inherited as an autosomal dominant character) and appears in early middle age.

dystrophy (**dystrophia**) (**dis**-trŏ-fi) *n.* a disorder of an organ or tissue, usually muscle, due to impaired nourishment of the affected part. *See also* muscular dystrophy.

dysuria (dis-**yoor**-iă) *n.* difficult or painful urination. This is usually associated with urgency and frequency of urination if due to cystitis or urethritis.

E

ear (eer) *n.* the sense organ concerned with hearing and balance. Sound waves, transmitted from the outside into the external auditory meatus, cause the eardrum (tympanic membrane) to vibrate. The small bones (ossicles) of the middle ear – the malleus, incus, and stapes – transmit the sound vibrations to the fenestra ovalis, which leads to the inner ear (*see* labyrinth). Inside the cochlea the sound vibrations are converted into nerve impulses. Pressure within the ear is released through the Eustachian tube. The semicircular canals, saccule, and utricle – also in the inner ear – are all concerned with balance.

Structure of the ear

earache (**eer**-ayk) *n. see* otitis, otalgia.

eardrum (**eer**-drum) *n. see* tympanic membrane.

earwax (**eer**-waks) *n. see* cerumen.

eburnation (ee-ber-**nay**-shŏn) *n.* the wearing down of the cartilage at the articulating surface of a bone, exposing the underlying bone. This is an end result of osteoarthritis.

ec- *prefix denoting* out of or outside.

ecbolic (ek-**bol**-ik) *n.* an agent, such as oxytocin, that induces childbirth by stimulating contractions of the womb.

ecchondroma (ek-kon-**droh**-mă) *n.* (*pl.* **ecchondromata**) a benign cartilaginous tumour (*see* chondroma) that protrudes beyond the margins of a bone. *Compare* enchondroma.

ecchymosis (eki-**moh**-sis) *n.* a bruise: an initially bluish-black mark on the skin, resulting from

the release of blood into the tissues either through injury or through the spontaneous leaking of blood from the vessels.

eccrine (**ek**-ryn) *adj.* describing sweat glands that are distributed all over the body. They are densest on the soles of the feet and the palms of the hands. *Compare* apocrine.

eccyesis (ek-sy-**ee**-sis) *n. see* ectopic pregnancy.

ecdysis (ek-**dy**-sis) *n.* the act of shedding skin; desquamation.

ECG *n. see* electrocardiogram.

echinococciasis (**echinococcosis**) (i-ky-noh-kŏ-ky-ă-sis) *n. see* hydatid disease.

Echinococcus (i-ky-nŏ-kok-ŭs) *n.* a genus of small parasitic tapeworms. Adults are found in the intestines of dogs, wolves, or jackals. If the eggs are swallowed by man, the resulting larvae may cause hydatid disease. Two species causing this condition are

E. granulosus and *E. multilocularis.*

echocardiography (ek-oh-kar-di-og-răfi) *n.* the use of ultrasound waves to investigate and display the action of the heart as it beats.

echoencephalography (ek-oh-en-sef-ă-log-răfi) *n.* investigation of structures within the skull by detecting the echoes of ultrasonic pulses.

echography (ek-og-răfi) *n.* the technique of using ultrasound waves to map out and study the internal structure of the body. *See also* ultrasonics.

echokinesis (ek-oh-ki-nee-sis) *n. see* echopraxia.

echolalia (ek-oh-lay-liă) *n.* pathological repetition of the words spoken by another person. It may be a symptom of language disorders, autism, catatonia, or Gilles de la Tourette syndrome.

echopraxia (echokinesis) (ek-oh-praks-iă) *n.* pathological imitation of the actions of another person. It may be a symptom of catatonia.

echotomography (ek-oh-tŏ-mog-răfi) *n. see* ultrasonotomography.

echovirus (ek-oh-vy-rŭs) *n.* one of a group of about 30 RNA-containing viruses originally isolated from the human intestinal tract. These viruses were termed *enteric cytopathic human orphan* viruses and are now thought to be the cause of nonspecific meningitis and many gastrointestinal and respiratory tract infections. *Compare* reovirus.

eclabium (ek-lay-biŭm) *n.* the turning outward of a lip.

eclampsia (i-klamp-siă) *n.* a rare and serious condition, affecting women either at the end of preg-

nancy or shortly after childbirth, in which the whole body is affected by convulsions and the patient eventually passes into a coma. It represents an advanced stage of toxaemia of pregnancy and can be prevented by regular antenatal examinations.

ecmnesia (ek-nee-ziă) *n.* loss of memory for recent events that does not extend to more remote ones: a common symptom of old age.

ecology (bionomics) (ee-kol-ŏji) *n.* the study of the relationships between man, plants and animals, and the environment. **—ecological** *adj.* **—ecologist** *n.*

écraseur (ay-kra-zer) *n.* a surgical device, resembling a snare, that is used to sever the base of a tumour during its surgical removal.

ecstasy (ek-stă-si) *n.* a sense of extreme well-being and bliss. While not necessarily pathological, it can be caused by epilepsy (especially of the temporal lobe) or by schizophrenia.

ECT *n. see* electroconvulsive therapy.

ect- (ecto-) *prefix denoting* outer or external.

ectasia (ectasis) (ek-tay-ziă) *n.* the dilatation of a tube, duct, or hollow organ.

ecthyma (ek-th'y-mă) *n.* a skin disease – an ulcerative type of impetigo – in which the infection spreads down to the lower layer of the skin (dermis) and causes scarring.

ectoderm (ek-toh-derm) *n.* the outer of the three germ layers of the early embryo. It gives rise to the nervous system and sense organs, the teeth and lining of the mouth, and the epidermis and its associated structures (hair, nails, etc.). **—ectodermal** *adj.*

ectomorphic (ek-toh-**mor**-fik) *adj.*
describing a body type that is
relatively thin, with a large skin
surface in comparison to weight.
—**ectomorph** *n.* —**ectomorphy** *n.*

-ectomy *suffix denoting* surgical removal of a segment or all of an
organ or part.

ectoparasite (ek-toh-**pa**-ră-syt) *n.* a
parasite that lives on the outer
surface of its host. *Compare* endoparasite.

ectopia (ek-**toh**-piă) *n.* **1.** the misplacement, due either to a congenital defect or injury, of a
bodily part. **2.** the occurrence of
something in an unnatural location (*see* ectopic beat, ectopic
pregnancy). —**ectopic** (ek-**top**-ik)
adj.

ectopic beat (**extrasystole**) *n.* a
heart beat due to an impulse
generated somewhere in the heart
outside the sinoatrial node. They
may be produced by any heart
disease, by nicotine from smoking, or by caffeine from excessive tea or coffee consumption;
they are common in normal individuals. *See* arrhythmia.

**ectopic pregnancy (extrauterine
pregnancy)** *n.* the development of
a fetus at a site other than in
the womb. The most common
type of ectopic pregnancy occurs in Fallopian tubes that become blocked or inflamed (*tubal*
or *oviducal pregnancy*). The
growth of the fetus may cause
the tube to burst and bleed. In
most cases the fetus dies within
three months of conception.
Medical name: **eccyesis.**

ectro- *prefix denoting* congenital
absence.

ectrodactyly (ek-troh-**dak**-ti-li) *n.*
congenital absence of all or part
of one or more fingers.

ectromelia (ek-troh-**mee**-liă) *n.*
congenital absence or gross
shortening (aplasia) of the long
bones of one or more limbs. *See
also* amelia, hemimelia, phocomelia.

ectropion (ek-**troh**-pi-ŏn) *n.* turning
out of the eyelid, away from the
eyeball.

eczema (**eks**-imă) *n.* a superficial
inflammation of the skin,
mainly affecting the epidermis.
Eczema causes itching, with a
red rash often accompanied by
small blisters that weep and become crusted. *atopic e.* a type
of endogenous eczema commonly
found in childhood and sometimes associated with a family
history of allergy. *discoid e.* a
type of endogenous eczema characterized by small well-defined
areas of eczema. *endogenous e.*
eczema that occurs without any
obvious external cause. *seborrhoeic e.* a type of endogenous
eczema in which scaly plaques
occur in areas of the greatest sebum production. *varicose e.* a
type of endogenous eczema that
develops on the legs in association with poor circulation. *See
also* dermatitis, pompholyx.
—**eczematous** (eks-**em**-ă-tŭs) *adj.*

edentulous (ee-**den**-choo-lŭs) *adj.*
lacking teeth: usually applied to
people who have lost their teeth.

edrophonium (ed-roh-**foh**-niŭm) *n.*
a drug that stimulates the
skeletal muscles (*see*
parasympathomimetic). It is administered by injection in a test
for diagnosis of myasthenia
gravis. Trade name: **Tensilon.**

EDTA (ethylenediamine tetraacetic acid) *n.* a compound used
as a chelating agent in the treatment of poisoning with several
different metals, such as lead
and strontium.

EEG (electroencephalogram) *n. see* electroencephalography.

effector (i-**fek**-ter) *n.* any structure or agent that brings about activity in a muscle or gland. The term is also used for the muscle or gland itself.

efferent (**ef**-er-ĕnt) *adj.* **1.** designating nerves or neurones that convey impulses from the brain or spinal cord to muscles, glands, and other effectors. **2.** designating vessels or ducts that drain fluid from an organ or part. *Compare* afferent.

effleurage (ef-ler-**ahz***h*) *n.* a form of massage in which the hands are passed continuously and rhythmically over a patient's skin in one direction only, with the aim of increasing blood flow in that direction and aiding the dispersal of any swelling due to oedema.

effort syndrome (**ef**-ert) *n.* a condition of marked anxiety about the condition of one's heart and circulatory system. This is accompanied by a heightened consciousness of heartbeat and respiration, which in turn is worsened by the anxiety it induces.

effusion (i-**few**-*zh*ŏn) *n.* **1.** the escape of pus, serum, blood, lymph, or other fluid into a body cavity. **2.** fluid that has escaped into a body cavity.

egg cell (eg) *n. see* ovum.

ego (**eg**-oh) *n.* (in psychoanalysis) the part of the mind that develops from a person's experience of the outside world and is most in touch with external realities.

Ehrlich's theory (**air**-liks) *n.* an early theory of antibody production, postulating that receptor groups with side chains were carried on cells and combined with antigens. The receptors were then thrown off the cell and became antibodies in the circulation. [P. Ehrlich (1854–1915), German bacteriologist]

eidetic (I-**det**-ik) *adj. see* imagery.

Eisenmenger reaction (I-zĕn-**meng**-er) *n.* a condition in which pulmonary hypertension is associated with a septal defect, so that blood flows from the right to the left side of the heart or from the pulmonary artery to the aorta. Oxygen-depleted blood enters the general circulation, resulting in cyanosis and polycythaemia. [V. Eisenmenger (1864–1932), German physician]

ejaculation (i-jak-yoo-**lay**-shŏn) *n.* the discharge of semen from the erect penis at the moment of sexual climax (orgasm) in the male.

elastic cartilage (i-**last**-ik) *n. see* cartilage.

elastic tissue *n.* strong extensible flexible connective tissue rich in yellow *elastic fibres.* Elastic tissue is found in the dermis of the skin, in arterial walls, and in the walls of the alveoli of the lungs.

elastin (i-**last**-in) *n.* protein forming the major constituent of elastic tissue fibres.

elation (exaltation) (i-**lay**-shŏn) *n.* a state of cheerful excitement and enthusiasm. Marked elation of mood is a characteristic of mania or hypomania.

elbow (**el**-boh) *n.* the joint in the arm formed between the ulna and part of the radius and the humerus.

Electra complex (i-**lek**-tră) *n.* the unconscious sexual feelings of a girl for her father, accompanied by aggressive feelings for her mother. *Compare* Oedipus complex.

P wave due to atrial contraction
Q,R, and T waves due to ventricular activity

Typical electrocardiograms

electrocardiogram (ECG) (i-lek-troh-**kar**-di-oh-gram) *n.* a recording of the electrical activity of the heart on a moving paper strip. The ECG tracing is recorded by means of an electrocardiograph (*see* electrocardiography). It aids in the diagnosis of heart disease, which may produce characteristic changes in the ECG.

electrocardiography (i-lek-troh-kar-di-**og**-răfi) *n.* a technique for recording the electrical activity of the heart. Electrodes connected to the recording apparatus (*electrocardiograph*) are placed on the skin of the four limbs and chest wall; the record itself is called an electrocardiogram (ECG).

electrocardiophonography (i-lek-troh-kar-di-oh-fŏ-**nog**-răfi) *n.* a technique for recording heart sounds and murmurs simultaneously with the ECG. The sound is picked up by a microphone placed over the heart. The tracing is a *phonocardiogram*.

electrocautery (galvanocautery) (i-lek-troh-**kaw**-ter-i) *n.* the destruction of diseased or unwanted tissue by means of a needle or snare that is electrically heated (*see* diathermy).

electrocoagulation (i-lek-troh-koh-ag-yoo-**lay**-shŏn) *n.* the coagulation of tissues by means of a high-frequency electric current concentrated at one point as it passes through them.

electroconvulsive therapy (ECT, electroplexy) (i-lek-troh-kŏn-**vul**-siv) *n.* a treatment for severe depression and occasionally for schizophrenia and mania. A convulsion is produced by passing an electric current through the brain; it is modified by giving a muscle relaxant drug and an anaesthetic.

electrode (i-lek-trohd) *n.* any part of an electrical conductor or recording device that is used to apply electric current to a part of the body or collect electrical activity (e.g. from the heart or brain).

electrodesiccation (i-lek-troh-dess-i-kay-shŏn) *n. see* fulguration.

electroencephalogram (EEG) (i-lek-troh-en-**sef**-ă-lŏ-gram) *n. see* electroencephalography.

elcctroencephalography (i-lek-troh-en-sef-ă-**log**-răfi) *n.* the technique for recording the electrical activity from different parts of the brain and converting it into a tracing called an *electroencephalogram* (*EEG*). The machine that records this activity is known as an *encephalograph*. Electroencephalography is used to detect and locate structural disease, such as tumours, in the brain; it is also used in the diagnosis and management of epilepsy.

electrolysis (i-lek-**trol**-i-sis) *n.* **1.** the chemical decomposition of a substance (*see* electrolyte) into positively and negatively charged ions (*see* anion, cation) when an electric current is passed through it. **2.** destruction of tissue, especially hair follicles (*see* epilation), by the passage of an electric current.

electrolyte (i-**lek**-trŏ-lyt) *n.* a solution that produces ions; for example, sodium chloride solution consists of free sodium and free chloride ions. In medical usage electrolyte usually means the ion itself; thus the *serum electrolyte level* is the concentration of separate ions (sodium, potassium, chloride, bicarbonate, etc.) in the circulating blood.

electromyography (i-lek-troh-my-og-răfi) *n.* continuous recording of the electrical activity of a muscle by means of electrodes inserted into the muscle fibres. The tracing is displayed on an oscilloscope.

electron (i-**lek**-tron) *n.* a negatively charged particle in an atom, one or more of which orbit around the positively charged nucleus of the atom.

electron microscope *n.* a microscope that uses a beam of electrons as a radiation source for viewing the specimen. The resolving power (ability to register fine detail) is a thousand times greater than that of an ordinary light microscope.

electrooculography (i-lek-troh-ok-yoo-**log**-răfi) *n.* an electrical method of recording eye movements by means of tiny electrodes attached to the skin at the inner and outer corners of the eye.

electroplexy (i-**lek**-troh-pleks-i) *n.* *see* electroconvulsive therapy.

electroretinography (i-lek-troh-ret-in-**og**-răfi) *n.* a method of recording changes in the electrical potential of the retina when it is stimulated by light. One electrode is placed on the eye in a contact lens and the other is usually attached to the back of the head.

electrotherapy (i-lek-troh-**th'e**-ră-pi) *n.* the passage of electric currents through the body's tissues to stimulate the functioning of nerves and the muscles that they supply. *See also* faradism, galvanism.

electuary (i-**lek**-tew-er-i) *n.* a pharmaceutical preparation in which the drug is made up into a paste with syrup or honey.

element (**el**-i-měnt) *n.* a substance, such as carbon, nitrogen, or oxygen, that cannot be decomposed into simpler substances. All the atoms of an element have the same number of protons. *See also* isotope.

elephantiasis (el-i-făn-**ty**-ă-sis) *n.* gross enlargement of the skin and underlying connective tissues caused by obstruction of the lymph vessels. Obstruction is commonly caused by the parasitic filarial worms *Wuchereria bancrofti* and *Brugia malayi*. The parts most commonly affected are the legs but the scrotum, breasts, and vulva may also be involved. *See also* filariasis.

elevator (el-i-vay-ter) *n.* **1.** an instrument that is used to raise a depressed broken bone. *periosteal e.* an instrument used in orthopaedics to strip the fibrous tissue (periosteum) covering bone. **2.** a lever-like instrument used to ease

a tooth out of its socket during extraction.

elimination (i-lim-i-**nay**-shŏn) *n.* (in physiology) the process of excretion of metabolic waste products from the blood by the kidneys and urinary tract.

elixir (i-**liks**-er) *n.* a preparation containing alcohol (ethanol) or glycerine, which is used as the vehicle for bitter or nauseous drugs.

elliptocytosis (i-lip-toh-sy-**toh**-sis) *n.* the presence of significant numbers of abnormal elliptical red cells (*elliptocytes*) in the blood.

em- *prefix. see* en-.

emaciation (i-may-si-**ay**-shŏn) *n.* wasting of the body, caused by such conditions as malnutrition or cancer.

emaculation (i-mak-yoo-**lay**-shŏn) *n.* the removal of spots, freckles, or similar marks from the skin, usually by surgery.

emasculation (i-mas-kew-**lay**-shŏn) *n.* strictly, surgical removal of the penis. The term is often used to mean loss of male characteristics, as a result of castration or emotional stress.

embalming (im-**bahm**-ing) *n.* the preservation of a dead body by the introduction of chemical compounds that delay putrefaction.

embolectomy (em-bŏ-**lek**-tŏmi) *n.* surgical removal of an embolus in order to relieve arterial obstruction.

embolism (em-**bŏl**-izm) *n.* the condition in which an embolus becomes lodged in an artery and obstructs its blood flow. Treatment is by anticoagulant therapy; major embolism is treated by embolectomy or streptokinase. *pulmonary e.* obstruction of the

amnion
fetal blood vessels
Fallopian tube
yolk sac
amniotic fluid
embryo

placenta
maternal blood vessels
chorion
cavity of uterus
umbilical cord
uterus lining
muscular wall of uterus
cervix

A developing embryo

pulmonary artery by an embolus, usually a blood clot derived from phlebothrombosis of the leg veins. Large emboli result in acute heart failure. *systemic e.* embolism affecting any artery except the pulmonary artery. The embolus is often a blood clot formed in the heart in mitral valve disease or following myocardial infarction. *See also* air embolism.

embolus (em-bŏ-lŭs) *n.* (*pl.* **emboli**) material, such as a blood clot, fat, air, amniotic fluid, or a foreign body, that is carried by the blood from one point in the circulation to lodge at another point (*see* embolism).

embrocation (em-broh-**kay**-shŏn) *n.* a lotion that is rubbed onto the body for the treatment of sprains.

embryo (em-bri-oh) *n.* an animal at an early stage of development, before birth. In man the term refers to the products of concep-

tion within the womb in the first eight weeks of development, during which time all the main organs are formed. *Compare* fetus. —**embryonic** (em-bri-**on**-ik) *adj.*

embryology (em-bri-**ol**-ŏji) *n.* the study of growth and development of the embryo and fetus from fertilization of the ovum until birth. —**embryological** *adj.*

embryotomy (em-bri-**ot**-ŏmi) *n.* the cutting up of a fetus during difficult birth by means of an instrument called an *embryotome*, in order to aid delivery and reduce the danger to the mother.

emesis (em-i-sis) *n. see* vomiting.

emetic (i-**met**-ik) *n.* an agent that causes vomiting, such as apomorphine, ipecacuanha, or common salt.

emetine (em-ĕ-teen) *n.* a drug administered by injection to treat infections of the liver, bowel, and intestine caused by amoebae, including amoebic dysentery.

eminence (**em**in-ĕns) *n.* a projection, often rounded, on an organ or tissue, particularly on a bone.

Emiscan (em-i-**skan**) *n.* trade name for computerized tomography: a development of diagnostic radiology for the examination of the soft tissues of the body. *See also* CT scanner.

emissary veins (**em**-iss-er-i) *pl. n.* a group of veins within the skull that drain blood from the venous sinuses of the dura mater to veins outside the skull.

emission (i-**mish**-ŏn) *n.* the flow of semen from the erect penis, usually occurring while the subject is asleep (*nocturnal e.*).

emmenagogue (i-**men**-ă-gog) *n.* an agent that stimulates menstruation.

emmetropia (em-i-**troh**-piă) *n.* the state of refraction of the normal eye, in which parallel light rays are brought to a focus on the retina with the accommodation relaxed. *Compare* ametropia, hypermetropia, myopia.

emollient (i-**mol**-iĕnt) *n.* an agent that soothes and softens the skin, such as lanolin or liquid paraffin. Emollients are used chiefly in skin preparations as a base for more active drugs, such as antibiotics.

emotion (i-**moh**-shŏn) *n.* a state of arousal that can be experienced as pleasant or unpleasant. Emotions can have three components: for example, fear can involve an unpleasant subjective experience, an increase in physiological measures such as heart rate, and a tendency to flee from the fear-provoking situation.

empathy (**em**-pă-thi) *n.* the ability to understand the thoughts and emotions of another person.

emphysema (em-fi-**see**-mă) *n.* air in the tissues. *pulmonary e.* emphysema in which the alveoli of the lungs are enlarged and damaged, which reduces the surface area for the exchange of oxygen and carbon dioxide. Severe emphysema causes breathlessness, which is made worse by infections. *surgical e.* emphysema in which air escapes into surrounding tissues through wounds or surgical incisions, usually into the tissues of the chest and neck from leaks in the lungs or oesophagus. Bacteria may form gas in soft tissues.

empirical (im-**pi**-ri-kăl) *adj.* describing a system of treatment based on experience or observation, rather than of logic or reason.

Employment Service Division (ESD) (im-**ploi**-mĕnt) *n.* an agency with responsibility for running public employment services, including the employment and training of the disabled.

empyema (pyothorax) (em-py-ee-mă) *n.* pus in the pleural cavity, usually secondary to infection in the lung or in the space below the diaphragm.

emulsion (i-**mul**-shŏn) *n.* a preparation in which fine droplets of one liquid (such as oil) are dispersed in another liquid (such as water). In pharmacy medicines are prepared in the form of emulsions to disguise the taste of an oil, which is dispersed in a flavoured liquid.

en- (em-) *prefix denoting* in; inside.

enamel (i-**nam**-ĕl) *n.* the insensitive and extremely hard outer covering of the crown of a tooth.

enanthema (en-an-**th'ee**-mă) *n.* an eruption occurring on a mucus-secreting surface, such as the inside of the mouth or vagina.

enarthrosis (en-arth-**roh**-sis) *n.* a ball-and-socket joint, e.g. the shoulder joint. Such a joint always involves a long bone, which is thus allowed to move in all planes.

encapsulated (in-**kaps**-yoo-layt-id) *adj.* (of an organ, tumour, etc.) enclosed in a capsule.

encephal- (encephalo-) *prefix denoting* the brain.

encephalin (enkephalin) (en-**sef**-ă-lin) *n.* either of two peptides occurring naturally in the brain and having effects resembling those of morphine or other opiates. *See also* endorphin.

encephalitis (en-sef-ă-**ly**-tis) *n.* inflammation of the brain. It may be caused by a viral or bacterial infection or it may be part of an allergic response to a systemic viral illness or vaccination (*see* encephalomyelitis). **e. lethargica** a form of viral encephalitis that is marked by headache and drowsiness, progressing to coma (hence its popular name – *sleepy sickness*). It can cause post-encephalitic parkinsonism.

encephalocele (en-**sef**-ă-loh-seel) *n.* protrusion of the brain through a defect in the bones of the skull. *See* neural tube defects.

encephalography (en-sef-ă-**log**-răfi) *n.* any of various techniques for recording the structure of the brain or the activity of the brain cells. *See* echoencephalography, electroencephalography, pneumoencephalography.

encephaloid (en-**sef**-ă-loid) *adj.* having the appearance of brain tissue: applied to certain tumours.

encephaloma (en-sef-ă-**loh**-mă) *n.* a brain tumour.

encephalomalacia (en-sef-ă-loh-mă-lay-shiă) *n.* softening of the brain.

encephalomyelitis (en-sef-ă-loh-my-ĕ-ly-tis) *n.* an acute inflammatory disease affecting the brain and spinal cord. *acute disseminated e.* a form of delayed tissue hypersensitivity provoked by a mild infection or vaccination 7–10 days earlier.

encephalomyelopathy (en-sef-ă-loh-my-ĕ-**lop**-ă-thi) *n.* any condition in which there is widespread disease of the brain and spinal cord.

encephalon (en-**sef**-ă-lon) *n. see* brain.

encephalopathy (en-sef-ă-**lop**-ă-thi) *n.* any of various diseases that affect the functioning of the brain. *See* hepatic (encephalopathy), Wernicke's encephalopathy.

enchondroma (en-kon-**droh**-mă) *n.* (*pl.* **enchondromata**) a benign cartilaginous tumour (*see* chondroma) occurring in the growing zone of a bone and not protruding beyond its margins. *Compare* ecchondroma.

encopresis (en-koh-**pree**-sis) *n.* incontinence of faeces. The term is used for faecal soiling associated with psychiatric disturbance.

encounter group (in-**kown**-ter) *n.* a form of group psychotherapy. The emphasis is on encouraging close relationships between group members and on the expression of feelings.

encysted (en-**sist**-id) *adj.* enclosed in a cyst.

end- (endo-) *prefix denoting* within or inner.

endarterectomy (end-ar-ter-ek-tŏmi) *n.* a surgical 're-bore' of an artery that has become obstructed by atheroma with or without a blood clot (thrombus); the former operation is known as *thromboendarterectomy*. The inner part of the wall is removed together with any clot that is present.

endarteritis (end-ar-ter-**I**-tis) *n.* chronic inflammation of the inner portion of the wall of an artery, which most often results from late syphilis. Thickening of the wall produces progressive arterial obstruction and symptoms from inadequate blood supply to the affected part.

end artery (end) *n.* the terminal branch of an artery, which does not communicate with other branches.

endaural (end-**or**-ăl) *adj.* within the ear, especially relating to the external auditory meatus of the outer ear.

endemic (en-**dem**-ik) *adj.* occurring frequently in a particular region or population: applied to diseases that are generally or constantly found among people in a particular area. *Compare* epidemic, pandemic.

endemic syphilis *n. see* bejel.

endemiology (en-dee-mi-ol-ŏji) *n.* the study of endemic disease.

endocarditis (en-doh-kar-**dy**-tis) *n.* inflammation of the endocardium and heart valves. It is most often due to rheumatic fever or bacterial infection (*bacterial e.*). The main features are fever, changing heart murmurs, heart failure, and embolism.

endocardium (en-doh-**kar**-diŭm) *n.* a delicate membrane that lines the heart and is continuous with the lining of arteries and veins. —**endocardial** *adj.*

endocervicitis (en-doh-ser-vi-sy-tis) *n.* inflammation of the membrane lining the neck of the womb, usually resulting from infection. The condition is accompanied by a white or yellow discharge.

endocervix (en-doh-**ser**-viks) *n.* the mucous membrane lining the cervix of the womb.

endochondral (en-doh-**kon**-drăl) *adj.* within the material of a cartilage.

endocrine gland (ductless gland) (**end**-oh-kryn) *n.* a gland that manufactures one or more hormones and secretes them directly into the bloodstream (and not through a duct to the exterior). Endocrine glands include the pituitary, thyroid, parathyroid, and adrenal glands, the ovary and testis, the placenta, and part of the pancreas.

endocrinology (en-doh-kri-**nol**-ŏji) *n.* the study of the endocrine glands and the hormones they secrete. —**endocrinologist** *n.*

endoderm (**end**-oh-derm) *n.* the inner of the three germ layers of the early embryo, which gives rise to the lining of most of the alimentary canal and its associated glands, the lining of the bronchi and alveoli of the lung, and most of the urinary tract.

endogenous (en-**doj**-in-ŭs) *adj.* arising within or derived from the body. *e. depression* depression arising from causes inside the body. *Compare* exogenous.

endolymph (**end**-oh-limf) *n.* the fluid that fills the membranous labyrinth of the ear.

endolysin (en-**dol**-i-sin) *n.* a substance within a cell that has a specific destructive action against bacteria.

endometriosis (en-doh-mee-tri-**oh**-sis) *n.* the presence of membranous material of the kind lining the womb (*see* endometrium) at other sites within the cavity of the pelvis.

endometritis (en-doh-mi-**try**-tis) *n.* inflammation of the endometrium. The condition, sometimes restricted to the neck of the womb, is a reaction to bacterial attack upon the membrane, possibly following physical damage.

endometrium (en-doh-**mee**-tri-ŭm) *n.* the mucous membrane lining the uterus. It becomes thicker and more vascular during the latter part of the menstrual cycle and much of it breaks down and is lost in menstruation. If pregnancy is established the endometrium becomes the decidua.

endomorphic (en-doh-**mor**-fik) *adj.* describing a body type that is relatively fat, with highly developed viscera and weak muscular and skeletal development. —**endomorph** *n.* —**endomorphy** *n.*

endomyocarditis (en-doh-my-oh-kar-**dy**-tis) *n.* an acute or chronic inflammatory disorder of the muscle and lining membrane of the heart. The principal causes are rheumatic fever and virus infections. There is enlargement of the heart, murmurs, embolism, and frequently arrhythmias.

endomysium (en-doh-**miz**-iŭm) *n.* the fine connective tissue sheath that surrounds a single muscle fibre.

endoneurium (en-doh-**newr**-iŭm) *n.* the layer of fibrous tissue that separates individual fibres within a nerve.

endoparasite (en-doh-**pa**-ră-syt) *n.* a parasite that lives inside its host, for example in the liver, lungs, gut, or other tissues of the body. *Compare* ectoparasite.

endophthalmitis (end-off-thal-**my**-tis) *n.* inflammation confined to the posterior chamber of the eye, i.e. the part behind the lens. *Compare* panophthalmitis.

endoplasmic reticulum (ER) (en-doh-**plaz**-mik) *n.* a system of membranes present in the cytoplasm of cells. It is the site of manufacture of proteins and lipids and is concerned with the transport of these products within the cell (*see also* Golgi apparatus).

end organ *n.* a specialized structure at the end of a peripheral nerve, such as the taste buds in the tongue, acting as a receptor for a particular sensation.

endorphin (en-**dor**-fin) *n.* one of a group of peptides that occur naturally in the brain and have pain-relieving properties similar to those of the opiates. *See also* encephalin.

endoscope (**end**-oh-skohp) *n.* any instrument, such as an auriscope or a gastroscope, used to obtain a view of the interior of the body. Most endoscopes consist of a tube with a light at the end and an optical system for transmitting an image to the examiner's eye. *See also* fibrescope. —**endoscopy** (en-**dos**-kŏ-pi) *n.*

endospore (**end**-oh-spor) *n.* the resting stage of certain bacteria, particularly species of the genera *Bacillus* and *Clostridium*.

endosteum (en-**dos**-tiŭm) *n.* the membrane that lines the marrow cavity of a bone.

endothelioma (en-doh-th'ee-li-oh-mă) *n.* any tumour arising from or resembling endothelium.

endothelium (en-doh-**th'ee**-li-um) *n.* the single layer of cells that lines the heart, blood vessels, and lymphatic vessels. It is derived from embryonic mesoderm. *Compare* epithelium.

endotoxin (en-doh-**toks**-in) *n.* a poison generally harmful to all body tissues, contained within a bacterium and released only when the bacterial cell is broken down or dies and disintegrates. *Compare* exotoxin.

endotracheal (en-doh-**tray**-ki-ăl) *adj.* within or through the trachea. *e. tube* a catheter inserted into the trachea to maintain a patent airway, administer oxygen or an anaesthetic, etc.

end-plate (**end**-playt) *n.* the area of muscle cell membrane immediately beneath the motor nerve ending at a neuromuscular junction.

enema (en-im-ă) *n.* (*pl.* **enemata** or **enemas**) a quantity of fluid infused into the rectum through a tube passed into the anus. *barium e.* an enema using barium sulphate, given to demonstrate the colon by X-ray. *evacuant e.* an enema using soap or olive oil to remove faeces. *therapeutic e.* an enema used to insert drugs into the rectum.

enervation (en-er-vay-shŏn) *n.* **1.** weakness; loss of strength. **2.** the surgical removal of a nerve.

enkephalin (en-**kef**-ă-lin) *n. see* encephalin.

enophthalmos (en-off-**thal**-mŏs) *n.* a condition in which the eye is abnormally sunken into the socket.

enostosis (en-os-**toh**-sis) *n.* a benign growth within a bone.

ensiform cartilage (en-si-form) *n. see* xiphoid process.

Entamoeba (ent-ă-**mee**-bă) *n.* a genus of widely distributed amoebae. *E. coli* a harmless intestinal parasite. *E. gingivalis* a species found between the teeth; it is associated with periodontal disease and gingivitis. *E. his-*

tolytica a species that invades the intestinal wall, causing dysentery and ulceration.

enter- (entero-) *prefix denoting* the intestine.

enteral (en-ter-ăl) *adj.* of or relating to the intestinal tract.

enteralgia (en-ter-al-jiă) *n. see* colic.

enterectomy (en-ter-ek-tŏmi) *n.* surgical removal of part of the intestine.

enteric (en-te-rik) *adj.* relating to or affecting the intestine. *e. fever see* paratyphoid fever, typhoid fever.

enteric-coated *adj.* describing tablets that are coated with a substance that enables them to pass through the stomach to the intestine unchanged.

enteritis (en-ter-**I**-tis) *n.* inflammation of the small intestine, usually causing diarrhoea. *infective e.* enteritis caused by viruses or bacteria. *radiation e.* enteritis caused by X-rays or radioactive isotopes. *See also* Crohn's disease (regional enteritis), gastroenteritis.

enterobiasis (oxyuriasis) (en-ter-oh-by-ă-sis) *n.* a disease, common in children throughout the world, caused by the parasitic nematode *Enterobius vermicularis* (*see* pinworm) in the large intestine. The worms do not cause any serious lesions of the gut wall although, rarely, they may provoke appendicitis. Enterobiasis responds well to treatment with piperazine compounds.

Enterobius (Oxyuris) (en-ter-oh-biŭs) *n. see* pinworm.

enterocele (en-ter-oh-seel) *n.* a hernia of part of the intestine.

enterocentesis (en-ter-oh-sen-tee-sis) *n.* a surgical procedure in which a hollow needle is pushed through the wall of the stomach or intestines to release an abnormal accumulation of gas or fluid.

enterococcus (en-ter-oh-**kok**-ŭs) *n.* any bacterium of the genus *Streptococcus* that inhabits the human intestine.

enterocolitis (en-ter-oh-kŏ-**ly**-tis) *n.* inflammation of the colon and small intestine. *See also* colitis, enteritis.

enterogenous (en-ter-**oj**-i-nŭs) *adj.* borne by or carried in the intestine.

enterokinase (en-ter-oh-**ky**-nayz) *n.* the former name for enteropeptidase.

enterolith (en-ter-oh-lith) *n.* a stone within the intestine. It usually builds up around a gallstone or a swallowed fruit stone.

enteron (en-ter-on) *n.* the intestinal tract.

enteropathy (en-ter-**op**-ă-thi) *n.* disease of the small intestine. *See also* coeliac disease (gluten-induced enteropathy).

enteropeptidase (en-ter-oh-**pep**-ti-dayz) *n.* an enzyme secreted by the glands of the small intestine that acts on trypsinogen to produce trypsin. It is part of the succus entericus.

enteroptosis (en-ter-op-**toh**-sis) *n.* a condition in which loops of intestine (especially transverse colon) are in a low anatomical position.

enterorrhaphy (en-ter-o-ră-fi) *n.* the surgical procedure of stitching an intestine that has either perforated or been divided during an operation.

enterospasm (en-ter-oh-spazm) *n.* powerful contraction of the intestine, usually accompanied by pain.

enterostomy (en-ter-ost-ŏmi) *n.* an operation in which the small intestine is brought through the abdominal wall and opened (*see* duodenostomy, jejunostomy, ileostomy) or is joined to the stomach (*gastroenterostomy*) or to another loop of small intestine (*enteroenterostomy*).

enterotomy (en-ter-ot-ŏmi) *n.* surgical incision into the intestine.

enterotoxin (en-ter-oh-**toks**-in) *n.* a poisonous substance that has a particularly marked effect upon the gastrointestinal tract, causing vomiting, diarrhoea, and abdominal pain.

enterovirus (en-ter-oh-vy-rŭs) *n.* any virus that enters the body through the gastrointestinal tract, multiplies there, and then (generally) invades the central nervous system. Enteroviruses include Coxsackie viruses, echoviruses, polioviruses, and rhinoviruses.

enterozoon (en-ter-oh-**zoh**-on) *n.* any animal species inhabiting or infecting the gut of another. *See also* endoparasite.

entropion (en-**troh**-pi-on) *n.* inturning of the eyelid towards the eyeball. The lashes may rub against the eye and cause irritation (*see* trichiasis).

enucleation (i-new-kli-ay-shŏn) *n.* a surgical operation in which an organ, tumour, or cyst is completely removed. In ophthalmology it is an operation in which the eyeball is removed but the other structures in the socket are left in place.

enuresis (en-yoor-ee-sis) *n.* the involuntary passing of urine, especially bedwetting at night (*nocturnal e.*). *See also* incontinence. —**enuretic** (en-yoor-et-ik) *adj.*

environment (in-vyr-ŏn-měnt) *n.* any or all aspects of the surroundings of an organism, both internal and external, which influence its growth, development, and behaviour.

Environmental Health Officer (EHO) (in-vyr-ŏn-**men**-tăl) *n.* a person, employed by local authorities, with special training in such aspects of environmental health and pollution as housing, sanitation, food, clean air, and water supplies (formerly known as a *Public Health Inspector*).

enzyme (**en**-zym) *n.* a protein that, in small amounts, speeds up the rate of a biological reaction without itself being used up in the reaction (i.e. it acts as a catalyst). Enzymes are essential for the normal functioning and development of the body. Failure in the production or activity of a single enzyme may result in metabolic disorders; such disorders are often inherited and some have serious effects. —**enzymatic** *adj.*

eonism (**ee**-ŏ-nizm) *n.* the adoption of female manners and dress by a man. *See* transsexualism, transvestitism.

eosin (**ee**-oh-sin) *n.* a red acidic dye, produced by the reaction of bromine and fluorescein, used to stain biological specimens for microscopical examination.

eosinopenia (ee-oh-sin-oh-**pee**-niă) *n.* a decrease in the number of eosinophils in the blood.

eosinophil (ee-oh-**sin**-ŏ-fil) *n.* a variety of white blood cell distinguished by the presence in its cytoplasm of coarse granules that stain orange-red with Romanowsky stains. Eosinophils are capable of ingesting foreign particles and are involved in allergic responses.

eosinophilia (ee-oh-sin-ŏ-**fil**-iă) *n.* an increase in the number of eosinophils in the blood. Eosi-

nophilia occurs in a variety of diseases, including allergies, parasitic infestations, and certain forms of leukaemia.

eparterial (ep-ar-**teer**-iăl) *adj.* situated on or above an artery.

ependyma (ep-en-dim-ă) *n.* the extremely thin membrane, composed of cells of the glia (*ependymal cells*), that lines the ventricles of the brain and the choroid plexuses. It is responsible for helping to form cerebrospinal fluid. —**ependymal** *adj.*

ependymoma (ep-en-di-**moh**-mă) *n.* a cerebral tumour derived from the glial ependymal cells. It may obstruct the flow of cerebrospinal fluid, causing a hydrocephalus.

ephebiatrics (i-fee-bi-**at**-riks) *n.* the branch of medicine concerned with the common disorders of children and adolescents. *Compare* paediatrics.

ephedrine (**ef**-i-drin) *n.* a drug that causes constriction of blood vessels and widening of the bronchial passages (*see* sympathomimetic). It is administered by mouth or by inhalation, mainly in the treatment of asthma and other allergic conditions and chronic bronchitis.

epi- *prefix denoting* above or upon.

epiblepharon (epi-**blef**-er-on) *n.* an abnormal fold of skin, present from birth, stretching across the eye just above the lashes of the upper eyelid or in front of them in the lower lid. It usually disappears within the first year of life.

epicanthus (epicanthic fold) (epi-**kanth**-ŭs) *n.* a vertical fold of skin from the upper eyelid that covers the inner corner of the eye. It occurs abnormally in certain congenital conditions, e.g.

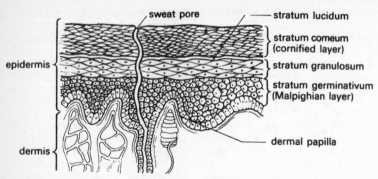

sweat pore — stratum lucidum

— stratum corneum (cornified layer)

epidermis — stratum granulosum

— stratum germinativum (Malpighian layer)

— dermal papilla

dermis

A section of epidermis

Down's syndrome. —**epicanthal**, **epicanthic** adj.

epicardium (epi-kar-diŭm) n. the outermost layer of the heart wall, enveloping the myocardium. It is a serous membrane that forms the inner layer of the serous pericardium. —**epicardial** adj.

epicondyle (epi-kon-dyl) n. the protuberance above a condyle at the end of an articulating bone.

epicranium (epi-kray-niŭm) n. the structures that cover the cranium, i.e. all layers of the scalp.

epicranius (epi-kray-ni-ŭs) n. the muscle of the scalp.

epicritic (epi-krit-ik) adj. describing or relating to sensory nerve fibres responsible for the fine degrees of sensation, as of temperature and touch. Compare protopathic.

epidemic (epi-dem-ik) n. a sudden outbreak of infectious disease that spreads rapidly through the population, affecting a large proportion of people. Compare endemic, pandemic. —**epidemic** adj.

epidemiology (epi-dee-mi-ol-ŏji) n. the study of epidemic disease, with a view to finding means of control and future prevention. It includes all forms of disease

that relate to the environment and ways of life.

epidermis (epi-der-mis) n. the outer layer of the skin, which is divided into four layers (see illustration). The top three layers are continually renewed as cells from the continuously dividing Malpighian layer are gradually pushed outwards and become progressively impregnated with keratin. —**epidermal** adj.

epidermolysis (epi-der-mol-i-sis) n. loosening of the epidermis, with the development of large blisters, occurring either spontaneously or after injury.

Epidermophyton (epi-der-mof-i-tŏn) n. a genus of fungi that grow on the skin and produce the skin infections athlete's foot and dhobie itch.

epidiascope (epi-dy-ă-skohp) n. an apparatus for projecting a greatly magnified image of an object, such as a specimen on a microscope slide, on to a screen.

epididymis (epi-did-i-mis) n. (pl. **epididymides**) a highly convoluted tube, about seven metres long, that connects the testis to the vas deferens. The spermatozoa are moved along the tube and are stored in the lower part until ejaculation. —**epididymal** *adj.*

epididymitis (epi-did-i-**my**-tis) *n.* inflammation of the epididymis. The usual cause is infection spreading down the vas deferens from the bladder or urethra. The inflammation may spread to the testicle (*epididymo-orchitis*).

epidural (**extradural**) (epi-**dewr**-ăl) *adj.* on or over the dura mater. *e. space* the space between the dura mater of the spinal cord and the vertebral canal. *See also* spinal anaesthesia.

epigastrium (epi-**gas**-tri-ŭm) *n.* the upper central region of the abdomen. —**epigastric** *adj.*

epigastrocele (epi-**gas**-troh-seel) *n.* a hernia through the upper central abdominal wall.

epiglottis (epi-**glot**-iss) *n.* a thin leaf-shaped flap of cartilage, covered with mucous membrane, situated immediately behind the root of the tongue. It covers the entrance to the larynx during swallowing.

epiglottitis (epi-glot-**I**-tis) *n.* inflammation of the mucous membrane of the epiglottis.

epilation (epi-**lay**-shŏn) *n.* the removal of a hair by its roots. This can be done mechanically or by electrolysis, which removes the hair permanently.

epilepsy (**ep**-i-lep-si) *n.* any one of a group of disorders of brain function characterized by recurrent attacks that have a sudden onset. *Focal* (or *symptomatic*) *e.* epilepsy caused by structural disease of the brain. *idiopathic e.* epilepsy that is not associated with structural damage to the brain. *See* grand mal, petit mal. *Jacksonian e.* focal epilepsy in which the epileptic discharge

spreads over the cerebral cortex, with the resulting manifestations spreading throughout the body. *temporal lobe* (or *psychomotor*) *e.* focal epilepsy caused by disease in the cortex of the temporal lobe or the adjacent parietal lobe of the brain. Its symptoms include hallucinations of smell, taste, sight, and hearing, paroxysmal disorders of memory, and automatism. —**epileptic** (epi-**lep**-tik) *adj.*, *n.*

epileptiform (epi-**lep**-ti-form) *adj.* resembling an epileptic attack.

epileptogenic (epi-lep-toh-**jen**-ik) *adj.* having the capacity to provoke epileptic fits.

epiloia (epi-**loi**-ă) *n. see* tuberous (sclerosis).

epimenorrhagia (epi-men-ŏ-**ray**-jiă) *n. see* menorrhagia.

epimenorrhoea (epi-men-ŏ-**ree**-ă) *n.* menstruation at shorter intervals than is normal.

epinephrine (epi-**nef**-rin) *n. see* adrenaline.

epineurium (epi-**newr**-iŭm) *n.* the outer sheath of connective tissue that encloses the bundles (fascicles) of fibres that make up a nerve.

epiphenomenon (epi-fin-**om**-inŏn) *n.* an unusual symptom or event that may occur simultaneously with a disease but is not necessarily directly related to it. *Compare* complication.

epiphora (i-**pif**-er-ă) *n.* watering of the eye, in which tears flow onto the cheek. It is due to some abnormality of the tear drainage system (*see* lacrimal (apparatus)).

epiphysis (i-**pif**-i-sis) *n.* **1.** the end of a long bone, which is initially separated by cartilage from the shaft (diaphysis) of the bone and develops separately. It eventually fuses with the diaphysis to form a complete bone. **2.** *see* pineal body.

epiphysitis (ep-ifi-sy-tis) *n.* inflammation of the epiphysis of a long bone.

epiplo- *prefix denoting* the omentum.

epiplocele (i-**pip**-loh-seel) *n.* a hernia that contains omentum.

epiploon (i-**pip**-loh-on) *n. see* omentum.

episcleritis (epi-skleer-**I**-tis) *n.* inflammation of the outermost layers of the sclera of the eyeball.

episio- *prefix denoting* the vulva.

episiorrhaphy (ep-izi-o-răfi) *n.* stitching together the margins of a tear in the tissues around the vaginal opening.

episiotomy (ep-izi-ot-ŏmi) *n.* an incision into the perineum during a difficult birth. The aim is to make delivery easier and to avoid extensive tearing of adjacent tissues.

epispadias (epi-**spay**-di-ăs) *n.* a congenital abnormality in which the opening of the urethra is on the dorsal (upper) surface of the penis. Surgical correction is carried out in infancy.

epispastic (epi-**spas**-tik) *n. see* vesicant.

epistaxis (epi-**staks**-iss) *n. see* nosebleed.

epithalaxia (epi-thal-**aks**-iă) *n.* loss of layers of epithelial cells from the skin or the lining of the intestine.

epithelialization (epi-th'ee-li-ă-ly-zay-shŏn) *n.* the growth of epithelium over the surface of a wound, which marks the final stage of healing.

epithelioma (epi-th'ee-li-oh-mă) *n.* a tumour of epithelium: a former term for carcinoma, but now also used to describe benign tumours.

epithelium (epi-**theel**-iŭm) *n.* the tissue that covers the external surface of the body and lines hollow structures (except blood and lymphatic vessels). Epithelium may be either *simple*, consisting of a single layer of cells; *stratified*, consisting of several layers; or *pseudostratified*, in which the cells appear to be arranged in layers but in fact share a common basement membrane. *See also* endothelium, mesothelium. —**epithelial** *adj.*

epituberculosis (epi-tew-ber-kew-loh-sis) *n.* enlargement of a lymph node in the thorax due to tuberculosis infection.

eponym (ep-ŏ-nim) *n.* a disease, structure, or species named after a particular person, usually the person who first discovered or described it. —**eponymous** (i-pon-i-mŭs) *adj.*

Epstein-Barr virus (ep-styn bar) *n.* the virus thought to be the causative agent of glandular fever. [M. A. Epstein (1921–), British pathologist; Y. M. Barr]

epulis (ep-**yoo**-lis) *n.* an old term for a swelling of the gum.

equi- *prefix denoting* equality.

equinia (i-kwin-iă) *n. see* glanders.

Erb's palsy (erbz) *n.* a partial paralysis of the arm caused by injury to a baby's brachial plexus during birth. The muscles of the shoulder and the flexors of the elbow are paralysed and the arm hangs at the side internally rotated at the shoulder. [W. H. Erb (1840–1921), German neurologist]

erectile (i-**rek**-tyl) *adj.* capable of causing erection or becoming erect. The penis is composed largely of erectile tissue.

Stratified squamous epithelium, surface view above and sectional view below

basement membrane

Simple cuboidal epithelium

goblet cell

Ciliated columnar epithelium

basement membrane

Pseudostratified ciliated epithelium

Types of epithelium

erection (i-**rek**-shŏn) *n.* the sexually active state of the penis, which becomes enlarged and rigid (due to the erectile tissue being swollen with blood). The term is also applied to the clitoris.

erepsin (i-**rep**-sin) *n.* a mixture of protein-digesting enzymes (*see* peptidase) secreted by the intestinal glands. It is part of the succus entericus.

erg- (ergo-) *prefix denoting* work or activity.

ergocalciferol (er-goh-kal-**sif**-er-ol) *n. see* vitamin D.

ergograph (er-gŏ-grahf) *n.* an apparatus for recording the work performed by the muscles of the body when undergoing activity.

ergometrine (er-goh-**met**-reen) *n.* a drug that stimulates contractions of the womb. It is administered by injection to assist labour and to control bleeding following delivery.

ergonomics (er-gŏ-**nom**-iks) *n.* the study of man in relation to his work and working surroundings.

ergosterol (er-**gos**-ter-ol) *n.* a plant sterol that, when irradiated with ultraviolet light, is converted to ergocalciferol (vitamin D_2). *See* vitamin D.

ergot (**er**-got) *n.* a fungus (*Claviceps purpurea*) that grows on rye. It produces several important alkaloids, including ergotamine and ergometrine. *See also* ergotism.

ergotamine (er-**got**-ă-meen) *n.* a drug that causes constriction of blood vessels and is used to relieve migraine. It is administered by mouth, injection, inhalation, or in suppositories. Trade names: **Femergin, Lingraine**.

ergotism (er-gŏ-tizm) *n.* poisoning caused by eating rye infected with the fungus ergot. The chief symptom is gangrene of the fingers and toes, with diarrhoea and vomiting, nausea, and headache.

erogenous (i-**roj**-in-ŭs) *adj.* describing certain parts of the body, the physical stimulation of which leads to sexual arousal.

erosion (i-roh-*zh*ŏn) *n.* an eating away of surface tissue by physical or chemical processes, including those associated with inflammation. *cervical e.* an abnormal area of epithelium that may develop at the neck of the womb due to tissue damage caused at childbirth or by attempts at abortion. *dental e.* absorption of the surface of the teeth, resembling caries.

erot- (eroto-) *prefix denoting* sexual desire or love.

eructation (i-ruk-**tay**-shŏn) *n.* belching: the sudden raising of gas from the stomach.

eruption (i-**rup**-shŏn) *n.* **1.** any lesion that appears at the surface of the skin and is characterized by its prominence and redness. **2.** (in dentistry) the emergence of a growing tooth from the gum into the mouth.

erysipelas (e-ri-**sip**-ilăs) *n.* an infection of the skin and underlying tissues with the bacterium *Streptococcus pyogenes*. The affected areas, usually the face and scalp, become inflamed and swollen, with the development of raised patches. The patient is ill, with a high temperature.

erysipeloid (erythema serpens) (e-ri-**sip**-i-loid) *n.* an infection of the skin and underlying tissues with the bacterium *Erysipelothrix*

rhusiopathiaè, developing usually in people handling fish, poultry, or meat. It is normally confined to a finger or hand, which becomes reddened; sometimes systemic illness develops.

erythema (e-ri-**theem**-ă) *n.* abnormal flushing of the skin caused by dilation of the blood capillaries. *e. multiforme* a disease caused by toxins in the blood in which circular or irregular red patches develop, commonly on the backs of the arms and hands. *e. nodosum* a disease of sudden onset, characterized by fever, joint pains, and an eruption of painful swellings on the legs.

erythr- (erythro-) *prefix denoting* **1.** redness. **2.** erythrocytes.

erythraemia (e-ri-**three**-miă) *n. see* polycythaemia (vera).

erythrasma (e-ri-**thraz**-mă) *n.* a chronic skin infection due to *Corynebacterium minutissimum*, occurring in such areas as the armpits, groin, and toes, where skin surfaces are in contact.

erythroblast (i-**rith**-roh-blast) *n.* any of a series of nucleated cells (*see* normoblast) that pass through a succession of stages of maturation to form red blood cells (erythrocytes). *See also* erythropoiesis.

erythroblastosis (i-**rith**-roh-blas-**toh**-sis) *n.* the presence in the blood of erythroblasts. *e. foetalis* a severe but rare haemolytic anaemia affecting newborn infants due to destruction of the infant's red blood cells by factors present in the mother's serum. It is usually caused by incompatibility of the rhesus blood groups between mother and infant (*see* rhesus factor).

erythrocyanosis (i-rith-roh-sy-ă-noh-sis) *n.* mottled purplish discoloration on the legs and thighs. The condition is worse in cold weather and there is no satisfactory treatment.

erythrocyte (red blood cell) (i-rith-roh-syt) *n.* a blood cell containing the pigment haemoglobin, the principal function of which is the transport of oxygen. There are normally about 5 × 10¹² erythrocytes per litre of blood.

erythrocyte sedimentation rate *n.* see ESR.

erythrocytosis (i-rith-roh-sy-toh-sis) *n.* an increase in the number of red blood cells (erythrocytes) in the blood. *See* polycythaemia.

erythroderma (exfoliative dermatitis) (i-rith-roh-der-mă) *n.* abnormal reddening, flaking, and thickening of the skin, typically affecting a wide area of the body.

erythroedema (i-rith-ri-dee-mă) *n.* see pink disease.

erythrogenesis (i-rith-roh-jen-i-sis) *n. see* erythropoiesis.

erythromycin (i-rith-roh-my-sin) *n.* an antibiotic used to treat infections caused by a wide range of bacteria and other microorganisms. It is administered by mouth or injection. Trade names: **Erycen, Erythromia, Erythropea, Ilotycin**.

erythropenia (i-rith-roh-pee-niă) *n.* a reduction in the number of red blood cells (erythrocytes) in the blood.

erythropoiesis (erythrogenesis) (i-rith-roh-poi-ee-sis) *n.* the process of red blood cell (erythrocyte) production, which normally occurs in the blood-forming tissue of the bone marrow. *See also* haemopoiesis.

erythropoietin (haemopoietin) (i-rith-roh-poi-ĕ-tin) *n.* a hormone secreted by certain cells in the kidney in response to a reduction in the amount of oxygen reaching the tissues. Erythropoietin increases and controls the rate of red cell production (erythropoiesis).

erythropsia (e-ri-throp-siă) *n.* red vision: a rare symptom sometimes experienced after removal of a cataract and also in snow blindness.

Esbach's albuminometer (ess-bahks) *n.* a graduated glass tube used for measuring the amount of albumin in a specimen of urine. [G. H. Esbach (1843–90), French physician]

eschar (ess-kar) *n.* a scab or slough, as produced by the action of heat or a corrosive substance on living tissue.

escharotic (ess-kă-rot-ik) *n.* a caustic agent that produces a dry scab, or slough, when applied to the skin.

Escherichia (esh-er-ik-iă) *n.* a genus of Gram-negative, generally motile, rodlike bacteria that are found in the intestines of man and many animals. *E. coli* a species that is usually not harmful but under certain conditions can cause infection of the urinogenital tract and diarrhoea in children.

eserine (ess-er-een) *n. see* physostigmine.

Esmarch's bandage (ess-marks) *n.* a rubber or elastic bandage that is wound tightly around a limb in order to force blood out from an area in which an operation is to be performed in a blood-free field. [J. F. A. von Esmarch (1823–1908), German surgeon]

esotropia (ess-oh-**troh**-piă) *n.* convergent strabismus: a type of squint.

espundia (mucocutaneous leishmaniasis) (ess-**puun**-diă) *n.* a disease of the skin and mucous membranes caused by the parasitic protozoan *Leishmania braziliensis* (*see* leishmaniasis), occurring in South and Central America.

ESR (erythrocyte sedimentation rate) *n.* the rate at which red blood cells (erythrocytes) settle out of suspension in blood plasma, measured under standardized conditions. The ESR increases in rheumatic diseases, chronic infections, and malignant disease, and thus provides a valuable screening test for the latter condition.

essence (ess-ĕns) *n.* a solution consisting of an essential oil dissolved in alcohol.

essential (i-sen-shăl) *adj.* describing a disorder that is not apparently attributable to an outside cause.

essential amino acid *n.* an amino acid that is essential for normal growth and development but cannot be synthesized by the body and must therefore be obtained from protein in the diet. *See* amino acid.

essential fatty acid *n.* one of a group of unsaturated fatty acids that are essential for growth but cannot be synthesized by the body. The essential fatty acids are *linoleic, linolenic,* and *arachidonic acids.*

essential oil *n.* a volatile oil derived from an aromatic plant. Essential oils are used in various pharmaceutical preparations.

ethacrynic acid (eth-ă-**krin**-ik) *n.* a diuretic administered by mouth or injection to treat fluid reten-tion (oedema), such as that associated with heart failure and kidney and liver disorders. Trade name: **Edecrin.**

ethambutol (eth-**am**-bew-tol) *n.* a drug administered by mouth in the treatment of tuberculosis, in conjunction with other drugs. Trade name: **Myambutol.**

ethamivan (eth-am-i-van) *n.* an analeptic drug that is administered by mouth or injection to treat reduced or abnormal breathing, particularly in newborn babies and in cases of drug overdosage. Trade name: **Clairvan.**

ethanol (ethyl alcohol) (eth-ă-nol) *n. see* alcohol.

ether (ee-ther) *n.* a volatile liquid formerly used as an anaesthetic administered by inhalation. It also has laxative action when administered by mouth.

ethical committee (eth-ikăl) *n.* (in Britain) a group of consultants and other experts set up (especially in a hospital) to monitor investigations, concerned with teaching or research, that involve the use of human subjects.

ethics (eth-iks) *n.* a code of principles governing correct behaviour, which in the nursing profession includes behaviour towards patients and their families, visitors, and colleagues.

ethinamate (eth-**in**-ă-mayt) *n.* a mild sedative administered by mouth to treat insomnia.

ethinyloestradiol (eth-i-nyl-ee-strǎ-dy-ol) *n.* a synthetic female sex hormone (*see* oestrogen) administered by mouth to treat symptoms of the menopause, to suppress lactation, and to treat cancer of the prostate gland. It is also used in oral contraceptives. Trade name: **Lynoral.**

ethionamide (eth-ee-**on**-a-myd) *n.* a drug used to treat tuberculosis, usually in conjunction with other drugs. It is administered by mouth or in suppositories. Trade name: **Trescatyl**.

ethisterone (eth-**iss**-ter-ohn) *n.* a synthetic female sex hormone (*see* progestogen) administered by mouth to treat menstrual disorders, particularly amenorrhoea.

ethmoid bone (**eth**-moid) *n.* a bone in the floor of the cranium that contributes to the nasal cavity and orbits. The part of the ethmoid forming the roof of the nasal cavity (the *cribriform plate*) is pierced with many small holes through which the olfactory nerves pass. *See also* nasal (concha), skull.

ethnology (eth-**nol**-ŏji) *n.* the study of the different races of mankind, concerned mainly with cultural and social differences between groups and the problems that arise from their particular ways of life. —**ethnic** (**eth**-nik) *adj.*

ethoglucid (eth-oh-**gloo**-sid) *n.* a drug that prevents the growth of tumours and is administered by injection to treat various cancers. Trade name: **Epodyl**.

ethopropazine (eth-oh-**proh**-pă-zeen) *n.* a drug that has effects similar to those of atropine and and is administered by mouth to treat parkinsonism. Trade name: **Lysivane**.

ethosuximide (eth-oh-**suks**-i-myd) *n.* an anticonvulsant drug administered by mouth to treat petit mal epileptic fits. Trade names: **Emeside, Zarontin**.

ethotoin (eth-oh-toh-in) *n.* an anticonvulsant drug administered by mouth, usually in conjunction with other anticonvulsants, to treat grand mal epileptic fits. Trade name: **Peganone**.

ethyl biscoumacetate (ee-thyl bis-koom-**ass**-it-ayt) *n.* an anticoagulant drug administered by mouth to prevent blood clotting. Trade name: **Tromexan**.

ethyl chloride (chloroethane) *n.* a volatile liquid used chiefly as a local anaesthetic applied topically to the skin before minor surgery. Formula: C_2H_5Cl.

ethyloestrenol (eth-il-ee-strĕ-nol) *n.* a steroid drug with anabolic properties, administered by mouth to treat conditions involving wasting of protein and bone, such as osteoporosis. Trade name: **Orabolin**.

ethynodiol (eth-I-noh-**dy**-ol) *n.* a synthetic female sex hormone (*see* progestogen) that is used to treat menstrual disorders and in oral contraceptives. It is administered by mouth, usually in combination with an oestrogen.

etiology (ee-ti-**ol**-ŏji) *n. see* aetiology.

eu- *prefix denoting* **1.** good, well, or easy. **2.** normal.

eucalyptol (yoo-kă-**lip**-tol) *n.* a volatile oil that has a mild irritant effect on the mucous membranes of the mouth and digestive system. It is taken as pastilles or inhaled as vapour to relieve catarrh.

eugenics (yoo-**jen**-iks) *n.* the science that is concerned with the improvement of the human race by means of the principles of genetics.

eunuch (**yoo**-nŭk) *n.* a male who has undergone castration.

eupepsia (yoo-**pep**-siă) *n.* the state of normal or good digestion.

euphoria (yoo-**for**-iă) *n.* a state of cheerfulness and well-being. A morbid degree of euphoria is characteristic of mania and hypomania. *See also* ecstasy, elation.

euplastic (yoo-**plast**-ik) *adj.* describing a tissue that heals quickly after injury.

Eustachian tube (pharyngotympanic tube) (yoo-**stay**-shŏn) *n.* the tube that connects the middle ear to the pharynx. It allows the pressure on the inner side of the eardrum to remain equal to the external pressure. [B. Eustachio (1520–74), Italian anatomist]

euthanasia (yooth-ăn-**ay**-ziă) *n.* the act of taking life to relieve suffering. This may be accomplished by active steps, usually the administration of a drug, or by the deliberate withholding of treatment. In no country is euthanasia legal.

euthyroid (yoo-**th'y**-roid) *adj.* having a normally functioning thyroid gland. *Compare* hyperthyroidism, hypothyroidism. **—euthyroidism** *n.*

eutocia (yoo-**toh**-siă) *n.* natural uncomplicated labour and childbirth.

evacuation (i-vak-yoo-**ay**-shŏn) *n.* removal of the contents of a cavity, especially the emptying of the bowels (defecation).

evacuator (i-**vak**-yoo-ay-ter) *n.* a device for sucking fluid out of a cavity. Evacuators may be used to empty the bladder of unwanted material during such operations as the removal of a calculus.

evaluation (i-val-yoo-**ay**-shŏn) *n.* the final stage of the nursing process, in which the effects of nursing interventions are compared with the goals or objectives set in the care plan. *See* expected outcome.

eventration (ee-ven-**tray**-shŏn) *n.* **1.**

protrusion of the intestines through the abdominal wall. **2.** abnormal elevation of part of the diaphragm due to a congenital weakness.

eversion (i-**ver**-shŏn) *n.* a turning outward. *e. of the cervix* a condition in which the edges of the neck of the womb turn outward after having been torn during childbirth.

evisceration (i-vis-er-**ay**-shŏn) *n.* (in ophthalmology) an operation in which the contents of the eyeball are removed, the empty outer envelope (sclera) being left behind. *Compare* enucleation.

evulsion (i-**vul**-shŏn) *n. see* avulsion.

Ewing's tumour (*or* sarcoma) (yoo-ingz) *n.* a malignant bone tumour arising in the bone marrow and usually affecting a long bone. It is most common in adolescents. [J. Ewing (1866–1943), US pathologist]

ex- (exo-) *prefix denoting* outside or outer.

exacerbation (eks-ass-er-**bay**-shŏn) *n.* an increase in the severity of a disorder, marked by an increase in the intensity of its symptoms and signs.

exaltation (eg-zawl-**tay**-shŏn) *n. see* elation.

exanthem (eks-**anth**-ĕm) *n.* **1.** a skin rash accompanying any eruptive disease or fever. **2.** any disease characterized by a skin rash. **—exanthematous** (eks-an-th'em-**ătŭs**) *adj.*

exchange transfusion (iks-**chaynj**) *n.* a technique for treating haemolytic disease in newborn infants. Rh positive blood is withdrawn from the baby (via the umbilical vein) and replaced by Rh negative donor blood, 20 ml at a time.

excise (ek-syz) *vb.* to cut out tissue, an organ, or a tumour from the body. —**excision** (ek-si-*zh*ŏn) *n.*

excitation (eks-i-**tay**-shŏn) *n.* (in neurophysiology) the triggering of a conducted impulse in the membrane of a muscle cell or nerve fibre.

excoriation (iks-kor-i-ay-shŏn) *n.* the destruction and removal of the surface of the skin or the covering of an organ by scraping, the application of a chemical, or other means.

excrescence (iks-**kress**-ĕns) *n.* an abnormal outgrowth on the surface of the body, such as a wart.

excreta (iks-**kree**-tă) *n.* any waste material discharged from the body, especially faeces.

excretion (iks-**kree**-shŏn) *n.* the removal of the waste products of metabolism from the body, mainly through the action of the kidneys. Excretion also includes the loss of water, salts, etc. through the sweat glands, the loss of carbon dioxide and water vapour from the lungs, and the egestion of faeces.

exenteration (eks-en-ter-ay-shŏn) *n.* (in ophthalmology) an operation in which all the contents of the eye socket (orbit) are removed, leaving only the bony walls intact.

exfoliation (eks-foh-li-ay-shŏn) *n.* **1.** flaking off of the upper layers of the skin. **2.** separation of a surface epithelium from the underlying tissue. —**exfoliative** *adj.*

exhalation (expiration) (eks-hă-lay-shŏn) *n.* the act of breathing air from the lungs out through the mouth and nose.

exhibitionism (eksi-**bish**-ŏn-izm) *n.* exposure of the genitals to another person, as a sexually deviant act. The word is often broadened to mean public flaunting of any quality of the individual.

exo- *prefix. see* ex-.

exocrine gland (eks-oh-kryn) *n.* a gland that discharges its secretion by means of a duct, which opens onto an epithelial surface. Examples of exocrine glands are the sebaceous and sweat glands. *See also* secretion.

exogenous (ek-**soj**-in-ŭs) *adj.* originating outside the body or part of the body: applied particularly to substances in the body that are derived from the diet rather than built up by the body's own processes of metabolism. *Compare* endogenous.

exomphalos (ek-**som**-fă-lŭs) *n.* an umbilical hernia.

exophthalmic goitre (Graves's disease) (eks-off-**thal**-mik) *n. see* thyrotoxicosis.

exophthalmos (eks-off-**thal**-mos) *n.* protrusion of the eyeballs in their sockets. This can result from injury or disease of the eyeball or socket but is most commonly associated with overactivity of the thyroid gland (*see* thyrotoxicosis). —**exophthalmic** *adj.*

exostosis (eks-os-**toh**-sis) *n.* a benign cartilaginous outgrowth from a bone. *See* osteoma.

exotic (ig-**zot**-ik) *adj.* describing a disease occurring in a region of the world far from where it might be expected.

exotoxin (eks-oh-**toks**-in) *n.* a highly potent poison, often harmful to only a limited range of tissues, that is produced by a bacterial cell and secreted into its surrounding medium. Exotoxins are produced by the bacteria causing botulism, diphtheria, and tetanus. *Compare* endotoxin.

exotropia (eks-oh-**troh**-piă) *n.* divergent strabismus: a type of squint.

expected outcome (iks-**pekt**-id) *n.* a statement in the care plan of what the nursing intervention is intended to achieve, usually described in terms of the patient's expected behaviour. *See* behavioural objective.

expectorant (iks-**pek**-ter-ănt) *n.* a drug that enhances the secretion of sputum by the air passages so that it is easier to cough up. Expectorants are used in cough mixtures; they act by increasing the bronchial secretion or make it less viscous (*see* mucolytic).

expectoration (iks-pek-ter-ay-shŏn) *n.* the act of spitting out material brought into the mouth by coughing.

experiential learning (iks-peer-i-en-shăl) *n.* learning by experiencing a situation or a simulated situation, as in role playing.

expiration (eks-per-ay-shŏn) *n.* **1.** the act of breathing out air from the lungs: exhalation. **2.** dying.

explant (eks-**plahnt**) **1.** *n.* live tissue transferred from the body (or any organism) to a suitable artificial medium for culture. **2.** *vb.* to transfer live tissue for culture outside the body. —**explantation** *n.*

exploration (eks-plŏ-**ray**-shŏn) *n.* (in surgery) an investigative operation to determine the cause of symptoms. —**exploratory** (iks-**plŏ**-ră-ter-i) *adj.*

expression (iks-**presh**-ŏn) *n.* **1.** the appearance of the face, reflecting the individual's physical or emotional state. **2.** expulsion by pressing or squeezing, as of milk from the breast after pregnancy

or the fetus or placenta from the womb at childbirth.

exsanguinate (iks-**sang**-win-ayt) *vb.* to deprive the body of blood; for example, as a result of an accident causing severe bleeding. —**exsanguination** *n.*

exsufflation (eks-suf-**lay**-shŏn) *n.* the forcible removal of secretions from the air passages by some form of suction apparatus.

extension (iks-**ten**-shŏn) *n.* **1.** the act of extending or stretching, especially the muscular movement by which a limb is straightened. **2.** the application of traction to a fractured or dislocated limb in order to restore it to its normal position.

extensor (iks-**ten**-ser) *n.* any muscle that causes the straightening of a limb or other part.

exteriorization (iks-teer-i-er-I-zay-shŏn) *n.* a surgical procedure in which an organ is brought from its normal site to the surface of the body, as in colostomy.

exteroceptor (eks-ter-oh-sep-ter) *n.* a sensory nerve, ending in the skin or a mucous membrane, that is responsive to stimuli from outside the body. *See also* chemoreceptor, receptor.

extinction (iks-**tink**-shŏn) *n.* (in psychology) the weakening of a conditioned reflex that takes place if it is not maintained by reinforcement.

extirpation (eks-ter-**pay**-shŏn) *n.* the complete surgical removal of tissue, an organ, or a growth.

extra- *prefix denoting* outside or beyond.

extracapsular (eks-tră-**kaps**-yoo-ler) *adj.* outside or not involving a capsule. *e. extraction* surgical removal of a cataract in which the capsule of the lens is left behind.

e. fracture a fracture, especially of the hip, that does not involve the joint capsule.

extracellular (eks-tră-**sel**-yoo-ler) *adj.* situated or occurring outside cells. *e. fluid* the fluid surrounding cells.

extract (**eks**-trakt) *n.* a preparation containing the pharmacologically active principles of a drug, made by evaporating a solution of the drug in water, alcohol, or ether.

extraction (iks-**trak**-shŏn) *n.* 1. the surgical removal of a part of the body. Extraction of teeth is usually achieved by applying extraction forceps to the root of the tooth to dislocate it from its socket. 2. the act of pulling out a baby from the body of its mother during childbirth.

extradural (eks-tră-**dewr**-ăl) *adj.* *see* epidural.

extraembryonic membranes (eks-tră-em-bree-**on**-ik) *pl. n.* the membranous structures that surround the embryo and contribute to the placenta and umbilical cord. They include the amnion, chorion, allantois, and yolk sac.

extrapleural (eks-tră-**ploor**-ăl) *adj.* relating to the tissues of the chest wall outside the parietal pleura.

extrapyramidal system (eks-tră-pi-**ram**-i-d'l) *n.* the system of nerve tracts and pathways connecting the cerebral cortex, basal ganglia, thalamus, cerebellum, reticular formation, and spinal neurones in complex circuits not included in the pyramidal system. The extrapyramidal system is mainly concerned with the regulation of stereotyped reflex muscular movements.

extrasystole (eks-tră-**sis**-tŏ-li) *n.* *see* ectopic beat.

extrauterine (eks-tră-**yoo**-teryn) *adj.* outside the womb.

extravasation (iks-trav-ă-**say**-shŏn) *n.* the leakage and spread of blood or fluid from vessels into the surrounding tissues, which follows injury, burns, inflammation, and allergy.

extraversion (eks-tră-**ver**-shŏn) *n.* *see* extroversion.

extrinsic factor (eks-**trin**-sik) *n.* an old name for vitamin B_{12}.

extrinsic muscle *n.* a muscle, such as any of those controlling movements of the eyeball, that has its origin some distance from the part it acts on.

extroversion (eks-trŏ-**ver**-shŏn) *n.* 1. (or **extraversion**) an enduring personality trait characterized by interest in the outside world rather than the self. People high in extroversion (*extroverts*) are gregarious and outgoing, prefer to change activities frequently, and are not susceptible to permanent conditioning. *Compare* introversion. 2. a turning inside out of a hollow organ, such as the womb (which sometimes occurs after childbirth).

extrovert (**eks**-trŏ-vert) *n.* *see* extroversion.

exudation (eks-yoo-**day**-shŏn) *n.* the slow escape of liquid (the *exudate*) containing proteins and white cells through the walls of intact blood vessels, usually as a result of inflammation. Exudation is a normal part of the body's defence mechanisms.

eye (I) *n.* the organ of sight: a three-layered roughly spherical structure specialized for receiving and responding to light (see illustration). Light enters the eye through the cornea, which refracts it through the aqueous humour onto the lens. By ac-

The eye (sagittal section)

commodation light is focused through the vitreous humour onto the retina. In the retina light-sensitive cells (*see* cone, rod) send nerve impulses to the brain via the optic nerve.

eyeball (I-bawl) *n.* the body of the eye, which is roughly spherical, is bounded by the sclera, and lies in the orbit. Its movements are controlled by three pairs of extrinsic eye muscles.

eyelid (I-lid) *n.* the protective covering of the eye. Each eye has two eyelids consisting of skin, muscle, and connective tissue. Each eyelid is lined with membrane (*see* conjunctiva) and fringed with eyelashes. Anatomical names: **blepharon, palpebra**.

eyestrain (I-strayn) *n.* a sense of fatigue brought on by use of the eyes for prolonged close work or in persons who have an uncorrected error of refraction. Symptoms are usually aching or burning of the eyes, accompanied by headache. Medical name: **asthenopia**.

eye tooth *n. see* canine.

F

F 1. *abbreviation of* Fahrenheit. **2.** *symbol for* farad.

facet (fas-it) *n.* a small flat surface on a bone, especially a surface of articulation.

facet syndrome *n.* a syndrome caused by dislocation of the articulating surface of the vertebrae, resulting in pain and muscle spasm.

facial nerve (fay-shăl) *n.* the seventh cranial nerve (VII): a mixed sensory and motor nerve that supplies the muscles of facial expression, the taste buds of the front part of the tongue, the sublingual salivary glands, and the lacrimal glands.

-facient *suffix denoting* causing or making.

facies (fay-shi-eez) *n.* facial expression, often a guide to a patient's state of health as well as his emotions. The typical facies seen in adenoids is the vacant look, with the mouth drooping open.

Hippocratic f. the sallow face, sagging and with listless staring eyes, that some read as the expression of approaching death.

Factory Inspectorate (fak-ter-i in-spek-ter-it) *n.* a statutory body responsible for monitoring the health and safety of factory workers. It is administered by the Department of Employment through the Health and Safety Commission under the terms of the Health and Safety at Work Act.

facultative (fak-ŭl-tă-tiv) *adj.* describing an organism, such as a parasite, that is not restricted to one way of life. *Compare* obligate.

faecalith (fee-kă-lith) *n.* a small hard mass of faeces, found particularly in the vermiform appendix: a cause of inflammation.

faeces (fee-seez) *n.* the waste material that is eliminated through the anus. It is formed in the colon and consists of a solid or semisolid mass of undigested food remains (chiefly cellulose), bacteria, various secretions (e.g. mucus), and some water. —**faecal** (fee-kăl) *adj.*

Fahrenheit temperature (fa-rěn-hyt) *n.* temperature expressed on a scale in which the melting point of ice is assigned a temperature of 32° and the boiling point of water a temperature of 212°. The formula for converting from Fahrenheit (F) to Celsius (C) is: $C = \frac{5}{9}(F - 32)$. *See also* Celsius temperature. [G. D. Fahrenheit (1686–1736), German physicist]

fainting (faynt-ing) *n. see* syncope.

Fairbank's splint (fair-banks) *n.* a splint used for the correction of Erb's palsy in infants. It immobilizes the affected arm with the shoulder abducted and externally rotated, the elbow bent at 90°, and the forearm and wrist held in a supine position. [T. J. Fairbank, British orthopaedic surgeon]

falciform ligament (fal-si-form) *n.* a fold of peritoneum separating the right and left lobes of the liver and attaching it to the diaphragm and the anterior abdominal wall as far as the umbilicus.

Fallopian tube (oviduct, uterine tube) (fă-loh-piăn) *n.* either of a pair of tubes that conduct ova from the ovary to the womb (*see* reproductive system). The ovarian end opens into the abdominal cavity via a funnel-shaped structure with fimbriae surrounding the opening. The ovum is fertilized near the ovarian end of the tube. [G. Fallopius (1523–63), Italian anatomist]

Fallot's tetralogy (fal-ohz) *n. see* tetralogy of Fallot.

falx (falx cerebri) (falks) *n.* a sickle-shaped fold of the dura mater that dips inwards from the skull in the midline, between the cerebral hemispheres.

familial (fă-mil-iăl) *adj.* describing a condition or character that is found in some families but not in others. It is often inherited.

family planning (fam-ili plan-ing) *n.* **1.** the use of contraception to limit or space out the numbers of children born to a couple. **2.** provision of contraceptive methods within a community or nation.

Family Practitioner Committee (FPC) *n.* (in Britain) an authority responsible for running general medical services (general practitioners, dentists, pharmacists, and opticians) for the population served by a District Health Authority.

Fanconi syndrome (fan-koh-ni) *n.* a disorder of the proximal kidney tubules, which may be inherited or acquired and is most common in children. It is characterized by the urinary excretion of large amounts of amino acids, glucose, and phosphates. Symptoms may include osteomalacia, rickets, muscle weakness, and cystinosis. [G. Fanconi (1892–), Swiss paediatrician]

fantasy (phantasy) (fan-tă-si) *n.* a complex sequence of imagination in which several imaginary elements are woven together into a story. An excessive preoccupation with one's own imaginings may be symptomatic of a difficulty in coping with reality.

farad (fa-răd) *n.* the SI unit of capacitance, equal to the capacitance of a capacitor between the plates of which a potential difference of 1 volt appears when it is charged with 1 coulomb of electricity. Symbol: F.

faradism (fa-ră-dizm) *n.* the use of induced rapidly alternating electric currents to stimulate nerve and muscle activity. *See also* electrotherapy.

farcy (far-si) *n. see* glanders.

farinaceous (fa-ri-nay-shŭs) *adj.* starchy; describing foods rich in starch (e.g. flour, bread, cereals) or diets based on these foods.

farmer's lung (far-merz) *n.* an occupational lung disease caused by allergy to fungal spores that grow in inadequately dried stored hay. An acute reversible form can develop a few hours after exposure; a chronic form, with the gradual development of irreversible breathlessness, occurs

with or without preceding acute attacks.

fascia (fash-iă) *n.* (*pl.* **fasciae**) connective tissue that forms sheaths for muscles and protective layers surrounding the softer or more delicate organs immediately beneath the skin.

fasciculation (fă-sik-yoo-lay-shŏn) *n.* brief spontaneous contraction of a few muscle fibres, which is seen as a flicker of movement under the skin. It is most often associated with disease of the motor neurones in the spinal cord or of the nerve fibres.

fasciculus (fascicle) (fă-sik-yoo-lŭs) *n.* a bundle, e.g. of nerve or muscle fibres.

Fasciola (fas-i-oh-lă) *n.* a genus of flukes. *F. hepatica* the liver fluke, which normally lives as a parasite of sheep and other herbivorous animals but sometimes infects man (*see* fascioliasis).

fascioliasis (fas-i-oh-ly-ă-sis) *n.* an infestation of the bile ducts and liver with the liver fluke, *Fasciola hepatica*. Symptoms include fever, dyspepsia, vomiting, loss of appetite, abdominal pain, and coughing; the liver may also be extensively damaged.

fastigium (fas-tij-iŭm) *n.* the highest point of a fever.

fat (neutral fat) (fat) *n.* a substance that consists chiefly of triglycerides and is the principal form in which energy is stored by the body (*see* adipose tissue). It also serves as an insulating material beneath the skin and around certain organs. *See also* fatty acid; lipid.

fatigue (fă-teeg) *n.* **1.** mental or physical tiredness, following prolonged or intense activity. Muscle fatigue may be due to the waste products of metabolism accumulating in the muscles faster than they can be removed by the venous blood. **2.** the inability of an organism, an organ, or a tissue to give a normal response to a stimulus until a certain recovery period has elapsed.

fatty acid (fat-i) *n.* an organic acid such as oleic acid or stearic acid. Fatty acids are the fundamental constituents of many important lipids, including triglycerides. Some fatty acids can be synthesized by the body; others (*see* essential fatty acid) must be obtained from the diet. *See also* fat.

fatty degeneration *n.* deterioration in the health of a tissue due to the deposition of abnormally large amounts of fat in its cells. It may be caused by incorrect diet, excessive alcohol consumption, or a shortage of oxygen in the tissues.

fauces (faw-seez) *n.* the opening leading from the mouth into the pharynx. It is surrounded by the *glossopalatine arch* (which forms the anterior pillars of the fauces) and the *pharyngopalatine arch* (the posterior pillars).

favism (fay-vizm) *n.* an inherited allergy to a chemical substance found in broad beans; it occurs in parts of the Mediterranean and Iran. Destruction of red blood cells may lead to severe anaemia, requiring blood transfusion.

favus (fay-vŭs) *n.* a type of ringworm of the scalp, caused by the fungus *Trichophyton schoenteini*. Favus, which is rare in Europe, is typified by yellow crusts forming honeycomb-like masses.

fear (feer) *n.* an emotional state evoked by threat of danger. It is usually characterized by unpleasant subjective experiences; physiological changes, such as increased heart rate and sweating; and behavioural changes, such as avoidance of fear-producing objects or situations. *See also* phobia.

febricula (fi-brik-yoo-lă) *n.* a fever of low intensity or short duration.

febrifuge (feb-ri-fewj) *n.* a treatment or drug that reduces or prevents fever. *See* antipyretic.

febrile (fee-bryl) *adj.* relating to or affected with fever.

feeblemindedness (fee-bŭl-mynd-idnis) *n.* a mild degree of mental subnormality, corresponding roughly to an intelligence quotient of 50–70.

feedback (feed-bak) *n.* the coupling of the output of a process to the input. Feedback mechanisms are important in regulating many physiological processes; for example, hormone output and enzyme-mediated reactions.

Fehling's solution (fay-lingz) *n.* a solution used for detecting the presence of sugar in urine. There are two components: Fehling's I (a copper sulphate solution) and Fehling's II (a solution of potassium sodium tartrate and sodium hydroxide). [H. von Fehling (1812–85), German chemist]

felon (fel-ŏn) *n. see* whitlow.

Felty's syndrome (fel-tiz) *n.* enlargement of the spleen (*see* hypersplenism) associated with rheumatoid arthritis, characterized by a decrease in the numbers of white blood cells and frequent infections. [A. R. Felty (1895–), US physician]

feminization (fem-i-ny-zay-shŏn) *n.* the development of female secondary sexual characteristics (enlargement of the breasts, loss of facial hair, and fat beneath the skin) in the male, either as a result of an endocrine disorder or of hormone therapy.

femoral (fem-er-ăl) *adj.* of or relating to the thigh or to the femur. *f. artery* an artery arising from the external iliac artery. It runs down the front medial aspect of the thigh, passing into the back of the thigh two-thirds of the way down. *f. nerve* the nerve that supplies the quadriceps muscle at the front of the thigh and receives sensation from the front and inner sides of the thigh. *f. triangle* (*Scarpa's triangle*) a triangular depression on the inner side of the thigh bounded by the sartorius and adductor longus muscles and the inguinal ligament. The pulse can be felt here as the femoral artery lies over the depression.

femur (thigh bone) (fee-mer) *n.* a long bone between the hip and the knee. The head of the femur articulates with the acetabulum of the hip bone; the lower end articulates with the tibia.

fenestra (fi-nes-trǎ) *n.* (in anatomy) an opening resembling a window. *f. ovalis* (*f. vestibuli*) the opening between the middle ear and the vestibule of the inner ear. *f. rotunda* (*f. cochleae*) the opening between the scala tympani of the cochlea and the middle ear.

fenestration (fen-i-stray-shŏn) *n.* a surgical operation in which a new opening is formed in the bony labyrinth of the inner ear as part of the treatment of deafness due to otosclerosis.

fenfluramine (fen-floor-ǎ-meen) *n.* a drug, similar to amphetamine, that reduces the appetite and is administered by mouth in the treatment of obesity. Trade name: **Ponderax**.

fenoprofen (fen-oh-proh-fĕn) *n.* an analgesic drug that also reduces inflammation and is administered by mouth to treat arthritic conditions. Trade name: **Fenopron**.

fermentation (fer-men-tay-shŏn) *n.* the biochemical process by which organic substances, particularly carbohydrates, are decomposed by the action of enzymes to provide chemical energy, as in the production of alcohol.

ferri- (ferro-) *prefix denoting* iron.

ferrous sulphate (fe-rǔs) *n.* an iron salt administered by mouth to treat or prevent iron-deficiency anaemia. Similar preparations used to treat anaemia include ferrous fumarate and ferrous succinate.

fertility rate (fer-til-iti) *n.* the number of live births occurring in a year per 1000 women of child-bearing age (usually 15 to 44 years of age).

fertilization (fer-ti-ly-zay-shŏn) *n.* the fusion of a spermatozoon and an ovum to form a zygote.

fester (fes-ter) *vb.* (of superficial wounds) to become inflamed, with the formation of pus.

festination (fes-ti-nay-shŏn) *n.* the short tottering steps that characterize the gait of a patient with parkinsonism.

fetishism (fet-i-shizm) *n.* sexual attraction to an inappropriate object (known as a *fetish*). This may be a part of the body, clothing, or other objects (e.g. leather handbags or rubber sheets). Treatment can involve psychotherapy or behaviour therapy. *See also* perversion.

feto- *prefix denoting* a fetus.

fetor (foetor) (fee-ter) *n.* an unpleasant smell. *f. oris* bad breath (*see* halitosis).

fetoscopy (fi-tos-kŏpi) *n.* a technique that enables the blood of a fetus to be examined for the prenatal diagnosis of blood disorders. A hollow needle is inserted through the abdomen of a pregnant woman and fetal blood is withdrawn from a blood vessel on the placenta.

fetus (foetus) (fee-tŭs) *n.* a mammalian embryo during the later stages of development within the womb, i.e. in humans from the beginning of the third month of pregnancy until birth. —**fetal** *adj.*

fever (pyrexia) (fee-ver) *n.* a rise in body temperature above the normal, i.e. above an oral temperature of 98.6°F (37°C) or a rectal temperature of 99°F (37.2°C), usually caused by bacterial or viral infection. Fever is generally accompanied by shivering, headache, nausea, constipation, or diarrhoea. *intermittent f.* a periodic rise and fall in body temperature, as in malaria. *remittent f.* a fever that diminishes daily, as in typhoid fever. *See also* relapsing fever.

fibr- (fibro-) *prefix denoting* fibres or fibrous tissue.

fibre (fy-ber) *n.* 1. (in anatomy) a threadlike structure, such as a muscle cell, a nerve fibre, or a collagen fibre. 2. (in dietetics) *see* dietary fibre. —**fibrous** (fy-brŭs) *adj.*

fibre optics *n.* the use of fibres for the transmission of light images. Synthetic fibres with special optical properties can be used in instruments to relay pictures of the inside of the body for direct ob-

servation or photography. *See* fibrescope.

fibrescope (fy-ber-skohp) *n.* an endoscope that uses fibre optics for the transmission of images from the interior of the body. Being flexible, fibrescopes can be introduced into relatively inaccessible cavities of the body.

fibril (fy-bril) *n.* a very small fibre or a constituent thread of a fibre. —**fibrillar, fibrillary** *adj.*

fibrillation (fy-bril-ay-shŏn) *n.* a rapid and chaotic beating of the many individual muscle fibres of the heart, which is consequently unable to maintain effective synchronous contraction. The affected part of the heart then ceases to pump blood. *atrial f.* a common type of arrhythmia that results in rapid and irregular heart and pulse rates. The main causes are atherosclerosis, chronic rheumatic heart disease, and hypertensive heart disease. *ventricular f.* fibrillation that causes the heart to stop beating (*see* cardiac arrest). It is most commonly the result of myocardial infarction.

fibrin (fib-rin) *n.* the final product of the process of blood coagulation, produced by the action of the enzyme thrombin on a soluble precursor fibrinogen. Fibrin molecules link together to give a fibrous meshwork that forms the basis of a blood clot.

fibrinogen (fi-brin-ŏ-jĕn) *n.* a substance (*see* coagulation factors), present in blood plasma, that is acted upon by the enzyme thrombin to produce the insoluble protein fibrin in the final stage of blood coagulation.

fibrinogenopenia (fi-brin-ŏ-jen-oh-pee-niă) *n. see* hypofibrinogenaemia.

fibrinolysin (fib-ri-**nol**-i-sin) *n. see* plasmin.

fibrinolysis (fib-ri-**nol**-i-sis) *n.* the process by which blood clots are removed from the circulation, involving digestion of the insoluble protein fibrin by the enzyme plasmin.

fibroadenoma (fy-broh-ad-in-**oh**-ma) *n. see* adenoma.

fibroblast (**fy**-broh-blast) *n.* a widely distributed cell in connective tissue that is responsible for the production of both the ground substance and the precursors of collagen, elastic fibres, and reticular fibres.

fibrocartilage (fy-broh-**kar**-ti-lij) *n.* a tough kind of cartilage in which there are dense bundles of fibres in the matrix.

fibrochondritis (fy-broh-kon-**dry**-tis) *n.* an inflammation of fibrocartilage.

fibrocyst (**fy**-broh-sist) *n.* a benign tumour of fibrous connective tissue containing cystic spaces. —**fibrocystic** (fy-broh-**sis**-tik) *adj.*

fibrocystic disease of the pancreas *n. see* cystic fibrosis.

fibrocyte (**fy**-broh-syt) *n.* an inactive cell present in fully differentiated connective tissue. It is derived from a fibroblast.

fibroelastosis (fy-broh-ee-las-**toh**-sis) *n.* overgrowth or disturbed growth of the yellow (elastic) fibres in connective tissue. *endocardial f.* overgrowth and thickening of the wall of the heart's left ventricle.

fibroid (**fy**-broid) **1.** *n.* (**fibromyoma, uterine fibroma**) a benign tumour of fibrous and muscular tissue, one or more of which may develop in the muscular wall of the womb. Fibroids often cause pain and excessive menstrual bleeding; they can be re-moved surgically. **2.** *adj.* resembling or containing fibres.

fibroma (fy-**broh**-mă) *n.* (*pl.* **fibromas** or **fibromata**) a nonmalignant tumour of connective tissue.

fibromyoma (fy-broh-my-**oh**-mă) *n. see* fibroid.

fibrosarcoma (fy-broh-sar-**koh**-mă) *n.* a malignant tumour of connective tissue, derived from fibroblasts. Fibrosarcomas may arise in soft tissue or bone; they can affect any organ but are most common in the limbs, particularly the leg.

fibrosis (fy-**broh**-sis) *n.* thickening and scarring of connective tissue, most often a consequence of inflammation or injury. *pulmonary interstitial f.* thickening and stiffening of the lining of the alveoli causing progressive breathlessness. *See also* cystic fibrosis.

fibrositis (fy-brŏ-sy-tis) *n.* inflammation of fibrous connective tissue, especially an acute inflammation of back muscles and their sheaths, causing pain and stiffness.

fibula (**fib**-yoo-lă) *n.* the long thin outer bone of the lower leg. The head of the fibula articulates with the tibia just below the knee; the lower end projects laterally and articulates with one side of the talus.

field of vision (feeld ŏv **vizh**-ŏn) *n. see* visual field.

filament (**fil**-ă-měnt) *n.* a very fine threadlike structure, such as a chain of bacterial cells. —**filamentous** (fil-ă-**ment**-ŭs) *adj.*

filaria (fil-**air**-iă) *n.* (*pl.* **filariae**) any of the long threadlike nematode worms that, as adults, are parasites of the connective and lymphatic tissues of man capable of causing disease. They include the genera *Brugia*, *Loa*, *Onchocerca*, and *Wuchereria*. *See also* microfilaria. —**filarial** *adj.*

filariasis (fil-er-I-ă-sis) *n.* a disease, common in the tropics and subtropics, caused by the presence in the lymph vessels of the filariae *Wuchereria bancrofti* and *Brugia malayi*. The lymph vessels eventually become blocked, causing the surrounding tissues to swell (*see* elephantiasis). Filariasis is treated with the drug diethylcarbamazine.

filiform (fil-i-form) *adj.* shaped like a thread. *f. papillae* threadlike papillae on the tongue.

filipuncture (fil-i-punk-cher) *n.* the insertion of a fine wire thread into an aneurysm in order to cause clotting of the blood within it.

filling (fil-ing) *n.* (in dentistry) the operation of inserting a specially prepared substance into a hole drilled in a carious tooth.

filtration (fil-tray-shŏn) *n.* the passage of a liquid through a porous filter in order to separate the solids or suspended particles within it.

filum (fy-lŭm) *n.* a threadlike structure. *f. terminale* the slender tapering terminal section of the spinal cord.

fimbria (fim-briă) *n.* (*pl.* **fimbriae**) a fringe or fringelike process, such as any of the finger-like projections that surround the opening of the ovarian end of the Fallopian tube.

fingerprint (fing-er-print) *n.* the distinctive pattern of minute ridges in the outer horny layer of the skin. Every individual has his or her own unique pattern. *See also* dermatoglyphics.

first aid (ferst) *n.* procedures used in an emergency to help a wounded or ill patient before the arrival of a doctor or admission to hospital.

first intention *n. see* intention.

fission (fish-ŏn) *n.* a method of asexual reproduction in which the body of a protozoan or bacterium splits into two equal parts (*binary f.*), as in the amoebae, or more than two equal parts (*multiple f.*).

fissure (fish-er) *n.* **1.** (in anatomy) a groove or cleft. **2.** (in pathology) a cleftlike defect in the skin or mucous membrane caused by some disease process. *anal f.* a break in the skin lining the anal canal.

fistula (fiss-tew-lă) *n.* an abnormal communication between two hollow organs or between a hollow organ and the exterior. Many fistulas are due to infection or injury, but there are a number of other causes. *anal f.* an opening between the anal canal and the surface of the skin that may develop after an abscess in the rectum has burst. *biliary f.* a fistula that may develop as a complication of gall bladder surgery. *gastrocolic f.* a fistula between the colon and the stomach that may result from malignant growth or ulceration. *rectovaginal f.* an opening between the rectum and vagina that occurs as a congenital abnormality.

fit (fit) *n.* a sudden attack. The term is usually reserved for the attacks of epilepsy but it is also used more generally, e.g. a fit of coughing.

fixation (fiks-ay-shŏn) *n.* **1.** (in psychoanalysis) a failure of psychological development, in which traumatic events prevent a child from progressing to the next developmental stage. *See also* psychosexual development. **2.** a procedure for the hardening and preservation of tissues or microorganisms to be examined under a microscope.

flaccid (flak-sid) *adj.* **1.** flabby and lacking in firmness. **2.** characterized by a decrease in muscle tone (e.g. *f. paralysis*). —**flaccidity** (flak-**sid**-iti) *n.*

flagellate (flaj-ĕl-ayt) *n.* a type of protozoan with one or more flagella projecting from its body surface, by means of which it is able to swim. Some flagellates are parasites of man. *See* trypanosomiasis, Leishmania, giardiasis, Trichomonas.

flagellum (flă-jel-ŭm) *n.* (*pl.* **flagella**) a fine long whiplike thread attached to certain types of cell (e.g. spermatozoa and flagellates). Flagella are responsible for the movement of the organisms to which they are attached.

flail chest (flayl) *n.* instability of the chest wall due to multiple fractures of the ribs, causing paradoxical breathing.

flap (flap) *n.* (in surgery) a strip of tissue dissected away from the underlying structures but left attached at one end so that it retains its blood and nerve supply. The flap is then used to repair a defect in another part of the body or to cover the end of a bone in an amputated limb. It is detached from its original site when it has healed into the new one.

flare (flair) *n.* **1.** reddening of the skin that spreads outwards from a focus of infection or irritation in the skin. **2.** the red outside part of an urticarial wheal – the skin's response in an allergic or hypersensitivity reaction (*see* urticaria).

flat-foot (flat-fuut) *n.* absence of the arching of the foot, so that the sole lies flat upon the ground. It may be present in infancy or be acquired in adult life. Medical name: **pes planus**.

flatulence (flat-yoo-lĕns) *n.* **1.** the expulsion of gas or air from the stomach through the mouth; belching. **2.** a sensation of abdominal distension. —**flatulent** *adj.*

flatus (flay-tŭs) *n.* intestinal gas, composed partly of swallowed air and partly of gas produced by bacterial fermentation of intestinal contents.

flatworm (**platyhelminth**) (flat-werm) *n.* any of the flatbodied worms, including the flukes and tapeworms. Both these groups contain many parasites of medical importance.

flav- (**flavo-**) *prefix denoting* yellow.

flea (flee) *n.* a small wingless bloodsucking insect with a laterally compressed body and long legs adapted for jumping. Adult fleas are temporary parasites on birds and mammals and those species that attack man (*Pulex*, *Xenopsylla*, and *Nosopsyllus*) may be important in the transmission of various diseases. Their bites may become a focus of infection.

flexibilitas cerea (fleks-i-**bil**-i-tas se-ri-ă) *n.* a disorder of posture in which a patient's limbs offer a continuous mild resistance to being moved passively by the examiner and remain for long periods in the position into which the examiner has moved them. It is a feature of catatonia. *See also* catalepsy.

flexion (flek-shŏn) *n.* the bending of a joint so that the bones forming it are brought towards each other. *plantar f.* the bending of the toes (or fingers) downwards, towards the sole· (or palm). *See also* dorsiflexion.

Flexner's bacillus (fleks-nerz) *n.* the bacterium *Shigella flexneri*, which causes a form of bacillary dysentery. [S. Flexner (1863– 1946), US pathologist]

flexor (fleks-er) *n.* any muscle that causes bending of a limb or other part.

flexure (flek-sher) *n.* a bend in an organ or part, such as the *hepatic* and *splenic flexures* of the colon.

floccillation (flok-si-lay-shŏn) *n. see* carphology.

flocculation (flok-yoo-lay-shŏn) *n.* a reaction in which normally invisible material leaves solution to form a coarse suspension or precipitate. *See also* agglutination.

flooding (flud-ing) *n.* **1.** excessive bleeding from the womb, as in menorrhagia or miscarriage. **2.** (also called **implosion**) a method of treating phobias in which the patient is exposed intensively and at length to the feared object, either in reality or fantasy.

floppy baby syndrome (flop-i) *n. see* amyotonia congenita.

flowmeter (floh-mee-ter) *n.* an instrument for measuring the flow of a liquid or gas.

fluctuation (fluk-tew-ay-shŏn) *n.* the characteristic feeling of a wave motion produced in a fluid-filled part of the body by an examiner's fingers. If fluctuation is present when a swelling is examined, this is an indication that there is fluid within.

fludrocortisone (floo-droh-kor-tiz-ohn) *n.* a synthetic corticosteroid administered by mouth to treat disorders of the adrenal glands. Trade name: **Florinef**.

flufenamic acid (floo-fĕ-nam-ik) *n.* an analgesic drug administered by mouth to relieve moderate pain, such as headache, rheumatic conditions, and toothache. Trade name: **Arlef**.

fluke (flook) *n.* any of the parasitic flatworms belonging to the group Trematoda. Adult flukes are parasites of man, occurring in the liver (*see* Fasciola), lungs (*see* paragonimiasis), gut (*see* heterophyiasis), and blood vessels (*see* Schistosoma) and often cause serious disease.

fluorescein sodium (floo-er-ess-i-in) *n.* a water-soluble dye that glows with a brilliant green colour when light is shone on it. A dilute solution is used to detect defects in the surface of the cornea, since it stains areas where the epithelium is not intact.

fluorescence (floo-er-ess-ĕns) *n.* the emission of light by a material as it absorbs radiation from outside. The radiation absorbed may be visible or invisible (e.g. ultraviolet rays or X-rays). *See* fluoroscope. —**fluorescent** *adj.*

fluoridation (floo-er-id-ay-shŏn) *n.* the addition of fluoride to drinking water in order to reduce dental caries. Drinking water with a fluoride content of one part per million is effective in reducing caries throughout life when given during the years of tooth development. *See also* fluorosis.

fluoride (floo-eryd) *n.* a compound of fluorine. The incorporation of fluoride ions in the enamel of teeth makes them more resistant to dental caries. Fluoride may be applied through fluoridation or topically in toothpaste or by a dentist.

fluoroscope (floo-er-ŏ-skohp) *n.* an instrument on which X-ray images may be viewed directly, without taking and developing X-ray photographs. It consists basically of a *fluorescent screen*, which is coated with chemicals that exhibit fluorescence when exposed to X-rays. Fluoroscopes are used for mass chest X-ray examinations.

fluorosis (floo-er-oh-sis) *n.* the effects of high fluoride intake. When the level of fluoride in the water supply is above 2 parts per million the enamel of teeth becomes mottled. At above 8 parts per million, calcification of ligaments occurs. *See also* fluoridation.

fluorouracil (floo-er-oh-**yoor**-ă-sil) *n.* a drug that prevents cell growth (*see* antimetabolite) and is used in the treatment of cancers of the digestive system and breast. It is administered by mouth or injection. Fluorouracil is also applied as a cream to treat certain skin conditions, including skin cancer.

fluphenazine (floo-**fen**-ă-zeen) *n.* a tranquillizer used to relieve anxiety and tension and to treat nausea and vomiting following anaesthesia. It is administered by mouth or injection. Trade names: **Modecate, Moditen.**

flurazepam (floor-**az**-ĕ-pam) *n.* a sedative drug administered by mouth to treat insomnia and sleep disturbances (*see* hypnotic). Trade name: **Dalmane.**

fluspirilene (floo-spy-ri-leen) *n.* a major tranquillizer administered by injection to treat schizophrenia. Trade name: **Redeptin.**

flutter (**flut**-er) *n.* a disturbance of normal heart rhythm, less rapid and less chaotic than fibrillation.

flux (fluks) *n.* an abnormally copious flow from an organ or cavity.

fly (fly) *n.* a two-winged insect belonging to the order Diptera. The mouthparts of flies are adapted for sucking and sometimes also for piercing and biting. Fly larvae (maggots) may infest human tissues and cause disease (*see* myiasis).

focal distance (foh-kăl) *n.* (of the eye) the distance between the lens and the point behind the lens at which light from a distant object is focused.

focus (foh-kŭs) **1.** *n.* the point at which rays of light converge after passing through a lens. **2.** *n.* the principal site of an infection or other disease. **3.** *vb.* (in ophthalmology) to accommodate (*see* accommodation).

foetus (fee-tŭs) *n. see* fetus.

folic acid (pteroylglutamic acid) (foh-lik) *n.* a B vitamin that is important in the synthesis of nucleic acids. The metabolic role of folic acid is interdependent with that of vitamin B_{12} (both are required by rapidly dividing cells) and a deficiency of one may lead to deficiency of the other. A deficiency of folic acid results in the condition of megaloblastic anaemia. Good sources of folic acid are liver and vegetables.

folie à deux (communicated insanity) (fol-i a der) *n.* a condition in which two people who are closely involved with each other share a system of delusions.

follicle (fol-ikŭl) *n.* a small secretory cavity, sac, or gland. *See also* Graafian follicle, hair (follifrontal bones

anterior
fontanelle

coronal
suture

sagittal
suture

parietal bone

posterior
fontanelle

occipital bone

Fontanelles in the skull of a
newborn infant (from above)

cle). **—follicular** (fŏ-**lik**-yoo-ler)
adj.

follicle-stimulating hormone (FSH)
n. a hormone (*see* gonadotrophin) synthesized and released
by the anterior pituitary gland.
FSH stimulates ripening of the
follicles in the ovary and formation of sperm in the testes. It is
injected to treat sterility.

folliculitis (fŏ-lik-yoo-ly-tis) *n.* inflammation of hair follicles in
the skin, commonly caused by
infection. *See also* sycosis.

fomentation (foh-men-**tay**-shŏn) *n.*
see poultice.

fomes (**foh**-meez) *n.* (*pl.* **fomites**)
any object that is used or handled by a person with a communicable disease and may therefore become contaminated with
the infective organisms and
transmit the disease to a subsequent user. Common fomites are
towels, bed-clothes, and cups.

fontanelle (fon-tă-**nel**) *n.* an opening in the skull of a fetus or
young infant due to incomplete
ossification of the cranial bones
and the resulting incomplete closure of the sutures. *anterior f.*

the opening at the junction of
the coronal, frontal, and sagittal
sutures. *posterior f.* the opening
at the junction of the sagittal
and lambdoidal sutures.

food poisoning (food) *n.* an illness
affecting the digestive system
that results from eating food
contaminated either by bacteria
or bacterial toxins or, less commonly, by poisonous chemicals
such as lead or mercury. It can
also be caused by eating poisonous fungi, berries, etc. Symptoms
include vomiting, diarrhoea, abdominal pain, and nausea. Foodborne infections are caused by
bacteria of the genus *Salmonella*
in foods of animal origin.
Toxin-producing bacteria causing
food poisoning include those of
the genus *Staphylococcus*, which
rapidly multiply in warm foods,
and the species *Clostridium
welchii*, which multiplies in
reheated cooked meals. *See also*
botulism, gastroenteritis.

foot drop (**fuut**-drop) *n.* inability
to keep the foot at right angles
to the leg, caused by paralysis of
the anterior leg muscles, pressure
of bedclothes, or insufficient support for the sole of the foot
when the leg is splinted.

foramen (fo-**ray**-men) *n.* (*pl.* **foramina**) an opening or hole, particularly in a bone. *apical f.* the
small opening at the apex of a
tooth. *f. magnum* a large hole in
the occipital bone through which
the spinal cord passes. *f. ovale*
the opening between the two
atria of the fetal heart, which allows blood to flow from the
right to the left side of the heart
by displacing a membranous
valve.

forceps (**for**-seps) *n.* a pincer-like
instrument designed to grasp an

bone-holding forceps

volsella

sinus forceps

dissecting forceps

dressing forceps

obstetrical forceps

dental extraction forceps

Types of forceps

object so that it can be held firm or pulled. Specially designed forceps are used by surgeons and dentists in operations (see illustration).

forebrain (for-brayn) *n.* the furthest forward division of the brain, consisting of the diencephalon and the two cerebral hemispheres.

foregut (for-gut) *n.* the front part of the embryonic gut, which gives rise to the oesophagus, stomach, and part of the small intestine.

forensic medicine (fer-en-sik) *n.* the branch of medicine concerned with the scientific investigation of the causes of injury and death in unexplained circumstances, particularly when criminal activity is suspected.

foreskin (for-skin) *n. see* prepuce.

forewaters (for-waw-terz) *n.* fluid that comes out of the vaginal opening when the bag (amnion) around the fetus bursts during labour.

formaldehyde (for-**mal**-di-hyd) *n.* the aldehyde derivative of formic acid, used as a vapour to sterilize and disinfect rooms and such items as mattresses and blankets. The toxic vapour is produced by boiling formalin in an open container or using it in a sealed autoclave.

formalin (for-mă-lin) *n.* a solution containing 40% formaldehyde in water, used as a sterilizing agent.

formication (for-mi-**kay**-shŏn) *n.* a prickling sensation said to resemble the feeling of ants crawling over the skin. It is a form of paraesthesiae and it is sometimes a symptom of drug intoxication.

formula (form-yoo-lă) *n.* 1. a representation of the structure of a chemical compound using symbols and subscript numbers for the atoms it contains (e.g. H_2O for water; CO_2 for carbon dioxide). 2. a prescription for a drug.

formulary (form-yoo-ler-i) *n.* a compendium of formulae used in

Colles'

greenstick

comminuted

impacted

compound

Pott's

Types of fracture

the preparation of medicinal drugs.

fornix (for-niks) *n.* (*pl.* **fornices**) an arched or vaultlike structure.

f. cerebri a triangular structure of white matter in the brain, situated between the hippocampus and hypothalamus. *f. of the vagina* any of three vaulted spaces at the top of the vagina, around the cervix of the womb.

fossa (fos-ă) *n.* (*pl.* **fossae**) a depression or hollow. *cubital f.* the triangular hollow at the front of the elbow joint. *iliac f.* the depression in the inner surface of the ilium. *pituitary f.* the hollow in the sphenoid bone in which the pituitary gland is situated.

Fothergill's operation (foth-er-gilz) *n.* an operation for prolapse of the womb in which the cervix is amputated and the vagina is sutured to reduce its laxity. [W. E. Fothergill (1865–1926), British gynaecologist]

fourchette (foor-**shet**) *n.* a thin fold of skin at the back of the vulva.

fovea (foh-viă) *n.* (in anatomy) a small depression, especially the shallow pit in the retina at the back of the eye. It contains a large number of cones and is therefore the area of greatest acuity of vision. *See also* macula (lutea).

fracture (frak-cher) *n.* breakage of a bone, either complete or incomplete. Treatment includes realignment of the bone ends and immobilization by external splints or internal fixation. *Colles' f.* fracture of the wrist, across the lower end of the radius. The hand and wrist below the fracture are displaced backwards. *comminuted f.* a fracture in which the bone is broken into more than two pieces. *compound f.* a fracture in which the bone end pierces the overlying skin. *greenstick f.* an incomplete break

in a long bone occurring in children. *impacted f.* a fracture in which the bone ends are driven into each other. *pathological f.* fracture of an already diseased bone that may occur after minor injuries. *Pott's f.* a fracture of the lower end of the fibula accompanied by a fracture of the malleolus of the tibia. *simple f.* a clean break with little damage to surrounding tissues.

fragilitas (fră-**jil**-i-tas) *n.* abnormal brittleness or fragility. *f. crinium* brittleness of the hair. *f. ossium* brittleness of the bones (*see* osteogenesis (imperfecta)).

framboesia (fram-**bee**-ziă) *n. see* yaws.

framycetin (fra-my-**see**-tin) *n.* an antibiotic used in the form of an ointment, cream, or solution to treat skin, eye, and ear infections. It is also administered by mouth to treat gastoenteritis and food poisoning. Trade names: **Framygen, Soframycin.**

fraternal twins (fră-**ter**-năl) *pl. n. see* twins.

free association (free) *n.* (in psychoanalysis) a technique in which the patient is encouraged to pursue a particular train of ideas as they enter consciousness. *See also* association of ideas.

Freiburg's disease (fry-bergz) *n.* osteochondritis affecting the head of the second metatarsal bone. [A. H. Freiburg (1868–1940), US orthopaedic surgeon]

Frei test (fry) *n.* a diagnostic test for the venereal disease lymphogranuloma venereum. [W. S. Frei (1885–1943), German dermatologist]

fremitus (**frem**-i-tŭs) *n.* vibrations or tremors in a part of the body, detected by palpation or auscultation. The term is most commonly applied to vibrations perceived through the chest when a patient breathes, speaks (*vocal f.*), or coughs.

frenulum (frenum) (fren-yoo-lŭm) *n.* **1.** any of the folds of mucous membrane under the tongue or between the gums and the upper or lower lips. **2.** any of several other structures of similar appearance.

frenum (free-nŭm) *n. see* frenulum.

Freudian (froi-di-ăn) *adj.* relating to or describing the work and ideas of Sigmund Freud (1856–1939): applied particularly to the school of psychiatry based on his teachings (*see* psychoanalysis).

friar's balsam (fry-erz) *n.* a tincture of benzoin, balsam of Tolu, storax, aloes, and various other plant extracts, the vapour of which is inhaled to relieve bronchitis.

friction murmur (friction rub) (frik-shŏn) *n.* a scratching sound, heard over the heart with the aid of the stethoscope, in patients who have pericarditis. It results from the two inflamed layers of the pericardium rubbing together during activity of the heart.

Friedländer's bacillus (freed-lenderz) *n.* a Gram-negative rodlike bacterium, *Klebsiella pneumoniae*, that causes a form of pneumonia. [K. Friedländer (1847–87), German pathologist]

Friedman's test (freed-manz) *n.* a pregnancy test in which a sample of the woman's urine is injected into an unmated female rabbit. After two days the rabbit is killed and its ovaries examined. If the woman is pregnant her urine will contain enough chorionic gonadotrophin to induce the development of corpora lutea in the ovaries of the rabbit. [M. H. Friedman (1903–), US physician]

Friedreich's ataxia (freed-ryks) *n. see* ataxia. [N. Friedreich (1825–82), German neurologist]

frigidity (fri-jid-iti) *n.* lack of sexual desire or inability to reach the climax of sexual excitement, especially in a woman.

fringe medicine (frinj) *n.* the various systems of healing, such as osteopathy and acupuncture, that are not regarded as part of orthodox treatment by the medical profession.

frog plaster (frog) *n.* a plaster of Paris splint used to maintain the legs in their correct position after a congenital dislocation of the hip has been corrected by manipulation.

Fröhlich's syndrome (frer-liks) *n.* a disorder of the hypothalamus affecting males: the boy is overweight with sexual development absent and disturbances of sleep and appetite. Medical name: **dystrophia adiposogenitalis**. [A. Fröhlich (1871–1953), Austrian neurologist]

frontal (frun-t'l) *adj.* **1.** of or relating to the forehead. *f. bone* the bone forming the forehead and the upper parts of the orbits. *f. sinuses see* paranasal sinuses. **2.** denoting the anterior part of a body or organ. *f. lobe* the anterior part of each cerebral hemisphere, extending as far back as the deep central sulcus of its upper and outer surface.

frostbite (frost-byt) *n.* damage to the tissues caused by freezing. The affected parts, usually the nose, fingers, or toes, become pale and numb. Ice forms in the tissues, which may thus be destroyed, and amputation may become necessary. Frostbitten skin is highly susceptible to bacterial infection.

frozen shoulder (froh-zĕn) *n.* chronic painful stiffness of the shoulder joint. This may follow injury, a stroke, or myocardial infarction or may gradually develop for no apparent reason. *See also* capsulitis.

fructose (fruk-tohz) *n.* a simple sugar found in honey and in such fruit as figs. Fructose is one of the two sugars in sucrose.

fructosuria (levulosuria) (fruk-tohz-yoor-iă) *n.* the presence of fructose (levulose) in the urine.

frusemide (frus-ĕ-myd) *n.* a diuretic administered by mouth or injection to treat fluid retention (oedema) associated with heart, liver, or kidney disease and also high blood pressure. Trade name: Lasix.

FSH *n. see* follicle-stimulating hormone.

fuchsin (magenta) (fook-sin) *n.* any one of a group of reddish to purplish dyes used in staining bacteria for microscopic observation and capable of killing various disease-causing microorganisms.

-fuge *suffix denoting* an agent that drives away, repels, or eliminates.

fugue (fewg) *n.* a period of memory loss during which the patient leaves his usual surroundings and wanders aimlessly or starts a new life elsewhere. It is often preceded by psychological conflict and depression, and may be associated with hysteria or organic mental disease. *See also* dissociation.

fulguration (electrodesiccation) (ful-gewr-ay-shŏn) *n.* the destruction with a diathermy instrument of warts, growths, or unwanted areas of tissue, particularly inside the bladder.

fulminating (fulminant, fulgurant) (ful-min-ayt-ing) *adj.* describing a condition or symptom that is of very sudden onset, severe, and of short duration.

fumigation (few-mig-ay-shŏn) *n.* the use of gases or vapours, such as formaldehyde or chlorine, to bring about disinfestation of clothing, buildings, etc.

functional disorder (funk-shŏn-ăl) *n.* a condition in which a patient complains of symptoms for which no physical cause can be found. Such a condition is frequently an indication of a psychiatric disorder. *Compare* organic (disorder).

fundus (fun-dŭs) *n.* **1.** the base of a hollow organ: the part farthest from the opening. **2.** part of the interior of the eye that is situated opposite the pupil.

fungicide (fun-ji-syd) *n.* an agent that kills fungi. *See also* antimycotic.

fungoid (fung-oid) **1.** *adj.* resembling a fungus. **2.** *n.* a fungus-like growth.

fungus (fung-ŭs) *n.* (*pl.* **fungi**) a simple plant that lacks the green pigment chlorophyll. Fungi include the yeasts, rusts, moulds, and mushrooms. Some species infect and cause disease in man (*see* blastomycosis). The yeasts are a good source of vitamin B and many antibiotics are obtained from the moulds (*see* penicillin). —**fungal** *adj.*

funiculitis (few-nik-yoo-ly-tis) *n.* inflammation of the spermatic cord.

funiculus (few-nik-yoo-lŭs) *n.* **1.** any of the three main columns of white matter found in each lateral half of the spinal cord. **2.**

a bundle of nerve fibres enclosed in a sheath. **3.** (formerly) the spermatic cord or umbilical cord.

funis (**few**-nis) *n.* (in anatomy) any cordlike structure, especially the umbilical cord.

funnel chest (**fun**-ĕl) *n.* a developmental abnormality in which the sternum is depressed and the ribs and costal cartilages curve inwards.

furfuraceous (fer-fewr-ay-shŭs) *adj.* describing scaling of skin in which the scales resemble bran or dandruff.

furor (**fewr**-or) *n.* indiscriminate violence and destructiveness, occurring especially during a period of mental confusion due to epilepsy.

furuncle (**fewr**-ung-kŭl) *n. see* boil.

furunculosis (fewr-unk-yoo-**loh**-sis) *n.* **1.** the occurrence of several boils (furuncles) at the same time. **2.** the recurrence of boils in the skin over a period of weeks or months.

fusiform (**few**-zi-form) *adj.* spindle-shaped; tapering at both ends.

fusion (**few**-*zh*ŏn) *n.* (in surgery) the joining together of two structures.

G

GABA *see* gamma aminobutyric acid.

gag (gag) *n.* (in medicine) an instrument that is placed between a patient's teeth to keep his mouth open.

gait (gayt) *n.* a manner of walking. *ataxic g.* an unsteady unco-ordinated walk due to disease of the sensory nerves or cerebellum. *See* ataxia. *cerebellar g.* a staggering walk due to disease of the

cerebellum. *spastic g.* a stiff shuffling walk in which the legs are held together.

galact- (**galacto-**) *prefix denoting* **1.** milk. **2.** galactose.

galactagogue (gă-**lak**-tă-gog) *n.* an agent that stimulates the secretion of milk or increases milk flow.

galactocele (gă-**lak**-toh-seel) *n.* **1.** a breast tumour containing milk, caused by closure cf a milk duct. **2.** an accumulation of milky liquid in the sac surrounding the testis (*see* hydrocele).

galactorrhoea (gă-lak-tŏ-**ree**-ă) *n.* **1.** abnormally copious milk secretion. **2.** secretion of milk after breast feeding has been stopped.

galactosaemia (gă-lak-toh-**see**-miă) *n.* an inborn inability to utilize the sugar galactose, which in consequence accumulates in the blood. Untreated, affected infants fail to thrive and become mentally retarded, but if galactose is eliminated from the diet growth and development may be normal.

galactose (gă-**lak**-tohz) *n.* a simple

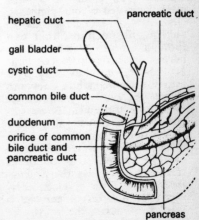

The gall bladder and pancreas

sugar and a constituent of the milk sugar lactose. Galactose is converted to glucose in the liver.

galea (gay-liă) *n.* 1. a helmet-shaped anatomical part. 2. a type of head bandage.

galenical (gă-len-ikăl) *n.* a pharmaceutical preparation of a drug of animal or plant origin.

gallamine (gal-ă-meen) *n.* a drug administered by injection to produce muscle relaxation during anaesthesia (*see* muscle relaxant). It is also used in a diagnostic test for myasthenia gravis. Trade name: **Flaxedil.**

gall bladder (gawl) *n.* a pear-shaped sac (7–10 cm long), lying underneath the right lobe of the liver, in which bile is stored (see illustration).

Gallie's operation (gal-iz) *n.* an operation in which strips of fascia taken from the thigh are used as suturing material to repair a hernia. [W. E. Gallie (1882–1959), Canadian surgeon]

gallipot (gal-i-pot) *n.* a small pot for holding lotions or ointments.

gallstone (gawl-stohn) *n.* a hard mass composed of bile pigments, cholesterol, and calcium salts, in varying proportions, that can form in the gall bladder. They may cause severe pain (*see* biliary (colic)) or they may pass into the common bile duct and cause obstructive jaundice or cholangitis. Treatment is by surgical removal of the gall bladder or the stones themselves.

galvanism (gal-vă-nizm) *n.* (formerly) any form of medical treatment using electricity. *interrupted g.* a form of electrotherapy in which direct current is used to stimulate the activity of nerves or the muscles they supply. *See also* faradism.

galvanocautery (gal-vă-noh-**kaw**-ter-i) *n. see* electrocautery.

galvanometer (gal-vă-**nom**-it-er) *n.* an instrument for measuring the strength of an electric current.

gamete (gam-eet) *n.* a mature sex cell: the ovum of the female or the spermatozoon of the male. Gametes are haploid, containing half the normal number of chromosomes.

gametocide (gam-i-toh-syd) *n.* a drug that kills gametocytes.

gametocyte (gă-**meet**-oh-syt) *n.* any of the cells that are in the process of developing into gametes by undergoing gametogenesis.

gametogenesis (gam-i-toh-**jen**-i-sis) *n.* the process by which spermatozoa and ova are formed. In both sexes the precursor cells undergo meiosis, which halves the number of chromosomes. *See* oogenesis, spermatogenesis.

gamgee tissue (gam-jee) *n.* a thick layer of absorbent cotton between two layers of gauze, used as a surgical dressing.

gamma aminobutyric acid (GABA) (gam-ă ă-meen-oh-bew-ti-rik) *n.* an amino acid found in the central nervous system, predominantly in the brain, where it acts as an inhibitory neurotransmitter.

gamma benzene hexachloride (heks-ă-**klor**-ryd) *n.* a drug used in creams, lotions, solutions, or shampoos to treat infestations caused by scabies, mites, and lice. Trade names: **Lorexane, Quellada.**

gamma camera *n.* a piece of apparatus for taking photographs of parts of the body into which radioactive isotopes that give off gamma rays have been introduced as tracers.

gamma globulin *n.* any of a class of proteins (*see* globulin) present in the blood plasma. Almost all gamma globulins are immunoglobulins.

gamma rays *pl. n.* electromagnetic radiation of wavelengths shorter than X-rays, given off by certain radioactive substances. Gamma rays are harmful to living tissues and can be used to sterilize certain materials. Carefully controlled doses are used in radiotherapy.

gamo- *prefix denoting* marriage.

gangli- (ganglio-) *prefix denoting* a ganglion.

ganglion (gang-li-ŏn) *n.* (*pl.* **ganglia**) **1.** (in neurology) any structure containing a collection of nerve cell bodies and often also numbers of synapses. Ganglia are found in the sympathetic and parasympathetic nervous systems. Within the central nervous system certain well-defined masses of nerve cells are called ganglia (*see* basal ganglia). **2.** an abnormal but harmless swelling (cyst) that sometimes forms in tendon sheaths, especially at the wrist.

ganglionectomy (gang-li-ŏn-ek-tŏmi) *n.* surgical removal of a ganglion cyst.

gangrene (gang-reen) *n.* death and decay of part of the body due to deficiency or cessation of blood supply. The causes include disease, injury, or atheroma in major blood vessels, frostbite or severe burns, and diseases such as diabetes mellitus and Raynaud's disease. *dry g.* death and withering of tissues caused simply by a cessation of local blood circulation. *moist g.* death and putrefactive decay of tissue caused by bacterial infection. *See also* gas gangrene.

Ganser state (pseudodementia) (gan-ser) *n.* a syndrome characterized by approximate answers, i.e. the patient gives absurdly false replies to questions, but the reply shows that the question has been understood. The condition is due to hysteria or to conscious malingering. [S. J. M. Ganser (1853–1931), German psychiatrist]

gargle (gar-gŭl) **1.** *n.* a medicated solution used for washing the mouth and throat. **2.** *vb.* to apply a gargle by holding it in the throat and exhaling through it.

gargoylism (gar-goil-izm) *n. see* Hurler's syndrome.

gas (gas) *n.* a fluid whose physical state is such that the forces of attraction between its constituent atoms and molecules are very weak. It therefore has no definite shape or volume. *laughing g. see* nitrous oxide.

gas gangrene *n.* death and decay of wound tissue infected by the soil bacterium *Clostridium welchii.* Toxins produced by the bacterium cause putrefactive decay of connective tissue with the generation of gas.

Gasserian ganglion (gas-eer-iǎn) *n.* a ganglion on the sensory root of the trigeminal nerve, deep within the skull. [J. L. Gasser (1723–65), Austrian anatomist]

gastr- (gastro-) *prefix denoting* the stomach.

gastralgia (gas-tral-jiǎ) *n.* pain in the stomach.

gastrectomy (gas-trek-tŏmi) *n.* a surgical operation in which the whole or a part of the stomach is removed. *partial* (or *subtotal*) *g.* an operation, usually carried out in severe cases of peptic ulcers, in which the upper third or half of the stomach is joined to the duodenum or small intestine. *See also* Billroth's operation. *total g.* an operation usually performed for stomach cancer, in which the oesophagus is joined to the duodenum.

gastric (**gas**-trik) *adj.* relating to or affecting the stomach. *g. glands* tubular glands in the mucous membrane of the stomach wall that secrete gastric juice. *g. juice* the liquid secreted by the gastric glands, containing hydrochloric acid, mucin, rennin, and pepsinogen. The acid acts on pepsinogen to produce the digestive enzyme pepsin. The acidity of the stomach contents also kills unwanted bacteria and other organisms that have been ingested with the food. *g. ulcer* an ulcer in the stomach, caused by the action of acid, pepsin, and bile on the stomach lining. Symptoms include vomiting and pain in the upper abdomen soon after eating, and such complications as bleeding, perforation, and obstruction due to scarring may occur.

gastrin (**gas**-trin) *n.* a hormone produced in the mucous membrane of the pyloric region of the stomach. Its secretion is stimulated by the presence of food. It is circulated in the blood to the rest of the stomach, where it stimulates the production of gastric juice.

gastritis (gas-**try**-tis) *n.* inflammation of the lining (mucosa) of the stomach. *acute g.* gastritis in which vomiting occurs, caused by ingesting excess alcohol or other irritating or corrosive substances. *atrophic g.* gastritis in which the stomach lining is atrophied. *chronic g.* gastritis that is associated with smoking

Gastrocnemius and soleus muscles

and chronic alcoholism and may be caused by bile entering the stomach from the duodenum. It has no definite symptoms, but the patient is liable to develop gastric ulcers.

gastrocele (**gas**-troh-seel) *n.* a hernia of the stomach.

gastrocnemius (gas-trok-**nee**-miŭs) *n.* a muscle that forms the greater part of the calf of the leg. It flexes the knee and foot (so that the toes point downwards).

gastrocolic reflex (gas-troh-**kol**-ik) *n.* a wave of peristalsis produced in the colon by introducing food into a fasting stomach.

gastroduodenostomy (gas-troh-dew-ŏ-di-**nost**-ŏmi) *n.* a surgical operation in which the duodenum is joined to an opening made in the stomach in order to bypass an obstruction or to facilitate the exit of food from the stomach after vagotomy. *See also* duodenostomy.

gastroenteritis (gas-troh-enter-**I**-tis) *n.* inflammation of the stomach and intestine. It is usually due to acute infection by viruses or bacteria or to food-poisoning toxins and causes vomiting and diarrhoea. Fluid loss is sometimes severe, especially in infants, and intravenous fluid replacement may be necessary.

gastroenterology (gas-troh-enter-ol-ŏji) *n.* the study of gastrointestinal disease, which includes disease of any part of the digestive tract and also of the liver, biliary tract, and pancreas.

gastroenterostomy (gas-troh-enter-ost-ŏmi) *n.* a surgical operation in which the small intestine is joined to an opening made in the stomach. The usual technique is gastroduodenostomy.

gastroileac reflex (gas-troh-il-i-ak) *n.* the relaxation of the ileocaecal valve caused by the presence of food in the stomach.

gastrojejunostomy (gas-troh-ji-joo-nost-ŏmi) *n.* a surgical operation in which the jejunum is joined to an opening made in the stomach.

gastrolith (gas-trŏ-lith) *n.* a stone in the stomach, which usually builds up around a bezoar.

gastropexy (gas-troh-peks-i) *n.* surgical attachment of the stomach to the abdominal wall.

gastroplasty (gas-troh-plasti) *n.* surgical treatment of a deformity of the stomach, e.g. a deformity due to peptic ulcers.

gastroptosis (gas-trop-toh-sis) *n.* a condition in which the stomach hangs low in the abdomen.

gastrorrhoea (gas-trŏ-ree-ă) *n.* excessive secretion of gastric juice. *See* hyperchlorhydria.

gastroscope (gas-trŏ-skohp) *n.* an illuminated optical instrument used to inspect the interior of the stomach. Fibreoptic gastro-scopes allow all areas of the stomach to be seen and photographed and specimens taken for microscopic examination. —**gastroscopy** (gas-tros-kŏ-pi) *n.*

gastrostomy (gas-trost-ŏmi) *n.* a surgical operation in which the stomach is brought through the abdominal wall and an opening made into it. It is usually performed to allow food and fluid to be poured directly into the stomach when swallowing is impossible because of disease or obstruction of the oesophagus.

gastrotomy (gas-trot-ŏmi) *n.* a procedure during abdominal surgery in which the stomach is opened, usually to allow inspection of the interior, to remove a foreign body, or to allow the oesophagus to be approached from below.

gastrula (gas-troo-lă) *n.* an early stage in the development of many animal embryos. It consists of a double-layered ball of cells formed by invagination and movement of cells in the preceding single-layered stage (blastula) in the process of *gastrulation*.

Gaucher's disease (goh-shayz) *n.* an inborn chemical defect causing accumulation of fatty compounds in the liver, spleen, lymph nodes, and nervous system. [P. C. E. Gaucher (1854–1918), French physician]

gauze (gawz) *n.* thin open-woven material used in several layers for the preparation of dressings and swabs.

gavage (gav-ahzh) *n.* forced feeding: any means used to get an unwilling or incapacitated patient to take in food by mouth, especially via a stomach tube.

Geiger counter (gy-ger kownt-er) *n.* a device for detecting and measuring the level of radioactivity of a substance. [H. Geiger (1882–1945), German physicist]

gel (jel) *n.* a colloidal suspension that has set to form a jelly. Some insoluble drugs are administered in the form of gels.

gelatin (jel-ă-tin) *n.* a jelly-like substance formed when tendons, ligaments, etc. containing collagen are boiled in water. Gelatin has been used in medicine as a source of dietary protein, in pharmacy for the manufacture of capsules and suppositories, and in bacteriology for preparing culture media.

gene (jeen) *n.* the basic unit of genetic material, which is carried at a particular place on a chromosome. Originally it was regarded as the unit of inheritance and mutation but is now usually defined as a piece of DNA or RNA that acts as the unit controlling the formation of a single polypeptide chain. In diploid organisms, including man, genes occur as pairs of alleles. *See also* dominant, recessive.

general paralysis of the insane (GPI) *n.* a late consequence of syphilitic infection. The symptoms are those of a dementia and spastic weakness of the limbs. Deafness, epilepsy, and dysarthria may occur.

general practitioner (GP) (jen-er-ăl prak-**tish**-ŏn-er) *n.* a doctor who is the main agent of *primary medical care*, through whom patients make first contact with health services for a new episode of illness or fresh developments of chronic diseases. Advice and treatment are provided for those who do not require the expertise of a consultant or other specialist services of hospitals (*secondary medical care*).

generic (jin-e-rik) *adj.* of or relating to a genus.

-genesis *suffix denoting* origin or development.

genetic code (ji-**net**-ik) *n.* the information carried by DNA and messenger RNA that determines the sequence of amino acids in every protein and thereby controls the nature of all proteins made by the cell.

genetics (ji-**net**-iks) *n.* the science of inheritance. It attempts to explain the differences and similarities between related organisms and the ways in which characters are passed from parents to their offspring. *See also* cytogenetics, Mendel's laws.

geni- (genio-) *prefix denoting* the chin.

-genic *suffix denoting* **1.** producing. **2.** produced by.

genicular (ji-**nik**-yoo-ler) *adj.* relating to the knee joint: applied to arteries that supply the knee.

genital (jen-i-t'l) *adj.* relating to the reproductive organs or to reproduction.

genitalia (jen-i-tay-liă) *pl. n.* the reproductive organs of either the male or the female, particularly the external parts of the reproductive system. *See also* vulva.

genito- *prefix denoting* the reproductive organs.

genitourinary (jen-i-toh-**yoor**-in-er-i) *adj.* of or relating to the organs of reproduction and excretion or to the branch of medicine concerned with them.

genome (jen-ohm) *n.* the basic haploid set of chromosomes of an organism. Man has a genome of 23 chromosomes.

genotype (jen-oh-typ) *n.* **1.** the genetic constitution of an individual or group, as determined by the particular set of genes it possesses. **2.** the genetic information carried by a pair of alleles, which determines a particular characteristic. *Compare* phenotype.

gentamicin (jen-tă-**my**-sin) *n.* an antibiotic used to treat infections caused by a wide range of bacteria. It can be administered by injection or applied in a cream to the skin or in drops to the ears and eyes. Trade names: **Cidomycin, Genticin.**

gentian violet (jen-shăn vy-ŏ-lit) *n.* see crystal violet.

genu (**jen**-yoo) *n.* **1.** the knee. *g. valgum* see knock-knee. *g. varum* see bow-legs. **2.** any bent anatomical structure resembling the knee. —**genual** *adj.*

genupectoral position (knee-chest position) (jen-yoo-**pek**-ter-ăl) *n.* the position of a patient in which the weight of the body is supported on the knees and chest. *See* position.

genus (**jen**-ŭs) *n.* (*pl.* **genera**) a category used in the classification of animals and plants. A genus consists of several closely related and similar species; for example the genus *Canis* includes the dog, wolf, and jackal.

ger- (gero-, geront(o)-) *prefix denoting* old age.

geriatrics (je-ri-**at**-riks) *n.* the branch of medicine concerned with the diagnosis and treatment of disorders that occur in old age and with the care of the aged. *See also* gerontology. —**geriatrician** (je-ri-ă-**trish**-ăn) *n.*

germ (jerm) *n.* any microorganism, especially one that causes disease. *See also* infection.

German measles (jer-măn) *n.* a mild highly contagious virus infection, mainly of childhood. Symptoms include headache, sore

throat, and slight fever, followed by swelling and soreness of the neck and the eruption of a rash of minute pink spots, spreading from the face and neck to the rest of the body. German measles can cause fetal malformations during early pregnancy. Medical name: **rubella.** *Compare* scarlet fever.

germ cell (gonocyte) *n.* **1.** any of the embryonic cells that have the potential to develop into spermatozoa or ova. **2.** a gamete.

germicide (**jerm**-i-syd) *n.* an agent that destroys microorganisms, particularly those causing disease. *See* antibiotic, antimycotic, antiseptic, disinfectant.

germinal (**jer**-min-ăl) *adj.* **1.** relating to the early developmental stages of an embryo or tissue. **2.** relating to a germ.

germ layer *n.* any of the three distinct types of tissue found in the very early stages of embryonic development (*see* ectoderm, endoderm, mesoderm).

gerontology (je-ron-**tol**-ŏji) *n.* the study of the changes in the mind and body that accompany ageing and the problems associated with them.

gestaltism (gĕsh-**talt**-izm) *n.* a school of psychology that regards mental processes as wholes (*gestalts*) that cannot be broken down into constituent parts. From this was developed *gestalt therapy*, which aims at achieving a suitable gestalt within the patient that includes all facets of functioning.

gestation (jes-**tay**-shŏn) *n.* the period during which a fertilized egg cell develops into a baby that is ready to be delivered. *See also* pregnancy.

Ghon's focus (gonz) *n.* the lesion produced in the lung of a previously uninfected person by tubercle bacilli. It is a small focus of granulomatous inflammation, which may become visible on a chest X-ray if it grows large enough or if it calcifies. [A. Ghon (1866–1936), Czech pathologist]

giant cell (jy-ănt) *n.* any large cell, such as a megakaryocyte. Giant cells may have one or many nuclei.

giant-cell arteritis *n. see* arteritis.

giardiasis (lambliasis) (jy-ar-dy-ă-sis) *n.* a disease caused by the parasitic protozoan *Giardia lamblia* in the small intestine. Symptoms include diarrhoea, nausea, bellyache, flatulence, and the passage of pale fatty stools (steatorrhoea). The disease is particularly common in children; it responds well to oral doses of quinacrine and metronidazole.

gibbus (gibbosity) (gib-ŭs) *n.* a sharply angled curvature of the backbone, resulting from collapse of a vertebra. Infection with tuberculosis was a common cause.

gigantism (jy-gan-tizm) *n.* abnormal growth causing excessive height, most commonly due to oversecretion during childhood of growth hormone (somatotrophin) by the pituitary gland. *See also* acromegaly.

Gilliam's operation (gil-i-ămz) *n.* an operation to correct retroversion of the womb in which the round ligaments are shortened. [D. T. Gilliam (1844–1923), US gynaecologist]

gingiv- (gingivo-) *prefix denoting* the gums.

gingiva (jin-jiv-ă) *n.* (*pl.* **gingivae**) the gum: the layer of dense connective tissue and overlying mucous membrane that covers the alveolar bone and necks of the teeth. —**gingival** *adj.*

gingivectomy (jin-ji-vek-tŏmi) *n.* the surgical removal of excess gum tissue.

gingivitis (jin-ji-vy-tis) *n.* inflammation of the gums, which become swollen and bleed easily, caused by plaque at the necks of the teeth.

ginglymus (hinge joint) (jing-li-mŭs) *n.* a form of diarthrosis that allows angular movement in one plane only. Examples are the knee joint and the elbow joint.

girdle (ger-d'l) *n.* (in anatomy) an encircling or arching arrangement of bones. *See also* pelvic girdle, shoulder girdle.

Girdlestone's operation (ger-d'l-stohnz) *n.* an operation in which the head of the femur and part of the acetabulum are removed and a mass of muscle is sutured between the bone ends. It is performed for osteoarthritis. [G. R. Girdlestone (1881–1950), British surgeon]

glabella (glă-bel-ă) *n.* the smooth rounded surface of the frontal bone in the middle of the forehead, between the two eyebrows.

gladiolus (glad-i-oh-lŭs) *n.* the middle and largest segment of the sternum.

gland (gland) *n.* an organ or group of cells that is specialized for synthesizing and secreting certain fluids, either for use in the body or for excretion. *See* endocrine gland, exocrine gland, secretion.

glanders (equinia) (glan-derz) *n.* an infectious disease of horses, donkeys, and mules that is caused by the bacterium *Actinobacillus mallei* and can be transmitted to man. Symptoms include fever and inflammation of the lymph nodes (a form of the disease known as *farcy*), skin, and nasal mucous membranes. Administration of sulphonamides or streptomycin is usually effective.

glandular fever (glan-dew-ler) *n.* an infectious disease, thought to be caused by the Epstein-Barr virus, that affects the lymph nodes in the neck, armpits, and groin; it mainly affects adolescents and young adults. Symptoms include swelling and tenderness of the lymph nodes, fever, headache, a sore throat, and loss of appetite. Glandular fever is diagnosed by the presence of large numbers of monocytes in the blood. Medical name: **infectious mononucleosis**.

glans (glans penis) (glanz) *n.* the acorn-shaped end part of the penis, formed by the expanded end of the corpus spongiosum. The term glans is also applied to the end of the clitoris.

glaucoma (glaw-koh-mă) *n.* a condition in which loss of vision occurs because of an abnormally high pressure in the eye. *acute congestive g.* primary glaucoma in which there is a sudden rise in pressure accompanied by pain and marked blurring of vision. *chronic simple g.* primary glaucoma in which the pressure increases gradually, usually without producing pain, and the visual loss is insidious. *primary g.* glaucoma that occurs without any other ocular disease. It is an important cause of blindness. *secondary g.* glaucoma that may occur when other ocular disease impairs the normal circulation of the aqueous humour and causes the intraocular pressure to rise.

gleet (gleet) *n.* a discharge of purulent mucus from the penis or vagina resulting from chronic gonorrhoea.

glenohumeral (glee-noh-**hew**-mer-ăl) *adj.* relating to the glenoid cavity and the humerus: the region of the shoulder joint.

glenoid cavity (glenoid fossa) (**glee**-noid) *n.* the socket of the shoulder joint: the pear-shaped cavity at the top of the scapula into which the head of the humerus fits.

gli- (glio-) *prefix denoting* 1. glia. 2. a glutinous substance.

glia (neuroglia) (glee-ă) *n.* the special connective tissue of the central nervous system. Glial cells outnumber the neurones by between five and ten to one, and make up some 40% of the total volume of the brain and spinal cord. —**glial** *adj.*

glibenclamide (gly-**ben**-klă-myd) *n.* a drug that reduces the level of sugar in the blood and is administered by mouth to treat diabetes. Trade name: **Daonil, Euglucon.**

glioblastoma (spongioblastoma) (gly-oh-blast-**oh**-mă) *n.* the most malignant type of brain tumour derived from glial tissue. Its rapid enlargement destroys normal brain cells, with a progressive loss of function, and raises the intracranial pressure, causing headache, vomiting, and drowsiness.

glioma (gly-**oh**-mă) *n.* any tumour of glial cells in the nervous system. The term is sometimes used for all tumours that arise in the central nervous system.

gliomyoma (gly-oh-my-**oh**-mă) *n.* a tumour composed of nervous and muscular tissue.

globin

globin (gloh-bin) *n.* a protein, found in the body, that can combine with iron-containing groups to form haemoglobin and myoglobin.

globulin (glob-yoo-lin) *n.* one of a group of simple proteins that are soluble in dilute salt solutions and can be coagulated by heat. *serum g.* any of the different globulins present in the blood, including gamma globulins. Some have important functions as antibodies (*see* immunoglobulin).

globulinuria (glob-yoo-lin-yoor-iă) *n.* the presence in the urine of globulins.

globus (gloh-bŭs) *n.* a spherical or globe-shaped anatomical structure. *g. hystericus* the sensation of having a lump in the throat that cannot be swallowed, sometimes occurring in anxiety states, emotional conflict, and hysteria.

glomangioma (gloh-man-ji-oh-mă) *n.* a harmless but often painful tumour usually occurring in the skin at the ends of the fingers and toes. It arises from nerve tissue in the blood vessels.

glomerulitis (glom-e-roo-ly-tis) *n.* any one of a variety of lesions of the glomeruli associated with acute or chronic kidney disease.

glomerulonephritis (glom-e-roo-loh-ni-fry-tis) *n.* a disease of the kidneys resulting in the syndrome of acute nephritis: the passage of blood in the urine and occasionally fluid retention and swelling. In most cases glomerulonephritis is thought to represent an abnormal allergic response following a streptococcal sore throat. The acute form of the disease usually settles completely; occasionally, it progresses to chronic glomerulonephritis and kidney failure.

glomerulus (glom-e-roo-lŭs) *n.* (*pl.* **glomeruli**) 1. the network of blood capillaries contained within the cuplike end (Bowman's capsule) of a nephron. It is the site of primary filtration of waste products from the blood into the kidney tubule. 2. any other small rounded mass.

gloss- (glosso-) *prefix denoting* the tongue.

glossa (glos-ă) *n. see* tongue.

glossectomy (glos-ek-tŏmi) *n.* surgical removal of the tongue, an operation usually carried out for cancer in this structure.

glossitis (glos-I-tis) *n.* inflammation of the tongue.

glossodynia (glos-oh-din-iă) *n.* pain in the tongue.

glossopharyngeal nerve (glos-oh-fa-rin-jee-ăl) *n.* the ninth cranial nerve (IX), which supplies motor fibres to part of the pharynx and to the parotid salivary glands and sensory fibres to the posterior third of the tongue and the soft palate.

glossoplegia (glos-oh-plee-jiă) *n.* paralysis of the tongue.

glottis (glot-iss) *n.* the space between the two vocal cords. The term is often applied to the vocal cords themselves or to that part of the larynx associated with the production of sound.

gluc- (gluco-) *prefix denoting* glucose.

glucagon (gloo-kă-gon) *n.* a hormone, produced by the pancreas, that causes an increase in the blood sugar level. Glucagon is administered by injection to counteract diabetic hypoglycaemia.

glucocorticoid (gloo-koh-kor-ti-koid) *n.* any of a group of corticosteroids, including cortisone, that are essential for the utilization of carbohydrate, fat, and protein by the body. Naturally occurring and synthetic glucocorticoids have very powerful anti-inflammatory effects.

gluconeogenesis (gloo-koh-nee-oh-jen-i-sis) *n.* the biochemical process in which glucose is synthesized from non-carbohydrate sources, such as amino acids, when carbohydrate is not available in sufficient amounts in the diet.

glucose (dextrose) (gloo-kohz) *n.* a simple sugar containing six carbon atoms (a hexose). Glucose, an important source of energy, is one of the constituents of both sucrose and starch, both of which yield glucose after digestion. It is stored in the body in the form of glycogen. If the blood-glucose concentration falls below the normal level of around 5 mmol/l, neurological and other symptoms may result (*see* hypoglycaemia). If the blood-glucose level is raised to 10 mmol/l, the condition of hyperglycaemia develops. This is a symptom of diabetes mellitus.

glucose tolerance test *n.* a test used in the diagnosis of diabetes mellitus. A quantity of glucose is administered and the concentration of sugar in the blood and urine is estimated at regular intervals afterwards.

glucoside (gloo-koh-syd) *n. see* glycoside.

glucuronic acid (gloo-kewr-on-ik) *n.* a sugar acid derived from glucose. Glucuronic acid is an important constituent of chondroitin sulphate (found in cartilage) and hyaluronic acid (found in synovial fluid).

glutamic acid (glutamate) (gloo-tam-ik) *n. see* amino acid.

glutamic oxaloacetic transaminase (GOT) *n.* an enzyme involved in the transamination of amino acids. Measurement of GOT in the serum (*SGOT*) may be used in the diagnosis of acute myocardial infarction and acute liver disease.

glutamic pyruvic transaminase (GPT) *n.* an enzyme involved in the transamination of amino acids. Measurement of GPT in the serum (*SGPT*) is of use in the diagnosis and study of acute liver disease.

glutaminase (gloo-tam-in-ayz) *n.* an enzyme, found in the kidney, that catalyses the breakdown of the amino acid glutamine to ammonia and glutamic acid: a stage in the production of urea.

glutamine (gloo-tă-meen) *n. see* amino acid.

gluten (gloo-těn) *n.* a mixture of the two proteins *gliadin* and *glutenin*. Gluten is present in wheat and rye and is important for its baking properties. Sensitivity to gluten leads to coeliac disease in children.

glutethimide (gloo-teth-i-myd) *n.* a drug administered by mouth to treat insomnia and other sleep disturbances (*see* hypnotic). Trade name: **Doriden.**

gluteus (gloo-tee-ŭs) *n.* one of three paired muscles of the buttocks (*g. maximus*, *g. medius*, and *g. minimus*). They are responsible for movements of the thigh. —**gluteal** *adj.*

glyc- (glyco-) *prefix denoting* sugar.

glycerin (glycerol) (glis-er-in) *n.* a clear viscous liquid obtained by hydrolysis of fats and mixed oils and produced as a by-product in the manufacture of soap. It is used as an emollient in many skin preparations, as a laxative (particularly in the form of suppositories), and as a sweetening agent in the pharmaceutical industry.

glyceryl trinitrate (nitroglycerin) (glis-er-il try-ny-trayt) *n.* a drug that dilates blood vessels and is administered by mouth to prevent and treat angina (*see* vasodilator). Trade names: **Nitrocontin, Sustac**.

glycine (gly-seen) *n. see* amino acid.

glycocholic acid (gly-koh-kol-ik) *n. see* bile acids.

glycogen (gly-koh-jĕn) *n.* a carbohydrate consisting of branched chains of glucose units. Glycogen is the principal form in which carbohydrate is stored in the body (in liver and muscles); it may be readily broken down to glucose.

glycogenesis (gly-koh-**jen**-i-sis) *n.* the biochemical process, occurring chiefly in the liver and in muscle, by which glucose is converted into glycogen.

glycogenolysis (gly-koh-jĕ-**nol**-i-sis) *n.* a biochemical process, occurring chiefly in the liver and in muscle, by which glycogen is broken down into glucose-1-phosphate. Glycogenolysis forms the first stage of glycolysis.

glycolysis (gly-**kol**-i-sis) *n.* the conversion of glucose, by a series of ten enzyme-catalysed reactions, to lactic acid, with the production of energy in the form of ATP.

glycoprotein (gly-koh-**proh**-teen) *n.* one of a group of compounds consisting of a protein combined with a carbohydrate (such as galactose or mannose). Examples of glycoproteins are certain enzymes, hormones, and antigens.

glycoside (gly-koh-syd) *n.* a compound formed by replacing the hydroxyl (–OH) group of a sugar by another group. (If the sugar is glucose the compound is known as a *glucoside*.) Glycosides found in plants include some pharmacologically important products (such as digitalis).

glycosuria (gly-kohs-**yoor**-iă) *n.* the presence of glucose in the urine in abnormally large amounts. Glycosuria may be associated with diabetes mellitus, kidney disease, and some other conditions.

glymidine (gly-mi-deen) *n.* a drug that reduces the level of sugar in the blood and is administered by mouth to treat diabetes. Trade name: **Gondafon**.

gnath- (gnatho-) *prefix denoting* the jaw.

gnathoplasty (**nath**-oh-plasti) *n.* plastic surgery of the jaw.

goal (gohl) *n.* a statement of what the nursing intervention is intended to achieve, usually expressed in terms of the patient's expected behaviour. *See* behavioural objective, expected outcome.

goblet cell (gob-lit) *n.* a column-shaped secretory cell found in the epithelium of the respiratory and intestinal tracts. Goblet cells secrete the principal constituents of mucus.

goitre (**goi**-ter) *n.* a swelling of the neck due to enlargement of the thyroid gland. This may be due to lack of dietary iodine, which is necessary for the production of thyroid hormone: the gland enlarges in an attempt to increase the output of hormone. *exophthalmic g.* (*Graves' disease*) *see* thyrotoxicosis. *sporadic g.* goitre due to simple overgrowth (hyperplasia) of the gland or to a tumour.

goitrogen (goi-troh-jen) *n.* any substance that causes goitre. —**goitrogenic** *adj.*

gold (gohld) *n.* (in pharmacology) any of several compounds of the metal gold, administered by injection in the treatment of rheumatoid arthritis. Trade name: **Myocrisin.**

Golgi apparatus (gol-ji) *n.* a collection of vesicles and folded membranes in a cell. It stores and later transports the proteins manufactured in the endoplasmic reticulum. [C. Golgi (1844–1926), Italian histologist]

Golgi cells *pl. n.* types of neurones (nerve cells) within the central nervous system. *Golgi type I neurones* have very long axons that connect different parts of the system; *Golgi type II neurones* have only short axons or sometimes none.

gomphosis (gom-**foh**-sis) *n.* a form of synarthrosis (immovable joint) in which a conical process fits into a socket.

gonad (**goh**-nad) *n.* a male or female reproductive organ, which produces the gametes. *See* ovary, testis.

gonadotrophin (gonadotrophic hormone) (gon-ă-doh-**troh**-fin) *n.* any of several hormones synthesized and released by the pituitary gland, such as follicle-stimulating hormone and luteinizing hormone, that act on the gonads to promote production of sex hormones and either sperm or ova. *See also* chorionic gonadotrophin.

gonagra (gon-**ag**-ră) *n.* gout in the knee.

goni- (gonio-) *prefix denoting* an anatomical angle or corner.

goniopuncture (goh-ni-oh-**punk**-cher) *n.* an operation for congenital glaucoma (*see* buphthalmos) to enable fluid to be drawn from the eye. *See* goniotomy.

gonioscope (goh-ni-oh-skohp) *n.* a special lens used for viewing the structures around the edge of the anterior chamber of the eye (in front of the lens).

goniotomy (trabeculotomy) (goh-ni-ot-ŏmi) *n.* an operation for congenital glaucoma (*see* buphthalmos) in which a fine knife is used to make an incision into Schlemm's canal from within the eye. It is the first stage of goniopuncture.

gonococcus (gon-oh-**kok**-ŭs) *n.* (*pl.* **gonococci**) the causative agent of gonorrhoea: the bacterium *Neisseria gonorrhoeae*. —**gonococcal** *adj.*

gonocyte (gon-oh-syt) *n. see* germ cell.

gonorrhoea (gon-ŏ-**ree**-ă) *n.* a venereal disease, caused by the bacterium *Neisseria gonorrhoeae*, that affects the genital mucous membranes of either sex. Symptoms include pain on passing water and discharge of gleet. In untreated cases, the infection may spread throughout the reproductive system, causing sterility; severe inflammation of the urethra in men can cause stricture. If a pregnant woman has gonorrhoea, her baby may contract ophthalmia neonatorum. Later complications include arthritis, endocarditis, and infection of the eyes, causing conjunctivitis. Treatment with sulphonamides, penicillin, or tetracycline in the early stages of the disease is usually effective.

A gouge

Compare syphilis. —**gonorrhoeal** *adj.*

Goodpasture's syndrome (guud-pas-cherz) *n.* a lung disorder resulting in the coughing up of blood and associated with glomerulonephritis. [E. W. Goodpasture (1886–1960), US pathologist]

goose flesh *n.* the reaction of the skin to cold or fear. The blood vessels contract and the small muscle attached to the base of each hair follicle also contracts, causing the hairs to stand up: this gives the skin an appearance of plucked goose skin. Medical name: **cutis anserina**.

Gordh needle (gord) *n.* an intravenous needle with an expanded base containing a rubber diaphragm, used to administer repeated injections. [T. Gordh, Swedish anaesthetist]

gorget (gor-jit) *n.* an instrument used in the operation for removal of stones from the bladder. It is a director or guide with a wide groove.

gouge (gowj) *n.* a curved chisel used in orthopaedic operations to cut and remove bone.

gout (gowt) *n.* a disease in which a defect in uric acid metabolism causes an excess of the acid and its salts (urates) to accumulate in the bloodstream and the joints. It results in attacks of acute gouty arthritis and chronic destruction of the joints and deposits of urates (tophi) in the skin and cartilage, especially of the ears. Treatment with uricosuric drugs or allopurinol has largely controlled the disease. *See also* podagra.

Graafian follicle (grah-fi-ăn) *n.* a mature follicle in the ovary prior to ovulation, containing a large fluid-filled cavity that distends the surface of the ovary. The oocyte develops inside the follicle, attached to one side. [R. de Graaf (1641–73), Dutch physician and anatomist]

Graefe's knife (gray-fiz) *n.* a knife with a narrow sharply pointed blade, used in operations for the removal of cataract. [A. von Graefe (1928–70), German ophthalmologist]

graft (grahft) **1.** *n.* any organ, tissue, or object used for transplantation to replace a faulty part of the body. *See also* keratoplasty, skin (graft), transplantation. **2.** *vb.* to transplant an organ or tissue.

grain (grayn) *n.* a unit of mass equal to 1/7000 of a pound (avoirdupois). 1 grain = 0.0648 gram.

gram (gram) *n.* a unit of mass equal to one thousandth of a kilogram. Symbol: g.

-gram *suffix denoting* a record; tracing.

gramicidin (gram-i-sy-din) *n.* an antibiotic that acts against a wide range of bacteria. It is used in ointments, solutions, or sprays for the treatment of infected ulcers, wounds, and burns.

Gram's stain (gramz) *n.* a method of staining bacterial cells, used as a primary means of identification. The bacterial cells are stained with a violet dye, treated with decolourizer (e.g. alcohol), and then counterstained with red dye. *Gram-negative* bacteria lose the initial stain but take up the counterstain, so that they appear red microscopically. *Gram-positive* bacteria retain the initial stain, appearing violet microscopically. [H. C. J. Gram (1853–1938), Danish physician]

grand mal (major epilepsy) (gron mal) *n.* an epileptic fit, sometimes called the *tonic-clonic fit*. The tonic phase begins when the patient falls to the ground unconscious with his muscles in a state of spasm. This is replaced by the convulsive movements of the clonic phase, when the tongue may be bitten and urinary incontinence may occur. *See also* epilepsy.

granular cast (gran-yoo-ler) *n.* a cellular cast derived from a kidney tubule. Such casts are shed from the kidney in certain kidney diseases, notably acute glomerulonephritis. Their presence in the urine indicates continued activity of the disease.

granulation (gran-yoo-lay-shŏn) *n.* the growth of small rounded outgrowths, made up of small blood vessels and connective tissue, on the healing surface of a wound (when the edges do not fit closely together) or an ulcer.

granulocyte (gran-yoo-loh-syt) *n.* any of a group of white blood cells that contain granules in their cytoplasm. They can be subclassified into neutrophils, eosinophils, and basophils.

granulocytopenia (gran-yoo-loh-sy-toh-**pee**-niă) *n.* a reduction in the number of granulocytes in the blood. *See* neutropenia.

granuloma (gran-yoo-**loh**-mă) *n.* (*pl.* **granulomas** or **granulomata**) a mass of granulation tissue produced in response to chronic infection, inflammation, a foreign body, or to unknown causes. **g.**

inguinale a venereal disease caused by the bacterium *Donovania granulomatis*, marked by a pimply rash on and around the genital organs, which develops into a granulomatous ulcer. —**granulomatous** *adj.*

granulomatosis (gran-yoo-loh-mă-toh-sis) *n.* any condition marked by multiple widespread granulomas.

granulopoiesis (gran-yoo-loh-poi-ee-sis) *n.* the process of production of granulocytes, which normally occurs in the blood-forming tissue of the bone marrow. *See also* haemopoiesis.

graph- (grapho-) *prefix denoting* handwriting.

-graph *suffix denoting* an instrument that records.

grattage (grat-ah*zh*) *n.* the process of brushing or scraping the surface of a slowly healing ulcer or wound to stimulate healing.

gravel (grav-ĕl) *n.* small stones formed in the urinary tract. The passage of gravel from the kidneys is usually associated with severe pain (ureteric colic) and may cause blood in the urine. *See also* calculus.

Graves' disease (exophthalmic goitre) (grayvz) *n. see* thyrotoxicosis. [R. J. Graves (1797–1853), Irish physician]

gravid (grav-id) *adj.* pregnant.

Grawitz tumour (grah-vits) *n. see* hypernephroma. [P. A. Grawitz (1850–1932), German pathologist]

green monkey disease *n. see* Marburg disease.

greenstick fracture (green-stik) *n. see* fracture.

grey matter (gray) *n.* the darker coloured tissues of the central nervous system, composed mainly of the cell bodies of neurones, branching dendrites, and glial cells. *Compare* white matter.

Griffith's types (grif-iths) *pl. n.* subdivisions of Lancefield group A streptococci (*see* Lancefield classification) on the basis of their agglutination reactions. [F. Griffith (1877–1941), British bacteriologist]

gripe (gryp) *n.* severe abdominal pain (*see* colic).

griseofulvin (griz-i-oh-**ful**-vin) *n.* an antibiotic administered by mouth to treat fungal infections of the hair, skin, and nails, such as ringworm. Trade names: **Fulcin, Grisovin.**

grocer's itch (groh-serz) *n.* dermatitis of the hands caused by frequent contact with flour and sugar.

groin (groin) *n.* the external depression on the front of the body that marks the junction of the abdomen with either of the thighs. *See also* inguinal.

ground substance (grownd) *n. see* connective tissue.

group therapy (groop) *n.* **1.** (**group psychotherapy**) psychotherapy involving at least two patients and a therapist. The patients are encouraged to understand and analyse their own and one another's problems. *See also* encounter group, psychodrama. **2.** therapy in which people with the same problem, such as alcoholism, meet and discuss together their difficulties and possible ways of overcoming them.

growth hormone (GH, somatotrophin) (grohth) *n.* a hormone, synthesized and stored in the anterior pituitary gland, that promotes growth of the long bones in the limbs and increases protein synthesis.

A tonsil guillotine

guanethidine (gwahn-**eth**-i-deen) *n.* a drug that is administered by mouth to reduce high blood pressure (*see* sympatholytic). Trade name: **Ismelin.**

guanine (**gwah**-neen) *n.* one of the nitrogen-containing bases (*see* purine) that occurs in the nucleic acids DNA and RNA.

gubernaculum (gew-ber-**nak**-yoo-lüm) *n.* (*pl.* **gubernacula**) either of a pair of fibrous strands of tissue that connect the gonads to the inguinal region in the fetus.

Guillain-Barré syndrome (gee-yan ba-ray) *n.* a disease of the peripheral nerves in which there is numbness and weakness in the limbs. It usually develops 10–20 days after a respiratory infection that provokes an allergic response in the peripheral nerves. [G. Guillain (1876–1961) and A. Barré (1880–1967), French neurologists]

guillotine (gil-ŏ-teen) *n.* a surgical instrument used for removing the tonsils.

guinea worm (ginn-i) *n.* a parasitic nematode worm, *Dracunculus medinensis.* The adult female lives in the connective tissues beneath the skin and releases its larvae into a large blister on the legs or arms. *See also* dracontiasis.

gullet (**gul**-it) *n. see* oesophagus.

gum (gum) *n.* (in anatomy) *see* gingiva.

gumboil (**gum**-boil) *n.* the opening on the surface of the gum of a chronic abscess at the root of a tooth. It may be accompanied by varying degrees of swelling, pain, and discharge.

gumma (**gum**-ă) *n.* a small soft tumour, characteristic of the tertiary stage of syphilis, that occurs in connective tissue, the liver, brain, testes, heart, or bone.

gustation (gus-**tay**-shŏn) *n.* the sense of taste or the act of tasting.

gustatory (**gus**-tă-ter-i) *adj.* relating to the sense of taste or to the organs of taste.

gut (gut) *n.* **1.** *see* intestine. **2.** *see* catgut.

Guthrie test (**guth**-ri) *n.* examination of blood obtained from a heel stab to exclude the presence of phenylketonuria. [R. Guthrie (1916–), US paediatrician]

gutta (**gut**-ă) *n.* (*pl.* **guttae**) (in pharmacy) a drop. Drops are the form in which medicines are applied to the eyes and ears.

gutta percha (**per**-chă) *n.* the juice of an evergreen Malaysian tree, which is hard at room temperature but becomes soft and elastic when heated in boiling water. On cooling gutta percha will retain any deformity imparted to it when hot; it is used in dentistry.

gutter splint (**gut**-er) *n.* a splint formed from a casting material, moulded to conform to the shape of the limb but not encircling it, in which the limb rests as in a gutter.

gyn- (**gyno-**, **gynaec(o)-**) *prefix denoting* women or the female reproductive organs.

gynaecology (gy-ni-**kol**-ŏji) *n.* the study of diseases of women and girls, particularly those affecting the female reproductive system. *Compare* obstetrics. **—gynaecological** *adj.* **—gynaecologist** *n.*

gynaecomastia (gy-ni-koh-**mas**-tiă) *n.* enlargement of the breasts in the male, due either to hormone imbalance or to hormone therapy.

gypsum (**jip**-sŭm) *n. see* plaster of Paris.

gyr- (**gyro-**) *prefix denoting* **1.** a gyrus. **2.** a ring or circle.

gyrus (**jy**-rŭs) *n.* (*pl.* **gyri**) a raised convolution of the cerebral cortex, between two sulci (clefts).

H

H *symbol for* hydrogen.

habit (**hab**-it) *n.* a constant, almost automatic, practice acquired by frequent repetition. *h. training* teaching psychiatric patients to relearn habits of personal hygiene by repetition and encouragement.

habituation (hă-bit-yoo-**ay**-shŏn) *n.* (in pharmacology) the condition of being psychologically dependent on a drug, following repeated consumption, marked by a craving for the drug if it is withdrawn. *See also* dependence.

haem (heem) *n.* an iron-containing compound (a porphyrin) that combines with the protein globin to form haemoglobin.

haem- (**haema-**, **haemo-**, **haemat(o)-**) *prefix denoting* blood.

haemangioma (heem-an-ji-**oh**-mă) *n.* a benign tumour of blood vessels. It often appears on the skin as a type of birthmark (*see* naevus). *See also* angioma.

haemarthrosis (heem-arth-roh-sis) *n.* joint pain and swelling caused by bleeding into a joint. This may follow injury or may occur spontaneously in a disease of the blood, such as haemophilia.

haematemesis (heem-ă-tem-i-sis) *n.* the act of vomiting blood. The blood may have been swallowed but more often arises from bleeding in the oesophagus, stomach, or duodenum. Common causes are gastric and duodenal ulcers, gastritis, and varicose veins in the oesophagus.

haematin (heem-ă-tin) *n.* a chemical derivative of haemoglobin formed by removal of the protein part of the molecule and oxidation of the iron atom from the ferrous to the ferric form.

haematinic (heem-ă-tin-ik) *n.* a drug that increases the amount of haemoglobin in the blood, e.g. ferrous sulphate and other iron-containing compounds. Haematinics are administered to prevent and treat anaemia due to iron deficiency, particularly during pregnancy.

haematocele (heem-ă-toh-seel) *n.* a swelling caused by leakage of blood into a cavity, especially that of the membrane overlying the front and sides of the testis. *parametric* (*pelvic*) *h.* a swelling near the womb formed by the escape of blood, usually from a Fallopian tube in ectopic pregnancy.

haematocolpos (heem-ă-toh-kol-pos) *n.* the accumulation of menstrual blood in the vagina because the hymen lacks an opening. *See* cryptomenorrhoea.

haematocrit (heem-ă-toh-krit) *n.* *see* packed cell volume.

haematocyst (heem-ă-toh-sist) *n.* a cyst containing blood.

haematogenous (haematogenic) (heem-ă-toj-in-ŭs) *adj.* **1.** relating to the production of blood or its constituents. **2.** produced by, originating in, or carried by the blood.

haematology (heem-ă-tol-ŏji) *n.* the study of blood and its disorders. —**haematological** *adj.* —**haematologist** *n.*

haematoma (heem-ă-toh-mă) *n.* an accumulation of blood within the tissues that clots to form a solid swelling. Injury, disease of the blood vessels, or a clotting disorder of the blood are the usual causative factors. *extradural h.* a haematoma caused by tearing of the middle meningeal artery, as a result of injury to the head. *intracerebral h.* a haematoma resulting from atherosclerosis of the cerebral arteries and high blood pressure or from severe head injury. *subdural h.* a haematoma caused by tearing of the veins where they cross the space beneath the dura. *See also* perianal haematoma.

haematometra (heem-ă-toh-mee-tră) *n.* **1.** accumulation of menstrual blood in the womb. **2.** abnormally copious bleeding in the womb.

haematomyelia (heem-ă-toh-my-ee-liă) *n.* bleeding into the tissue of the spinal cord.

haematopoiesis (heem-ă-toh-poi-ee-sis) *n. see* haemopoiesis.

haematoporphyrin (heem-ă-toh-por-fi-rin) *n.* a type of porphyrin produced during the metabolism of haemoglobin.

haematosalpinx (haemosalpinx) (heem-ă-toh-sal-pinks) *n.* the accumulation of menstrual blood in the Fallopian tubes.

haematoxylin (heem-ă-toks-i-lin) *n.*
a colourless crystalline compound
extracted from logwood (*Haema-toxylon campechianum*) and used
in various histological stains.

haematozoon (heem-ă-toh-**zoh**-on)
n. (*pl.* **haematozoa**) any animal
parasite living in the blood.

haematuria (heem-ă-**tewr**-iă) *n.* the
presence of blood in the urine.
The blood may come from the
kidneys, one or both ureters, the
bladder, or the urethra, as a re-sult of injury or disease.

haemin (**heem**-in) *n.* a chemical
derivative of haemoglobin formed
by removal of the protein part
of the molecule, oxidation of the
iron atom, and combination with
an acid to form a salt. *Compare*
haematin.

haemo- *prefix. see* haem-.

haemochromatosis (bronze diabe-tes, iron-storage disease) (heem-
ŏ-kroh-mă-**toh**-sis) *n.* a hereditary
disorder in which there is exces-sive absorption and storage of
iron. This leads to damage of
many organs, including the liver,
pancreas, and endocrine glands.
The main features are a bronze
colour of the skin, diabetes, and
liver failure. *Compare* haemo-siderosis.

haemoconcentration (hee-moh-kon-
sĕn-**tray**-shŏn) *n.* an increase in
the proportion of red blood cells
relative to the plasma, brought
about by a decrease in the vol-ume of plasma. *Compare*
haemodilution.

haemocytometer (hee-moh-sy-
tom-it-er) *n.* a special glass
chamber of known volume into
which diluted blood is intro-duced. The numbers of the vari-ous blood cells present are then
counted visually, through a mi-croscope.

haemodialysis (hee-moh-dy-**al**-i-sis)
n. a technique of removing waste
materials or poisons from the
blood using the principle of dial-ysis. Haemodialysis is performed
on patients whose kidneys have
ceased to function; the process
takes place in an *artificial kid-ney*, or *dialyser*.

haemodilution (hee-moh-dy-
lew-shŏn) *n.* a decrease in the
proportion of red blood cells rel-ative to the plasma, brought
about by an increase in the total
volume of plasma. *Compare*
haemoconcentration.

haemoglobin (hee-moh-**gloh**-bin) *n.*
a substance contained within the
red blood cells (erythrocytes) and
responsible for their colour, com-posed of the pigment haem
linked to the protein globin.
Haemoglobin is the medium by
which oxygen is transported
within the body. Blood nor-mally contains 12–18 g/dl of
haemoglobin. *See also* ox-yhaemoglobin.

haemoglobinaemia (heem-ŏ-gloh-
bin-ee-miă) *n.* the presence of
haemoglobin in the blood
plasma.

haemoglobinometer (heem-ŏ-gloh-
bin-**om**-it-er) *n.* an instrument for
determining the concentration of
haemoglobin in a sample of
blood.

haemoglobinopathy (heem-ŏ-gloh-
bin-**op**-ă-thi) *n.* any of a group
of inherited diseases, including
thalassaemia and sickle-cell dis-ease, in which there is an abnor-mality in the production of
haemoglobin.

haemoglobinuria (heem-ŏ-gloh-bin-
yoor-iă) *n.* the presence in the
urine of free haemoglobin. The
condition sometimes follows
strenuous exercise. It is also as-

sociated with certain infectious diseases, ingestion of certain chemicals, and injury.

haemogram (hee-moh-gram) *n.* the results of a routine blood test, including an estimate of the blood haemoglobin level, packed cell volume, and blood count.

haemolysin (hi-mol-i-sin) *n. see* lysin.

haemolysis (hi-mol-i-sis) *n.* the destruction of red blood cells (erythrocytes). Within the body, haemolysis may result from poisoning, infection, or the action of antibodies in mismatched blood transfusions and it leads to anaemia. *See also* laking.

haemolytic (hee-moh-lit-ik) *adj.* causing, associated with, or resulting from destruction of red blood cells (erythrocytes). *h. anaemia see* anaemia.

haemolytic disease of the newborn *n.* the condition resulting from destruction (haemolysis) of the red blood cells of the fetus by antibodies in the mother's blood passing through the placenta. This most commonly happens when the red blood cells of the fetus are Rh positive (*see* rhesus factor) but the mother's red cells are Rh negative. The fetal cells are therefore incompatible in her circulation and evoke the production of antibodies. This may result in very severe anaemia of the fetus or severe jaundice after birth. A blood test early in pregnancy enables the detection of antibodies in the mother's blood and the adoption of various precautions for the infant's safety. *See also* anti D.

haemopericardium (heem-ŏ-pe-ri-kar-diŭm) *n.* the presence of blood within the pericardium, which may result from injury, tumours, rupture of the heart, or a leaking aneurysm.

haemoperitoneum (heem-ŏ-pe-ri-tŏn-ee-ŭm) *n.* the presence of blood in the peritoneal cavity, between the lining of the abdomen or pelvis and the membrane covering the organs within.

haemophilia (hee-moh-fil-iă) *n.* a hereditary disorder in which the blood clots very slowly, due to a deficiency of one of the coagulation factors (antihaemophilic factor or Factor VIII). Prolonged bleeding follows any injury or wound, and in severe cases there is spontaneous bleeding into muscles and joints. Bleeding in haemophilia may be treated by transfusions of plasma or administration of concentrated Factor VIII. Haemophilia is almost exclusively restricted to males: women can carry the disease without being affected themselves. —**haemophiliac** *n.* —**haemophilic** *adj.*

Haemophilus (hi-mof-i-lŭs) *n.* a genus of Gram-negative aerobic nonmotile parasitic rodlike bacteria frequently found in the respiratory tract. Most species are pathogenic. *H. influenzae* a species associated with acute and chronic respiratory infections and a common secondary cause of influenza infections.

haemophthalmia (heem-off-thal-miă) *n.* bleeding into the vitreous humour of the eye.

haemopneumothorax (**pneumohaemothorax**) (heem-ŏ-new-moh-thor-aks) *n.* blood and air in the pleural cavity, usually as a result of injury. *See also* haemothorax.

haemopoiesis (hee-moh-poi-ee-sis) *n.* the process of production of blood cells and platelets which continues throughout life, replacing aged cells (which are removed from the circulation). In healthy adults, haemopoiesis is confined to the bone marrow. *See also* erythropoiesis, leucopoiesis, thrombopoiesis. —**haemopoietic** *adj.*

haemopoietin (hee-moh-poi-**ee**-tin) *n. see* erythropoietin.

haemoptysis (hi-**mop**-ti-sis) *n.* the coughing up of blood.

haemorrhage (bleeding) (**hem**-er-ij) *n.* the escape of blood from a ruptured blood vessel, externally or internally. Arterial blood is bright red and emerges in spurts, venous blood is dark red and flows steadily, while damage to minor vessels may produce only an oozing. Rupture of a major blood vessel such as the femoral artery can lead to the loss of several litres of blood in a few minutes, resulting in shock, collapse, and death, if untreated. *primary h.* haemorrhage occurring immediately after injury or surgery. *secondary h.* haemorrhage occurring some time after injury, usually due to sepsis. *See also* haematemesis, haematuria, haemoptysis.

haemorrhagic (hem-er-**aj**-ik) *adj.* associated with or resulting from blood loss. *See* haemorrhage.

haemorrhagic disease of the newborn *n.* a transient disorder of newborn infants in which prolonged bleeding may result from the slightest injury. It is caused by deficiency of vitamin K and therefore of prothrombin, which is necessary for blood clotting.

haemorrhoidectomy (hem-er-oid-ek-**tŏmi**) *n.* the surgical operation for removing haemorrhoids, which are tied and then excised. The operation is usually performed only for second- or third-degree haemorrhoids.

haemorrhoids (piles) (**hem**-er-oidz) *pl. n.* enlarged (varicose) veins in the wall of the anus (*internal h.*), usually a consequence of prolonged constipation or, occasionally, diarrhoea. The main symptom is bleeding. *external h.* prolapsed internal haemorrhoids or perianal haematomas. *first-degree h.* haemorrhoids that never appear at the anus but cause bleeding at the end of defaecation. *second-degree h.* haemorrhoids that protrude beyond the anus as an uncomfortable swelling but return spontaneously. *third-degree h.* haemorrhoids that remain outside the anus and need to be returned by pressure. They often require surgery (*see* haemorrhoidectomy), especially if they become strangulated (producing severe pain and further enlargement).

haemosalpinx (hee-moh-**sal**-pinks) *n. see* haematosalpinx.

haemosiderosis (heem-ŏ-sid-er-**oh**-sis) *n.* a disorder caused by excessive deposition of iron, which results from excessive intake or administration of iron. It results in damage to various organs, including the heart and liver. *Compare* haemochromatosis.

haemostasis (hee-moh-**stay**-sis) *n.* the arrest of bleeding, involving the physiological processes of blood coagulation and the contraction of damaged blood vessels. The term is also applied to various surgical procedures used to stop bleeding.

haemostatic (styptic) (hee-moh-**stat**-ik) *n.* an agent that stops of prevents haemorrhage; for example, phytomenadione and thromboplastin.

haemothorax (hee-moh-**thor**-aks) *n.* blood in the pleural cavity, usually due to injury.

hair (hair) *n.* a threadlike keratinized outgrowth of the epidermis of the skin. The root of the hair, beneath the surface of the skin, is expanded at its base to form the bulb, which contains a matrix of dividing cells. As new cells are formed the older ones are pushed upwards and become keratinized to form the root and shaft. *h. follicle* a sheath of epidermal cells and connective tissue that surrounds the root of a hair. *h. papilla* a projection of the dermis that is surrounded by the base of the hair bulb. It contains the capillaries that supply blood to the growing hair.

half-life (hahf-lyf) *n.* **1.** the time taken for half the atoms of a radioactive isotope to decay: a measure of the radioactivity of the isotope. **2.** (in pharmacology) the time taken for the body to excrete half a given amount of a drug.

halibut liver oil (**hal**-i-bŭt) *n.* an oil extracted from the liver of halibut. It is rich in vitamins A and D.

halitosis (hal-i-**toh**-sis) *n.* bad breath. Causes of temporary halitosis include recently eaten strongly flavoured food; more long-lasting causes include periodontal disease and infective conditions of the nose, throat, and lungs.

hallucination (hă-loo-sin-**ay**-shŏn) *n.* a false perception of something that is not really there. Hallucinations may be provoked by psychological illness (such as schizophrenia) or physical disor-

ders in the brain or they may be caused by drugs or sensory deprivation. *Compare* illusion.

hallucinogen (hă-**loo**-sin-ŏ-jen) *n.* a drug that produces hallucinations, e.g. cannabis and lysergic acid diethylamide. Hallucinogens were formerly used to treat certain types of mental illness. —**hallucinogenic** *adj.*

hallux (**hal**-ŭks) *n.* (*pl.* **halluces**) the big toe. *h. valgus* a deformity in which the big toe is displaced towards the other toes. It is usually associated with a bunion.

halogen (**hal**-ŏ-jen) *n.* any one of the related elements fluorine, chlorine, bromine, or iodine.

haloperidol (hal-oh-**pe**-ri-dol) *n.* a tranquillizer administered by mouth or injection to relieve anxiety and tension in the treatment of schizophrenia and other psychiatric disorders. Trade names: **Haldol, Serenace**.

halothane (**hal**-oh-thayn) *n.* a potent general anaesthetic administered by inhalation, used for inducing and maintaining anaesthesia in all types of surgical operations. Trade name: **Fluothane**.

hamate bone (unciform bone) (**ham**-ayt) *n.* a hook-shaped bone of the wrist (*see* carpus). It articulates with the pisiform and triquetral bones behind and with the fourth and fifth metacarpal bones in front.

hammer (**ham**-er) *n.* (in anatomy) *see* malleus.

hammer toe *n.* a deformity of a toe, most often the second, caused by fixed flexion of the first joint. A corn often forms over the deformity, which may be painful.

hamstring (**ham**-string) *n.* any of the tendons at the back of the knee. *h. muscles* the biceps femoris, semitendinosus, and semimembranosus, attached by the hamstrings to their insertions in the tibia and fibula.

handicap (han-di-kap) *n.* partial or total inability to perform a social, occupational, or other activity.

Hand-Schüller-Christian disease (hand shew-ler kris-chăn) *n. see* reticuloendotheliosis. [A. Hand (1868–1949), US paediatrician; A. Schüller (1874–1958), Austrian neurologist; H. A. Christian (1876–1951), US physician]

Hansen's bacillus (han-sěnz) *n. see* Mycobacterium. [G. H. A. Hansen (1841–1912), Norwegian physician]

haploid (monoploid) (hap-loid) *adj.* describing cells, nuclei, or organisms with a single set of unpaired chromosomes. In man the gametes are haploid following meiosis. *Compare* diploid, triploid. **—haploid** *n.*

hapt- (hapto-) *prefix denoting* touch.

hapten (hap-tĕn) *n.* a substance that becomes antigenic by combining with and modifying the body's own proteins.

harelip (hair-lip) *n.* the congenital deformity of a cleft in the upper lip, on one or both sides of the midline. It is often associated with a cleft palate. Medical name: **cheiloschisis.**

Harrison's sulcus (ha-ri-sŏnz) *n.* a depression on both sides of the chest wall of a child between the pectoral muscles and the lower margin of the ribcage. It develops in conditions in which the airways are partially obstructed or when the lungs are abnormally congested due to some congenital abnormality of the heart. [E. Harrison (1789–1838), British physician]

Harris's operation (ha-ris-ěz) *n.* an operation in which the prostate gland is removed through an incision above the pubic bone and through the bladder. *See* prostatectomy. [S. H. Harris (1880–1936), Australian surgeon]

Hartmann's solution (hart-manz) *n.* a solution containing sodium, potassium, and calcium chlorides and sodium lactate, administered by infusion to treat dehydration. [A. Hartmann (1898–), US physician]

Hartnup disease (hart-nup) *n.* a hereditary defect in the metabolism of the amino acid tryptophan, leading to mental retardation, thickening and roughening of the skin, and lack of muscular coordination.

Hashimoto's disease (hash-i-moh-tohz) *n.* chronic thyroiditis due to the formation of autoantibodies against normal thyroid tissue. Its features include a firm swelling of the thyroid and partial or total failure of secretion of thyroid hormones; often there are autoantibodies to other organs, such as the stomach. [H. Hashimoto (1881–1934), Japanese surgeon]

hashish (hash-eesh) *n. see* cannabis.

haustrum (how-strum) *n.* one of the pouches on the external surface of the colon.

Haversian canal (ha-ver-si-ăn) *n.* one of the small canals that ramify throughout compact bone. *See also* bone. [C. Havers (1650–1702), English anatomist]

Haversian system *n. see* bone.

hay fever (hay) *n.* a form of allergy due to pollen, characterized by inflammation of the membrane lining the nose and sometimes of the conjunctiva. The symptoms of sneezing, running or blocked nose, and watering eyes often respond to treatment with antihistamines. Medical name: **allergic rhinitis.**

HCG *n. see* chorionic gonadotrophin.

head (hed) *n.* **1.** the part of the body that contains the brain and the organs of sight, hearing, smell, and taste. **2.** the rounded portion of a bone, which fits into a groove of another to form a joint.

headache (hed-ayk) *n.* pain felt deep within the skull. Most headaches are caused by emotional stress or fatigue but some are symptoms of serious intracranial disease. *See also* migraine.

healing (heel-ing) *n. see* intention.

health-care delivery (helth-kair) *n.* the services provided by nurses and others in the health service.

health centre *n.* (in Britain) a building, owned or leased by a District Health Authority, that houses personnel and/or services from one or several sections of the National Health Service.

health education *n.* persuasive methods used to encourage people to adopt life styles that the educators believe will improve health and to reject habits regarded as harmful to health.

health service commissioner (ombudsman) *n.* an official responsible to Parliament and appointed to protect the interests of patients in relation to administration of the National Health Service. He can investigate complaints and allegations of maladministration but not of professional negligence.

health visitor *n.* a trained nurse with experience in midwifery and special training in preventive medicine (including health education). All births are notified to the appropriate health visitor, most of whose work is concerned with routine visiting of selected preschool children (though the elderly and chronic sick also receive routine visits).

hearing aid (heer-ing) *n.* an electronic device to enable a deaf person to hear, consisting of a miniature sound receiver, an amplifier, and either an earpiece or a vibrator to transfer the amplified sound to the ear.

heart (hart) *n.* a hollow muscular cone-shaped organ, lying between the lungs, with the apex directed downwards, forwards, and to the left. It is divided by a septum into separate right and left halves, each of which is divided into an upper atrium and a lower ventricle (see illustration). Deoxygenated blood is pumped to the lungs via the right atrium and ventricle; newly oxygenated blood is pumped out to the body via the left atrium and ventricle. The direction of blood flow within the heart is controlled by valves.

heart attack *n. see* myocardial infarction.

heart block *n.* a condition in which conduction of the electrical impulses generated by the sinoatrial node is impaired, so that the pumping action of the heart is slowed down. Heart block may be congenital or it may be due to heart disease, myocarditis, cardiomyopathy, and disease of the valves. Symptoms may be abolished by the use of an artificial pacemaker. *first de-*

semilunar valve — pulmonary artery
superior vena cava — aorta
— pulmonary vein
inferior vena cava —
right atrium — left atrium
tricuspid valve — bicuspid valve
— chorda tendina (tendon)
right ventricle — left ventricle
— ➤ direction of blood
septum — flow through the heart

Vertical section through the heart

gree h. b. heart block in which conduction between atria and ventricles is delayed. *second degree h. b.* heart block in which not all the impulses are conducted from the atria to the ventricles. *third degree h. b.* heart block in which no impulses are conducted and the ventricles beat at their own slow intrinsic rate (20–40 per minute).

heartburn (pyrosis) (hart-bern) *n.* discomfort or pain, usually burning in character, that is felt behind the breastbone. It may be accompanied by the appearance of acid or bitter fluid in the mouth and is usually caused by regurgitation of the stomach contents into the gullet or by oesophagitis.

heart failure *n.* a condition in which the pumping action of the ventricle of the heart is inadequate. This results in back pressure of blood, with congestion of the lungs and liver, and oedema. There is a reduced flow of arterial blood from the heart, which in extreme cases results in peripheral circulatory failure (cardi-

ogenic shock). Heart failure may result from any condition that overloads, damages, or reduces the efficiency of the heart muscle, such as coronary thrombosis or hypertension. Treatment consists of rest, a low salt diet, diuretic drugs (e.g. frusemide), and digitalis derivatives (e.g. digoxin).

heart-lung machine *n.* an apparatus for taking over temporarily the functions of both the heart and the lungs during heart surgery. It incorporates a pump, to maintain the circulation, and equipment to oxygenate the blood.

heat exhaustion (heet) *n.* fatigue and collapse due to the low blood pressure and blood volume that result from loss of body fluids and salts after prolonged or unaccustomed exposure to heat.

heat rash *n. see* prickly heat.

heatstroke (sunstroke) (heet-strohk) *n.* raised body temperature (pyrexia), absence of sweating, and eventual loss of consciousness due to failure or exhaustion of the temperature-regulating mechanism of the body.

hebephrenia (hee-bi-free-niă) *n.* a form of schizophrenia. It is typically a chronic condition, and the most prominent features are disordered thinking; inappropriate emotions with thoughtless cheerfulness, apathy, or querulousness; and silly behaviour. It typically starts in adolescence or young adulthood. —**hebephrenic** *adj.*

Heberden's node (hee-ber-děnz) *n.* a lump of cartilage-covered bone arising at the terminal joint of a finger in osteoarthritis. It is often inherited. [W. Heberden (1710–1801), British physician]

hebetude (heb-i-tewd) *n.* apathy and emotional dullness. This is not a symptom specific to any one condition; extreme degrees are found in schizophrenia and dementia.

hectic (hek-tik) *adj.* occurring regularly. *h. fever* a fever that typically develops in the afternoons, in cases of pulmonary tuberculosis.

hecto- *prefix denoting* a hundred.

heel (heel) *n.* the part of the foot that extends behind the ankle joint. *See* calcaneus.

Hegar's sign (hay-garz) *n.* an indication of pregnancy that may be detectable during the second and third months. If fingers of one hand are inserted into the vagina and those of the other are placed over the pelvic cavity, the lower part of the womb, including the neck, can easily be compressed between the two hands. *See also* Jacquemier's sign. [A. Hegar (1830–1914), German gynaecologist]

helc- (helco-) *prefix denoting* an ulcer.

helcoplasty (hel-koh-plasti) *n.* the surgical repair of ulcers by skin grafting. *See* skin (graft).

helio- *prefix denoting* the sun.

heliotherapy (hee-li-oh-th'e-ră-pi) *n.* the use of sunlight to promote healing; sunbathing.

helium (hee-li-ŭm) *n.* a colourless inert gas that is used in combination with oxygen in respiratory tests and therapy and to prevent decompression sickness in deepsea divers. Symbol: He.

helix (hee-liks) *n.* the outer curved fleshy ridge of the pinna of the outer ear.

Heller's operation (hel-erz) *n. see* cardiomyotomy. [E. Heller (1877–1964), German surgeon]

Heller's test *n.* a test for the presence of protein (albumin) in the urine. [J. F. Heller (1813–71), Austrian pathologist]

helminth (hel-minth) *n.* any of the various parasitic worms, including the flukes, tapeworms, and roundworms.

helminthiasis (hel-min-th'y-ă-sis) *n.* the diseased condition resulting from an infestation with parasitic worms (helminths).

helminthology (hel-min-thol-ŏji) *n.* the study of parasitic worms.

heloma (hee-loh-mă) *n.* a callosity or corn on the foot or hand.

hemeralopia (hem-er-ă-loh-piă) *n. see* day blindness.

hemi- *prefix denoting* (in medicine) the right or left half of the body.

hemianopia (hemi-an-oh-piă) *n.* absence of half of the normal field of vision.

hemiballismus (hemi-bal-iz-mŭs) *n.* a violent involuntary movement usually restricted to one arm and primarily involving the proximal muscles. It is a symptom of disease of the basal ganglia.

hemicolectomy (hemi-koh-**lek**-tŏmi) *n.* surgical removal of about half the colon, usually the right section (*right h.*) with subsequent joining of the ileum to the transverse colon. This is performed for such diseases as Crohn's disease or cancer.

hemicrania (hemi-**kray**-niă) *n.* **1.** a headache affecting only one side of the head, usually migraine. **2.** absence of half of the skull in a developing fetus.

hemimelia (hemi-**mee**-liă) *n.* congenital absence or gross shortening (aplasia) of the distal portion of the arms or legs. *See also* ectromelia.

hemiparesis (hemi-pă-**ree**-sis) *n. see* hemiplegia.

hemiplegia (hemiparesis) (hemi-**plee**-jiă) *n.* paralysis of one side of the body. Movements of the face and arm are often more severely affected than those of the leg. It is caused by disease of the opposite (contralateral) hemisphere of the brain.

hemisphere (**hem**-iss-feer) *n.* one of the two halves of the cerebrum, not in fact hemispherical but more nearly quarter-spherical.

hemlock (**hem**-lok) *n.* the plant *Conium maculatum*, found in Britain and central Europe. It is a source of the poisonous alkaloid coniine.

hemp (hemp) *n. see* cannabis.

Henle's loop (**hen**-liz) *n.* the part of a kidney tubule that forms a loop extending towards the centre of the kidney. It is surrounded by blood capillaries, which reabsorb water and selected soluble substances back into the bloodstream. [F. G. J. Henle (1809–85), German anatomist]

Henoch's purpura (**hen**-ohks) *n. see* Schönlein-Henoch purpura.

hepar (**hee**-par) *n.* the liver.

heparin (**hep**-er-in) *n.* an anticoagulant produced in liver cells, some white blood cells, and certain other sites, which acts by inhibiting the action of the enzyme thrombin in the final stage of blood coagulation. An extracted purified form of heparin is widely used for the prevention of blood coagulation both in patients with thrombosis and similar conditions and in blood collected for examination.

hepat- (hepato-) *prefix denoting* the liver.

hepatalgia (hep-ă-**tal**-jiă) *n.* pain in or over the liver. It is caused by liver inflammation or swelling.

hepatectomy (hep-ă-**tek**-tŏmi) *n.* the operation of removing the liver. *partial h.* the removal of one or more lobes of the liver; it may be carried out after severe injury or to remove a tumour localized in one part of the liver.

hepatic (hip-**at**-ik) *adj.* relating to the liver. *h. duct see* bile duct. *h. encephalopathy* (*portosystemic encephalopathy*) a condition in which brain function is impaired by the presence of toxic substances, absorbed from the colon, which are normally removed or detoxified by the liver. *h. flexure* the bend in the colon, just underneath the liver, where the ascending colon joins the transverse colon. *h. vein* one of several veins that drain blood from the liver directly into the inferior vena cava.

hepaticostomy (hip-at-i-**kost**-ŏmi) *n.* a surgical operation in which a temporary or permanent opening is made into the main duct carrying bile from the liver.

hepatitis (hep-ă-**ty**-tis) *n.* inflammation of the liver due to a virus infection or such diseases as amoebic dysentery and lupus. *infectious h.* (*epidemic h.*, *epidemic jaundice*) hepatitis transmitted by contaminated food or drink. After an incubation period of 15–40 days, the patient develops fever and sickness. Yellow discoloration of the skin (*see* jaundice) appears about a week later and persists for up to three weeks. *serum h.* hepatitis transmitted by infected blood or blood products contaminating hypodermic needles, blood transfusions, etc. Symptoms, which develop suddenly after an incubation period of 1–6 months, include headache, fever, chills, general weakness, and jaundice. Patients may be detected by identification of the Australia antigen in their blood.

hepatization (hep-ă-ty-**zay**-shŏn) *n.* the conversion of lung tissue, which normally holds air, into a solid liver-like mass during the course of acute lobar pneumonia.

hepato- *prefix. see* hepat-.

hepatoblastoma (hep-ă-toh-blas-toh-mă) *n.* a malignant tumour of the liver occurring in children, made up of embryonic liver cells.

hepatocele (hip-**at**-oh-seel) *n.* a hernia of the liver.

hepatocellular (hep-ă-toh-**sel**-yoo-ler) *adj.* relating to or affecting the cells of the liver.

hepatocirrhosis (hep-ă-toh-si-**roh**-sis) *n.* cirrhosis of the liver. *See* cirrhosis.

hepatoma (hep-ă-toh-mă) *n.* a malignant tumour of the liver, originating in mature liver cells. In Western countries it often develops in patients with cirrhosis. The term hepatoma is often,

though incorrectly, used to include malignant tumours arising in the bile duct (*cholangiocarcinomas*).

hepatomegaly (hep-ă-toh-**meg**-ă-li) *n.* enlargement of the liver to such an extent that it can be felt below the rib margin. This may be due to congestion, inflammation, infiltration (e.g. by fat), or tumour.

hepatotoxic (hep-ă-toh-**toks**-ik) *adj.* damaging or destroying liver cells. Drugs such as paracetamol and phenacemide can be hepatotoxic at high doses or with prolonged use.

hept- (**hepta-**) *prefix denoting* seven.

heptabarbitone (hep-tă-**bar**-bit-ohn) *n.* a barbiturate administered by mouth to treat insomnia. Trade name: **Medomin**.

hereditary (hi-**red**-it-er-i) *adj.* transmitted from parents to their offspring; inherited.

heredity (hi-**red**-iti) *n.* the process that causes the biological similarity between parents and their offspring. Genetics is the study of heredity.

heredo- *prefix denoting* heredity.

Hering-Breuer reflexes (h'e-ring **broi**-er) *pl. n.* the reflexes that maintain the normal rhythm of inflation and deflation of the lungs. [K. E. K. Hering (1834–1918), German physiologist; J. Breuer (1842–1925), German physician]

hermaphrodite (her-**maf**-rŏ-dyt) *n.* an individual in which both male and female sex organs are present or in which the sex organs contain both ovarian and testicular cells. —**hermaphroditism** *n.*

hernia (her-niă) *n.* the protrusion of an organ or tissue out of the body cavity in which it normally lies. *diaphragmatic h.* the protrusion of an abdominal organ through the diaphragm into the chest cavity. *femoral h.* the protrusion of part of the bowel at the top of the thigh, through the point at which the femoral artery passes from the abdomen to the thigh. *hiatus h.* the most common type of diaphragmatic hernia, in which the stomach passes partly or completely into the chest cavity through the oesophageal opening. *incarcerated h.* a hernia that is swollen and fixed within its sac. *inguinal h.* (or *rupture*) the protrusion of a sac of peritoneum, containing fat or part of the bowel, through the lower abdominal wall. *irreducible h.* a hernia that cannot be returned to its normal site. *strangulated h.* a hernia that is cut off from its blood supply, becoming painful and eventually gangrenous. *umbilical h.* the protrusion of part of the bowel at the navel, most common in young children.

hernio- *prefix denoting* a hernia.

hernioplasty (**her**-ni-oh-plasti) *n.* the surgical operation to repair a hernia, in which the abnormal opening is sewn up and/or the weakness strengthened with suture material.

herniorrhaphy (her-ni-o-**rǎ**-fi) *n.* surgical repair of a hernia.

herniotomy (her-ni-ot-ŏmi) *n.* an operation to repair a hernia that involves cutting the sac that contains it.

heroin (diamorphine) (**h'e**-roh-in) *n.* a white crystalline powder derived from morphine but with a shorter duration of action. Like morphine it is a powerful narcotic analgesic whose continued use leads to dependence.

herpangina (herp-an-jy-nǎ) *n.* a viral infectious disease of sudden onset that causes fever, blisters, and ulceration of the soft palate and tonsillar area.

herpes (**her**-peez) *n.* inflammation of the skin caused by viruses and characterized by collections of small blisters. *h. simplex* a type of herpes that affects the mouth (*cold sore*) and conjunctiva (type 1) or the genitals (*genital h.*; type 2). The disease may recur. *h. zoster* (*shingles*) a type of herpes that usually starts with pain along the distribution of a nerve (often in the face, chest, or abdomen), followed by the development of vesicles. The virus that causes herpes zoster can also cause chickenpox in children.

herpesvirus (her-peez-vy-rǔs) *n.* one of a group of DNA-containing viruses causing latent infections in man and animals. The herpesviruses are the causative agents of herpes simplex, herpes zoster, and chickenpox. *See also* cytomegalovirus.

heter- (hetero-) *prefix denoting* difference; dissimilarity.

heterochromia (het-er-oh-**kroh**-miǎ) *n.* colour difference in the iris of the eye, which is usually congenital but is occasionally secondary to inflammation of the iris.

heterogenous (het-er-oj-in-ǔs) *adj.* derived from a different source: describing tissue used for grafting, vaccines, etc.

heterograft (xenograft) (**het**-er-oh-grahft) *n.* a living tissue graft that is made from one animal species to another.

heterophoria (het-er-oh-**for**-iǎ) *n.* a tendency to squint. Under normal circumstances both the eyes work together, but if one eye is covered it will move out of alignment with the object the other eye is still viewing. When the cover is removed the eye immediately returns to its normal position. *See also* strabismus.

heterophyiasis (het-er-oh-fi-**I**-ă-sis) *n.* an infestation of the small intestine with the parasitic fluke *Heterophyes heterophyes*. Man becomes infected on eating raw or salted fish that contains the larval stage of the fluke. Symptoms include abdominal pain and diarrhoea; if the eggs reach the brain, spinal cord, and heart they produce serious lesions.

heteroplasty (**het**-er-oh-plasti) *n.* the grafting of tissue from an animal of one species to another.

heteropsia (het-er-**op**-siă) *n.* different vision in each eye.

heterosexuality (het-er-oh-seks-yoo-**al**-iti) *n.* the pattern of sexuality in which sexual behaviour and thinking are directed towards people of the opposite sex. —**heterosexual** *adj., n.*

heterosis (het-er-**oh**-sis) *n.* hybrid vigour: the increased sturdiness, resistance to disease, etc., of individuals whose parents are of different races or species.

heterotopia (heterotopy) (het-er-oh-**toh**-piă) *n.* the displacement of an organ or part of the body from its normal position.

heterotropia (het-er-oh-**troh**-piă) *n.* *see* strabismus.

heterozygous (het-er-oh-zy-gŭs) *adj.* describing an individual in whom the members of a pair of genes determining a particular characteristic are dissimilar. *See* allele. *Compare* homozygous. —**heterozygote** *n.*

hex- (hexa-) *prefix denoting* six.

hexachlorophane (heks-ă-**klor**-ŏ-fayn) *n.* a disinfectant similar to phenol, formerly used in soaps and creams to treat skin disorders. Its use in medicinal products was limited by law in 1973 because of the toxic effects it might produce when absorbed into the body.

hexamine (methenamine) (heks-ă-meen) *n.* an antiseptic with a wide range of antibacterial activity, used to treat infections and inflammation of the urinary tract, such as cystitis. Trade names: **Hiprex, Mandelamine**.

hexobarbitone (heks-oh-**bar**-bit-ohn) *n.* an intermediate-acting barbiturate administered by mouth to treat insomnia.

hexose (**heks**-ohz) *n.* a simple sugar with six carbon atoms. Hexose sugars are the sugars most frequently found in food. The most important hexose is glucose.

Hg *symbol for* mercury.

hiatus (hy-**ay**-tŭs) *n.* an opening or aperture. For example, the diaphragm contains hiatuses for the oesophagus and aorta. *h. hernia see* hernia.

hiccup (**hik**-up) *n.* abrupt involuntary lowering of the diaphragm and closure of the sound-producing folds at the upper end of the trachea, producing a characteristic sound as the breath is drawn in. Hiccups, which usually occur repeatedly, may be caused by indigestion or more serious disorders, such as alcoholism. Medical name: **singultus**.

hidr- (hidro-) *prefix denoting* sweat.

hidradenitis (hidrosadenitis) (hy-drad-ě-**ny**-tis) *n.* inflammation of the sweat glands, usually occurring when the glands become blocked. This may occur in the armpit, around the nipple or umbilicus, or in the groin.

hidroa (hid-**roh**-ă) *n. see* hydroa.

hidrosis (hid-**roh**-sis) *n.* **1.** the excretion of sweat. **2. excessive sweating.**

hidrotic (hid-**rot**-ik) *n.* an agent that causes sweating. Parasympathomimetic drugs are hidrotics.

Higginson's syringe (**hig**-in-sŏnz) *n.* a rubber syringe with a bulb in the centre that is compressed to force liquid in one direction to irrigate a body cavity. [A. Higginson (1808–84), British surgeon]

hilum (**hy**-lŭm) *n.* (*pl.* **hila**) a hollow situated on the surface of an organ, at which structures such as blood vessels and nerve fibres enter or leave it. −**hilar** *adj.*

hindbrain (**hynd**-brayn) *n.* the part of the brain comprising the cerebellum, pons, and medulla oblongata.

hindgut (**hynd**-gut) *n.* the back part of the embryonic gut, which gives rise to part of the large intestine, the rectum, bladder, and urinary ducts. *See also* cloaca.

hinge joint (hinj) *n. see* ginglymus.

hip (hip) *n.* the region of the body where the thigh bone (femur) articulates with the pelvis: the region on each side of the pelvis. *h. bone* (*innominate bone*) a bone formed by the fusion of the ilium, ischium, and pubis. It articulates with the femur by the acetabulum. *h. girdle see* pelvic girdle.

hippocampal formation (hip-oh-kam-păl) *n.* a curved band of cortex lying within each cerebral hemisphere. It forms a portion of the limbic system and is involved in the complex physical aspects of behaviour governed by emotion and instinct.

hippocampus (hip-oh-**kam**-pŭs) *n.* a swelling in the floor of the lateral ventricle of the brain. It contains complex foldings of cortical tissue and is involved in the workings of the limbic system. −**hippocampal** *adj.*

Hippocratic oath (hip-ŏ-**krat**-ik) *n.* the oath taken by a doctor that binds him to observe the code of behaviour and practice followed by the Greek physician Hippocrates (460–370 BC), called the 'Father of Medicine'.

Hirschsprung's disease (**heersh**-spruungz) *n.* a congenital condition in which the rectum and sometimes part of the lower colon have failed to develop a normal nerve network. The affected portion does not expand or conduct the contents of the bowel, which accumulate in and distend the upper colon. *See also* megacolon. [H. Hirschsprung (1830–1916), Danish physician]

hirsutism (**herss**-yoo-tizm) *n.* excessive hairiness, particularly in women.

hirudin (hi-**roo**-din) *n.* an anticoagulant, present in the salivary glands of leeches and in certain snake venoms, that prevents blood coagulation by inhibiting the action of the enzyme thrombin.

Hirudo (hi-**roo**-doh) *n.* a genus of leeches. *See* leech.

hist- (**histio-**, **histo-**) *prefix denoting* tissue.

histamine (**hist**-ă-meen) *n.* a compound derived from the amino acid histidine, found in nearly all tissues of the body. Histamine causes dilation of blood vessels and contraction of smooth muscle; it is an important mediator of inflammation and is released in large amounts after skin damage, producing flushing, a flare, and a wheal. Histamine is also released in anaphylactic reactions. *See also* anaphylaxis.

histidine (hist-i-deen) *n.* an amino acid from which histamine is derived.

histiocyte (hist-i-ŏ-syt) *n.* a fixed macrophage, i.e. one that is stationary within connective tissue.

histiocytoma (hist-i-oh-sy-toh-mă) *n.* a tumour that contains macrophages or histiocytes.

histiocytosis (hist-i-oh-sy-toh-sis) *n.* any of a group of diseases, such as Gaucher's disease and Letterer-Siwe disease, in which there are abnormalities in certain large phagocytic cells (histiocytes), leading to biochemical defects.

histocompatibility (hist-oh-kŏm-pat-i-bil-iti) *n.* the form of compatibility that depends upon tissue components, mainly specific glycoprotein antigens in cell membranes. A high degree of histocompatibility is necessary for a tissue graft or organ transplant to be successful. —**histocompatible** *adj.*

histogenesis (hist-oh-jen-i-sis) *n.* the formation of tissues.

histoid (hist-oid) *adj.* **1.** resembling normal tissue. **2.** composed of one type of tissue.

histology (hiss-tol-ŏji) *n.* the study of the structure of tissues by means of special staining techniques combined with light and electron microscopy. —**histological** *adj.*

histolysis (hiss-tol-i-sis) *n.* disintegration of tissue.

histone (hist-ohn) *n.* a simple protein that combines with a nucleic acid to form a nucleoprotein.

histoplasmin (hist-oh-plaz-min) *n.* a preparation of antigenic material from a culture of the fungus *Histoplasma capsulatum*, used to test for the presence of histoplasmosis by subcutaneous injection.

histoplasmosis (hist-oh-plaz-moh-sis) *n.* an infection caused by inhaling spores of the fungus *Histoplasma capsulatum.* The primary pulmonary form usually produces no symptoms or harmful effects. Occasionally, progressive histoplasmosis, which resembles tuberculosis, develops. Symptomatic disease is treated with intravenous amphotericin-B.

histotoxic (hist-oh-toks-ik) *adj.* poisonous to tissues: applied to certain substances and conditions.

hives (hyvz) *n. see* urticaria.

HL-A system *n.* histocompatibility lymphocyte-A system: a group of eight antigens that are the most important of the 20 or more antigens responsible for histocompatibility. Successful tissue transplantation requires a minimum number of HL-A differences between donor's and recipient's tissues.

hobnail liver (hob-nayl) *n.* the liver of a patient with cirrhosis, which has a knobbly appearance caused by regenerating nodules separated by bands of fibrous tissue.

Hodgkin's disease (hoj-kinz) *n.* a malignant disease of lymphatic tissues, usually characterized by painless enlargement of one or more groups of lymph nodes in the neck, armpits, groin, chest, or abdomen; the spleen, liver, bone marrow, and bones may also be involved. Treatment may include surgery, radiotherapy, drug therapy (using drugs such as procarbazine and prednisone), or a combination of these. [T. Hodgkin (1798–1866), British physician]

holistic (hoh-**list**-ik) *adj.* describing an approach to patient care in which the physical, mental, and social factors in the patient's condition are taken into account, rather than just the diagnosed disease.

holo- *prefix denoting* complete or entire.

holocrine (**hol**-ŏ-kryn) *adj.* describing a gland or type of secretion in which the entire cell disintegrates when the product is released.

Homans' sign (hoh-**mănz**) *n.* pain felt in the calf when the foot is flexed backwards: a sign of phlebothrombosis. [J. Homans (1877–1954), US physician]

home nurse (district nurse) (hohm) *n.* (in Britain) a trained nurse with special training in domiciliary services. Formerly all home nurses were State Registered, but in recent years increasing numbers of State Enrolled Nurses are working in this field. Normally day care only is provided but under special circumstances out of hours nursing can be arranged.

homeo- (homoeo-) *prefix denoting* similar; like.

homeopathic (homoeopathic) (hoh-mi-ŏ-**path**-ik) *adj.* **1.** of or relating to homeopathy. **2.** infinitesimally small, as applied to the dose of a drug.

homeopathy (homoeopathy) (hoh-mi-**op**-ă-thi) *n.* a system of medicine based on the theory that 'like cures like'. The patient is treated with extremely small quantities of drugs that are themselves capable of producing symptoms of his particular disease. The system was founded by Samuel Hahnemann (1755–1843). *See also* fringe medicine. —**homeopathist** *n.*

homeostasis (hoh-mi-oh-**stay**-sis) *n.* the physiological process by which the internal systems of the body are maintained at equilibrium, despite variations in the external conditions. —**homeostatic** *adj.*

homo- *prefix denoting* the same or common.

homoeopathy (hoh-mi-**op**-ă-thi) *n.* *see* homeopathy.

homogenize (hŏ-**moj**-i-nyz) *vb.* to reduce material to a uniform consistency, e.g. by crushing and mixing. —**homogenization** *n.*

homogentisic acid (hoh-moh-jen-**tis**-ik) *n.* a product formed during the metabolism of the amino acids phenylalanine and tyrosine. In normal individuals homogentisic acid is oxidized by the enzyme *homogentisic acid oxidase.* In rare cases this enzyme is lacking and alcaptonuria results.

homograft (allograft) (hom-ŏ-grahft) *n.* a living tissue or organ graft between two members of the same species. Such grafts will not survive unless the recipient is treated to suppress his body's automatic rejection of the foreign tissue.

homoiothermic (hoh-moi-ŏ-**therm**-ik) *adj.* warm-blooded: able to maintain a constant body temperature independently of, and despite variations in, the temperature of the surroundings. *Compare* poikilothermic. —**homoiothermy** *n.*

homolateral (hoh-moh-**lat**-er-ăl) *adj.* *see* ipsilateral.

homologous (hoh-**mol**-ŏ-gŭs) *adj.* **1.** (in anatomy) describing organs or parts that have the same basic structure and evolutionary origin, but not necessarily the same function or superficial structure. *Compare* analogous. **2.** (in genetics) describing a pair of chromosomes of similar shape and size and having identical gene loci.

homoplasty (hoh-moh-plasti) *n.* surgical repair of defective or damaged tissues or organs with a homograft.

homosexuality (hoh-moh-seks-yoo-al-iti) *n.* the condition of being sexually attracted, covertly or overtly, by members of one's own sex: it can affect either sex (*see also* lesbianism). Homosexuality is no longer generally regarded as a psychological disorder but therapy may be offered to individuals wishing to change their sexual orientation. —**homosexual** *adj.*, *n.*

homozygous (hoh-moh-zy-gǔs) *adj.* describing an individual in whom the members of a pair of genes determining a particular characteristic are identical. *See* allele. *Compare* heterozygous. —**homozygote** *n.*

hook (huuk) *n.* a surgical instrument with a bent or curved tip, used to hold, lift, or retract tissue at operation.

hookworm (huuk-werm) *n.* either of two nematode worms, *Necator americanus* or *Ancylostoma duodenale*, which live as parasites in the intestine of man. *h. disease* a condition resulting from an infestation of the small intestine by hookworms. Heavy hookworm infections may cause considerable damage to the wall of the intestine, leading to severe anaemia. Bephenium hydroxynaphthoate is used in treatment.

hordeolum (hor-dee-ŏ-lum) *n. see* stye.

hormone (hor-mohn) *n.* a substance that is produced by an endocrine gland in one part of the body, passes into the bloodstream, and is carried to other (distant) organs or tissues, where it acts to modify their structure or function. Examples of hormones are corticosteroids, growth hormone, and androgens.

horn (horn) *n.* (in anatomy) a process, outgrowth, or extension of an organ or other structure. It is often paired.

Horner's syndrome (hor-nerz) *n.* a group of symptoms that are due to a disorder of the sympathetic nerves in the cervical (neck) region. The syndrome consists of a constricted pupil, ptosis, and an absence of sweating over the affected side of the face. [J. F. Horner (1831–86), Swiss ophthalmologist]

horseshoe kidney (hors-shoo) *n.* an anatomical variation in kidney development whereby the lower poles of both kidneys are joined together. This usually causes no trouble but it may be associated with impaired drainage of urine from the kidney by the ureters.

Horton's syndrome (hor-t'nz) *n.* a severe headache caused by the release of histamine. [B. T. Horton (1895–), US physician]

hospice (hos-pis) *n.* an institution that specializes in the care of terminally ill patients, especially in the care of the dying.

hospital (hos-pi-t'l) *n.* an institution offering residential, investigatory, and/or therapeutic care regarded as too complex or specialized for provision as a domiciliary service. *day h.* a hospital at which patients are cared for during the day, returning home at night. *general h.* a hospital that provides sufficient basic services for the population of a Health District.

host (hohst) *n.* an animal or plant in or upon which a parasite lives. *intermediate h.* a host in which the parasite passes its larval or asexual stages. *definitive h.* a host in which the parasite develops to its sexual stage.

hourglass contraction (ow-er-glahs) *n.* constriction of an organ at its centre as a result of abnormal muscular contraction. Hourglass contraction may be a complication of labour, tending to trap the placenta in the upper part of the constricted womb and possibly leading to excessive blood loss after delivery.

housemaid's knee (howss-maydz) *n.* a fluid-filled swelling of the bursa in front of the kneecap, often resulting from frequent kneeling. *See also* bursitis.

human chorionic gonadotrophin (HCG) (hew-măn) *n. see* chorionic gonadotrophin.

humectant (hew-mek-tănt) **1.** *n.* a substance that is used for moistening. **2.** *adj.* causing moistening.

humerus (hew-mer-ŭs) *n.* the bone of the upper arm. The head of the humerus articulates with the scapula at the shoulder joint. At the lower end of the shaft the trochlea articulates with the ulna and part of the radius.

humour (hew-mer) *n.* a body fluid. *See* aqueous humour, vitreous humour.

hunger pain (hung-er) *n.* pain in the upper abdomen that is relieved by taking food. It is associated with a duodenal ulcer.

Huntington's chorea (hunt-ing-tŏnz) *n. see* chorea. [G. Huntington (1850–1916), US physician]

Hurler's syndrome (hoor-lerz) *n.*

an inborn defect of metabolism causing the accumulation of mucopolysaccharides and lipids in the cells of the body. This leads to mental retardation, enlargement of the liver and spleen, deformities of the bones, and coarsening and thickening of the features (gargoylism). [G. Hurler, Austrian paediatrician]

Hutchinson's teeth (huch-in-sŏnz) *pl. n.* narrowed and notched permanent incisor teeth: a sign of congenital syphilis. [J. Hutchinson (1828–1913), British surgeon]

hyal- (hyalo-) *prefix denoting* **1.** glassy; transparent. **2.** hyalin. **3.** the vitreous humour of the eye.

hyalin (hy-ă-lin) *n.* a clear glassy material produced as the result of degeneration in certain tissues, particularly connective tissue and epithelial cells.

hyaline cartilage (hy-ă-lin) *n. see* cartilage.

hyaline membrane disease *n. see* respiratory distress syndrome.

hyalitis (hy-ă-ly-tis) *n.* inflammation of the vitreous body of the eye. *asteroid h.* a degenerative condition in which the vitreous contains many small white opacities.

hyaloid membrane (hy-ă-loid) *n.* the transparent membrane that surrounds the vitreous humour of the eye, separating it from the retina.

hyaluronidase (hy-ăl-yoor-on-i-dayz) *n.* an enzyme that increases the permeability of connective tissue. Hyaluronidase is found in the testes, in semen, and in other tissues.

hybrid (hy-brid) *n.* the offspring of a cross between two genetically unlike individuals. A hybrid, whose parents are usually of different species or varieties, is often sterile.

hydatid (hy-dă-tid) *n.* a bladder-like cyst formed in various human tissues following the growth of the larval stage of an *Echinococcus* tapeworm. *alveolar h.* an aggregate of small cysts, which enlarge by budding off external daughter cysts. *unilocular h.* a single large fluid-filled cyst, bound by a fibrous capsule, that gives rise internally to smaller daughter cysts. *See also* hydatid disease.

hydatid disease (hydatidosis, echinococciasis, echinococcosis) *n.* a condition resulting from the presence in the liver, lungs, or brain of hydatid cysts. Alveolar hydatids form malignant tumours; unilocular hydatids exert pressure as they grow and thereby damage surrounding tissues.

hydatidiform mole (hydatid mole, vesicular mole) (hy-dă-**tid**-i-form) *n.* a collection of fluid-filled sacs that develop when the chorion degenerates in early pregnancy. The embryo dies, the womb enlarges, and there is a discharge of pinkish liquid and cysts from the vagina. A malignant condition may subsequently develop (*see* chorionepithelioma).

hydatidosis (hy-dă-tid-oh-sis) *n. see* hydatid disease.

hydr- (hydro-) *prefix denoting* water or a watery fluid.

hydraemia (hy-**dree**-miă) *n.* the presence in the blood of more than the normal proportion of water.

hydragogue (**hy**-dră-gog) *n.* an agent that produces a watery discharge, particularly a laxative that produces watery stools.

hydrallazine (hy-**dral**-ă-zeen) *n.* a drug that lowers blood pressure and is administered by mouth or injection, usually in conjunction with diuretics, to treat hypertension. Trade name: **Apresoline**.

hydramnios (hydramnion) (hy-**dram**-ni-ŏs) *n.* the presence of an abnormally large amount of amniotic fluid surrounding the fetus from about the fifth month of pregnancy.

hydrargyria (hy-drar-**jy**-riă) *n. see* mercurialism.

hydrarthrosis (hy-drar-**throh**-sis) *n.* swelling at a joint caused by excessive synovial fluid. The condition usually involves the knees and may be recurrent.

hydrate (**hy**-drayt) **1.** *vb.* to undergo treatment or impregnation with water. **—hydration** *n.* **2.** *n.* a chemical compound in which one or more molecules of water are combined with a molecule of another substance.

hydroa (hidroa) (hid-**roh**-ă) *n.* an eruption of small blisters accompanied by intense itching, occurring (usually in preadolescent boys) on skin surfaces exposed to sunlight. Hydroa is a severe form of light-sensitive dermatitis.

hydrocele (**hy**-droh-seel) *n.* the accumulation of watery liquid in a sac, usually the sac surrounding the testes. This condition is characterized by painless enlargement of the scrotum.

hydrocephalus (hy-droh-**sef**-ă-lŭs) *n.* an abnormal increase in the amount of cerebrospinal fluid within the ventricles of the brain. In childhood, before the sutures of the skull have fused, hydrocephalus makes the head enlarge. In adults, hydrocephalus raises the intracranial pressure with consequent drowsiness and vomiting. Spina bifida is commonly associated with hydrocephalus.

hydrochloric acid (hy-drŏ-**klor**-ik) *n*. a strong acid present, in a very dilute form, in gastric juice. The secretion of excess hydrochloric acid by the stomach results in the condition hyperchlorhydria.

hydrochlorothiazide (hy-drŏ-klor-oh-**th'y**-ă-zyd) *n*. a diuretic administered by mouth to treat fluid retention (oedema) and high blood pressure. Trade names: **Direma**, **Esidrex**, **Hydrosaluric**.

hydrocolpos (hy-droh-**kol**-pŏs) *n*. a cyst containing watery liquid or mucus formed in the vagina.

hydrocortisone (cortisol) (hy-droh-**kor**-tiz-ohn) *n*. a steroid hormone: the major glucocorticoid synthesized and released by the human adrenal cortex. It is important for normal carbohydrate metabolism and for the normal response to any stress. Hydrocortisone is used to treat adrenal failure (Addison's disease) and inflammatory, allergic, and rheumatic conditions (including rheumatoid arthritis, colitis, and eczema). It may be given by mouth, by injection, or in the form of a cream or ointment.

hydrocyanic acid (prussic acid) (hy-droh-sy-**an**-ik) *n*. an intensely poisonous volatile acid that can cause death within a minute if inhaled. It smells of bitter almonds. See cyanide.

hydroflumethiazide (hy-droh-floo-meth-**I**-ă-zyd) *n*. a diuretic administered by mouth to treat fluid retention (oedema) and high blood pressure. Trade name: **Hydrenox**.

hydrogen (hy-drŏ-**jĕn**) *n*. a colourless gas that is combined with oxygen to form water (H_2O) and with various other molecules (chiefly carbon and oxygen) to form all organic compounds. Symbol: H. *h. ion concentration see* pH.

hydrogen peroxide (per-ok-syd) *n*. a colourless liquid used as a disinfectant for cleansing wounds and, diluted, as a deodorant mouthwash or as ear drops for removing wax. Formula: H_2O_2.

hydrolysis (hy-**drol**-i-sis) *n*. any chemical reaction in which a compound and water react together to produce other compounds.

hydroma (hy-**droh**-mă) *n. see* hygroma.

hydrometer (hy-**drom**-it-er) *n*. an instrument for measuring the density or relative density of liquids. —**hydrometry** *n*.

hydrometra (hy-droh-**mee**-tră) *n*. an abnormal accumulation of watery fluid in the womb.

hydronephrosis (hy-droh-ni-**froh**-sis) *n*. distension and dilatation of the pelvis of the kidney. This is due to an obstruction to the free flow of urine from the kidney. Surgical relief by pyeloplasty is advisable to avoid the back pressure atrophy of the kidney and the complications of infection and stone formation. —**hydronephrotic** *adj*.

hydropericarditis (hy-droh-pe-ri-kar-**dy**-tis) *n. see* hydropericardium.

hydropericardium (hy-droh-pe-ri-kar-di-ŭm) *n*. accumulation of a clear serous fluid within the membranous sac surrounding the heart. It occurs in many cases of pericarditis (*hydropericarditis*).

hydroperitoneum (hy-droh-pe-ri-tŏn-**ee**-ŭm) *n. see* ascites.

hydrophobia (hy-drŏ-**foh**-biă) *n. see* rabies.

hydrophthalmos (hy-drof-**thal**-mŏs) *n. see* buphthalmos.

hydropneumoperitoneum (hy-droh-new-moh-pe-ri-tŏn-**ee**-ŭm) *n.* the presence of fluid and gas in the peritoneal cavity.

hydropneumothorax (pneumohydrothorax) (hy-droh-new-moh-**thor**-aks) *n.* air and fluid in the pleural cavity. An effusion of serous fluid commonly complicates a pneumothorax, and must be drained.

hydrops foetalis (hy-drops fee-**tah-**lis) *n.* the state of certain infants severely affected by haemolytic disease. Fluid accumulates in the body cavities, especially in the peritoneal and pleural cavities, and the liver becomes enlarged: these are features of chronic heart failure due to profound anaemia.

hydrorrhachis (hy-**dror**-ră-kis) *n.* an abnormal accumulation of watery fluid in the space surrounding the spinal cord.

hydrorrhoea (hy-drŏ-**ree**-ă) *n.* a watery discharge. *h. gravidarum* excessive secretion by the glands of the womb during pregnancy leading to a discharge from the vagina.

hydrosalpinx (hydrops tubae) (hy-droh-**sal**-pinks) *n.* the accumulation of watery fluid in one of the Fallopian tubes, which becomes swollen.

hydrotherapy (hy-droh-**th'e**-ră-pi) *n.* the use of water in the treatment of disorders: today restricted in orthodox medicine to exercises in remedial swimming pools for the rehabilitation of ar-thritic or partially paralysed patients.

hydrothorax (hy-droh-**thor**-aks) *n.* fluid in the pleural cavity. *See also* hydropneumothorax.

hydroureter (hy-droh-yoor-**ee**-ter) *n.* an accumulation of urine in one of the ureters, usually resulting from obstruction of the ureter by a stone or a misplaced artery.

hydrovarium (hy-droh-**vair**-iŭm) *n.* the accumulation of watery fluid in an ovary.

hydroxocobalamine (hy-droks-oh-koh-**bal**-ă-min) *n.* a cobalt-containing drug administered by injection to treat conditions involving vitamin B_{12} deficiency, such as pernicious anaemia. Trade names: **Cobalin-H, Neo-Cytamen**.

hydroxychloroquine (hy-droks-i-**klor**-ŏ-kwin) *n.* a drug similar to chloroquine, used mainly to treat lupus erythematosus and rheumatoid arthritis. Trade name: **Plaquenil**.

hydroxyprogesterone (hy-droks-i-proh-**jes**-ter-ohn) *n.* a synthetic female sex hormone (*see* progestogen) administered by injection to prevent miscarriage and to treat menstrual disorders. Trade name: **Primolut**.

hydroxyproline (hy-droks-i-**proh-**leen) *n.* a compound, similar in structure to the amino acids, found only in collagen.

hydroxystilbamidine (hy-droks-i-stil-**bam**-i-deen) *n.* a drug administered by injection to treat infections caused by fungi and protozoa, such as blastomycosis.

hydroxytryptamine (hy-droks-i-**trip**-tă-meen) *n. see* serotonin.

hydroxyurea (hy-droks-i-yoor-**ee**-ă) *n.* a drug that prevents cell growth and is administered by mouth to treat some types of leukaemia. Hydroxyurea may lower the white cell content of the blood due to its effects on the bone marrow. Trade name: **Hydrea**.

hydroxyzine (hy-**droks**-i-zeen) *n.* an antihistamine drug with sedative properties, administered by mouth to relieve anxiety, tension, and agitation and to treat nausea and vomiting. Trade name: **Atarax**.

hygiene (hy-jeen) *n.* the science of health and the study of ways of preserving it, particularly by promoting cleanliness.

hygr- (hygro-) *prefix denoting* moisture.

hygroma (hydroma) (hy-**groh**-mǎ) *n.* a type of cyst. It may develop from a lymphangioma (*cystic h.*) or from the liquified remains of a subdural haematoma (*subdural h.*).

hymen (hy-měn) *n.* the membrane that covers the opening of the vagina at birth but usually perforates spontaneously before puberty.

hymenectomy (hy-měn-**ek**-tŏmi) *n.* surgical removal of the hymen to enlarge the vaginal opening.

hymenorrhaphy (hy-měn-o-rǎ-fi) *n.* a tissue-grafting operation on the hymen in order to partially or completely close the vagina.

hymenotomy (hy-měn-**ot**-ŏmi) *n.* incision of the hymen. This operation may be performed in cases of imperforate hymen.

hyo- *prefix denoting* the hyoid bone.

hyoid bone (hy-oid) *n.* a small isolated U-shaped bone in the neck, below and supporting the tongue. It is held in position by muscles and ligaments between it and the styloid process of the temporal bone.

hyoscine (scopolamine) (hy-ŏ-seen) *n.* a drug that prevents muscle spasm (*see* parasympatholytic). It is used in the treatment of gastric or duodenal ulcers, to relax the womb in labour, for preoperative medication, and for travel sickness. It is administered by mouth or injection. Trade names: **Buscospan, Pamine**.

hyoscyamine (hy-ŏ-sy-ǎ-meen) *n.* a drug with similar activity to hyoscine, administered by mouth to treat muscle spasm. Trade name: **Peptard**.

hyp- (hypo-) *prefix denoting* **1.** deficiency, lack, or small size. **2.** (in anatomy) below; beneath.

hypaemia (hy-**pee**-miǎ) *n.* a decrease in the blood supply to an organ or tissue. *Compare* hyperaemia.

hypalgesia (hy-pal-**jeez**-iǎ) *n.* an abnormally low sensitivity to pain.

hyper- *prefix denoting* **1.** excessive; abnormally increased. **2.** (in anatomy) above.

hyperacidity (hy-per-ǎ-**sid**-iti) *n.* an abnormally increased concentration of acid, especially in the stomach (*see* hyperchlorhydria).

hyperactivity (hy-per-ak-**tiv**-iti) *n.* *see* hyperkinesia.

hyperacusis (hy-per-ǎ-**kew**-sis) *n.* abnormally acute hearing or painful sensitivity to sounds.

hyperadrenalism (hy-per-ǎ-**dren**-ǎ-lizm) *n.* overactivity of the adrenal glands. *See* Cushing's syndrome.

hyperaemia (hy-per-**ee**-miǎ) *n.* the presence of excess blood in the vessels supplying a part of the body. *active h.* (*arterial h.*) hyperaemia that occurs when the arterioles are relaxed and there is an increased blood flow. *passive h.* hyperaemia that occurs when the blood flow from the affected part is obstructed.

hyperaesthesia (hy-per-ees-**theez**-iă) *n.* excessive sensibility, especially of the skin.

hyperalgesia (hy-per-al-**jeez**-iă) *n.* an abnormal state of increased sensitivity to painful stimuli.

hyperbaric (hy-per-**ba**-rik) *adj.* at a pressure greater than atmospheric pressure. *h. oxygenation* a technique for exposing a patient to oxygen at high pressure. It is used to treat carbon monoxide poisoning, gas gangrene, and acute breathing difficulties.

hypercalcaemia (hy-per-kal-**see**-miă) *n.* the presence in the blood of an abnormally high concentration of calcium. *idiopathic h.* hypercalcaemia that affects infants who have received too much vitamin D, leading to mental disorder. *Compare* hypocalcaemia.

hypercalcinuria (hypercalcuria) (hy-per-kal-sin-**yoor**-iă) *n.* the presence in the urine of an abnormally high concentration of calcium.

hypercapnia (hypercarbia) (hy-per-**kap**-niă) *n.* the presence in the blood of an abnormally high concentration of carbon dioxide.

hypercatabolism (hy-per-kă-**tab**-ŏl-izm) *n.* an abnormally increased rate of metabolic breakdown of substances in the body. *See* catabolism. —**hypercatabolic** *adj.*

hyperchloraemia (hy-per-klor-ee-miă) *n.* the presence in the blood of an abnormally high concentration of chloride.

hyperchlorhydria (hy-per-klor-hy-driă) *n.* a greater than normal secretion of hydrochloric acid by the stomach, usually associated with a duodenal ulcer.

hyperchromatism (hy-per-**kroh**-mă-

tizm) *n.* the property of the nuclei of certain cells (for example, those of tumours) to stain more deeply than normal. —**hyperchromatic** *adj.*

hyperdactylism (polydactylism) (hy-per-**dak**-til-izm) *n.* the condition of having more than the normal number of fingers or toes.

hyperdynamia (hy-per-dy-**nay**-miă) *n.* excessive activity of muscles.

hyperemesis (hy-per-**em**-i-sis) *n.* severe vomiting. *h. gravidarum* hyperemesis affecting pregnant women: the stomach contents and bile are vomited, and the acidity of the arterial blood increases. *h. lactentium* vomiting by babies at the breast-feeding stage.

hyperextension (hy-per-iks-ten-shŏn) *n.* excessive and forceful extension of a limb beyond the normal limits, usually as part of an orthopaedic procedure to correct deformity.

hyperflexion (hy-per-**flek**-shŏn)˙ *n.* excessive and forceful flexion of a limb or other part.

hyperglycaemia (hy-per-gly-see-miă) *n.* an excess of glucose in the bloodstream. It may occur in a variety of diseases, most notably in diabetes mellitus.

hyperidrosis (hyperhidrosis) (hy-per-id-**roh**-sis) *n.* excessive sweating, which may occur in certain diseases, such as fevers or thyrotoxicosis, or following the use of certain drugs.

hyperinsulinism (hy-per-**ins**-yoo-lin-izm) *n.* **1.** excessive secretion of the hormone insulin by the islet cells of the pancreas. **2.** metabolic disturbance due to administration of too much insulin.

hyperinvolution (superinvolution) (hy-per-in-vŏ-**loo**-shŏn) *n.* **1.** excessive shrinkage of the womb

focusing point is beyond the retina

Uncorrected

Corrected

convex lens converges light rays falling on the eye

Hypermetropia (long-sightedness)

and associated structures after childbirth. **2.** excessive reduction in the size of any organ after it has attained an extremely large size.

hyperkalaemia (hy-per-kal-ee-miă) *n.* the presence in the blood of an abnormally high concentration of potassium. *See* electrolyte.

hyperkeratosis (hy-per-ke-ră-toh-sis) *n.* thickening of the outer horny layer of the skin. It may occur as an inherited disorder, affecting the palms and soles.

hyperkinesia (hyperactivity) (hy-per-ki-neez-iă) *n.* a state of overactive restlessness in children. *See* hyperkinetic syndrome. —**hyperkinetic** (hy-per-ki-net-ik) *adj.*

hyperkinetic syndrome *n.* a mental disorder, usually of children, characterized by a grossly excessive level of activity and a marked impairment of the ability to attend, resulting in aggressive disruptive behaviour. Treatment

usually involves drugs (such as amphetamines or haloperidol) and behaviour therapy.

hyperlipaemia (hy-per-lip-ee-miă) *n.* the presence in the blood of an abnormally high concentration of fats.

hypermetropia (long-sightedness) (hy-per-mi-troh-piă) *n.* the condition in which parallel light rays are brought to a focus behind the retina when the accommodation is relaxed. Normal vision can be restored by wearing spectacles with convex lenses. *Compare* emmetropia, myopia.

hypermotility (hy-per-moh-til-iti) *n.* excessive movement or activity, especially of the stomach or intestine.

hypernatraemia (hy-per-nă-tree-miă) *n.* the presence in the blood of an abnormally high concentration of sodium. *See also* electrolyte.

hypernephroma (Grawitz tumour, renal cell carcinoma) (hy-per-ni-froh-mă) *n.* a malignant tumour of kidney cells. It may be present for some years before giving rise to symptoms, which include fever, loin pain, and blood in the urine. Treatment is by surgery but tumours are apt to recur locally.

hyperopia (hy-per-oh-piă) *n.* the usual US term for hypermetropia.

hyperostosis (hy-per-os-toh-sis) *n.* excessive enlargement of the outer layer of a bone. It commonly affects the frontal bone of the skull (*h. frontalis*).

hyperparathyroidism (hy-per-pa-ră-th'y-roid-izm) *n.* overactivity of the parathyroid glands. *See* von Recklinghausen's disease.

hyperphagia (hy-per-**fay**-jiă) *n.* excessive overeating. *See* bulimia.

hyperpiesia (hy-per-py-**ee**-ziă) *n.* see hypertension.

hyperpituitarism (hy-per-pit-**yoo**-iter-izm) *n.* overactivity of the pituitary gland, resulting in acromegaly or gigantism.

hyperplasia (hy-per-**play**-ziă) *n.* the increased production and growth of normal cells in a tissue or organ. *Compare* hypertrophy, neoplasm.

hyperpnoea (hy-perp-**nee**-ă) *n.* an increase in the rate of breathing that is proportional to an increase in metabolism; for example, on exercise. *Compare* hyperventilation.

hyperpyrexia (hy-per-py-**reks**-iă) *n.* a rise in body temperature above 106°F (41.1°C). *See* fever.

hypersecretion (hy-per-si-**kree**-shŏn) *n.* excessive secretion, as of hydrochloric acid by the stomach (*see* hyperchlorhydria).

hypersensitive (hy-per-**sen**-si-tiv) *adj.* prone to respond abnormally to the presence of a particular antigen, which may cause a variety of tissue reactions ranging from serum sickness to an allergy (such as hay fever) or, at the severest, to anaphylactic shock (*see* anaphylaxis). *See also* allergy, immunity. —**hypersensitivity** *n.*

hypersplenism (hy-per-**splen**-izm) *n.* a decrease in the numbers of red cells, white cells, and platelets in the blood resulting from destruction or pooling of these cells by an enlarged spleen.

hypertension (hy-per-**ten**-shŏn) *n.* high blood pressure, i.e. elevation of the arterial blood pressure above the normal range expected in a particular age group. Hypertension may be of unknown cause (*essential h.* or *hyperpiesia*). It may also result from disease (*secondary* or *symptomatic h.*), as of the kidneys (*renal h.*), endocrine system, or arteries. Complications that may arise from hypertension include atherosclerosis, heart failure, cerebral haemorrhage, and kidney failure. Most cases of hypertension depend upon long-term drug therapy to lower the blood pressure and maintain it within the normal range. The drugs used include thiazide diuretics, beta blockers, methyldopa, and many others. *See also* portal hypertension, pulmonary (hypertension).

hyperthermia (hyperthermy) (hy-per-**therm**-iă) *n.* **1.** exceptionally high body temperature (about 41°C or above). *See* fever. **2.** treatment of disease by inducing fever. *Compare* hypothermia.

hyperthyroidism (hy-per-**th'y**-roid-izm) *n.* overactivity of the thyroid gland, either due to a tumour, overgrowth of the gland, or Graves's disease. *See* thyrotoxicosis.

hypertonia (hypertonicity) (hy-per-**toh**-niă) *n.* exceptionally high tension in muscles.

hypertonic (hy-per-**tonn**-ik) *adj.* **1.** describing a solution that has a greater osmotic pressure than another solution. *See* osmosis. **2.** describing muscles that demonstrate an abnormal increase in tonicity.

hypertrichosis (hy-per-trik-**oh**-sis) *n.* excessive growth of hair.

hypertrophy (hypertrophia) (hy-per-**trŏ**-fi) *n.* increase in the size of a tissue or organ brought about by the enlargement of its cells rather than by cell multiplication. *Compare* hyperplasia.

hypertropia (hy-per-**troh**-piă) *n.* strabismus in which one eye looks upwards.

hyperuricaemia (lithaemia) (hy-per-yoor-i-**see**-miă) *n.* the presence in the blood of an abnormally high concentration of uric acid. *See* gout.

hyperuricuria (lithuria) (hy-per-yoor-ik-**yoor**-iă) *n.* the presence in the urine of an abnormally high concentration of uric acid.

hyperventilation (hy-per-ven-ti-lay-shŏn) *n.* breathing at an abnormally rapid rate at rest. This causes unconsciousness by lowering the carbon dioxide concentration in the blood.

hypervitaminosis (hy-per-vit-ă-min-**oh**-sis) *n.* the condition resulting from excessive consumption of vitamins. The fat-soluble vitamins A and D are toxic if taken in excessive amounts.

hypervolaemia (hy-per-vŏ-**lee**-miă) *n.* an increase in the volume of circulating blood.

hyphaema (hy-**fee**-mă) *n.* bleeding into the chamber of the eye that lies in front of the lens.

hypn- (hypno-) *prefix denoting* **1.** sleep. **2.** hypnosis.

hypnosis (hip-**noh**-sis) *n.* a sleep-like state, artificially induced by a *hypnotist*, in which the mind is more than usually receptive to suggestion. Hypnotic suggestion has been used for a variety of purposes in medicine, for example as a cure for addiction and in other forms of psychotherapy.

hypnotic (soporific) (hip-**not**-ik) *n.* a drug that produces sleep by depressing brain function. Hypnotics include barbiturates, chloral hydrate, methaqualone, and nitrazepam. They often cause hangover effects in the morning and the barbiturate

hypnotics can lead to dependence.

hypnotism (**hip**-nŏ-tizm) *n.* the induction of hypnosis.

hypo- *prefix. see* hyp-.

hypoaesthesia (hy-poh-ees-**theez**-iă) *n.* a condition in which the sense of touch is diminished. This may rarely be extended to include other forms of sensation.

hypocalcaemia (hy-poh-kal-see-miă) *n.* the presence in the blood of an abnormally low concentration of calcium. *See* tetany. *Compare* hypercalcaemia.

hypocapnia (hy-poh-**kap**-niă) *n.* the presence in the blood of an abnormally low concentration of carbon dioxide.

hypochloraemia (hy-poh-klor-ee-miă) *n.* the presence in the blood of an abnormally low concentration of chloride.

hypochlorhydria (hy-poh-klor-hy-driă) *n.* reduced secretion of hydrochloric acid by the stomach. *See* achlorhydria.

hypochlorite (hy-poh-**klor**-ryt) *n.* any salt of hypochlorous (chloric(I)) acid (HClO). Hypochlorites have antiseptic and disinfectant properties, e.g. Milton (sodium hypochlorite).

hypochondria (hy-poh-**kon**-driă) *n.* preoccupation with the physical functioning of the body and with fancied ill health. In the most severe form there are delusions of ill health, usually due to underlying depression. **–hypochondriac** *adj., n.*

hypochondrium (hy-poh-kon-dri-ŭm) *n.* the upper lateral portion of the abdomen, situated beneath the lower ribs. **–hypochondriac** *adj.*

hypochromic (hy-poh-**kroh**-mik) *adj.* **1.** deficient in pigmentation.

2. (of red blood cells) deficient in haemoglobin.

hypodermic (hy-poh-**derm**-ik) *adj.* beneath the skin: usually applied to subcutaneous injections. The term is also applied to the syringe used for such injections.

hypodermoclysis (hy-poh-der-**mok**-li-sis) *n.* the continuous infusion under the skin of saline or other medicated solution to clean away blood, pus, and foreign matter from a wound.

hypofibrinogenaemia (fibrinogenopenia) (hy-poh-fi-brin-oh-jĕ-nee-miă) *n.* a deficiency of the clotting factor fibrinogen in the blood, which results in an increased tendency to bleed. It may occur as an inherited disorder or it may be acquired.

hypogammaglobulinaemia (hy-poh-gam-ă-glob-yoo-lin-**ee**-miă) *n.* a deficiency of the protein gamma globulin in the blood, resulting in an increased susceptibility to infections. It may occur in a variety of inherited disorders or as an acquired defect.

hypogastrium (hy-poh-**gas**-triŭm) *n.* that part of the central abdomen situated below the region of the stomach. —**hypogastric** *adj.*

hypoglossal nerve (hy-poh-**glos**-ăl) *n.* the twelfth cranial nerve (XII), which supplies the muscles of the tongue and is therefore responsible for the movements of talking and swallowing.

hypoglycaemia (hy-poh-gly-**see**-miă) *n.* a deficiency of glucose in the bloodstream, causing muscular weakness and incoordination, mental confusion, and sweating. If severe it may lead to *hypoglycaemic coma.* Hypoglycaemia most commonly occurs in diabetes mellitus. It is treated by administration of glucose. —**hypoglycaemic** *adj.*

hypoidrosis (hypohidrosis) (hy-poh-id-**roh**-sis) *n.* the production of an abnormally small amount of sweat.

hypoinsulinism (hy-poh-**ins**-yoo-lin-izm) *n.* a deficiency of insulin due either to inadequate secretion of the hormone by the pancreas or to inadequate treatment of diabetes mellitus.

hypokalaemia (hy-poh-kal-**ee**-miă) *n.* the presence of abnormally low levels of potassium in the blood: occurs in dehydration. *See* electrolyte.

hypomania (hy-poh-**may**-niă) *n.* a mild degree of mania. Elated mood leads to faulty judgment; behaviour lacks the usual social restraints and the sexual drive is increased; speech is rapid and animated; the individual is energetic but not persistent and tends to be irritable. —**hypomanic** (hy-poh-**man**-ik) *adj., n.*

hypomenorrhoea (hy-poh-men-ŏ-**ree**-ă) *n.* the release of an abnormally small quantity of blood at menstruation.

hypomotility (hy-poh-moh-**til**-iti) *n.* decreased movement or activity, especially of the stomach or intestine.

hyponatraemia (hy-poh-nă-**tree**-miă) *n.* the presence in the blood of an abnormally low concentration of sodium: occurs in dehydration. *See* electrolyte.

hypoparathyroidism (hy-poh-pa-ră-th'y-roid-izm) *n.* subnormal activity of the parathyroid glands, causing a fall in the blood concentration of calcium and muscular spasms (*see* tetany).

hypophysectomy (hy-pof-i-**sek**-tŏmi) *n.* the surgical removal or destruction of the pituitary gland (hypophysis) in the brain.

hypophysis (hy-**pof**-i-sis) *n. see* pituitary gland.

hypopiesis (hy-poh-py-**ee**-sis) *n.* abnormally reduced blood pressure (*see* hypotension) in the absence of organic disease.

hypopituitarism (hy-poh-pit-**yoo**-iter-izm) *n.* subnormal activity of the pituitary gland, causing dwarfism in childhood and a syndrome of impaired sexual function, pallor, and premature ageing in adult life (*see* Simmond's disease).

hypoplasia (hy-poh-**play**-ziă) *n.* underdevelopment of an organ or tissue.

hypopnoea (hy-poh-**nee**-ă) *n.* a decrease in breathing rate, which indicates that the body is attempting to compensate for metabolic disturbances due to disease in nonrespiratory organs.

hypoproteinaemia (hy-poh-proh-ti-**nee**-miă) *n.* a decrease in the quantity of protein in the blood, resulting in oedema and increased susceptibility to infections. It may result from malnutrition, impaired protein production, or increased loss of protein from the body. *See also* hypogammaglobulinaemia.

hypoprothrombinaemia (hy-poh-proh-throm-bin-**ee**-miă) *n.* a deficiency of the clotting factor prothrombin in the blood, which results in an increased tendency to bleed.

hypopyon (hy-**poh**-pi-ŏn) *n.* pus in the chamber of the eye that lies in front of the lens.

hyposecretion (hy-poh-si-**kree**-shŏn) *n.* decreased secretion.

hyposensitive (hy-poh-**sen**-si-tiv) *adj.* less than normally responsive to the presence of antigenic material. *Compare* hypersensitive. —**hyposensitivity** *n.*

hyposensitization (hy-poh-sen-si-ty-zay-shŏn) *n. see* desensitization.

hypospadias (hy-poh-**spay**-di-ăs) *n.* a congenital abnormality in which the opening of the urethra is on the underside of the penis: either on the glans penis (*glandular h.*), at the junction of the glans with the shaft (*coronal h.*), or on the shaft itself (*penile h.*).

hypostasis (hy-**pos**-tă-sis) *n.* accumulation of fluid or blood in a dependent part of the body in cases of poor circulation. *Hypostatic pneumonia* results from hypostatic congestion of the lung bases in debilitated patients who are confined to bed. —**hypostatic** (hy-poh-**stat**-ik) *adj.*

hyposthenia (hy-pos-**th'ee**-niă) *n.* a state of physical weakness or abnormally low muscular tension.

hypotension (hy-poh-**ten**-shŏn) *n.* a condition in which the arterial blood pressure is abnormally low. It occurs after excessive fluid or blood loss. Other causes include myocardial infarction, pulmonary embolism, Addison's disease, severe infections, allergic reactions, arrhythmias, and acute abdominal conditions (e.g. pancreatitis). *orthostatic h.* temporary hypotension experienced when rising from a horizontal position.

hypothalamus (hy-poh-**thal**-ă-mŭs) *n.* the region of the forebrain in the floor of the third ventricle, linked with the thalamus above and the pituitary gland below. It contains several important centres controlling body temperature, thirst, hunger, and eating, water balance, and sexual function. It also functions as a centre for the integration of hormonal

and autonomic nervous activity.
—hypothalamic *adj.*

hypothenar (hy-**poth**-i-nar) *adj.*
describing or relating to the
fleshy prominent part of the
palm of the hand below the little
finger. *Compare* thenar.

hypothermia (hy-poh-**therm**-iă) *n.*
1. accidental reduction of body
temperature below the normal
range. It is particularly liable to
occur in babies and the elderly.
2. deliberate lowering of body
temperature for therapeutic purposes. This may be done during
surgery, in order to reduce the
patient's requirement for oxygen.

hypothyroidism (hy-poh-**th'y**-roid-
izm) *n.* subnormal activity of the
thyroid gland. If present at birth
and untreated it leads to cretinism. In adult life it causes myxoedema. The condition can be
treated by administration of thyroxine.

hypotonia (hy-poh-**toh**-niă) *n.* a
state of reduced tension in muscle.

hypotonic (hy-poh-**tonn**-ik) *adj.* **1.**
describing a solution that has a
lower osmotic pressure than another solution. *See* osmosis. **2.**
describing muscles that demonstrate diminished tonicity.

hypotrichosis (hy-poh-trik-**oh**-sis)
n. a condition in which less hair
develops than normal.

hypotropia (hy-poh-**troh**-piă) *n.*
strabismus in which one eye
looks downwards.

hypoventilation (hy-poh-ven-ti-
lay-shŏn) *n.* breathing at an abnormally slow rate, which results
in an increased amount of carbon dioxide in the blood.

hypovitaminosis (hy-poh-vit-ă-min-
oh-sis) *n.* a deficiency of a vitamin caused either through lack
of the vitamin in the diet or

from an inability to absorb or
utilize it.

hypovolaemia (oligaemia) (hy-poh-
vŏ-**lee**-miă) *n.* a decrease in the
volume of circulating blood. *See*
shock.

hypoxaemia (hy-poks-**ee**-miă) *n.*
the presence in the blood of an
abnormally low concentration of
oxygen. *See also* anoxia.

hypoxia (hy-**poks**-iă) *n.* a deficiency of oxygen in the tissues.
See also anoxia, hypoxaemia.

hyster- (hystero-) *prefix denoting*
1. the womb. **2.** hysteria.

hysteralgia (hysterodynia, uteralgia)
(hiss-ter-**al**-jiă) *n.* pain in the
womb.

hysterectomy (hiss-ter-**ek**-tŏmi) *n.*
the surgical removal of the
womb, either through an incision
in the abdominal wall or through
the vagina. *subtotal h.* removal of
the body of the womb, leaving
the neck (cervix) in place. *total
h.* removal of the entire womb.

hysteria (hiss-**teer**-iă) *n.* **1.** a neurosis whose principal features
consist of emotional instability,
repression, dissociation, physical
symptoms, and vulnerability to
suggestion. *conversion h.* hysteria
characterized mainly by physical
symptoms, such as paralysis. *dis-
sociative h.* hysteria in which patients show changes in thinking,
such as multiple personality
states or amnesia. *See also* hysterical. **2.** a state of great emotional excitement.

hysterical (hiss-**te**-ri-kăl) *adj.* **1.**
describing a symptom that is not
due to organic disease, is produced unconsciously, and from
which the individual derives
some gain. **2.** describing a kind
of personality disorder characterized by instability and shallow-
ness of feelings.

hysterocele (uterocele) (**hiss**-ter-oh-seel) *n.* hernia (rupture) of the womb, usually during pregnancy.

hysterocleisis (hiss-ter-oh-**kly**-sis) *n.* surgical closure of the passage from the womb to the vagina at the mouth of the womb.

hysteropexy (**hiss**-ter-oh-peks-i) *n.* stitching the womb to the abdominal wall to prevent its downward displacement. *See* prolapse.

hysteroptosis (hiss-ter-op-**toh**-sis) *n.* prolapse of the womb. *See* prolapse.

hysterorrhaphy (hiss-ter-o-răfi) *n.* stitching the womb. *See also* hysteropexy.

hysterorrhexis (metrorrhexis) (hiss-ter-oh-**reks**-iss) *n.* rupture of the womb.

hysterosalpingography (hiss-ter-oh-sal-ping-**og**-răfi) *n. see* uterosalpingography.

hysteroscope (uteroscope) (**hiss**-ter-oh-skohp) *n.* a tubular instrument with a light source for observing the interior of the womb. *See also* endoscope.

hysterotomy (hiss-ter-**ot**-ŏmi) *n.* incision of the womb, either through the abdominal wall or the vagina. *See* Caesarean section.

hysterotrachelorrhaphy (hiss-ter-oh-tray-kĕl-o-răfi) *n.* the operation of stitching a tear in the cervix of the womb.

I

-iasis *suffix denoting* a diseased condition.

iatro- *prefix denoting* 1. medicine. 2. doctors.

iatrogenic (I-at-roh-**jen**-ik) *adj.* describing a condition that has resulted from treatment, as either an unforeseen or inevitable side-effect.

ibuprofen (I-**bew**-proh-fen) *n.* an analgesic that relieves inflammation, administered by mouth in the treatment of arthritic conditions. Trade name: **Brufen**.

ichor (I-kor) *n.* a watery material oozing from wounds or ulcers.

ichthammol (ik-**tham**-ol) *n.* a sulphur-containing drug with antibacterial properties, used in the form of an ointment for treating certain skin diseases.

ichthyosis (ik-thi-**oh**-sis) *n.* a congenital condition, usually present at birth, in which the skin is dry, rough, and scaly because of a defect in keratinization.

ICSH (interstitial-cell-stimulating hormone) *n. see* luteinizing hormone.

icterus (ik-ter-ŭs) *n. see* jaundice.

ictus (ik-tŭs) *n.* a stroke or any sudden attack. The term is often used for an epileptic fit.

id (id) *n.* (in psychoanalysis) a part of the unconscious mind governed by the instinctive forces of libido and the death wish.

-id *suffix denoting* relationship or resemblance to.

ideation (I-di-ay-shŏn) *n.* the process of thinking or of having imagery or ideas.

identical twins (I-**den**-tik-ăl) *pl. n. see* twins.

identification (I-den-ti-fi-**kay**-shŏn) *n.* (in psychological development) the process of adopting other people's characteristics more or less permanently. Identification with a parent is important in personality formation.

ideo- *prefix denoting* 1. the mind or mental activity. 2. ideas.

ideomotor (I-di-ŏ-**moh**-ter) *adj.* describing or relating to a motor action that is evoked by an idea. *i. apraxia* the inability to translate the idea of a complex behaviour into action.

idio- *prefix denoting* peculiarity to the individual.

idiocy (**id**-i-ŏ-si) *n.* a profound degree of intellectual subnormality. The term is now obsolete, but roughly corresponds to an intelligence quotient of less than 20.

idiopathic (idi-oh-**path**-ik) *adj.* denoting a disease or condition the cause of which is not known or that arises spontaneously. —**idiopathy** (idi-**op**-ă-thi) *n.*

idiosyncrasy (idi-oh-**sink**-răsi) *n.* an unusual and unexpected sensitivity exhibited by an individual to a particular drug or food. —**idiosyncratic** (idi-oh-sin-**krat**-ik) *adj.*

idiot savant (eed-**yoh** sa-**vahn**) *n.* an individual whose overall functioning is at the level of mental subnormality but who has one or more special intellectual abilities that are advanced to a high level.

idioventricular (idi-oh-ven-**trik**-yooler) *adj.* affecting or peculiar to the ventricles of the heart. *i. rhythm* the very slow beat of the ventricles under the influence of their own natural subsidiary pacemaker.

idoxuridine (I-doks-**yoor**-i-deen) *n.* an iodine-containing drug that inhibits the growth of viruses and is administered in eye drops or ointment to treat viral infections of the eye (such as keratitis). Trade names: **Dendrid, Kerecid.**

ile- (**ileo-**) *prefix denoting* the ileum.

ileal conduit (**il**-i-ăl) *n.* a segment of small intestine (ileum) used to convey urine from the ureters to the exterior into an appliance. The ureters are implanted into an isolated segment of bowel, one end of which is brought through the abdominal wall to the skin surface.

ileectomy (ili-**ek**-tŏmi) *n.* surgical removal of the ileum or part of the ileum.

ileitis (ili-**I**-tis) *n.* inflammation of the ileum. It may be caused by Crohn's disease, tuberculosis, or typhoid or it may occur in association with ulcerative colitis.

ileocaecal (ili-oh-**see**-kăl) *adj.* relating to the ileum and caecum. *i. valve* a valve at the junction of the small and large intestines consisting of two membranous folds that close to prevent the backflow of food from the colon and caecum to the ileum.

ileocolitis (ili-oh-kŏ-**ly**-tis) *n.* inflammation of the ileum and the colon. The commonest causes are Crohn's disease and tuberculosis.

ileocolostomy (ili-oh-kŏ-**lost**-ŏmi) *n.* a surgical operation in which the ileum is joined to some part of the colon.

ileoproctostomy (ileorectal anastomosis) (ili-oh-prok-**tost**-ŏmi) *n.* a surgical operation in which the ileum is joined to the rectum, usually after surgical removal of the colon (*see* colectomy).

ileorectal (ili-oh-**rek**-t'l) *adj.* relating to the ileum and rectum.

ileosigmoidostomy (ili-oh-sig-moid-**ost**-ŏmi) *n.* an operation in which an opening is created between the ileum and the sigmoid colon.

ileostomy (ili-**ost**-ŏmi) *n.* a surgical operation in which the ileum is brought through the abdominal wall to create an artificial opening (*stoma*) through which the intestinal contents can discharge, thus bypassing the colon. Various types of bag may be worn to collect the effluent.

ileum (il-iŭm) *n.* the lowest of the three portions of the small intestine. It runs from the jejunum to the ileocaecal valve. —**ileal, ileac** *adj.*

ileus (il-i-ŭs) *n.* intestinal obstruction, usually obstruction of the small intestine (ileum). *paralytic* or *adynamic i.* functional obstruction of the ileum due to loss of peristalsis, which may be caused by abdominal surgery, spinal injuries, hypokalaemia, or peritonitis. Treatment consists of intravenous administration of fluid and nutrients and removal of excess stomach secretions by tube until peristalsis returns.

ili- (**ilio-**) *prefix denoting* the ilium.

iliac (il-i-ak) *adj.* relating to the ilium. *i. arteries* the arteries that supply most of the blood to the lower limbs and pelvic region. *i. fossa* a concave depression on the inside of the pelvis. The right iliac fossa provides space for the vermiform appendix. *i. veins* the veins draining most of the blood from the lower limbs and pelvic region.

iliacus (i-lee-ă-kŭs) *n.* a flat triangular muscle situated in the area of the groin. This muscle acts in conjunction with the psoas muscle to flex the thigh.

iliococcygeal (ili-oh-kok-sij-iăl) *adj.* relating to the ilium and the coccyx.

iliopsoas (ili-oh-soh-ăs) *n.* a composite muscle made up of the iliacus and psoas muscles, which have a common tendon.

ilium (il-iŭm) *n.* the haunch bone: a wide bone forming the upper part of each side of the hip bone (*see also* pelvis). —**iliac** *adj.*

illusion (i-loo-zhŏn) *n.* a false perception due to misinterpretation of the stimuli arising from an object. Illusions may occur in almost any psychiatric syndrome, especially depression. *Compare* hallucination. *optical i.* a perception that does not agree with the actual object in the external world. Optical illusions are produced by deceptive qualities of the stimulus and are in no way pathological.

image (im-ij) *n.* **1.** (in physiology) an optical reproduction of an object formed on the retina when light is refracted through the eye. **2.** (in psychology) a mental representation resulting from thought rather than from sensory perception. *See* body image, imagery.

imagery (im-ij-er-i) *n.* the production of vivid mental representations by the normal processes of thought. *eidetic i.* the production of images of exceptional clarity, which may be recalled long after being first experienced.

imago (i-may-goh) *n.* (in psychoanalysis) the internal unconscious representation of an important person in the individual's life, particularly a parent.

imbecility (imbi-sil-iti) *n.* a moderate to severe degree of intellectual subnormality that falls short of idiocy. The term is now obsolete, but roughly corresponds to an intelligence quotient of between 20 and 50.

imipramine (i-mip-ră-meen) *n.* a drug administered by mouth or injection to treat depression (*see* antidepressant). Trade names: **Berkomine, Dimipressin, Tofranil.**

immersion foot (i-mer-shŏn) *n. see* trench foot.

immiscible (i-mis-ibŭl) *adj.* incapable of being mixed to form a homogeneous substance. Oil and water are immiscible.

immobilization (i-moh-bi-ly-zay-shŏn) *n.* the procedure of making a normally movable part of the body, such as a joint, immovable. This helps an infected, diseased, or injured tissue (bone, joint, or muscle) to heal.

immune (i-mewn) *adj.* protected against a particular infection by the presence of specific antibodies against the organisms concerned. *i. response* the reaction of the body to the presence of foreign tissues, bacteria, etc., which are attacked and destroyed by antibodies. *See* antibody, antigen, immunity.

immunity (i-**mewn**-iti) *n.* the body's ability to resist infection, afforded by the presence of circulating antibodies and white blood cells. *active i.* immunity that arises when the body's own cells produce, and remain able to produce, appropriate antibodies following an attack of a disease or deliberate stimulation (*see* immunization). *passive i.* temporary immunity that may be provided by injecting ready-made antibodies in antiserum taken from another person or animal already immune. Babies have passive immunity, conferred by antibodies from the maternal blood and colostrum, to common diseases for several weeks after birth.

immunization (im-yoo-ny-zay-shŏn) *n.* the production of immunity by artificial means. Passive immunity may be conferred by the injection of an antiserum, but the production of active immu-

nity calls for the use of a vaccine (*see* vaccination).

immuno- *prefix denoting* immunity or immunological response.

immunoglobulin (Ig) (im-yoo-noh-**glob**-yoo-lin) *n.* one of a group of structurally related proteins (gamma globulins) that act as antibodies.

immunological tolerance (im-yoo-nŏ-**loj**-ik-ăl) *n.* a failure of the body to distinguish between materials that are 'self', and therefore to be tolerated, and those that are 'not self', against which antibodies should be produced.

immunology (im-yoo-**nol**-ŏji) *n.* the study of immunity and all of the phenomena connected with the defence mechanisms of the body. —**immunological** *adj.*

immunophoresis (im-yoo-noh-fer-ee-sis) *n.* a technique, relying upon the precipitin reaction, for identifying an unknown antigen or testing for an antibody in a serum.

immunosuppressive (im-yoo-noh-sŭ-**pres**-iv) *n.* a drug, such as azathioprine, mustine, or cyclophosphamide, that reduces the body's resistance to infection and other foreign bodies by suppressing the immune system. Immunosuppressives are used to maintain the survival of organ and tissue transplants and to treat various autoimmune diseases.

immunotransfusion (i-mew-noh-trans-**few**-zhŏn) *n.* the transfusion of an antiserum to treat or give temporary protection against a disease.

impacted (im-**pak**-tid) *adj.* firmly wedged. *i. faeces* faeces that are so hard and dry that they cannot pass through the anus without special measures being taken (*see* constipation). *i. fracture see* fracture. *i. tooth* a tooth, usually a wisdom tooth, that cannot erupt into a normal position because it is obstructed by other tissues. —**impaction** *n.*

impalpable (im-**palp**-ăbŭl) *adj.* describing a structure within the body that cannot be detected by feeling with the hand.

imperforate (im-**per**-fer-it) *adj.* lacking an opening. *i. anus* (*proctatresia*) partial or complete obstruction of the anus: a condition, discovered at birth, due to failure of the anus to develop normally in the embryo. Most mild cases of imperforate anus can be treated by a simple operation. *i. hymen* a condition in which the hymen completely closes the vagina and thus impedes the flow of menstrual blood.

impetigo (imp-i-**ty**-goh) *n.* a bacterial skin infection usually caused by staphylococci, though occasionally by streptococci. The infection, which spreads quickly over the body, starts as a red patch and develops into small pustules that join together, forming crusty yellow sores. Impetigo is very contagious, especially in communities of children. The condition usually responds to treatment with antibiotics.

implant (im-plahnt) *n.* a substance (such as a drug) or a tissue graft inserted into the skin.

implantation (im-plahn-**tay**-shŏn) *n.* **1.** (*or* **nidation**) the attachment of the early embryo to the lining of the womb, which occurs six to eight days after ovulation. **2.** the placing of a substance (e.g. a drug) or an object (e.g. an artificial pacemaker) within a tissue.

3. the surgical replacement of damaged tissue with healthy tissue (*see* transplantation).

implosion (im-**ploh**-zhŏn) *n. see* flooding.

impotence (im-pŏ-tĕns) *n.* inability in a man to have sexual intercourse. Impotence may be *erectile*, in which the penis does not become firm enough to enter the vagina, or *ejaculatory*, in which penetration occurs but there is no ejaculation of semen (orgasm).

impregnate (im-preg-nayt) *vb.* **1.** to make pregnant. **2.** to saturate with another substance. —**impregnation** *n.*

impression (im-**presh**-ŏn) *n.* (in dentistry) a moulding, made in plastic material, of the teeth and gums or roof of the mouth. An impression is used in the construction of orthodontic appliances, restorations, and dentures.

impulse (im-puls) *n.* (in neurology) *see* nerve impulse.

in- (**im-**) *prefix denoting* **1.** not. **2.** in; within; into.

inaccessible (in-ak-**ses**-ibŭl) *adj.* (in psychiatry) unresponsive to words and similar stimuli: describing the mental state of certain patients, e.g. schizophrenics. —**inaccessibility** *n.*

inanition (in-ă-**nish**-ŏn) *n.* a condition of exhaustion caused by lack of nutrients in the blood. This may arise through starvation, malnutrition, or intestinal disease.

in articulo mortis (in ar-tik-yoo-loh **mor**-tis) Latin: at the moment of death.

inbreeding (in-breed-ing) *n.* the production of offspring by parents who are closely related. *Compare* outbreeding.

incarcerated (in-**kar**-ser-ayt-id) *adj.* confined or constricted so as to be immovable: applied particularly to a type of hernia.

incest (in-sest) *n.* sexual intercourse between close relatives, e.g. brother and sister or father and daughter.

incipient (in-**sip**-iĕnt) *adj.* coming into existence: describing a stage in a disease.

incision (in-si*zh*-ŏn) *n.* **1.** the surgical cutting of soft tissues, such as skin or muscle, with a knife or scalpel. **2.** the cut so made.

incisor (in-sy-zer) *n.* any of the four front teeth in each jaw, two on each side of the midline. *See also* dentition.

inclusion bodies (in-**kloo**-*zh*ŏn) *pl. n.* particles occurring in the nucleus and cytoplasm of cells usually as a result of virus infection. Their presence can sometimes be used to diagnose such an infection.

incompatibility (in-kŏm-pat-i-**bil**-iti) *n.* lack of compatibility. In cases of severe incompatibility, there are likely to be swift immune reactions to transplanted organs or tissues.

incompetence (in-**kom**-pi-tĕns) *n.* impaired function of the valves of the heart or veins, which allows backward leakage of blood. *See* aortic regurgitation, mitral incompetence, varicose veins.

incontinence (in-**kon**-ti-nĕns) *n.* **1.** the inappropriate involuntary passage of urine. *stress i.* the leak of urine on coughing and straining. It is common in women in whom the muscles of the pelvic floor are weakened after childbirth. *overflow i.* leakage from a full bladder, which occurs most commonly in old men with bladder outflow obstruction. *urge i.* leakage of urine that accompanies an intense desire to pass water with failure of restraint. *See also* enuresis. **2.** inability to control bowel movements (*faecal i.*).

incoordination (in-koh-or-din-ay-shŏn) *n.* (in neurology) an impairment in the performance of precise rapid movements. Incoordination may result from a disorder in any part of the nervous system. *See* apraxia, ataxia, dyssynergia.

incubation (in-kew-**bay**-shŏn) *n.* **1.** the process of development of an egg or a culture of bacteria. **2.** the care of a premature baby in an incubator.

incubation period (latent period) *n.* the interval between exposure to an infection and the appearance of the first symptoms.

incubator (**ink**-yoo-bay-ter) *n.* a transparent container for keeping premature babies in controlled conditions and protecting them from infection. Other forms of incubator are used for cultivating bacteria and for hatching eggs.

incus (**ink**-ŭs) *n.* a small anvil-shaped bone in the middle ear that articulates with the malleus and the stapes. *See* ossicle.

independent nursing function (indi-**pend**-ĕnt) *n.* any aspect of nursing practice for which the nurse alone is responsible, acting on her own initiative and without instructions from any other discipline.

Inderal (**in**-der-al) *n. see* propranolol.

indican (**in**-di-kăn) *n.* a compound excreted in the urine as a detoxification product of indoxyl.

indicanuria (in-di-kăn-**yoor**-iă) *n.* the presence in the urine of an abnormally high concentration of indican. This may be a sign that the intestine is obstructed.

indication (indi-**kay**-shŏn) *n*. (in medicine) a strong reason for believing that a particular course of action is desirable. *Compare* contraindication.

indigenous (in-**dij**-in-ŭs) *adj*. occurring naturally in a particular area, region, or country. Certain diseases are indigenous to particular regions.

indigestion (indi-**jes**-chŏn) *n. see* dyspepsia.

indigo carmine (in-dig-oh **kar**-myn) *n*. a blue dye that is administered by injection to test for kidney function.

individualized nursing care (indi-**vid**-yoo-ă-lyzd) *n*. care that is planned to meet the particular needs of one patient, as opposed to a routine applied to all patients suffering from the same disease.

indole (**in**-dohl) *n*. a derivative of the amino acid tryptophan, excreted in the urine and faeces.

indolent (**in**-dŏl-ĕnt) *adj*. describing a disease process that is failing to heal or has persisted. The term is applied particularly to ulcers of skin or mucous membrane.

indomethacin (in-doh-**meth**-ă-sin) *n*. an analgesic that relieves inflammation, administered by mouth or in suppositories in the treatment of arthritic conditions. Trade names: **Imbrilon, Indocid**.

indoxyl (in-**doks**-il) *n*. an alcohol derived from indole by bacterial action. It is excreted in the urine as indican.

induction (in-**duk**-shŏn) *n*. **1**. (in obstetrics) the artificial starting of childbirth, e.g. by injecting oxytocin or puncturing the amnion, when pregnancy has con-

tinued considerably beyond the expected date of birth or if there is a risk to the health of mother or infant. **2**. (in anaesthetics) initiation of anaesthesia. General anaesthesia is usually induced by injecting certain drugs, usually barbiturates, into the bloodstream.

induration (in-dewr-ay-shŏn) *n*. abnormal hardening of a tissue or organ. *See also* sclerosis.

industrial disease (in-**dus**-tri-ăl) *n*. an occupational disease associated with a particular industry or group of industries.

inertia (in-**er**-shă) *n*. (in physiology) sluggishness or absence of activity in certain smooth muscles. *uterine i.* inertia of the muscular wall of the womb during labour, making the process excessively long. It may be present from the start of labour or it may develop because of exhaustion following strong contractions.

in extremis (in iks-**tree**-mis) Latin: at the point of death.

infant (**in**-fănt) *n*. a child incapable of any form of independence from its mother: a child under one year of age, especially a newborn child. *i. mortality rate* the number of deaths of infants per 1000 live births in a given year. Included are the *neonatal death rate* (calculated from deaths occurring in the first four weeks of life) and *postneonatal death rate* (from deaths in the remainder of the first year).

infanticide (in-**fant**-i-syd) *n*. (in Britain) under the terms of the Infanticide Act (1938), the felony of child destruction by the natural mother within 12 months of birth when the balance of her mind is disturbed because she has not fully recovered from childbirth and/or lactation.

infantile (in-**făn**-tyl) *adj.* **1.** denoting conditions occurring in adults that are recognizable in childhood, e.g. poliomyelitis (*i. paralysis*). **2.** of, relating to, or affecting infants. *i.* spasms a serious brain disorder of infants, usually under the age of six months, characterized by involuntary flexing movements of the arms, legs, neck, and trunk. It may be arrested by treatment with corticosteroids and ACTH.

infantilism (in-**fant**-il-izm) *n.* persistence of childlike physical or psychological characteristics into adult life.

infarct (in-**farkt**) *n.* a small localized area of dead tissue produced as a result of an inadequate blood supply.

infarction (in-**fark**-shŏn) *n.* the death of part or the whole of an organ that occurs when the artery carrying its blood supply is obstructed by a blood clot (thrombus) or an embolus. *See also* myocardial infarction.

infection (in-**fek**-shŏn) *n.* invasion of the body by harmful organisms (pathogens), such as bacteria, fungi, protozoa, rickettsiae, or viruses. The infective agent may be transmitted by a patient or carrier in airborne droplets or by direct contact; by animal or insect vectors; by ingestion of contaminated food or drink; or from an infected mother to the fetus. After an incubation period symptoms appear, usually consisting of either localized inflammation and pain or more remote effects. Treatment with drugs is usually effective against all but the viral infections.

infectious disease (in-**fek**-shŭs) *n.* *see* communicable disease.

infectious mononucleosis *n.* *see* glandular fever.

inferior (in-**feer**-i-er) *adj.* (in anatomy) lower in the body in relation to another structure or surface.

inferiority complex (in-feer-i-o-riti) *n.* **1.** an unconscious exaggeration of feelings of inferiority, which is shown by compensatory behaviour, such as aggression. **2.** (in psychoanalysis) a complex resulting from the conflict between Oedipal wishes (*see* Oedipus complex) and the reality of the child's lack of power. This gives rise to repressed feelings of personal inferiority.

infertility (in-fer-**til**-iti) *n.* inability in a woman to conceive or in a man to induce conception.

infestation (in-fes-**tay**-shŏn) *n.* the presence of animal parasites either on the skin or inside the body.

infiltration (in-fil-**tray**-shŏn) *n.* the abnormal entry of a substance (*infiltrate*) into a cell, tissue, or organ. Examples of infiltrates are blood cells, cancer cells, fat, or starch.

inflammation (in-flă-**may**-shŏn) *n.* the body's response to injury. *acute i.* the immediate defensive reaction of tissue to injury, which may be caused by infection, chemicals, or physical agents. It involves pain, heat, redness, swelling, and loss of function of the affected part. *chronic i.* the response that ensues when acute inflammation does not heal.

influenza (in-floo-**en**-ză) *n.* a highly contagious virus infection that affects the respiratory system. Symptoms include headache, fever, loss of appetite, weakness, and general aches and pains. After bed rest and aspirin most patients recover, but a secondary infection of the lungs is a common serious complication.

infra- *prefix denoting* below.

infrared radiation (in-fră-**red**) *n.* the band of electromagnetic radiation that is longer in wavelength than the red of the visible spectrum and is responsible for the transmission of radiant heat. It may be used in physiotherapy to warm tissues, reduce pain, and improve circulation.

infundibulum (in-fun-**dib**-yoo-lŭm) *n.* any funnel-shaped channel or passage, particularly the hollow conical stalk that extends downwards from the hypothalamus and is continuous with the posterior lobe of the pituitary gland.

infusion (in-**few**-zhŏn) *n.* **1.** a slow injection of a substance (e.g. saline or dextrose) into a vein or subcutaneous tissue. **2.** the process whereby the active principles are extracted from plant material by steeping it in boiling water (as in the making of tea). **3.** the solution produced by this process.

ingesta (in-**jes**-tă) *pl. n.* food and drink that is taken into the alimentary canal through the mouth.

ingestion (in-**jes**-chŏn) *n.* the process by which food is taken into the alimentary canal. It involves chewing and swallowing.

ingrowing toenail (**in**-groh-ing) *n.* a toenail whose free margin grows or is pressed into the skin at the side of the nail, causing inflammation.

inguinal (**ing**-win-ăl) *adj.* relating to or affecting the region of the groin (inguen). *i. canal* either of a pair of openings that connect the abdominal cavity with the scrotum in the male fetus. *i. hernia see* hernia. *i. ligament* (*Poupart's ligament*) a ligament in the groin that extends from the anterior superior iliac spine to the pubic tubercle. It is part of the aponeurosis of the external oblique muscle of the abdomen.

INH *n. see* isoniazid.

inhalation (in-hă-**lay**-shŏn) *n.* **1.** (*or* **inspiration**) the act of breathing air into the lungs through the mouth and nose. *See* breathing. **2.** a gas, vapour, or aerosol breathed in for the treatment of conditions of the respiratory tract.

inherent (in-**heer**-ěnt) *adj.* inborn; innate.

inhibition (in-hib-**ish**-ŏn) *n.* **1.** (in physiology) the prevention or reduction of the functioning of an organ, muscle, etc., by the action of certain nerve impulses. **2.** (in psychoanalysis) an inner command that prevents one from doing something forbidden. **3.** (in psychology) a tendency not to carry out a specific action, produced each time the action is carried out.

inhibitor (in-**hib**-it-er) *n.* a substance that prevents the occurrence of a given process or reaction. *See also* MAO inhibitor.

injected (in-**jekt**-id) *adj.* congested.

injection (in-**jek**-shŏn) *n.* introduction into the body of drugs or other fluids by means of a syringe. Common routes for injection are into the skin (*intracutaneous* or *intradermal*); below the skin (*subcutaneous*); into a muscle (*intramuscular*), for drugs that are slowly absorbed; and into a vein (*intravenous*), for drugs to be rapidly absorbed. Enemas are also regarded as injections.

inlay (**in**-lay) *n.* a substance or piece of tissue inserted to replace a defect in a tissue.

innate (**in**-ayt) *adj.* describing a condition or characteristic that is present in an individual at birth and is inherited from his parents. *See also* congenital.

inner ear (**in**-er) *n. see* labyrinth.

innervation (in-er-**vay**-shŏn) *n.* the nerve supply to an area or organ of the body.

innocent (**in**-ŏ-sĕnt) *adj.* (of a tumour) benign; not malignant.

innominate artery (brachiocephalic artery) (in-**om**-in-it) *n.* a short artery originating as the first large branch of the aortic arch, which divides at the lower neck into the right common carotid and the right subclavian arteries.

innominate bone *n. see* hip (bone).

innominate vein (brachiocephalic vein) *n.* either of two veins, one on each side of the neck, formed by the junction of the external jugular and subclavian veins. The two veins join to form the superior vena cava.

ino- *prefix denoting* 1. fibrous tissue. 2. muscle.

inoculation (in-ok-yoo-**lay**-shŏn) *n.* the introduction of a small quantity of vaccine in the process of immunization: a more general name for vaccination.

inoculum (in-**ok**-yoo-lŭm) *n.* any material that is used for inoculation.

inorganic (in-or-**gan**-ik) *adj.* 1. not of animal or vegetable origin. 2. (in chemistry) describing or relating to compounds that do not contain carbon.

inositol (in-**oh**-sit-ol) *n.* a compound similar to a hexose sugar,

present in the bran of cereal grain. It is sometimes classified as a vitamin but it can be synthesized by most animals and there is no evidence that it is essential to man.

inotropic (in-ŏ-**trop**-ik) *adj.* affecting the contraction of heart muscle. Drugs such as digitalis have positive inotropic action, stimulating heart muscle contractions. Beta-blocker drugs, such as propranolol, have negative inotropic action.

in-patient (**in**-pay-shĕnt) *n.* a patient who is admitted to a bed in a hospital ward and remains there for a period of time for treatment, examination, or observation. *Compare* out-patient.

inquest (**in**-kwest) *n.* an official judicial enquiry into the cause of a person's death: carried out when the death is sudden or takes place under suspicious circumstances. *See also* autopsy.

insanity (in-**san**-iti) *n.* a degree of mental illness such that the affected individual is not responsible for his actions. The term is used in legal rather than medical contexts.

insect (**in**-sekt) *n.* a member of a large group of mainly land-dwelling arthropods. Insects of medical importance include various bloodsucking insects transmitting tropical diseases; lice, whose bites can cause intense irritation and bacterial infection; and flies, which transmit organisms causing diarrhoea and dysentery to food. *See also* myiasis.

insecticide (in-**sekt**-i-syd) *n.* a preparation used to kill destructive or disease-carrying insects. Some insect powders contain organic phosphorus compounds and fluorides; when ingested accidentally they may cause damage to the nervous system. The use of such compounds is generally under strict control. *See also* DDT.

insemination (in-sem-i-**nay**-shŏn) *n.* introduction of semen into the vagina. *See also* artificial insemination.

insertion (in-**ser**-shŏn) *n.* (in anatomy) the point of attachment of a muscle (e.g. to a bone) that is relatively movable when the muscle contracts. *Compare* origin.

insidious (in-**sid**-iŭs) *adj.* describing a disease that develops gradually and imperceptibly.

insight (**in**-syt) *n.* (in psychology) knowledge of oneself. The term is applied particularly to a patient's recognition that he has psychological problems; in this sense absence of insight is a feature of psychosis.

in situ (in **sit**-yoo) *adj.* **1.** in the natural or original position. **2.** describing a cancer that has not undergone metastasis to invade surrounding tissue.

insolation (in-soh-**lay**-shŏn) *n.* exposure to the sun's rays. *See also* heatstroke.

insomnia (in-**som**-niă) *n.* inability to fall asleep or to remain asleep for an adequate length of time. Insomnia may be associated with disease, but is more often caused by worry.

inspiration (in-spi-**ray**-shŏn) *n. see* inhalation.

inspissated (in-**spis**-ayt-id) *adj.* thickened or hardened by absorption or evaporation. *i. sputum* a thick sputum produced in whooping cough, which is difficult to cough up.

instillation (in-stil-**ay**-shŏn) *n.* **1.** the application of liquid medica-

tion drop by drop, as into the eye. **2.** the medication applied in this way.

instinct (**in**-stinkt) *n.* **1.** a complex pattern of behaviour innately determined, which is characteristic of all individuals of the same species. **2.** an innate drive that urges the individual towards a particular goal.

insufficiency (in-sŭ-**fish**-ĕn-si) *n.* inability of an organ or part, such as the heart or kidney, to carry out its normal function.

insufflation (in-suf-**lay**-shŏn) *n.* the act of blowing gas or a powder, such as a medication, into a body cavity.

insulin (**ins**-yoo-lin) *n.* a protein hormone, produced in the pancreas by the beta cells of the islets of Langerhans, that is important for regulating the amount of sugar (glucose) in the blood. Lack of this hormone gives rise to diabetes mellitus, in which large amounts of sugar are present in the blood and urine. This condition may be treated successfully by insulin injections.

insulinase (**ins**-yoo-lin-ayz) *n.* an enzyme, found in such tissues as the liver and kidney, that is responsible for the normal breakdown of insulin in the body.

insulinoma (ins-yoo-lin-**oh**-mă) *n.* an insulin-producing tumour of the beta cells in the islets of Langerhans of the pancreas. Symptoms include sweating, faintness, and other features of hypoglycaemia.

Intal (**in**-tal) *n. see* cromolyn sodium.

integument (in-**teg**-yoo-mĕnt) *n.* **1.** the skin. **2.** a membrane or layer of tissue covering any organ of the body.

intelligence quotient (IQ) (in-tel-i-jĕns **kwoh**-shĕnt) *n.* an index of intellectual development. In childhood and adult life it represents intellectual ability relative to the rest of the population; in children it can also represent rate of development (mental age as a percentage of chronological age).

intelligence test *n.* a standardized assessment procedure for the determination of intellectual ability. The score produced is usually expressed as an intelligence quotient. Scores on intelligence tests are used for such purposes as the diagnosis of subnormality and the assessment of intellectual deterioration.

intensive care (in-**ten**-siv) *n.* constant and specialized health care provided for critically ill patients by trained staff in a specially designed hospital unit (*i. c. unit*).

intention (in-**ten**-shŏn) *n.* a process of healing. *first i.* healing in which the edges of a wound are brought together under aseptic conditions and granulation tissue forms.

intention tremor *n. see* tremor.

inter- *prefix denoting* between.

intercalated (inter-kă-**layt**-id) *adj.* describing structures, tissues, etc., that are inserted or situated between other structures.

intercellular (inter-**sel**-yoo-ler) *adj.* situated or occurring between cells.

intercostal muscles (inter-**kos**-t'l) *pl. n.* muscles that occupy the spaces between the ribs and are responsible for controlling some of the movements of the ribs.

intercurrent (inter-**ku**-rĕnt) *adj.* going on at the same time: applied to an infection contracted by a patient who is already suffering from an infection or other disease.

interferon (inter-**feer**-on) *n.* a substance that is produced by cells infected with a virus and has the ability to inhibit viral growth. Particular interferons are effective only in the species that produces them.

interkinesis (inter-ky-**nee**-sis) *n.* **1.** the resting stage between the two divisions of meiosis. **2.** *see* interphase.

intermenstrual (inter-**men**-stroo-ăl) *adj.* between the menstrual periods.

intermittent claudication (inter-mit-ĕnt) *n. see* claudication.

intermittent fever *n.* a fever that rises, subsides, then returns again. *See* malaria.

International Classification of Diseases (inter-**nash**-ŏn-ăl) *n.* a list of all known diseases and syndromes published by the World Health Organization every ten years (approximately).

interoceptor (inter-oh-**sep**-ter) *n.* any receptor organ composed of sensory nerve cells that respond to and monitor changes within the body, such as the stretching of muscles or the acidity of the blood.

interosseous (inter-**oss**-i-ŭs) *adj.* between two bones.

interparietal bone (inca bone, incarial bone) ´(inter-pă-ry-i-t'l) *n.* the bone lying between the parietal bones, at the back of the skull.

interphase (interkinesis) (**in**-ter-fayz) *n.* the period when a cell is not undergoing division (mitosis), during which activities such as DNA synthesis occur.

intersex (**in**-ter-seks) *n.* an individual who shows anatomical characteristics of both sexes. *See* her-

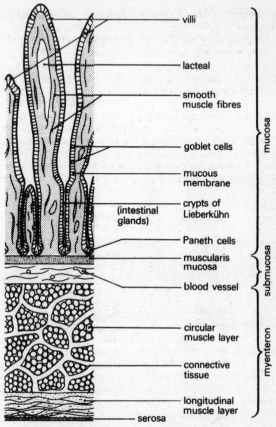

villi

lacteal

smooth
muscle fibres

goblet cells

mucous
membrane

(intestinal
glands)

crypts of
Lieberkühn

Paneth cells

muscularis
mucosa

blood vessel

circular
muscle layer

connective
tissue

longitudinal
muscle layer

serosa

mucosa

submucosa

myenteron

Longitudinal section through the ileum

maphrodite. —**intersexuality** *n.*

interstice (in-**ter**-stiss) *n.* a small
space in a tissue or between
parts of the body. —**interstitial**
(inter-**stish**-ăl) *adj.*

interstitial cells (**Leydig cells**) *pl.*
n. the cells interspersed between
the seminiferous tubules of the
testis. They secrete androgens in
response to stimulation by luteinizing hormone.

interstitial-cell-stimulating hormone
n. see luteinizing hormone.

intertrigo (in-ter-**try**-goh) *n.* superficial inflammation (dermatitis)
of two skin surfaces that are in
contact. The dermatitis is caused
by friction, warmth, moisture,
and sweat.

intervertebral disc (inter-ver-tib-răl)
n. the flexible plate of fibrocartilage that connects any two adjacent vertebrae in the backbone.
The intervertebral discs act as
shock absorbers, protecting the
brain and spinal cord from the

impact produced by running and other movements. *See also* prolapsed intervertebral disc.

intestinal flora (in-test-in-ăl) *pl. n.* bacteria normally present in the intestinal tract. Some are responsible for the synthesis of vitamin K.

intestinal juice *n. see* succus (entericus).

intestine (bowel, gut) (in-test-in) *n.* the part of the alimentary canal that extends from the stomach to the anus. *large i.* the part of the intestine that consists of the caecum, vermiform appendix, colon, and rectum. It is largely concerned with the absorption of water from the material passed from the small intestine. *small i.* the part of the intestine that consists of the duodenum, jejunum, and ileum. It is here that most of the processes of digestion and absorption of food take place. −**intestinal** *adj.*

intima (tunica intima) (in-tim-ă) *n.* **1.** the inner layer of the wall of an artery or vein. It is composed of a lining of endothelial cells and an elastic membrane. **2.** the inner layer of various other organs or parts.

intolerance (in-tol-er-ăns) *n.* the inability of a patient to tolerate a particular drug, manifested by various adverse reactions.

intoxication (in-toks-i-kay-shŏn) *n.* the symptoms of poisoning due to ingestion of any toxic material, including alcohol.

intra- *prefix denoting* inside; within.

intra-articular (intră-ar-tik-yoo-ler) *adj.* within or into a joint.

intracellular (intră-sel-yoo-ler) *adj.* situated or occurring inside a cell or cells.

intracranial (intră-kray-ni-ăl) *adj.* within the skull.

intradermal (intră-derm-ăl) *adj.* within the skin.

intradural (intră-dewr-ăl) *adj.* within or beneath the dura mater.

intramedullary (intră-mi-dul-er-i) *adj.* within the bone marrow.

intramuscular (intră-mus-kew-ler) *adj.* within a muscle. *See also* injection.

intraocular (intră-ok-yoo-ler) *adj.* of or relating to the area within the eyeball.

intrathecal (intră-th'ee-kăl) *adj.* within the meninges of the spinal cord.

intrauterine device (intră-yoo-teryn) *n. see* IUD.

intravenous (intră-vee-nŭs) *adj.* into or within a vein. *See also* injection. *i. pyelography see* pyelography.

intraversion (intră-ver-shŏn) *n. see* introversion.

intra vitam (in-tră vy-tam) Latin: during life.

intrinsic (in-trin-sik) *adj.* exclusive to a part or body.

intrinsic factor *n.* a glycoprotein secreted in the stomach. The secretion of intrinsic factor is necessary for the absorption of vitamin B_{12}; a failure of secretion leads to a deficiency of the vitamin and the condition of pernicious anaemia.

intro- *prefix denoting* in; into.

introitus (in-troh-it-ŭs) *n.* (in anatomy) an entrance into a hollow organ or cavity.

introjection (intrŏ-jek-shŏn) *n.* (in psychoanalysis) the process of adopting, or of believing that one possesses, the qualities of another person. This can be a form of defence mechanism. *See also* identification.

introspection (intrŏ-**spek**-shŏn) *n.* the study by an individual of his own mental processes, reactions, etc. —**introspective** *adj.*

introversion (intrŏ-**ver**-shŏn) *n.* **1.** (*or* **intraversion**) an enduring personality trait characterized by interest in the self rather than the outside world. People high in introversion (*introverts*) tend to have a small circle of friends, like to persist in activities once they have started, and are highly susceptible to permanent conditioning. *Compare* extroversion. **2.** a turning inwards of a hollow organ (such as the womb) on itself.

introvert (**in**-trŏ-vert) *n. see* introversion.

intubation (in-tew-**bay**-shŏn) *n.* the introduction of a tube into part of the body for the purpose of diagnosis or treatment. *gastric i.* intubation performed to remove a sample of the stomach contents for analysis or to administer drugs directly into the stomach.

intumescence (in-tew-**mes**-ĕns) *n.* a swelling or an increase in the volume of an organ.

intussusception (in-tŭs-sŭ-**sep**-shŏn) *n.* the telescoping (*invagination*) of one part of the bowel into another, resulting in intestinal obstruction. It is most common in young children under the age of four. Symptoms include intermittent pain, vomiting, and the passing of red jelly with the stools; if the condition does not receive prompt surgical treatment, shock from gangrene of the bowel may result.

inulin (**in**-yoo-lin) *n.* a carbohydrate with a high molecular weight that is filtered from the bloodstream by the kidneys. *i.*

clearance a test of kidney function in which inulin is injected into the blood. By measuring the amount that appears in the urine over a given period, it is possible to calculate how much filtrate the kidneys are producing.

inunction (in-**unk**-shŏn) *n.* the rubbing in with the fingers of an ointment or liniment.

invagination (in-vaj-i-**nay**-shŏn) *n.* **1.** the infolding of the wall of a solid structure to form a cavity. **2.** *see* intussusception.

invasion (in-**vay**-zhŏn) *n.* **1.** the onset of a disease. **2.** the entry of bacteria into the body. **3.** the destruction of healthy tissue by a malignant tumour.

inversion (in-**ver**-shŏn) *n.* **1.** the turning inwards or inside-out of a part or organ: commonly applied to the state of the womb after childbirth when its upper part is pulled through the cervical canal. **2.** a chromosome mutation in which a block of genes within a chromosome are in reverse order.

invertase (in-**ver**-tayz) *n.* an enzyme in intestinal juice that digest sugars.

in vitro (in **vee**-troh) Latin: describing biological phenomena that are made to occur outside the living body (traditionally in a test-tube).

in vivo (in **vee**-voh) Latin: describing biological phenomena that occur within the bodies of living organisms.

involucrum (in-vŏ-**loo**-krŭm) *n.* a growth of new bone that sometimes surrounds a mass of infected and dead bone in osteomyelitis.

involuntary muscle (in-**vol**-ŭn-ter-i) *n.* muscle that is not under conscious control, such as the muscle of the gut, stomach, blood vessels, and heart. *See also* cardiac muscle, smooth muscle.

involution (in-vŏ-**loo**-shŏn) *n.* **1.** the shrinking of the womb to its normal size after childbirth. **2.** atrophy of an organ in old age. —**involutional** (in-vŏ-**loo**-shŏn-ăl) *adj.*

involutional melancholia *n.* a severe depression, usually psychotic, appearing for the first time in the involutional period of middle life (approximately 40–55 for women, 50–65 for men). Characteristic features include agitation; delusions of ill-health, poverty, and sin; and preoccupations with death and loss. *See* manic-depressive psychosis.

iodine (I-ŏ-din) *n.* an element required in small amounts for healthy growth and development. The thyroid gland requires iodine to synthesize thyroid hormones; a deficiency of the element leads to goitre. Radioactive isotopes of iodine (usually *iodine-131*) are used in the diagnosis and treatment of diseases of the thyroid gland. Iodine is also used as an antiseptic. Symbol: I.

iodism (I-ŏ-dizm) *n.* iodine poisoning. The main features are a characteristic staining of the mouth and odour on the breath. Emergency treatment includes administration of starch or flour in water and lavage with sodium thiosulphate solution.

ion (I-ŏn) *n.* an atom or group of atoms that conducts electricity. *See* anion, cation, electrolyte.

ionization (I-ŏ-ny-zay-shŏn) *n.* **1.** the dissociation of a substance into ions. **2.** *see* iontophoresis.

iontophoresis (ionization) (I-on-toh-fer-ee-sis) *n.* the technique of introducing through the skin, by means of an electric current, charged particles of a drug, so that it reaches a deep site. *See also* cataphoresis.

iopanoic acid (I-oh-pă-**noh**-ik) *n.* a radio-opaque iodine-containing compound used in cholecystography. It is administered by intravenous injection.

iophendylate (I-oh-**fen**-di-layt) *n.* a radio-opaque iodine-containing compound that is sometimes used in myelography. It is injected through a lumbar puncture needle.

ipecacuanha (ipi-kak-yoo-**an**-ă) *n.* a plant extract used in small doses, usually in the form of tinctures and syrups, as an expectorant to relieve coughing and to induce vomiting.

iprindole (i-**prin**-dohl) *n.* a drug administered by mouth for the treatment of depression (*see* antidepressant). Trade name: **Prondol.**

iproniazid (ip-roh-ny-ă-zid) *n.* a drug administered by mouth to treat all types of depression (*see* antidepressant). Trade name: **Marsilid.**

ipsilateral (ipselateral, homolateral) (ip-si-**lat**-er-ăl) *adj.* on or affecting the same side of the body. *Compare* contralateral.

IQ *n. see* intelligence quotient.

irid- (irido-) *prefix denoting* the iris.

iridectomy (i-ri-**dek**-tŏmi) *n.* an operation on the eye in which a part of the iris is removed.

iridocele (i-**rid**-oh-seel) *n.* the protrusion of part of the iris through a wound in the cornea.

iridocyclitis (i-ri-doh-sy-**kly**-tis) *n.* inflammation of the iris and ciliary body of the eye. *See* uveitis.

iridodialysis (i-ri-doh-dy-**al**-i-sis) *n.* a tear, caused by injury to the eye, in the attachment of the iris to the ciliary body.

iridoplegia (i-ri-doh-**plee**-jiă) *n.* paralysis of the iris, which is usually associated with cycloplegia and results from injury, inflammation, or the use of drugs in the eye.

iridoptosis (i-ri-**dop**-tŏ-sis) *n.* prolapse of the iris.

iridotomy (i-ri-**dot**-ŏmi) *n.* an operation on the eye in which an incision is made in the iris.

iris (**I**-ris) *n.* the part of the eye that regulates the amount of light that enters. It forms a coloured muscular diaphragm across the front of the lens; light enters through a central opening (the pupil). Contraction of different sets of muscles of the iris causes the pupil to dilate in dim light and to contract in bright light. *i. bombé* an abnormal condition of the eye in which the iris bulges forward towards the cornea.

iritis (**I**-**ry**-tis) *n.* inflammation of the iris. *See* uveitis.

iron (**I**-ern) *n.* an element essential to life. The body of an adult contains on average 4 g of iron, over half of which is contained in haemoglobin in the red blood cells. Iron is an essential component in the transfer of oxygen in the body; a deficiency of iron may lead to anaemia. Many preparations of iron are used to treat iron-deficiency anaemia. Symbol: Fe.

iron dextran *n.* a drug containing iron and dextran, administered by intramuscular or intravenous injection to treat iron-deficiency anaemia. Trade name: **Imferon**.

iron lung *n. see* respirator.

iron-storage disease *n. see* haemochromatosis.

irradiation (i-ray-di-ay-shŏn) *n.* the therapeutic application of electromagnetic radiation (usually alpha, beta, gamma, or X-rays) to a particular structure. *See* radiotherapy.

irreducible (i-ri-**dew**-sibŭl) *adj.* unable to be replaced in a normal position: applied particularly to a type of hernia.

irrigation (i-ri-**gay**-shŏn) *n.* the process of washing out a wound or hollow organ with a continuous flow of water or medicated solution.

irritability (i-ri-tă-**bil**-iti) *n.* (in physiology) the property of certain kinds of tissue that enables them to respond in a specific way to outside stimuli.

irritable bowel syndrome (spastic colon, mucous colitis) (i-ri-tăbŭl) *n.* a common condition in which recurrent abdominal pain with constipation and/or diarrhoea continues for years without any general deterioration in health or detectable structural disease.

irritant (i-ri-tănt) *n.* any material that causes irritation of a tissue.

isch- (ischo-) *prefix denoting* suppression or deficiency.

ischaemia (isk-**ee**-miă) *n.* an inadequate flow of blood to a part of the body, caused by constriction or blockage of the blood vessels supplying it.

ischi- (ischio-) *prefix denoting* the ischium.

ischiorectal abscess (isk-i-oh-rek-t'l) *n.* an abscess in the space between the sheet of muscle that assists in control of the rectum and the pelvic bone. Symptoms are severe throbbing pain near the anus with swelling and fever.

Pus is drained from the abscess by surgical incision.

ischium (isk-iŭm) *n.* a bone forming the lower part of each side of the hip bone (*see also* pelvis). —**ischiac, ischial** *adj.*

ischuria (isk-**yoor**-iă) *n.* retention or suppression of the urine. *See* anuria, retention.

islets of Langerhans (I-lits ŏv **lang**-er-hans) *pl. n.* small groups of cells, scattered through the material of the pancreas, that secrete the hormones insulin and glucagon. *See also* alpha cells, beta cells. [P. Langerhans (1847–88), German pathologist]

iso- *prefix denoting* equality, uniformity, or similarity.

isoaminile (I-soh-**am**-i-nyl) *n.* a drug administered in capsules and linctuses to suppress coughs (*see* antitussive). Trade name: **Dimyril.**

isoantibody (I-soh-**an**-ti-bodi) *n.* an antibody that occurs naturally against the components of foreign tissues from an individual of the same species.

isoantigen (I-soh-**an**-ti-jĕn) *n.* an antigen that forms a natural component of an individual's tissues.

isograft (isogenic graft, syngraft) (I-soh-grahft) *n.* a graft of tissue from one identical twin to another or between animals that are genetically identical.

isoimmunization (I-soh-im-yoo-ny-zay-shŏn) *n.* the development of antibodies (isoantibodies) within an individual against antigens from another individual of the same species.

isolation (I-sŏ-lay-shŏn) *n.* **1.** the separation of a person with an infectious disease from noninfected people. *See also* quarantine. **2.** (in surgery) the

separation of a structure from surrounding structures by the use of instruments.

isolator (I-sŏ-lay-ter) *n.* a large transparent plastic bag in which a patient can be nursed or operated upon without the danger of contamination by infective agents.

isoleucine (I-soh-**loo**-seen) *n.* an essential amino acid. *See also* amino acid.

isometric exercises (isometrics) (I-soh-**met**-rik) *pl. n.* a system of exercises based on the principle of *isometric contraction* of muscles. This can be induced in muscles that are used when a limb is made to pull or push against something that does not move. The exercises increase fitness and build muscle.

isomorphism (I-soh-**mor**-fizm) *n.* the condition of two or more objects being alike in shape or structure. —**isomorphic, isomorphous** *adj.*

isoniazid (isonicotinic acid hydrazide, INH) (I-soh-**ny**-ă-zid) *n.* a drug used in the treatment of tuberculosis, usually taken by mouth. Because tuberculosis bacteria soon become resistant to isoniazid, it is usually given in conjunction with streptomycin or PAS.

isoprenaline (I-soh-**pren**-ă-leen) *n.* a sympathomimetic drug used to dilate the air passages in asthma and other bronchial conditions. It also stimulates the heart and is used to treat some heart conditions involving reduced heart activity. It is administered by inhalation, by mouth, by injection, or in suppositories. Trade names: **Aleudrin, Lomupren, Medihaler-Iso, Prenomiser.**

isosthenuria (I-sos-thĕn-**yoor**-iă) *n.* inability of the kidneys to produce either a concentrated or a dilute urine. This occurs in the final stages of renal failure.

isotonic (I-soh-**ton**-ik) *adj.* **1.** describing solutions that have the same osmotic pressure. *See* osmosis. **2.** describing muscles that have equal tonicity.

isotope (I-sŏ-tohp) *n.* any one of the different forms of an element, having the same atomic number but different atomic weights. Radioactive isotopes decay into other isotopes or elements, emitting alpha, beta, or gamma radiation. Artificially produced radioactive isotopes (*see* nuclide) are used extensively in radiotherapy for the treatment of cancer.

isoxuprine (I-**soks**-yoo-preen) *n.* a drug that dilates blood vessels and is administered by mouth or injection to improve blood flow in such conditions as cerebrovascular disease and arteriosclerosis and to inhibit contractions in premature labour. Trade names: **Duvalidan, Defencin.**

isthmus (iss-mŭs) *n.* a constricted or narrowed part of an organ or tissue.

itch (ich) *n.* local discomfort or irritation of the skin, prompting the sufferer to scratch or rub the affected area. *See* pruritis.

itch mite *n. see* Sarcoptes.

-itis *suffix denoting* inflammation of an organ, tissue, etc.

IUD (intrauterine device) *n.* a plastic or metal coil, spiral, or other shape, about 25 mm long, that is inserted into the cavity of the womb to prevent conception. Its exact mode of action is unknown but it is thought to inter-fere with implantation of the embryo.

ixodiasis (iks-oh-**dy**-ă-sis) *n.* any disease caused by the presence of ticks.

J

Jacksonian epilepsy (jak-**sohn**-iăn) *n. see* epilepsy. [J. H. Jackson (1835–1911), British neurologist]

Jacquemier's sign (Spiegelberg's sign) (z*h*ak-mi-ayz) *n.* a bluish or purplish coloration of the membrane lining the vagina: a possible indication of pregnancy. [J. M. Jacquemier (1806–79), French obstetrician]

jactitation (jak-ti-**tay**-shŏn) *n.* restless tossing and turning of a person suffering from a severe disease, frequently one with a high fever.

jamais vu (zha-may-vew) *n.* one of the manifestations of temporal lobe epilepsy, in which there is a sudden feeling of unfamiliarity with everyday surroundings.

jaundice (**jawn**-dis) *n.* a yellowing of the skin or whites of the eyes, indicating excess bilirubin in the blood. *haemolytic j.* jaundice that occurs when there is excessive destruction of red cells in the blood (*see* haemolysis). *hepatocellular j.* jaundice due to disease of the liver cells, such as hepatitis. *obstructive j.* jaundice that occurs when bile made in the liver fails to reach the intestine due to obstruction of the bile ducts (e.g. by gallstones) or to cholestasis. Medical name: **icterus.**

jaw (jaw) *n.* either the maxilla (upper jaw) or the mandible (lower jaw).

jejun- (jejuno-) *prefix denoting* the jejunum.

jejunal ulcer (ji-**joo**-năl) *n. see* peptic (ulcer), Zollinger-Ellison syndrome.

jejunectomy (ji-joo-**nek**-tŏmi) *n.* surgical removal of the jejunum or part of the jejunum.

jejunoileostomy (ji-joo-noh-ili-**ost**-ŏmi) *n.* an operation in which the jejunum is joined to the ileum (small intestine), when either the end of the jejunum or the beginning of the ileum has been removed or is to be bypassed.

jejunostomy (ji-joo-**nost**-ŏmi) *n.* a surgical operation in which the jejunum is brought through the abdominal wall and opened.

jejunotomy (ji-joo-**not**-ŏmi) *n.* a surgical incision into the jejunum in order to inspect the interior or remove something from within it.

jejunum (ji-**joo**-nŭm) *n.* part of the small intestine. It comprises about two-fifths of the whole small intestine and connects the duodenum to the ileum. **—jejunal** *adj.*

jerk (jerk) *n.* the sudden contraction of a muscle in response to a nerve impulse. **knee j.** *see* patellar reflex.

joint (joint) *n.* the point at which two or more bones are connected. The opposing surfaces of bone are lined with cartilaginous, fibrous, or soft (synovial) tissue. *See also* amphiarthrosis, diarthrosis, synarthrosis.

joule (jool) *n.* the SI unit of work or energy, equal to the work done when the point of application of a force of 1 newton is displaced through a distance of 1 metre in the direction of the force. Symbol: J. *See also* calorie.

jugular (**jug**-yoo-ler) *adj.* relating to or supplying the neck or throat. **j. vein** any one of several veins in the neck. **internal j.** a very large paired vein running vertically down the side of the neck and draining blood from the brain, face, and neck into the subclavian vein.

junction (**junk**-shŏn) *n.* (in anatomy) the point at which two different tissues or structures are in contact. *See also* neuromuscular junction.

juxta- *prefix denoting* proximity to.

K

Kahn reaction (kahn) *n.* a test for syphilis, in which antibodies specific to the disease are detected in a sample of the patient's blood by means of a precipitin reaction. The test is not as reliable as the Wassermann reaction, but is useful as confirmation. [R. L. Kahn (1887–), US bacteriologist]

kala-azar (visceral leishmaniasis, Dumdum fever) (kah-lă-ă-zar) *n.* a tropical disease caused by the parasitic protozoan *Leishmania donovani*, which is transmitted to man by sandflies. Symptoms include enlargement and subsequent lesions of the liver and spleen; anaemia; a low leucocyte count; weight loss; and irregular fevers.

kanamycin (kan-ă-my-sin) *n.* an antibiotic used to treat a wide range of bacterial infections. It is administered mainly by injection but is given by mouth for infections of the intestine and by inhalation for respiratory infections. Trade name: **Kantrex**.

kaolin (kay-ŏ-lin) *n.* a white clay that contains aluminium and silicon and is purified and powdered for use as an adsorbent. It is taken by mouth to treat diarrhoea and vomiting. Kaolin is also used in dusting powders and poultices.

Kaposi's sarcoma (kap-oh-siz) *n.* a cancer of the reticuloendothelial system, principally affecting the skin with the formation of soft brownish nodules. Formerly rare and restricted to certain racial groups, it has become more widespread with the growing incidence of AIDS, with which it is associated. *See* AIDS. [M. Kaposi (1837–1902), Austrian dermatologist]

kary- (**karyo-**) *prefix denoting* a cell nucleus.

karyokinesis (ka-ri-oh-ky-**nee**-sis) *n.* division of the nucleus of a cell, which occurs during cell division before division of the cytoplasm (*cytokinesis*). *See* mitosis.

karyotype (**ka**-ri-ŏ-typ) *n.* **1.** the chromosome set of an individual or species described in terms of both the number and structure of the chromosomes. **2.** the representation of the chromosome set in a diagram.

katathermometer (kat-ă-ther-**mom**-it-er) *n.* a thermometer used to measure the cooling power of the air surrounding it.

Kayser-Fleischer ring (**ky**-zer fly-sher) *n.* a brownish-yellow ring in the outer rim of the cornea of the eye. It is a deposit of copper granules and is diagnostic of Wilson's disease. [B. Kayser (1869–1954), German ophthalmologist; B. Fleischer (1848–1904), German physician]

Keller's operation (kel-erz) *n.* a surgical operation to correct hallux valgus, in which the base of the first phalanx of the big toe is excised. [W. L. Keller (1874–1959), US surgeon]

keloid (**cheloid**) (**kee**-loid) *n.* hard prominent irregular scar tissue in the skin that often increases in size. It often forms where healing injuries or surgical incisions are under tension.

kerat- (**kerato-**) *prefix denoting* **1.** the cornea. **2.** horny tissue, especially of the skin.

keratectasia (ke-ră-tek-**tay**-ziă) *n.* bulging of the cornea at the site of scar tissue (which is thinner than normal corneal tissue).

keratectomy (ke-ră-**tek**-tŏmi) *n.* an operation in which a part of the cornea is removed, usually a superficial layer.

keratin (**ke**-ră-tin) *n.* a fibrous protein that forms the body's horny tissues, such as fingernails.

keratinization (**cornification**) (ke-ră-tin-I-**zay**-shŏn) *n.* the process by which cells become horny due to the deposition of keratin within them. It occurs in the epidermis of the skin and associated structures (hair, nails, etc.).

keratitis (ke-ră-**ty**-tis) *n.* inflammation of the cornea of the eye. The eye waters and is very painful and vision is blurred. It may be due to physical or chemical agents or result from infection. *interstitial k.* inflammation within the layers of the cornea, caused by syphilis, leprosy, or tuberculosis.

keratoconjunctivitis (ke-ră-toh-kŏn-junk-ti-**vy**-tis) *n.* combined inflammation of the cornea and conjunctiva of the eye.

keratoconus (ke-ră-toh-**koh**-nŭs) *n.* conical cornea: an abnormal condition of the eye in which the cornea, instead of having a regular curvature, comes to a rounded apex towards its centre.

keratoglobus (megalocornea) (ke-ră-toh-**gloh**-bŭs) *n.* a congenital disorder of the eye in which the whole cornea bulges forward in a regular curve. *Compare* keratoconus.

keratolytic (ke-ră-toh-**lit**-ik) *n.* an agent, such as salicylic acid, that breaks down the outer horny layer of epidermis and is used for treating warts.

keratoma (ke-ră-toh-mă) *n. see* keratosis.

keratomalacia (ke-ră-toh-mă-lay-shiă) *n.* a progressive disease of the eye due to vitamin A deficiency. The cornea softens and may become perforated. *See also* xerophthalmia.

keratome (ke-ră-tohm) *n.* any instrument designed for cutting the cornea.

keratometer (ophthalmometer) (ke-ră-**tom**-it-er) *n.* an instrument for measuring the radius of curvature of the cornea. It is used for assessing the degree of abnormal curvature of the cornea in astigmatism. —**keratometry** *n.*

keratoplasty (corneal graft) (ke-ră-toh-plasti) *n.* an eye operation in which any diseased parts of the cornea are replaced by clear corneal tissue from a donor.

keratoscope (Placido's disc) (ke-ră-toh-skohp) *n.* an instrument for detecting abnormal curvature of the cornea. It consists of a black disc marked with concentric white rings. The examiner looks at the reflection of the rings in the patient's cornea; a cornea that is abnormally curved (for example in keratoconus) or scarred reflects distorted rings.

keratosis (keratoma) (ke-ră-toh-sis) *n.* any horny growth of the skin. *actinic k.* a well-defined red or skin-coloured warty growth, usually occurring in middle or old age, caused by overexposure to the sun. *seborrhoeic k.* (or *warts*) yellow or brown oval spots with clearly marked perimeters and raised surfaces, developing in middle age.

keratotomy (ke-ră-**tot**-ŏmi) *n.* an incision into the cornea.

kerion (keer-iŏn) *n.* a soft inflammatory swelling covered with pustules, caused by a ringworm fungus infection.

kernicterus (ker-**nik**-ter-ŭs) *n.* staining and subsequent damage of the brain by bile pigment (bilirubin), which may occur in severe cases of haemolytic disease of the newborn.

Kernig's sign (ker-nigz) *n.* a symptom of meningitis in which the patient is unable to extend his legs at the knee when the thighs are held at a right angle to the body. [V. Kernig (1840–1917), Russian physician]

ketogenesis (kee-toh-**jen**-i-sis) *n.* the production of ketone bodies. These are normal products of lipid metabolism and can be used to provide energy.

ketogenic diet (kee-toh-**jen**-ik) *n.* a diet that promotes the formation of ketone bodies in the tissues, in which the principal energy source is fat rather than carbohydrate.

ketonaemia (kee-toh-**nee**-miă) *n.* the presence in the blood of ketone bodies.

ketone (kee-tohn) *n.* any member of a group of organic compounds consisting of a carbonyl

diaphragm
aorta
inferior vena cava
left kidney
renal vein
renal artery
ureter
bladder
urethra

Position of the kidneys

cortex
medulla
renal vein
renal artery
pelvis
ureter
pyramid

Section through a kidney

group (=CO) flanked by two alkyl groups. *k. bodies* (*acetone bodies*) the ketones acetoacetic acid, acetone, and β-hydroxybutyrate, produced during the metabolism of fats. *See also* ketosis.

ketonuria (acetonuria) (kee-tohn-**yoor**-iă) *n.* the presence in the urine of ketone bodies. This may occur in diabetes mellitus, starvation, or after persistent vomiting and results from the partial oxidation of fats.

ketoprofen (kee-toh-**proh**-fen) *n.* an analgesic that reduces inflammation, administered by mouth to treat various arthritic and rheumatic diseases. Trade name: **Orudis**.

ketosis (kee-**toh**-sis) *n.* raised levels of ketone bodies in the body tissues, resulting from an imbalance in fat metabolism. Ketosis may result in severe acidosis. *See also* ketonuria.

ketosteroid (kee-toh-**steer**-oid) *n.* a steroid that contains one or more ketone groups ($-C=O$). 17-ketosteroids (having the oxygen at carbon 17) are normally excreted in the urine; excess 17-ketosteroids in the urine indicates overactivity of the adrenal glands and gonads.

kidney (**kid**-ni) *n.* either of the pair of organs responsible for the excretion of nitrogenous wastes, principally urea, from the blood (see illustration). The active units of the kidney are the nephrons, which filter the blood under pressure and then reabsorb water and selected substances back into the blood. The urine thus formed is conducted via the renal tubules to the ureter, which leads to the bladder.

Killian's operation (kil-iänz) *n.* a surgical operation in which part of the frontal bone is removed to allow drainage of the frontal sinus (*see* paranasal sinuses), when this is filled with pus. [G. Killian (1860–1921), German otorhinolaryngologist]

kilo- *prefix denoting* a thousand.

kilogram (kil-ŏ-gram) *n.* the SI unit of mass equal to 1000 grams. Symbol: kg.

Kimmelstiel-Wilson disease (kim-ĕl-steel wil-sŏn) *n.* a disease in which diabetes mellitus is associated with the nephrotic syndrome resulting from breakdown of the glomeruli of the kidneys. [P. Kimmelstiel (1900–), German-born pathologist; C. Wilson (1906–), British physician]

kin- (kine-) *prefix denoting* movement.

kinaesthesia (kin-iss-theez-iă) *n.* the sense that enables the brain to be constantly aware of the position and movement of muscles in different parts of the body.

kinanaesthesia (kin-anis-theez-iă) *n.* inability to sense the positions and movements of parts of the body, with consequent disordered physical activity.

kinase (ky-nayz) *n.* **1.** an agent that can convert the inactive form of an enzyme (*see* proenzyme) to the active form. **2.** an enzyme that catalyses the transfer of phosphate groups.

kinematics (kin-i-mat-iks) *n.* the study of motion and the forces required to produce it. This includes the different forces at work during the movement of a single part of the body, and more complex movements such as running and climbing.

kineplasty (kin-i-plasti) *n.* a method of amputation in which the muscles and tendons of the affected limb are arranged so that they can be integrated with a specially made artificial replacement.

-kinesis *suffix denoting* movement.

kinetochore (ky-nee-toh-kor) *n. see* centromere.

kinin (ky-nin) *n.* one of a group of naturally occurring polypeptides that are powerful vasodilators, which lower blood pressure, and cause contraction of smooth muscle.

Kirschner's wire (keersh-nerz) *n.* a wire that can be inserted into a bone to exert skeletal traction or to fix fractures. [M. Kirschner (1879–1942), German surgeon]

kiss of life *n.* emergency artificial respiration, performed mouth-to-mouth, by blowing air into the victim's lungs to inflate them and then allowing exhalation to occur automatically.

Klebsiella (kleb-si-el-ă) *n.* a genus of Gram-negative rodlike nonmotile mostly lactose-fermenting bacteria found in the respiratory, intestinal, and urinogenital tracts of animals and man.

Klebs-Loeffler bacillus (klebz-lerf-ler) *n. see* Corynebacterium. [T. Klebs (1834–1913) and F. A. J. Loeffler (1852–1915), German bacteriologists]

klepto- *prefix denoting* stealing.

kleptomania (kleptŏ-**may**-niă) n. a pathologically strong impulse to steal, often in the absence of any desire for the stolen object(s). It is sometimes associated with depression.

Klinefelter's syndrome (klyn-fel-terz) n. a genetic disorder in which there are three sex chromosomes, XXY, rather than the normal XX or XY. Affected individuals are apparently male, but have small testes, enlarged breasts, and absence of facial and body hair. [H. F. Klinefelter (1912–), US physician]

Klumpke's paralysis (kluump-kĕz) n. a partial paralysis of the arm caused by injury to a baby's brachial plexus during birth. It results in weakness and wasting of the muscles of the hand. [A. Klumpke (1859–1927), French neurologist]

kneading (**need**-ing) n. see petrissage.

knee (nee) n. the hinge joint between the femur and the tibia. k. jerk see patellar reflex.

kneecap (**nee**-kap) n. see patella.

knock-knee (**nok**-nee) n. abnormal in-curving of the legs, resulting in a gap between the feet when the knees are in contact. Medical name: **genu valgum**.

Koch's bacillus (koks) n. see Mycobacterium. [R. Koch (1843–1910), German bacteriologist]

Köhler's disease (**ker**-lerz) n. inflammation of the navicular bone of the foot (see osteochondritis). It occurs in children, causing pain and limping. [A. Köhler (1874–1947), German physician]

koilonychia (koi-loh-**nik**-iă) n. the development of brittle spoon-shaped nails, a common disorder that can occur with anaemia due to iron deficiency.

Koplik's spots (**kop**-liks) pl. n. small red spots with bluish-white centres that often appear on the mucous membranes of the mouth in measles. [H. Koplik (1858–1927), US paediatrician]

Korsakoff's syndrome (**Korsakoff's psychosis**) (kor-**sak**-offs) n. an organic disorder affecting the brain that results in impaired memory for recent events, disorientation for time and place, and confabulation. The commonest cause of the condition is alcoholism, especially when this has led to deficiency of thiamin (vitamin B_1). [S. S. Korsakoff (1854–1900), Russian neurologist]

kraurosis (kraw-**roh**-sis) n. shrinking of a body part, usually the vulva in elderly women (k. vulvae).

Krebs cycle (**citric acid cycle**) (krebz) n. a complex cycle of enzyme-catalysed reactions, occurring within the cells of all living animals, in which acetate is broken down to produce energy in the form of ATP and carbon dioxide. The cycle is the final step in the oxidation of carbohydrates, fats, and proteins. [Sir H. A. Krebs (1900–81), German-born biochemist]

Krukenberg tumour (**kroo**-kĕn-berg) n. a rapidly developing malignant growth in one or (more often) both ovaries: a type of fibrosarcoma. The tumour usually arises following the development of a similar growth in the stomach or intestine. [F. E. Krukenberg (1871–1946), German pathologist]

krypton-81m (**krip**-ton) n. a radioactive gas that is the shortest-lived isotope in medical use (half-life 13 seconds). It can be used to investigate the function

Küntscher nail

of the lungs. *See also* rubidium-81.

Küntscher nail (koont-sher) *n.* a
long steel nail that is inserted
down the long axis of a long
bone, into the marrow, in order
to fix a fracture. [G. Küntscher
(1902–), German orthopaedic
surgeon]

Kupffer's cells (kuup-ferz) *pl. n.*
phagocytic cells that line the si-
nusoids of the liver (*see* macrophage). They are particularly
concerned with the formation of
bile. [K. W. von Kupffer (1829–
1902), German anatomist]

kwashiorkor (kwash-i-**or**-ker) *n.* a
form of malnutrition due to a
diet deficient in protein and en-
ergy-producing foods, common
among young children in certain
African tribes. The symptoms are
oedema, loss of appetite, diarrhoea, general discomfort, and
apathy; the child fails to thrive
and there is usually associated
gastric infection.

kymograph (ky-mŏ-grahf) *n.* an instrument for recording the flow
and varying pressure of the
blood within blood vessels. **–ky-
mography** *n.*

kypho- *prefix denoting* a hump.

kyphos (ky-fos) *n.* a sharply localized forward angulation of the
spine, resulting in the appearance
of a lump (the deformity of the
traditional hunchback).

kyphoscoliosis (ky-foh-skoh-li-
oh-sis) *n.* abnormal curvature of
the spine both forwards and
sideways: kyphosis combined
with scoliosis.

kyphosis (ky-**foh**-sis) *n.* excessive
outward curvature of the spine,
causing hunching of the back. It
may result from bad posture or
muscle weakness (*mobile k.*) or
from diseases such as osteochondritis or ankylosing spondylitis
(*fixed k.*). Treatment depends on
the cause, and may include physiotherapy, bracing, and spinal osteotomy in severe cases. *See also*
kyphos, kyphoscoliosis.

L

labial (lay-bi-ăl) *adj.* relating to
the lips or to a labium.

labile (lay-byl) *adj.* unstable. The
term is applied to drugs and
other chemicals that readily undergo change in solution, when
subjected to heat, etc., and also
to emotions when there are rapid
mood swings.

labio- *prefix denoting* the lip(s).

labioplasty (cheiloplasty) (lay-bi-
oh-plasti) *n.* surgical repair of injury or deformity of the lips.

labium (lay-bi-ŭm) *n.* (*pl.* **labia**) a
lip-shaped structure, especially either of the two pairs of skin
folds that enclose the vulva. The

uterus

cervix

vagina

The mechanism of labour

larger outer pair are known as the *labia majora* and the smaller inner pair the *labia minora* (or *nymphae*).

labour (lay-ber) *n*. the sequence of actions by which a baby and the afterbirth are expelled from the womb at childbirth. The process usually starts spontaneously about 266 days after conception, but it may be started by artificial means (*see* induction). In the first stage the muscular wall of the womb begins contracting while the cervix expands. The amnion bursts, releasing amniotic fluid to the exterior. In the second stage the baby passes through the vagina, assisted by contractions of the abdominal muscles and conscious pushing by the mother. When the whole infant has been eased clear of the vagina, the umbilical cord is cut. In the final stage the placenta and membranes are pushed

lacrimal gland

lacrimal canaliculus

lacrimal sac

nasal cavity

excretory ducts of lacrimal glands

punctum

nasolacrimal duct

The lacrimal apparatus

out by the continuing contraction of the womb. *See also* Caesarean section.

labrum (lay-brŭm) *n.* (*pl.* **labra**) a lip or liplike structure; occurring, for example, around the margins of the acetabulum.

labyrinth (inner ear) (lab-er-inth) *n.* a convoluted system of cavities and ducts comprising the organs of hearing and balance. *bony l.* the bony canals and chambers, embedded in the petrous part of the temporal bone, that surround the membranous labyrinth. *membranous l.* the membranous canals and chambers comprising the semicircular canals, utricle, saccule, and cochlea.

labyrinthitis (lab-er-inth-I-tis) *n.* see otitis (interna).

laceration (las-er-ay-shŏn) *n.* a tear in the flesh producing a wound with irregular edges.

lacrimal (lak-rim-ăl) *adj.* relating to tears. *l. apparatus* the structures that produce and drain away fluid from the eye (see illustration). *l. bone* either of a pair of small rectangular bones that contribute to the orbits. *l. gland* the gland that secretes tears, which drain away through

small openings (*puncta*) at the inner corner of the eye.

lacrimation (lak-ri-may-shŏn) *n.* the production of excess tears; crying.

lacrimator (lak-rim-ay-ter) *n.* an agent that irritates the eyes, causing excessive secretion of tears.

lact- (**lacti-**, **lacto-**) *prefix denoting* 1. milk. 2. lactic acid.

lactalbumin (lak-tal-bew-min) *n.* a milk protein present in milk at a lower concentration than casein.

lactase (lak-tayz) *n.* an enzyme, secreted by the glands of the small intestine, that converts lactose (milk sugar) into glucose and galactose during digestion.

lactate (lak-tayt) 1. *n.* any salt of lactic acid. 2. *vb.* to secrete milk (*see* lactation).

lactation (lak-tay-shŏn) *n.* the secretion of milk by the mammary glands of the breasts, which usually begins at the end of pregnancy. Lactation is controlled by hormones (*see* prolactin, oxytocin); it stops when the baby is no longer fed at the breast.

lacteal (lak-ti-ăl) *n.* a blind-ended lymphatic vessel that extends into a villus of the small intestine. Digested fats are absorbed into the lacteals.

lactic acid (lak-tik) *n.* a simple sugar that forms in the cells as the end-product of glucose metabolism in the absence of oxygen (*see* glycolysis). Lactic acid (owing to its low pH) is an important food preservative.

lactiferous (lak-tif-er-ŭs) *adj.* transporting or secreting milk, as the ducts (*l. ducts*) of the breast.

lactifuge (lak-ti-fewj) *n.* a drug that reduces the secretion of milk. Oestrogenic drugs, such as chlorotrianisene and dienoestrol, have this effect.

Lactobacillus (lak-toh-bă-**sil**-ŭs) *n.* a genus of Gram-positive non-motile rodlike bacteria capable of producing lactic acid from the fermentation of carbohydrates. They are found in fermenting animal and plant products, especially dairy products, and in the alimentary tract and vagina.

lactogenic hormone (lak-tŏ-jen-ik) *n. see* prolactin.

lactometer (lak-**tom**-it-er) *n.* an instrument for measuring the relative density (specific gravity) of milk.

lactose (milk sugar) (lak-tohz) *n.* a sugar, consisting of one molecule of glucose and one of galactose, found only in milk. *l. intolerance* inability to absorb lactose, caused by absence or low activity of the enzyme lactase.

lactosuria (lak-tohs-**yoor**-iă) *n.* the presence of lactose in the urine. This often occurs during pregnancy and breast-feeding or if the milk flow is suppressed.

lacuna (lă-**kew**-nă) *n. (pl.* **lacunae**) (in anatomy) a small cavity or depression.

Laënnec's cirrhosis (la-en-**neks**) *n.* alcoholic cirrhosis: the commonest type of cirrhosis. [R. T. H. Laënnec (1781–1826), French physician]

laevo- *prefix. see* levo-.

laevocardia (lee-voh-**kar**-di-ă) *n.* the normal position of the heart, in which its apex is directed towards the left. *Compare* dextrocardia.

laking (**layk**-ing) *n.* the physical or chemical treatment of blood to abolish the structure of the red cells and thus form a homogeneous solution. Laking is an im-portant preliminary step in the analysis of haemoglobin or enzymes present in red cells.

-lalia *suffix denoting* a condition involving speech.

lallation (lalling) (la-**lay**-shŏn) *n.* **1.** unintelligible speechlike babbling, as heard from infants. **2.** the immature substitution of one consonant for another (e.g. *l* for *r*).

lambda (**lam**-dă) *n.* the point on the skull at which the lambdoidal and sagittal sutures meet.

lambdoidal suture (lam-doi-d'l) *n.* the immovable joint between the parietal and occipital bones (*see* skull).

lambliasis (lam-**bly**-ă-sis) *n. see* giardiasis.

lamella (lă-**mel**-ă) *n. (pl.* **lamellae**) **1.** a thin layer, membrane, scale, or platelike tissue or part. **2.** a thin gelatinous medicated disc used to apply drugs to the eye. The disc is placed on the eyeball; the gelatinous material dissolves and the drug is absorbed.

lamina (**lam**-in-ă) *n. (pl.* **laminae**) a thin membrane or layer of tissue.

laminectomy (rachiotomy) (lam-in-ek-tŏmi) *n.* surgical cutting into the backbone to obtain access to the spinal cord. The operation is performed to remove tumours or prolapsed intervertebral discs or to relieve pressure on a spinal nerve.

lanatoside (lă-**nat**-oh-syd) *n.* a drug similar to digitalis, administered by mouth or injection in the treatment of heart failure. Trade name: **Cedilanid.**

Lancefield classification (lans-feeld) *n.* a classification of the *Streptococcus* bacteria based on the presence or absence of antigenic carbohydrate on the cell surface. Species are classified into the groups A–P. Most species causing disease in man belong to group A. [R. C. Lancefield (1895–), US bacteriologist]

lancet (**lahn**-sit) *n.* a broad two-edged surgical knife with a sharp point.

lancinating (**lahn**-sin-ayt-ing) *adj.* describing a sharp stabbing or cutting pain.

Landry's paralysis (lahn-**dreez**) *n.* a rapidly progressive form of the Guillain-Barré syndrome. [J. B. O. Landry (1826–65), French physician]

Lange curve (**lahng**-ĕ) *n.* a method of detecting excess globulins in the protein of the cerebrospinal fluid. It is useful in the diagnosis of neurosyphilis and multiple sclerosis. [F. A. Lange (1883–), German physician]

lanolin (**lan**-ŏ-lin) *n.* a fatty substance obtained from sheep's wool, used as an emollient and as a base for ointments.

lanugo (lă-**new**-goh) *n.* fine hair covering the body and limbs of the human fetus.

laparo- *prefix denoting* the loins or abdomen.

laparoscope (peritoneoscope) (**lap**-er-ŏ-skohp) *n. see* laparoscopy.

laparoscopy (peritoneoscopy, abdominoscopy) (lap-er-os-kŏpi) *n.* examination of the abdominal structures by means of an illuminated tubular instrument (*laparoscope*) passed through a small incision in the wall of the abdomen. Laparoscopy is often used for examining the ovaries and Fallopian tubes as well as for performing one method of sterilization.

laparotomy (lap-er-**ot**-ŏmi) *n.* a surgical incision into the abdominal cavity. The operation is done

to examine the abdominal organs as a help to diagnosis.

lardaceous (lar-**day**-shŭs) *adj.* resembling lard: often applied to tissue infiltrated with the starchlike substance amyloid (*see* amyloidosis).

larva (**lar**-vă) *n.* (*pl.* **larvae**) the preadult or immature stage hatching from the egg of some animal groups, e.g. insects and nematodes, which may be markedly different from the sexually mature adult. *l. migrans see* creeping eruption. —**larval** *adj.*

laryng- (laryngo-) *prefix denoting* the larynx.

laryngeal reflex (la-rin-**jee**-ăl) *n.* a cough produced by irritating the larynx.

laryngectomy (la-rin-**jek**-tŏmi) *n.* surgical removal of the whole or a part of the larynx.

laryngismus (la-rin-**jiz**-mŭs) *n.* closure of the vocal cords by sudden contraction of the laryngeal muscles, followed by a noisy indrawing of breath. It occurs in young children when a foreign body has lodged in the larynx or in croup; in the past it was associated with low-calcium rickets.

laryngitis (la-rin-**jy**-tis) *n.* inflammation of the larynx and vocal cords, due to infection or irritation. The voice becomes husky or is lost completely; breathing is harsh and difficult (*see* stridor); and the cough is painful. Obstruction of the airways may occasionally be serious, especially in children (*see* croup).

laryngofissure (lă-ring-oh-**fish**-er) *n. see* laryngotomy.

laryngology (la-ring-**ol**-ŏji) *n.* the study of diseases of the larynx and vocal cords. —**laryngologist** *n.*

lateral

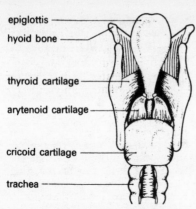

epiglottis
hyoid bone
thyroid cartilage
arytenoid cartilage
cricoid cartilage
trachea

Cartilages of the larynx

laryngopharynx (lă-ring-oh-**fa**-rinks) *n.* the part of the pharynx that lies below the hyoid bone.

laryngoscope (lă-**ring**-ŏ-skohp) *n.* an instrument for examining the larynx.

laryngospasm (lă-**ring**-oh-spazm) *n.* closure of the larynx, obstructing the flow of air to the lungs. It usually occurs as part of an allergic reaction.

laryngostenosis (lă-ring-oh-sti-**noh**-sis) *n.* narrowing of the cavity of the larynx.

laryngotomy (laryngofissure) (la-ring-**ot**-ŏmi) *n.* surgical incision of the larynx. *inferior l.* surgical incision of the cricothyroid membrane beneath the larynx; a life-saving operation when there is obstruction to breathing at or above the larynx.

laryngotracheobronchitis (lă-ring-oh-trak-i-oh-brong-ky-tis) *n.* a severe infection of the respiratory tract, especially of young children, in whom there may be a dangerous degree of obstruction either at the larynx (*see* croup) or bronchi.

larynx (**la**-rinks) *n.* the organ re-sponsible for the production of vocal sounds, also serving as an air passage conveying air from the pharynx to the lungs. It is situated in the front of the neck, above the trachea. It is made up of a framework of nine cartilages, bound together by ligaments and muscles and lined with mucous membrane, and contains a pair of vocal cords. —**laryngeal** *adj.*

laser (**lay**-zer) *n.* a device that produces a very thin beam of light in which high energies are concentrated. In surgery lasers can be used to operate on small areas of abnormality (for example, in the retina of the eye) without damaging delicate surrounding tissue.

Lassa fever (**las**-ă) *n.* a serious virus disease confined to Central West Africa. Symptoms include headache, high fever, and severe muscular pains; difficulty in swallowing often arises. Death from kidney or heart failure occurs in over 50% of cases. Treatment with plasma from recovered patients is the best therapy.

Lassar's paste (**las**-arz) *n.* an ointment containing zinc oxide, starch, and salicylic acid in a soft paraffin base, used in the treatment of eczema and similar skin diseases. [G. Lassar (1849–1907), German dermatologist]

latent heat (**lay**-těnt) *n.* the quantity of heat absorbed or released when a substance changes state (e.g. from solid to liquid or from liquid to vapour) without any change in temperature.

lateral (**lat**-er-ăl) *adj.* **1.** situated at or relating to the side of an organ or organism. **2.** (in anatomy) relating to the region or parts of the body that are furthest from the median plane. 3. (in radiology) in the sagittal plane.

lateroversion (lat-er-oh-ver-shŏn) *n.* a turning or displacement of an organ, for example the womb (*uterine l.*), to one side.

laudanum (lawd-nŭm) *n.* a hydroalcoholic solution containing 1% morphine, prepared from macerated raw opium. It was formerly widely used as a narcotic analgesic, taken by mouth.

laughing gas (lahf-ing) *n. see* nitrous oxide.

lavage (lav-ah*zh*) *n.* washing out a body cavity, such as the colon or stomach, with water or a medicated solution.

laxative (cathartic, purgative) (laks-ă-tiv) *n.* a drug used to stimulate or increase the frequency of bowel evacuation (e.g. castor oil, senna) or to encourage a softer or bulkier stool (e.g. magnesium sulphate, methylcellulose).

L-dopa *n. see* levodopa.

lead (led) *n.* a soft bluish-grey metallic element that forms several poisonous compounds. Acute lead poisoning causes abdominal pains, vomiting, diarrhoea, and sometimes encephalitis. In chronic poisoning a characteristic blue mark on the gums (*l. line*) is seen and the peripheral nerves are affected; there is also anaemia. Treatment is with EDTA. The use of lead in paints is now strictly controlled. Symbol: Pb.

LE cells *pl. n. see* lupus (erythematosus).

lecithin (les-i-thin) *n.* one of a group of phospholipids that are important constituents of cell membranes and are involved in the metabolism of fat by the liver. An example is *phosphatidylcholine*.

lecithinase (les-i-thin-ayz) *n.* an enzyme from the small intestine that breaks lecithin down into its constituents (i.e. glycerol, fatty acids, phosphoric acid, and choline).

Ledermycin (led-er-my-sin) *n. see* demethylchlortetracycline.

leech (leech) *n.* a type of worm that possesses suckers at both ends of its body. Certain parasitic species suck blood from animals and man, causing irritation and, occasionally, infection. Leeches were formerly used in bloodletting.

Legg-Calvé-Perthes disease (Perthes disease, pseudocoxalgia) (leg kal-vay per-tĕz) *n.* inflammation of the heads of the femurs, resulting in loss of the blood supply and death of the outer layer of bone (*see* osteochondritis). It occurs most commonly in boys between the ages of 5 and 10, and causes aching and a limp. [A. T. Legg (1874–1939), US surgeon; J. Calvé (1875–1954), French orthopaedist; G. C. Perthes (1869–1927), German surgeon]

legionnaires' disease (lee-jŏn-airz) *n.* a bacterial infection of the lungs. Symptoms include malaise and muscle pain, succeeded by a fever, dry cough, chest pain, and breathlessness. Erythromycin provides the most effective therapy.

legumin (lig-yoo-min) *n.* a protein (a globulin) obtained from the seeds of plants of the family Leguminosae, such as beans and peas.

leio- *prefix denoting* smoothness.

leiomyoma (ly-oh-my-oh-mă) *n.* a benign tumour of smooth muscle. Such tumours occur most commonly in the uterus (*see* fibroid) but can also arise in the digestive tract, walls of blood vessels, etc.

leiomyosarcoma (ly-oh-my-oh-sar-koh-mă) *n.* a malignant tumour of smooth muscle, most commonly found in the womb, stomach, small bowel, and at the base of the bladder.

Leishman-Donovan body (leesh-măn don-ŏ-văn) *n.* *see* Leishmania. [Sir W. B. Leishman (1865–1926), British surgeon; C. Donovan (1863–1951), Irish physician]

Leishmania (leesh-**may**-niă) *n.* a genus of parasitic flagellate protozoans, several species of which cause disease in man (*see* leishmaniasis). In man, especially in kala-azar patients, the parasite is a small rounded structure called a *Leishman-Donovan body*, which is found within the cells of the lymphatic system, spleen, and bone marrow.

leishmaniasis (leesh-mă-**ny**-ă-sis) *n.* a disease, common in the tropics and subtropics, caused by parasitic protozoans of the genus *Leishmania*, which are transmitted by the bite of sandflies. *cutaneous l.* leishmaniasis that affects the tissues of the skin. *See* espundia, oriental sore. *visceral l.* leishmaniasis in which the cells of various internal organs are affected. *See* kala-azar.

Lembert's suture (lahm-**bairz**) *n.* a suture used for closing wounds in the intestine in which the edges are turned inwards and stitched down to the level of the submucosa. [A. Lembert (1802–51), French surgeon]

lens (lenz) *n.* **1.** (in anatomy) the transparent crystalline structure situated behind the pupil of the eye. It helps to refract incoming light and focus it onto the retina. *See also* accommodation. **2.** (in optics) a piece of glass shaped to refract rays of light in a particular direction. Lenses are worn to correct faulty eyesight. *See also* bifocal lenses, contact lenses, multifocal lenses.

lenticular (len-**tik**-yoo-ler) *adj.* relating to or shaped like a lens.

lenticular nucleus (lentiform nucleus) *n.* *see* basal ganglia.

lentigo (len-ty-goh) *n.* a brown roundish flat spot on the skin caused by excess development of melanin.

leontiasis (lee-on-ty-ă-sis) *n.* overgrowth of the skull bones, said to resemble the appearance of a lion's head: a rare feature of untreated Paget's disease. Medical name: **leontiasis ossea.**

lepidosis (lep-i-**doh**-sis) *n.* any skin eruption that causes scaling.

leproma (lep-**roh**-mă) *n.* a lump on the skin characteristic of leprosy.

leprosy (Hansen's disease) (lep-rŏ-si) *n.* a chronic disease, caused by the bacterium *Mycobacterium leprae*, that affects the skin, mucous membranes, and nerves. It is confined mainly to the tropics and is transmitted by direct contact. Symptoms mainly involve the skin and nerves. Leprosy can be controlled with sulphone drugs. *lepromatous l.* a contagious steadily progressive form of the disease characterized by the development of widely distributed lumps on the skin, thickening of the skin and nerves, and in serious cases by severe numbness of the skin, muscle weakness, and paralysis leading to disfigurement and deformity. Tuberculosis is a common complication. *tuberculoid l.* a benign, often self-limiting, form of leprosy causing discoloration and disfiguration of patches of skin associated with localized numbness.

lept- (lepto-) *prefix denoting* 1. slender; thin. 2. small. 3. mild; slight.

leptocyte (lep-toh-syt) *n.* a red blood cell (erythrocyte) that is abnormally thin. Leptocytes are seen in certain types of anaemia.

leptomeninges (lep-toh-min-**in**-jeez) *pl. n.* the inner two meninges: the arachnoid and pia mater.

leptomeningitis (lep-toh-men-in-jy-tis) *n.* inflammation of the leptomeninges. *See also* meningitis.

Leptospira (lep-toh-**spy**-ră) *n.* a genus of spirochaete bacteria, commonly bearing hooked ends. *L. icterohaemorrhagiae* a parasite that is the main causative agent of leptospirosis.

leptospirosis (Weil's disease) (lep-toh-spy-**roh**-sis) *n.* an infectious disease, caused by bacteria of the genus *Leptospira*, that is transmitted from rodents, dogs, and other mammals to man. The disease begins with a fever and may affect the liver (causing jaundice) or meninges (resulting in meningitis); in some cases the kidneys are involved.

leresis (ler-ee-sis) *n.* rambling speech, immature both in syntax and pronunciation. It is a feature of dementia.

lesbianism (lez-bi-ăn-izm) *n.* the condition in which a woman is sexually attracted to, or engages in sexual behaviour with, another woman (*see also* homosexuality). **–lesbian** *adj., n.*

lesion (lee-zhŏn) *n.* a zone of tissue with impaired function as a result of damage by disease or wounding.

lethal gene (lee-thăl) *n.* a gene that, under certain conditions, causes the death of the individual carrying it. Lethal genes are usually recessive: an individual will die only if both his parents carry the gene.

lethargy (leth-er-ji) *n.* mental and physical sluggishness: a degree of inactivity and unresponsiveness approaching or verging on the unconscious.

Letterer-Siwe disease (let-er-er sy-wě) *n. see* reticuloendotheliosis. [E. Letterer (1895–) and S. A. Siwe (1897–), German physicians]

leuc- (leuco-, leuk-, leuko-) *prefix denoting* 1. lack of colour; white. 2. leucocytes.

leucine (loo-seen) *n.* an essential amino acid. *See also* amino acid.

leucocidin (loo-koh-sy-din) *n.* a bacterial exotoxin that selectively destroys white blood cells (leucocytes).

leucocyte (white blood cell) (loo-kŏ-syt) *n.* any blood cell that contains a nucleus. In health there are three major subdivisions: granulocytes, lymphocytes, and monocytes, which are involved in protecting the body against foreign substances and in antibody production. In disease, a variety of other types may appear in the blood.

leucocytolysis (loo-koh-sy-tol-i-sis) *n.* destruction of white blood cells.

leucocytosis (loo-koh-sy-toh-sis) *n.* an increase in the number of leucocytes in the blood. *See* basophilia, eosinophilia, lymphocytosis, monocytosis.

leucoderma (loo-koh-der-mă) *n. see* vitiligo.

leucolysin (loo-**kol**-i-sin) *n. see* lysin.

leucoma (loo-**koh**-mă) *n.* a white opacity in the cornea. Most leucomas result from scarring after corneal inflammation or ulceration.

leuconychia (loo-koh-**nik**-iă) *n.* white discoloration of the nails, which may be total or partial. The cause is unknown.

leucopenia (loo-koh-**pee**-niă) *n.* a reduction in the number of leucocytes in the blood. *See* eosinopenia, lymphopenia, neutropenia.

leucoplakia (leukoplakia) (loo-koh-**play**-kiă) *n.* thickened white patches on membranes, such as the mouth lining or vulva, due to an overgrowth of the tissues. Leucoplakia can occasionally become malignant.

leucopoiesis (loo-koh-poi-**ee**-sis) *n.* the process of the production of leucocytes, which normally occurs in the blood-forming tissue of the bone marrow. *See also* granulopoiesis, haemopoiesis, lymphopoiesis, monoblast.

leucorrhoea (whites) (loo-kŏ-**ree**-ă) *n.* a whitish or yellowish discharge of mucus from the vaginal opening. An abnormally large discharge may indicate infection of the lower reproductive tract.

leucotomy (loo-**kot**-ŏmi) *n.* the surgical operation of interrupting the pathways of white nerve fibres within the brain: it involves stereotaxy to make selective lesions in small areas of the brain. The operation is used for intractable pain, severe depression, obsessional neurosis, and chronic anxiety. **prefrontal l.** (*lobotomy*) the original form of the operation, which involved cutting

through the nerve fibres connecting the frontal lobe with the thalamus and the association fibres of the frontal lobe.

leukaemia (loo-**kee**-miă) *n.* any of a group of malignant diseases in which increased numbers of certain immature or abnormal leucocytes are produced. This leads to increased susceptibility to infection, anaemia, and bleeding. Other symptoms include enlargement of the spleen, liver, and lymph nodes. Leukaemias may be *acute* or *chronic* depending on the rate of progression of the disease. They are also classified according to the type of white cell that is proliferating abnormally (*see* lymphoblast, myeloblast, myeloid (leukaemia)). Leukaemias are treated with radiotherapy or cytotoxic drugs.

leukoplakia (loo-koh-**play**-kiă) *n. see* leucoplakia.

levallorphan (lev-ă-**lor**-fan) *n.* a drug that counteracts the depression in breathing caused by narcotic analgesics such as morphine without affecting their pain-relieving effects. It is administered by injection. Trade name: **Lorfan.**

levator (li-**vay**-ter) *n.* **1.** a surgical instrument used for levering up displaced bone fragments in a depressed fracture of the skull. **2.** any muscle that lifts the structure into which it is inserted.

levo (laevo-) *prefix denoting* **1.** the left side. **2.** (in chemistry) levorotation.

levodopa (L-dopa) (lee-voh-**doh**-pă) *n.* a naturally occurring amino acid administered by mouth to treat parkinsonism. Trade names: **Berkdopa, Brocadopa, Larodopa, Veldopa.**

levorphanol (li-vor-fă-nol) *n.* a narcotic analgesic, similar to morphine, administered by mouth or injection to relieve severe pain. Trade name: **Dromoran.**

levulosuria (lev-yoo-lohs-yoor-iă) *n.* *see* fructosuria.

Leydig cells (ly-dig) *pl. n. see* interstitial cells. [F. von Leydig (1821–1908), German anatomist]

LH *n. see* luteinizing hormone.

Lhermitte's sign (lair-mits) *n.* a tingling shocklike sensation passing down the arms or trunk when the neck is flexed. It is a nonspecific indication of disease in the cervical (neck) region of the spinal cord. [J. Lhermitte (1877–1959), French neurologist]

libido (lib-ee-doh) *n.* the sexual drive: the term is often used to refer to the intensity of sexual desires. In psychoanalytic theory, the libido is one of the fundamental sources of energy for all mental life.

Librium (lib-riŭm) *n. see* chlordiazepoxide.

lice (lys) *pl. n. see* louse.

lichen (ly-kĕn) *n.* any of several types of skin disease in which small round hard lesions occur close together. *l. planus* an inflammatory condition in which wide flat mauve pimples are found mainly on the forearms, neck, and between the thighs.

lichenification (ly-ken-i-fi-kay-shŏn) *n.* the thickening of certain cell layers in the epidermis causing exaggeration of the normal creases with lozenge-shaped flat-topped shiny areas. The cause is abnormal scratching or rubbing of the skin.

lichenoid (ly-kĕn-oid) *adj.* describing any skin disease that resembles lichen.

Lieberkühn's glands (crypts of

Lieberkühn) (lee-ber-koonz) *pl. n.* simple tubular glands in the mucous membrane of the intestine. They are lined with columnar epithelium in which various types of secretory cells are found. [J. N. Lieberkühn (1711–56), German anatomist]

lien (ly-ĕn) *n. see* spleen.

lien- (lieno-) *prefix denoting* the spleen.

lienculus (ly-enk-yoo-lŭs) *n.* an accessory spleen.

lientery (ly-ĕn-ter-i) *n.* diarrhoea with the passage of undigested food in the faeces.

ligament (lig-ă-mĕnt) *n.* **1.** a tough band of white fibrous connective tissue that links two bones together at a joint. Ligaments are inelastic but flexible; they strengthen the joint and limit its movements to certain directions. **2.** a sheet of peritoneum that supports or links together abdominal organs.

ligation (li-gay-shŏn) *n.* the application of a ligature.

ligature (lig-ă-cher) *n.* any material – for example, nylon, silk, catgut, or wire – that is tied firmly round a blood vessel or duct to prevent bleeding, the passage of materials, etc.

light adaptation (lyt) *n.* reflex changes in the eye to enable vision either in normal light after being in darkness or in very bright light after being in normal light. *See* iris. *Compare* dark adaptation.

lightening (ly-t'n-ing) *n.* the descent of the womb into the pelvic cavity at a late stage of pregnancy, usually two to three weeks before labour begins. Lightening occurs when the head of the fetus turns down towards the vagina.

lightning pains (lyt-ning) *pl. n.* severe stabbing pains in the legs experienced in tabes dorsalis.

light reflex *n. see* pupillary reflex.

lignocaine (lig-nŏ-kayn) *n.* a local anaesthetic administered by injection or by direct application to mucous membranes for minor surgery and dental procedures. Lignocaine is also injected to treat conditions involving abnormal heart rhythm, particularly myocardial infarction. Trade names: **Xylocaine, Xylotox.**

limbic system (lim-bik) *n.* a complex system of nerve pathways and networks in the brain that is involved in the expression of instinct and mood in activities of the endocrine and motor systems of the body. Among the brain regions involved are the amygdala, hippocampal formation, and hypothalamus.

limbus (lim-bŭs) *n.* (in anatomy) an edge or border. *l. sclerae* the junction of the cornea and sclera of the eye.

limen (ly-men) *n.* (in anatomy) a border or boundary.

lime water (lym) *n.* an aqueous solution of calcium hydroxide used in skin preparations, as an antacid, and as an astringent.

liminal (lim-in-ăl) *adj.* (in physiology) relating to the threshold of perception.

lincomycin (link-oh-my-sin) *n.* an antibiotic administered by mouth or injection to treat infections caused by a narrow range of bacteria, including osteomyelitis. Trade names: **Lincocin, Mycivin.**

linctus (link-tŭs) *n.* a syrupy liquid medicine, particularly one used in the treatment of irritating coughs.

linea (lin-iă) *n.* (*pl.* **lineae**) (in anatomy) a line, narrow streak, or stripe. *l. alba* a tendinous line, extending from the xiphoid process to the pubic symphysis, where the flat abdominal muscles are attached. *l. nigra* a pigmented line, seen on the abdomen in pregnancy, extending from the umbilicus to the pubis.

lingual (ling-wăl) *adj.* relating to, situated close to, or resembling the tongue (lingua).

lingula (ling-yoo-lă) *n.* a thin tonguelike projection of bone or other tissue.

liniment (lin-i-měnt) *n.* a medicinal preparation that is rubbed onto the skin or applied on a surgical dressing. Liniments often contain camphor and alcohol.

linoleic acid (lin-oh-lee-ik) *n. see* essential fatty acid.

linolenic acid (lin-oh-len-ik) *n. see* essential fatty acid.

lint (lint) *n.* a material used in surgical dressings, made of scraped linen or a cotton substitute. It is usually fluffy one side and smooth the other.

liothyronine (ly-oh-th'y-rŏ-neen) *n.* a hormone produced by the thyroid gland that is similar to thyroxine and is administered by mouth or injection to treat conditions of thyroid deficiency.

lip- (lipo-) *prefix denoting* **1.** fat. **2.** lipid.

lipaemia (lip-ee-miă) *n.* the presence in the blood of an abnormally large amount of fat, such as cholesterol.

lipase (steapsin) (lip-ayz) *n.* an enzyme, produced by the pancreas and the glands of the small intestine, that breaks down fats into glycerol and fatty acids during digestion.

lipid (lip-id) *n.* one of a group of naturally occurring compounds that are soluble in solvents such as chloroform or alcohol, but insoluble in water. Lipids are important dietary constituents. The group includes fats, steroids, phospholipids, and glycolipids.

lipidosis (lipoidosis) (lip-i-**doh**-sis) *n.* (*pl.* -ses) any disorder of lipid metabolism within the cells of the body.

Lipiodol (lip-I-ŏ-dol) *n. Trademark.* a preparation of poppyseed oil and iodine, used as a contrast medium in X-ray examination of the bronchi, sinuses, and other cavities.

lipochondrodystrophy (lip-oh-kon-droh-**dis**-trŏ-fi) *n.* multiple congenital defects affecting lipid (fat) metabolism, cartilage and bone, skin, and the major internal organs, leading to mental retardation, dwarfism, and deformities of the bones.

lipodystrophy (lip-oh-**dis**-trŏ-fi) *n.* any disturbance of fat metabolism or of the distribution of fat in the body.

lipogenesis (lip-oh-**jen**-i-sis) *n.* the process by which glucose and other substances, derived from carbohydrate in the diet, are converted to fatty acids in the body.

lipoid (lip-oid) *n.* a substance, such as cholesterol, that resembles a lipid. *l. factor* one of the substances involved in the clotting of blood, important for the activation of plasma thromboplastin.

lipoidosis (lip-oi-**doh**-sis) *n. see* lipidosis.

lipolysis (lip-**ol**-i-sis) *n.* the process by which lipids are broken down into their constituent fatty acids in the body by the enzyme lipase. —**lipolytic** *adj.*

lipoma (lip-oh-mă) *n.* a common

benign tumour composed of well-differentiated fat cells.

lipomatosis (lip-oh-mă-**toh**-sis) *n.* **1.** the presence of an abnormally large amount of fat in the tissues. **2.** the presence of multiple lipomas.

lipoprotein (lip-oh-**proh**-teen) *n.* one of a group of proteins, found in blood plasma and lymph, that are combined with fats or other lipids (such as cholesterol). Lipoproteins are important for the transport of lipids in the blood and lymph.

liposarcoma (lip-oh-sar-**koh**-mă) *n.* a malignant tumour of fat cells. It is most commonly found in the thigh and is rare under the age of 30 years.

lipotropic (lip-oh-**trop**-ik) *adj.* describing a substance that promotes the transport of fatty acids from the liver to the tissues or accelerates the utilization of fat in the liver itself.

lipping (**lip**-ing) *n.* overgrowth of bone as seen in X-rays near a joint margin. This is a characteristic sign of degenerative or inflammatory joint disease, particularly osteoarthritis. *See also* osteophyte.

lipuria (adiposuria) (lip-**yoor**-iă) *n.* the presence of fat or oil droplets in the urine.

liquor (**lik**-er) *n.* (in pharmacy) any solution, usually an aqueous solution.

lith- (litho-) *prefix denoting* a calculus (stone).

-lith *suffix denoting* a calculus (stone).

lithaemia (lith-**ee**-miă) *n. see* hyperuricaemia.

lithagogue (**lith**-ă-gog) *n.* an agent that promotes the removal of stones (calculi), such as kidney stones in the urine.

lithiasis (lith-I-ă-sis) *n.* formation of stones (*see* calculus) in an internal organ.

lithium (lithium carbonate) (lith-iŭm) *n.* a drug given by mouth to prevent and treat schizophrenia and similar psychiatric disorders. Trade names: **Camcolit, Priadel.**

litholapaxy (lithotripsy) (lith-ol-ă-paks-i) *n.* the operation of crushing a stone in the bladder, using an instrument called a *lithotrite.* The small fragments of stone can then be removed by irrigation and suction.

lithonephrotomy (lith-oh-ni-frot-ŏmi) *n.* surgical removal of a stone from the kidney. *See* nephrolithotomy, pyelolithotomy.

lithopaedion (lith-oh-**pee**-di-ŏn) *n.* a fetus that has died in the womb or abdominal cavity and has become calcified.

lithotomy (lith-ot-ŏmi) *n.* the surgical removal of a stone (calculus) from the urinary tract. *See* nephrolithotomy, pyelolithotomy, ureterolithotomy.

lithotripsy (lith-ŏ-trip-si) *n. see* litholapaxy.

lithotrite (lith-ŏ-tryt) *n. see* litholapaxy.

lithuresis (lith-yoor-ee-sis) *n.* the passage of small stones or gravel in the urine.

lithuria (lith-**yoor**-iă) *n. see* hyperuricuria.

litmus (lit-mŭs) *n.* a pigment used as an indicator of acids and alkalis. In the presence of acids it turns red; with alkalis it turns blue.

litre (lee-ter) *n.* a unit of volume equal to the volume occupied by 1 kilogram of pure water at 4°C and 760 mmHg pressure.

Little's disease (li-t'lz) *n.* a form of cerebral palsy involving both

The microscopic structure of the liver

sides of the body and affecting the legs more severely than the arms. [W. J. Little (1810–94), British surgeon]

livedo (liv-**ee**-doh) *n.* a discoloured area or spot on the skin, often caused by local congestion of the circulation.

liver (liv-er) *n.* the largest gland of the body, weighing 1200–1600 g. Situated in the top right portion of the abdominal cavity, the liver has a number of important functions. It synthesizes bile, which drains into the gall bladder before being released into the duodenum. The liver is an important site of metabolism of carbohydrates, proteins, and fats. It regulates the amount of blood sugar, removes excess amino acids, and stores and metabolizes fats. The liver also synthesizes fibrinogen, prothrombin, and heparin, and has an important role in the detoxification of poisonous substances.

liver spot *n.* a local brown discoloration on the skin known medically as *senile lentigo*.

livid (liv-id) *adj.* denoting a bluish colour of the skin, such as that produced locally by a bruise or of the general complexion in cyanosis.

Loa (loh-ă) *n.* a genus of parasitic nematode worms (*see* filaria). *L. loa* the eye worm, which lives within the tissues beneath the skin and causes loiasis.

lobe (lohb) *n.* a major division of an organ or part of an organ, especially one having a rounded form and often separated from other lobes by fissures or bands of connective tissue. —**lobar** *adj.*

lobectomy (loh-bek-tŏmi) *n.* the surgical removal of a lobe of an organ or gland, such as the lung, thyroid, or brain.

lobeline (loh-bĕ-leen) *n.* a drug administered by injection to stimulate breathing or given by mouth as a smoking deterrent.

lobotomy (prefrontal leucotomy) (loh-**bot**-ŏmi) *n. see* leucotomy.

lobule (lob-yool) *n.* a subdivision of a part or organ, such as the liver or lung, that can be distinguished from the whole by boundaries, such as septa, that are visible with or without a microscope.

localized (loh-kă-lyzd) *adj.* (of a lesion, eruption, etc.) restricted to a particular part of the body; not widespread.

lochia (lok-iă) *n.* the material eliminated from the womb through the vagina after the completion of labour. The first discharge consists largely of blood (*l. rubra*). This is followed by a brownish mixture of blood and mucus (*l. serosa*), and finally a yellowish or whitish discharge containing microbes and cell fragments (*l. alba*). Each stage may last for several days. —**lochial** *adj.*

lockjaw (lok-jaw) *n. see* tetanus.

locomotor ataxia (loh-kŏ-**moh**-ter) *n. see* tabes dorsalis.

loculated (lok-yoo-layt-id) *adj.* divided into many cavities.

loculus (lok-yoo-lŭs) *n.* (in anatomy) a small space or cavity.

locum tenens (locum) (loh-kŭm teen-enz) *n.* a doctor who stands in temporarily for a colleague who is absent or ill.

locus (loh-kŭs) *n.* **1.** (in anatomy) a region or site. **2.** (in genetics) the region of a chromosome occupied by a particular gene.

log- (logo-) *prefix denoting* words; speech.

logopaedics (log-ŏ-pee-diks) *n.* the scientific study of defects and disabilities of speech and of the methods used to treat them; speech therapy.

-logy (-ology) *suffix denoting* field of study.

loiasis (loh-I-ă-sis) *n.* a disease, occurring in West and Central Africa, caused by the eye worm *Loa loa*. The adult worms live and migrate within the skin tissues, causing inflammation and swellings, and often migrate across the eyeball just beneath the conjunctiva, producing irritation and congestion. Loiasis is treated with diethylcarbamazine.

loin (loin) *n.* the region of the back and side of the body between the lowest rib and the pelvis.

long-sightedness (long-syt-id-nis) *n. see* hypermetropia.

loop (loop) *n.* **1.** a bend in a tubular organ. **2.** one of the patterns of dermal ridges in fingerprints.

lorazepam (lor-az-ĕ-pam) *n.* a tranquillizer administered by mouth to relieve moderate or severe anxiety and tension and to treat insomnia. Trade name: **Ativan.**

lordosis (lor-**doh**-sis) *n.* inward curvature of the spine. A certain degree of lordosis is normal in the lumbar and cervical regions of the spine. Exaggerated lordosis may occur in adolescence, through faulty posture or as a result of disease. *Compare* kyphosis.

lotion (loh-shŏn) *n.* a medicinal solution for external use. Lotions usually have a cooling, soothing, or antiseptic action.

loupe (loop) *n.* a small magnifying hand lens used for examining the front part of the eye.

louse (lowss) *n.* (*pl.* **lice**) a small wingless bloodsucking insect that is an external parasite of man and may transmit disease. Lice attach themselves to hair and clothing; they thrive in overcrowded and unhygienic conditions. *See also* Pediculus, Phthirus.

lozenge (loz-inj) *n.* a medicated tablet containing sugar.

LSD *n.* *see* lysergic acid diethylamide.

lubb-dupp (lub-**dup**) *n.* a representation of the normal heart sounds as heard through the stethoscope. The first coincides with closure of the mitral and tricuspid valves; the second with closure of the aortic and pulmonary valves.

Ludwig's angina (luud-vigz) *n.* severe inflammation caused by bacterial infection of the floor of the mouth, resulting in massive swelling of the neck. [W. F. von Ludwig (1790–1865), German surgeon]

lues (loo-eez) *n.* a serious infectious disease such as bubonic plague or syphilis.

Lugol's solution (loo-golz) *n.* an aqueous solution of iodine and potassium iodide. [J. G. A. Lugol (1786–1851), French physician]

lumbago (lum-**bay**-goh) *n.* low backache, of any cause or description. Severe lumbago, of sudden onset, can be due either to a slipped disc or to a strained muscle or ligament.

lumbar (lum-ber) *adj.* relating to the loin. *l. puncture* a procedure in which cerebrospinal fluid is withdrawn for diagnostic purposes by means of a hollow needle inserted into the subarachnoid space in the region of the lower back (usually between the third and fourth lumbar vertebrae). *See also* Queckenstedt test. *l. vertebrae* the five bones of the backbone that are situated between the thoracic vertebrae and the sacrum, in the lower part of the back. *See also* vertebra.

lumbo- *prefix denoting* the loin; lumbar region.

lumbosacral (lum-boh-say-krăl) *adj.* relating to the part of the spine composed of the lumbar vertebrae and the sacrum.

lumen (loo-min) *n.* **1.** the space within a tubular or saclike part. **2.** the SI unit of luminous flux. Symbol: lm.

lunate bone (loo-nayt) *n.* a bone of the wrist (*see* carpus). It articulates with the capitate bone in

The lungs and main air passages

Details of the alveoli

front and with the radius and ulna behind.

lung (lung) *n.* one of the pair of organs of respiration, situated in the chest cavity on either side of the heart. The lungs communicate with the atmosphere through the trachea, which opens into the pharynx. The trachea divides into two bronchi, which enter the lungs and branch into bronchioles. These divide further and terminate in minute air sacs (*see* alveolus), the sites of gaseous exchange. Atmospheric oxygen is absorbed and carbon dioxide from the blood of the pulmonary capillaries is released into the lungs (*see* (pulmonary) circulation).

lung cancer *n.* cancer arising in the epithelium of the air passages (*bronchial cancer*) or lung. It is strongly associated with cigarette smoking and exposure to industrial air pollutants (including asbestos). Treatment includes surgical removal of the affected lobe or lung, radiotherapy, and chemotherapy.

lunula (loon-yoo-lă) *n.* the whitish crescent-shaped area at the base of a nail.

lupus (loo-pŭs) *n.* any of several chronic skin diseases. *l. erythematosus* (*LE*) an inflammatory disease of connective tissue, affecting the skin and various internal organs. Typically, there is a red scaly rash on the nose and cheeks; arthritis; and progressive damage to the kidneys. Often the heart, lungs, and brain are also affected. LE is regarded as an autoimmune disease and can be diagnosed by a test that reveals characteristic white blood cells (*LE cells*). The disease is treated with corticosteroids. *l. verrucosus* a tuberculous infection of the skin – commonly the arm or hand – typified by warty lesions. It occurs in those who have been reinfected with tuberculosis. *l. vulgaris* a tuberculous infection of the skin that often starts in childhood, with dark red patches on the nose or cheek. Unless treated with antituberculous drugs lupus vulgaris spreads, ulcerates, and causes extensive scarring.

lutein (loo-ti-in) *n.* 1. *see* xanthophyll. 2. the yellow pigment of the corpus luteum.

luteinizing hormone (LH) (loo-ti-i-nyz-ing) *n.* a hormone (*see* gonadotrophin), synthesized and released by the anterior pituitary gland, that stimulates ovulation, corpus luteum formation, progesterone synthesis by the ovary, and androgen synthesis by the testes. Also called: **interstitial-cell-stimulating hormone (ICSH)**.

luteo- *prefix denoting* 1. yellow. 2. the corpus luteum.

luteotrophic hormone (luteotrophin) (loo-ti-oh-trof-ik) *n.* *see* prolactin.

luxation (luks-ay-shŏn) *n.* *see* dislocation.

lymph (limf) *n.* the fluid present within the vessels of the lymphatic system, which is derived from the fluid that bathes the tissues. Lymph is similar in composition to plasma, but contains less protein and some cells, mainly lymphocytes. *l. node* one of a number of small swellings found at intervals along the lymphatic system. Groups of nodes occur in the groin and armpit, behind the ear, and in many other parts. They act as filters for the lymph and produce lymphocytes.

lymphaden- (lymphadeno-) *prefix denoting* lymph node(s).

lymphadenectomy (lim-fad-in-ek-tŏmi) *n.* surgical removal of lymph nodes.

lymphadenitis (lim-fad-in-I-tis) *n.* inflammation of lymph nodes, which become swollen, painful, and tender. The most commonly affected lymph nodes are those in the neck, in association with tonsillitis.

lymphadenoma (lim-fad-in-oh-mă) *n.* an obsolete term for lymphoma.

lymphangi- (lymphangio-) *prefix denoting* a lymphatic vessel.

lymphangiectasis (lim-fan-ji-ek-tă-sis) *n.* dilatation of the lymphatic vessels, which is usually congenital. It may also be caused by obstruction of the lymphatic vessels (*see* lymphoedema).

lymphangiography (lim-fan-ji-og-răfi) *n.* X-ray examination of the lymphatic vessels and lymph nodes after a contrast medium has been injected into them (*see* angiography).

lymphangioma (lim-fan-ji-oh-mă) *n.* a localized collection of distended lymphatic vessels, which may result in a large cyst in the neck or armpit (cystic hygroma).

lymphangioplasty (lim-fan-ji-oh-plasti) *n.* the surgical creation of artificial lymph channels when the lymphatic vessels are obstructed.

lymphangiosarcoma (lim-fan-ji-oh-sar-koh-mă) *n.* a malignant tumour of the lymphatic vessels. It is most commonly seen in the arms of women who have had a mastectomy for breast cancer.

lymphangitis (lim-fan-jy-tis) *n.* inflammation of the lymphatic vessels, which can be seen most commonly as red streaks in the skin adjacent to a focus of streptococcal infection.

lymphatic (lim-fat-ik) **1.** *n.* a lymphatic vessel. *See* lymphatic system. **2.** *adj.* relating to or transporting lymph.

lymphatic system *n.* a network of vessels that conveys electrolytes, water, proteins, etc. – in the form of lymph – from the tissue fluids to the bloodstream. Lymph passes through fine capillaries into the lymphatic vessels, which have valves to prevent backflow of lymph. The lymphatics lead to two large channels – the *thoracic duct* and the *right lymphatic duct* – which return the lymph to the bloodstream via the innominate veins.

lympho- *prefix denoting* lymph or the lymphatic system.

lymphoblast (lim-foh-blast) *n.* an abnormal cell present in the blood and blood-forming organs in a type of leukaemia (*lymphoblastic leukaemia*). —**lymphoblastic** *adj.*

lymphocyte (lim-foh-syt) *n.* a variety of white blood cell (leucocyte), present also in the lymph nodes, spleen, thymus gland, gut wall, and bone marrow. They are involved in immunity and can be subdivided into *B-lymphocytes*, which produce antibodies, and *T-lymphocytes*, which are involved in graft rejection, etc. —**lymphocytic** *adj.*

lymphocytopenia (lim-foh-sy-toh-pee-niă) *n. see* lymphopenia.

lymphocytosis (lim-foh-sy-toh-sis) *n.* an increase in the number of lymphocytes in the blood.

lymphoedema (lim-fee-dee-mă) *n.* an accumulation of lymph in the tissues, producing swelling. It may be due to a congenital abnormality of the lymphatic vessels or result from obstruction of the lymphatic vessels by a tumour, parasites, inflammation, or injury.

lymphogranuloma venereum (lim-foh-gran-yoo-**loo**-mă vi-**neer**-iŭm) *n.* a venereal disease that is caused by a virus and is most common in tropical regions. An initial lesion on the genitals is followed by swelling and inflammation of the lymph nodes in the groin. Early treatment with sulphonamides or tetracyclines is usually effective.

lymphography (lim-**fog**-răfi) *n.* the technique of injecting radio-opaque material into the lymphatic system in a particular region of the body so that X-ray photographs may be taken of the lymph vessels and nodes.

lymphoid tissue (lim-foid) *n.* a tissue responsible for the production of lymphocytes and antibodies. It occurs in the form of the lymph nodes, tonsils, thymus, and spleen, and also as diffuse groups of cells.

lymphoma (lim-**foh**-mă) *n.* any malignant tumour of lymph nodes, excluding Hodgkin's disease. Disease is usually widespread, but in some cases is confined to a single area, such as the tonsil. Treatment is with drugs such as chlorambucil or combinations of cyclophosphamide, vincristine, and prednisone.

lymphopenia (**lymphocytopenia**) (lim-foh-**pee**-niă) *n.* a decrease in the number of lymphocytes in the blood.

lymphopoiesis (lim-foh-poi-**ee**-sis) *n.* the process of the production of lymphocytes, which occurs in the bone marrow as well as in the lymph nodes, spleen, thymus gland, and gut wall.

lymphorrhagia (lim-fŏ-**ray**-jiă) *n.* the escape of the lymph from lymphatic vessels that have been injured.

lymphosarcoma (lim-foh-sar-**koh**-mă) *n.* an old term for certain types of lymphoma.

lymphuria (limf-**yoor**-iă) *n.* the presence in the urine of lymph.

lynoestrenol (lin-ees-trĕ-nol) *n.* a synthetic female sex hormone (*see* progestogen) used mainly in oral contraceptives, together with an oestrogen. It is also used to treat menstrual disorders.

lyophilization (ly-ofi-ly-**zay**-shŏn) *n.* preservation of biological material (e.g. plasma, serum, skin) by rapid freezing followed by dehydration.

lys- (lysi-, lyso-) *prefix denoting* lysis; dissolution.

lysergic acid diethylamide (LSD) (ly-**ser**-jik **ass**-id dy-eth-il-ay-myd) *n.* a psychedelic drug that is also a hallucinogen. It has been used to aid treatment of psychological disorders. Alterations in sight, hearing, and other senses occur, psychotic effects, depression, and confusion are common, and tolerance to the drug develops rapidly. Because of these toxic effects, LSD is used only to treat severe cases.

lysin (ly-sin) *n.* a protein component in the blood that is capable of bringing about the destruction (lysis) of whole cells. *Haemolysin* attacks red blood cells, *leucolysin* white cells, and a *bacteriolysin* bacterial cells.

lysine (ly-seen) *n.* an essential amino acid. *See also* amino acid.

lysis (ly-sis) *n.* **1.** the destruction of cells through damage or rupture of the plasma membrane, allowing escape of the cell contents. *See also* autolysis, lysozyme. **2.** gradual remission of the symptoms of a disease.

-lysis *suffix denoting* lysis; dissolution.

lysosome (ly-sŏ-sohm) *n.* a particle in the cytoplasm of cells that contains enzymes responsible for breaking down substances in the cell. Lysosomes are especially abundant in liver and kidney cells.

lysozyme (ly-sŏ-zym) *n.* an enzyme found in tears and egg white. It catalyses the destruction of the cell walls of certain bacteria.

M

maceration (mas-er-ay-shŏn) *n.* **1.** the softening of a solid by leaving it immersed in a liquid. **2.** (in obstetrics) the natural breakdown of a dead fetus within the womb.

Mackenrodt's ligaments (mahk-ĕn-rohts) *pl. n. see* cardinal ligaments. [A. K. Mackenrodt (1859–1925), German gynaecologist]

macr- (macro-) *prefix denoting* large size.

macrocephaly (megalocephaly) (mak-roh-sef-ăli) *n.* abnormal largeness of the head. *Compare* microcephaly.

macrocheilia (mak-roh-ky-liă) *n.* hypertrophy of the lips: a congenital condition in which the lips are abnormally large. *Compare* microcheilia.

macrocyte (megalocyte) (mak-roh-syt) *n.* an abnormally large red blood cell (erythrocyte). *See also* macrocytosis. —**macrocytic** *adj.*

macrocytosis (mak-roh-sy-toh-sis) *n.* the presence of macrocytes in the blood. Macrocytosis is a fea-

ture of certain anaemias (*macrocytic anaemias*), including those due to deficiency of vitamin B_{12} or folic acid.

macrodactyly (mak-roh-dak-tili) *n.* abnormally large size of one or more of the fingers or toes.

macrogenitosoma (mak-roh-jen-it-oh-soh-mă) *n.* excessive bodily growth with marked enlargement of the genitalia.

macroglobulin (immunoglobulin M) (mak-roh-glob-yoo-lin) *n.* a protein of the globulin series that is present in the blood and functions as an antibody, forming an effective first-line defence against bacteria in the bloodstream. *See also* immunoglobulin.

macroglossia (mak-roh-glos-iă) *n.* an abnormally large tongue. It may be due to a congenital defect, to infiltration of the tongue with amyloid or a tumour, or to obstruction of the lymph vessels.

macrognathia (mak-roh-nay-thiă) *n.* marked overgrowth of one jaw relative to the growth of the other.

macromastia (mak-roh-mas-tiă) *n.* abnormally large size of the breasts.

macromelia (mak-roh-mee-liă) *n.* abnormally large size of the arms or legs. *Compare* micromelia.

macrophage (clasmocyte) (mak-roh-fayj) *n.* a large scavenger cell (*see* phagocyte) present in connective tissue and many major organs and tissues, including the bone marrow, spleen, lymph nodes, liver, and the central nervous system. *See also* histiocyte, reticuloendothelial system.

macropsia (mak-rop-siă) *n.* a condition in which objects appear larger than they really are. It is usually due to disease of the retina.

macroscopic (mak-roh-**skop**-ik) *adj.* visible to the naked eye. *Compare* microscopic.

macula (**mak**-yoo-lă) *n.* (*pl.* **maculae**) **1.** a small anatomical area that is distinguishable from the surrounding tissue. *m. lutea* the yellow spot on the retina at the back of the eye, which surrounds the greatest concentration of cones (*see* fovea). **2.** *see* macule.

macule (**macula**) (**mak**-yool) *n.* a spot, discoloration, or thickening of the skin that forms a distinct area from the surrounding normal surface. *Compare* papule.

maculopapular (mak-yoo-loh-**pap**-yoo-ler) *adj.* describing a rash that consists of both macules and papules.

Madura foot (mă-**dewr**-ă) *n.* an infection of the tissues and bones of the foot producing chronic inflammation (mycetoma), occurring in the tropics. Medical name: **maduromycosis.**

Madurella (mad-yoo-**rel**-ă) *n.* a genus of widely distributed fungi. The species *M. grisea* and *M. mycetomi* cause the tropical infection Madura foot.

maduromycosis (mă-dewr-oh-my-**koh**-sis) *n. see* Madura foot.

Magendie's foramen (ma-**jen**-deez) *n.* an opening in the roof of the fourth ventricle of the brain through which cerebrospinal fluid passes to the subarachnoid space. [F. Magendie (1783–1855), French physiologist]

magenta (mă-**jen**-tă) *n. see* fuchsin.

maggot (**mag**-ŏt) *n.* the wormlike larva of a fly, which occasionally infests human tissues (*see* myiasis).

magnesium (mag-**nee**-ziŭm) *n.* a metallic element essential to life. Magnesium is necessary for the proper functioning of muscle and nervous tissue. Symbol: Mg. *m. carbonate* a weak antacid used to relieve indigestion and also pain due to stomach and duodenal ulcers; it is also used as a mild laxative. *m. hydroxide* a magnesium salt with effects and uses similar to those of magnesium carbonate. Trade name: **Milk of Magnesia.** *m. sulphate* a magnesium salt given in mixtures or enemas to treat constipation (*see* laxative). It is also administered by injection to treat magnesium deficiency. *m. trisilicate* a compound of magnesium with antacid and absorbent properties, used in the treatment of peptic ulcers and other digestive disorders.

mal (mal) *n.* illness or disease. *See also* grand mal, petit mal.

mal- *prefix denoting* disease, disorder, or abnormality.

malabsorption (mal-ăb-**sorp**-shŏn) *n.* a state in which absorption by the small intestine of one or more substances, such as fat, vitamins, or amino acids, is reduced. Symptoms (depending on the substances involved) include weight loss, diarrhoea, anaemia, swelling (oedema), and vitamin deficiencies. The commonest causes are coeliac disease, pancreatitis, cystic fibrosis, stagnant-loop syndrome, or surgical removal of a length of small intestine.

malacia (mă-**lay**-shiă) *n.* abnormal softening of a part, organ, or tissue, such as bone (*see* osteomalacia).

-malacia *suffix denoting* abnormal softening of a tissue.

malaise (mal-ayz) *n.* a general feeling of being unwell. The feeling may be accompanied by identifiable physical discomfort and may indicate the presence of disease.

malar bone (may-ler) *n. see* zygomatic bone.

malaria (**ague, marsh fever, periodic fever, paludism**) (mă-lair-iă) *n.* an infectious disease due to the presence of parasitic protozoa of the genus *Plasmodium* within the red blood cells. The disease is transmitted by the *Anopheles* mosquito and is confined mainly to tropical and subtropical areas. After an incubation period varying from 12 days to 10 months parasites invade, multiply within, and eventually destroy the red blood cells, releasing new parasites. This causes a short bout of shivering, fever, and sweating, and the loss of healthy red cells results in anaemia. When the next batch of parasites is released symptoms reappear. The interval between fever attacks varies in different types of malaria (*see* quartan fever, quotidian fever, tertian fever). Preventative and curative treatment relies on such drugs as chloroquine, mepacrine, and proguanil.

malarial therapy (mă-lair-iăl) *n.* a treatment for neurosyphilis in which a high fever is induced by infecting the patient with malaria parasites.

malformation (mal-for-may-shŏn) *n.* any variation from the normal physical structure, due either to congenital or developmental defects or to disease or injury.

malignant (mă-lig-nănt) *adj.* **1.** describing a tumour that invades and destroys the tissue in which it originates and can spread to other sites in the body. If untreated such tumours cause progressive deterioration and death. *See* cancer. **2.** describing any disorder that becomes progressively worse if untreated. *Compare* benign.

malignant pustule *n. see* anthrax.

malingering (mă-ling-er-ing) *n.* pretending to be ill, usually in order to avoid work or gain attention. It may be a sign of mental disorder (*see* Munchhausen's syndrome).

malleolus (mă-lee-ŏ-lŭs) *n.* either of the two protuberances on each side of the ankle: at the lower end of the fibula (*lateral m.*) and at the lower end of the tibia (*medial m.*).

malleus (**mal**-iŭs) *n.* a hammer-shaped bone in the middle ear that articulates with the incus and is attached to the eardrum. *See* ossicle.

malnutrition (mal-new-**trish**-ŏn) *n.* the condition caused by an improper balance between what an individual eats and what he requires to maintain health. This can result from eating too little (*subnutrition* or *starvation*) but may also imply dietary excess or an incorrect balance of basic foodstuffs.

malocclusion (mal-ŏ-kloo-zhŏn) *n.* the condition in which the upper and lower teeth are abnormally related.

Malpighian body (mal-**pig**-iăn) *n.* the part of a nephron comprising the blood capillaries of the glomerulus and its surrounding Bowman's capsule. [M. Malpighi (1628–94), Italian anatomist]

Malpighian layer *n.* the stratum germinativum: one of the layers of the epidermis.

malposition (mal-pŏ-**zish**-ŏn) *n*. abnormal location of any part of the body.

malpractice (mal-**prak**-tis) *n*. professional misconduct: treatment falling short of the standards of skill and care that can reasonably be expected from a qualified medical practitioner.

malpresentation (mal-prez-ĕn-tay-shŏn) *n*. arrival of the fetus at the opening from the womb other than in the normal head-first position (*see* presentation).

malt (mawlt) *n*. a mixture of carbohydrates, predominantly maltose, produced by the breakdown of starch contained in barley or wheat grains. Malt is used for brewing and distilling; it has been used as a source of nutrients in wasting diseases.

Malta fever (**mawl**-tă) *n. see* brucellosis.

maltase (**mawl**-tayz) *n*. an enzyme, present in saliva and pancreatic juice, that converts maltose into glucose during digestion.

maltose (**mawl**-tohz) *n*. a sugar consisting of two molecules of glucose. Maltose is formed from the digestion of starch and glycogen.

malunion (mal-**yoon**-yŏn) *n*. deformity of a bone resulting from union of a fracture in which the bone ends are poorly aligned. Osteotomy may be needed to correct the deformity.

mamilla (mă-**mil**-ă) *n. see* nipple.

mamma (**mam**-ă) *n. see* breast.

mammary gland (**mam**-er-i) *n*. the milk-producing gland of female mammals. *See* breast.

mammography (mam-og-**răfi**) *n*. the making of X-ray or infra-red ray photographs of the breast: used for the early detection of abnormal growths. *See also* radiography, thermography.

mammoplasty (**mam**-ŏ-plasti) *n*. plastic surgery of the breasts, in order to alter their shape or increase or decrease their size.

mammothermography (mam-oh-ther-**mog**-răfi) *n*. the technique of examining the breasts for the presence of tumours or other abnormalities by thermography.

mandible (**man**-dib-ŭl) *n*. the lower jawbone. It consists of a horseshoe-shaped body, the upper surface of which bears the lower teeth, and two vertical branches (rami). *See also* temporo-mandibular joint. —**mandibular** (man-**dib**-yoo-ler) *adj*.

manganese (mang-ă-neez) *n*. a greyish metallic element, the oxide of which, when inhaled by miners in under-ventilated mines, causes brain damage. Symbol: Mn.

mania (**may**-niă) *n*. a state of mind characterized by excessive cheerfulness and increased activity. The mood is euphoric and changes rapidly to irritability. Thought and speech are rapid to the point of incoherence and the connections between ideas may be impossible to follow. Treatment is usually with drugs such as lithium or phenothiazines. *See* manic-depressive psychosis. —**manic** (**man**-ik) *adj*.

-mania *suffix denoting* obsession, compulsion, or exaggerated feeling for.

manic-depressive psychosis (man-ik-di-**pres**-iv) *n*. a severe mental illness causing repeated episodes of depression, mania, or both. Treatment is with phenothiazine drugs for mania and with antidepressant drugs or electroconvulsive therapy for depression.

Lithium can prevent or reduce the frequency and severity of attacks, and the sufferer is usually well in the intervals between them.

manipulation (mă-nip-yoo-**lay**-shŏn) *n.* the use of the hands to produce a desired movement or therapeutic effect in part of the body.

mannitol (**man**-i-tol) *n.* a diuretic administered by injection to supplement other diuretics in the treatment of fluid retention (oedema), to treat some kidney disorders, and to relieve pressure in brain injuries.

mannomustine (man-oh-**must**-een) *n.* a drug that prevents the growth of cancer cells and is administered by mouth or injection in the treatment of some types of leukaemia and other cancers. Trade name: **Degranol**.

manometer (mă-**nom**-it-er) *n.* a device for measuring pressure in a gas. *See also* sphygmomanometer.

Mantoux test (man-**too**) *n.* a test for immunity to tuberculosis. Tuberculin is injected beneath the skin and a patch of inflammation appearing in the next 18 – 24 hours indicates that a degree of immunity is present. [C. Mantoux (1877 – 1947), French physician]

manubrium (mă-**new**-bri-ŭm) *n.* (*pl.* **manubria**) 1. the upper section of the breastbone (*see* sternum). It articulates with the clavicles and the first costal cartilage. 2. the handle-like part of the malleus, attached to the eardrum. —**manubrial** *adj.*

MAO *n. see* monoamine oxidase.

MAO inhibitor *n.* any drug, such as iproniazid or phenelzine, that prevents the activity of the en-

zyme monoamine oxidase (MAO) in brain tissue and therefore affects mood. MAO inhibitors are antidepressants; their side-effects include interactions with other drugs and foods containing tyramine (e.g. cheese) to produce a sudden increase in blood pressure.

maple syrup urine disease (**may**-pŭl si-**rŭp**) *n.* an inborn defect of amino acid metabolism causing an excess of valine, leucine, isoleucine, and alloisoleucine in the urine, which has an odour like maple syrup. Untreated it leads to mental retardation and death in infancy.

maprotiline (mă-**proh**-til-een) *n.* a drug administered by mouth to treat all types of depression, including that associated with anxiety (*see* antidepressant). It is administered by mouth and may cause drowsiness, dizziness, and tremor. Trade name: **Ludiomil**.

marasmus (mă-**raz**-mŭs) *n.* severe wasting in infants, when body weight is below 75% of that expected for age. The infant looks 'old', pallid, apathetic, lacks skin fat, and has subnormal temperature. The condition may be due to malabsorption, wrong feeding, metabolic disorders, repeated vomiting, diarrhoea, or disease.

marble-bone disease (mar-bŭl bohn) *n. see* osteopetrosis.

Marburg disease (green monkey disease) (mar-berg) *n.* a virus disease of vervet (green) monkeys transmitted to man by contact with blood or tissues from an infected animal. Symptoms include fever, malaise, severe headache, vomiting, diarrhoea, and bleeding from mucous membranes. Treatment with antiserum and measures to reduce the bleeding are sometimes effective.

Marfan's syndrome (mar-**fahnz**) *n.* an inherited disorder of connective tissue characterized by excessive height, abnormally long and slender fingers and toes (*arachnodactyly*), heart defects, and partial dislocation of the lenses of the eyes. [B. J. A. Marfan (1858–1942), French physician]

marihuana (ma-ri-**hwah**-nǎ) *n. see* cannabis.

marrow (**ma**-roh) *n. see* bone marrow.

marsupialization (mar-soo-piǎl-I-zay-shŏn) *n.* an operative technique for curing a cyst. The cyst is opened, its contents removed, and the edges then stitched to the skin incision.

Marzine (**mar**-zeen) *n. see* cyclizine.

masculinization (mas-kew-lin-I-zay-shŏn) *n.* development of excess body and facial hair, deepening of the voice, and increase in muscle bulk in a female due to a hormone disorder or to hormone therapy. *See also* virilism, virilization.

Maslow's hierarchy of human needs (**maz**-lohz) *n.* a listing of human needs in order of priority, from basic physiological needs (e.g. eating and drinking) to self-actualization. It is held that the individual does not consider meeting each level of need until the previous level has been at least partly satisfied. *See* self-actualization. [A. H. Maslow (1908–70), US psychologist]

masochism (**mas**-ŏ-kizm) *n.* sexual pleasure derived from the experience of pain. *See* perversion. —**masochist** *n.* —**masochistic** *adj.*

massage (mas-ah*zh*) *n.* manipula-tion of the soft tissues of the body with the hands. Massage is used to improve circulation, prevent adhesions in tissues after injury, and reduce muscular spasm. *See also* effleurage, petrissage, tapotement.

masseter (ma-**see**-ter) *n.* a thick muscle in the cheek extending from the zygomatic arch to the outer corner of the mandible. It is important for mastication and acts by closing the jaws.

mast- (masto-) *prefix denoting* the breast.

mastalgia (mas-**tal**-jiǎ) *n.* pain in the breast.

mastatrophy (mastatrophia) (mas-tat-rŏfi) *n.* atrophy of the breasts.

mast cell (mahst) *n.* a large cell in connective tissue. Mast cells contain heparin, histamine, and serotonin, which are released during inflammation and allergic responses.

mastectomy (mas-**tek**-tŏmi) *n.* surgical removal of a breast. *radical m.* surgical removal of the breast itself, the lymph nodes in the nearest armpit, and the muscles linking the upper part of the chest with the shoulder, to combat cancer.

mastication (mas-ti-**kay**-shŏn) *n.* the process of chewing food.

mastitis (mas-**ty**-tis) *n.* inflammation of the breast, usually caused by bacterial infection through damaged nipples. *cystic m.* chronic mastitis in which the breast feels lumpy due to the presence of cysts. *puerperal m.* acute mastitis that develops during the period of breast-feeding.

mastoid (**mas**-toid) *adj.* relating to the mastoid process. *m. antrum* an air-filled channel connecting the mastoid process to the cavity of the middle ear. *m. cells* air spaces in the mastoid process. *m. process* a nipple-shaped process on the temporal bone that extends downward and forward behind the ear canal.

mastoidectomy (mas-toi-**dek**-tŏmi) *n.* an operation to remove some or all of the mastoid cells when they have become infected (*see* mastoiditis).

mastoiditis (mas-toi-**dy**-tis) *n.* inflammation of the mastoid process and antrum, usually caused by bacterial infection that spreads from the middle ear. *See* otitis (media).

mastoidotomy (mas-toi-**dot**-ŏmi) *n.* surgical incision of the mastoid bone, usually done to treat infection (*see* mastoidectomy).

masturbation (mas-ter-**bay**-shŏn) *n.* physical stimulation of the male or female external genital organs in order to produce sexual pleasure, which may result in orgasm.

materia medica (mă-**teer**-iă **med**-ikă) *n.* the study of drugs used in medicine, including pharmacognosy, pharmacy, pharmacology, and therapeutics.

maternal deprivation (mă-**ter**-năl) *n.* the condition said to result if infants are deprived of the opportunity to form a close relationship with a single parental figure, who may or may not be the child's natural parent. It is characterized by distress and depression, leading to an inability to form lasting relationships.

maternal mortality rate *n.* the number of deaths due to complications of pregnancy, childbirth, and the puerperium expressed as a proportion of all births (i.e. including stillbirths). The rate is usually expressed per 100,000 births.

matrix (**may**-triks) *n.* the substance of a tissue or organ in which more specialized structures are embedded.

mattress suture (**mat**-ris) *n.* a suture in which a loop is made on each side of the incision, which may be parallel with the incision (*horizontal m. s.*) or at right angles to it (*vertical m. s.*).

maturation (mat-yoor-**ay**-shŏn) *n.* the process of attaining full development.

maxilla (maks-**il**-ă) *n.* (*pl.* **maxillae** or **maxillas**) 1. (loosely) the upper jaw. 2. either of the pair of bones contributing to the upper jaw, the orbits, the nasal cavity, and the roof of the mouth (*see* palate). —**maxillary** (maks-**il**-er-i) *adj.*

maxillary sinus *n. see* paranasal sinuses.

mazindol (mă-**zin**-dol) *n.* a drug that reduces the appetite and is administered by mouth in the treatment of obesity. Trade name: **Teronac**.

McBurney's point (măk-**ber**-niz) *n.* the point on the abdomen that overlies the anatomical position of the appendix and is the site of maximum tenderness in acute appendicitis. [C. McBurney (1845–1913), US surgeon]

mean (**arithmetic mean**) (meen) *n.* the average of a group of observations calculated by adding their values and dividing by the number in the group.

measles (**mee**-zŭlz) *n.* a highly infectious virus disease that mainly affects children. Early symptoms are those of a cold accompanied by a high fever, and Koplik's spots may appear on the inside of the cheeks. On the third to fifth day a blotchy slightly elevated pink rash develops; it lasts 3–5 days. The patient is infectious throughout this period. In most cases the symptoms soon subside but patients are susceptible to pneumonia and middle ear infections. Medical names: **rubeola, morbilli.**

meat- (meato-) *prefix denoting* a meatus.

meatus (mee-ay-tŭs) *n.* (in anatomy) a passage or opening. *external auditory m.* the passage leading from the pinna of the outer ear to the eardrum. *nasal m.* one of three groovelike parts of the nasal cavity beneath each of the nasal conchae. *urethral m.* the external opening of the urethra.

mecamylamine (mek-ă-mil-ă-meen) *n.* a drug administered by mouth to lower high blood pressure. Trade name: **Inversine.**

mechanism of labour (mek-ă-nizm) *n.* the sum of the forces that act to expel a fetus from the womb together with those that resist its expulsion and affect its position during birth. *See* labour.

mechanotherapy (mek-ă-noh-th'e-ră-pi) *n.* the use of mechanical equipment during physiotherapy to produce regularly repeated movements in part of the body.

Meckel's diverticulum (mek-ĕlz) *n.* see diverticulum. [J. F. Meckel (1781–1833), German anatomist]

meclozine (mek-lŏ-zeen) *n.* an antihistamine drug administered by mouth to prevent and treat nausea and vomiting, particularly in travel sickness, and also to relieve allergic reactions.

meconism (mek-oh-nizm) *n.* poisoning from the effects of eating or smoking opium or the products derived from it, especially morphine.

meconium (mi-koh-niŭm) *n.* the first stools of a newborn baby, which are sticky and dark green and composed of cellular debris, mucus, and bile pigments. *m. ileus* obstruction of the ileum caused by thickened meconium in babies with cystic fibrosis.

media (tunica media) (meed-iă) *n.* **1.** the middle layer of the wall of a vein or artery. **2.** the middle layer of various other organs or parts.

medial (mee-di-ăl) *adj.* relating to or situated in the central region of an organ, tissue, or the body.

median (mee-di-ăn) *adj.* (in anatomy) situated in or towards the plane that divides the body into right and left halves.

mediastinitis (mee-di-asti-ny-tis) *n.* inflammation of the mediastinum, usually complicating a rupture of the oesophagus (gullet).

mediastinum (mee-di-ă-sty-nŭm) *n.* the space in the thorax between the two pleural sacs. The mediastinum contains the heart, aorta, trachea, oesophagus, and thymus gland.

medical (med-ik-ăl) *adj.* **1.** of or relating to the science or practice of medicine. **2.** of or relating to conditions that require the attention of a physician rather than a surgeon.

medical certificate *n.* a certificate stating a doctor's diagnosis of a patient's medical condition, disability, or fitness to work.

medical jurisprudence *n.* the study or practice of the legal aspects of medicine. *See* forensic medicine.

medical social worker *n.* a person with some medical training, employed to assist patients with domestic problems that may arise through illness.

medicated (med-i-kayt-id) *adj.* containing a medicinal drug: applied to lotions, soaps, sweets, etc.

medication (med-i-kay-shŏn) *n.* 1. a substance administered by mouth, applied to the body, or introduced into the body for the purpose of treatment. *See also* premedication. 2. treatment of a patient using drugs.

medicine (med-sin) *n.* 1. the science or practice of the diagnosis, treatment, and prevention of disease. 2. the science or practice of nonsurgical methods of treating disease. 3. any drug or preparation used for the treatment or prevention of disease, particularly a preparation that is taken by mouth.

medicochirurgical (med-i-koh-ky-rer-jik-ăl) *adj.* of or describing matters that are related to both medicine and surgery.

Mediterranean fever (med-it-er-ay-ni-ăn) *n.* 1. *see* brucellosis. 2. *see* polyserositis.

medium (meed-iŭm) *n.* 1. any substance, usually a broth, agar, or gelatin, used for the culture of microorganisms or tissue cells. 2. *see* contrast medium.

medroxyprogesterone (med-roks-i-proh-jes-ter-ohn) *n.* a synthetic female sex hormone (*see* progestogen) used to treat menstrual disorders, to prevent miscarriage, and in oral contraceptives. It is administered by mouth or injection. Trade name: **Provera**.

medulla (mi-dul-ă) *n.* 1. the inner region of any organ or tissue, particularly the inner part of the kidney, adrenal glands, or lymph nodes. *m. oblongata* (*myelencephalon*) the extension within the skull of the upper end of the spinal cord, containing centres responsible for the regulation of the heart and blood vessels, respiration, salivation, and swallowing. 2. the myelin layer of certain nerve fibres. —**medullary** *adj.*

medullated (myelinated) nerve fibre (med-ŭl-ayt-id) *n. see* myelin.

medulloblastoma (mi-dul-oh-blas-toh-mă) *n.* a cerebral tumour that occurs during childhood, usually developing adjacent to the fourth ventricle. It causes an unsteady gait and shaky limb movements.

mefenamic acid (me-fen-am-ik) *n.* an analgesic that also reduces inflammation and fever and is administered by mouth to treat headache, toothache, rheumatic pain, and similar conditions. Trade name: **Ponstan**.

mega- *prefix denoting* 1. large size or abnormal enlargement or distention. 2. a million.

megacolon (meg-ă-koh-lŏn) *n.* dilatation, and sometimes lengthening, of the colon. It is caused by obstruction of the colon, Hirschsprung's disease, or longstanding constipation.

megakaryocyte (meg-ă-ka-ri-oh-syt) *n.* a cell in the bone marrow that produces platelets. *See also* thrombopoiesis.

megal- (**megalo-**) *prefix denoting* abnormal enlargement.

megaloblast (meg-ă-loh-blast) *n.* an abnormal form of erythroblast. Megaloblasts are unusually large and their nuclei fail to mature in the normal way; they are seen in the bone marrow in certain anaemias (*megaloblastic anaemias*) due to deficiency of vitamin B_{12} or folic acid. —**megaloblastic** *adj.*

megalocephaly (meg-ă-loh-sef-ăli) *n.* 1. *see* macrocephaly. 2. overgrowth and distortion of skull bones (*see* leontiasis).

megalocyte (meg-ă-loh-syt) *n. see* macrocyte.

megalomania (meg-ă-loh-**may**-niă) *n.* delusions of grandeur. It may be a feature of a schizophrenic or manic illness or of cerebral syphilis.

-megaly *suffix denoting* abnormal enlargement.

megaureter (meg-ă-yoor-ee-ter) *n.* gross dilatation of the ureter. This occurs above the site of a longstanding obstruction in the ureter, which blocks the free flow of urine from the kidney.

megestrol (mi-jes-trohl) *n.* a synthetic female sex hormone (*see* progestogen) that is used in oral contraceptives.

meibomian cyst (my-**boh**-mi-ăn) *n. see* chalazion. [H. Meibom (1638–1700), German anatomist]

meibomian glands (tarsal glands) *pl. n.* small sebaceous glands that lie under the conjunctiva of the eyelids.

Meigs' syndrome (megz) *n.* the accumulation of fluid in the pleural and peritoneal cavities associated with a benign tumour of the ovary. [J. V. Meigs (1892–1963), US surgeon]

meiosis (reduction division) (my-**oh**-sis) *n.* a type of cell division that produces four daughter cells, each having half the number of chromosomes of the original cell. It occurs before the formation of sperm and ova and the normal (diploid) number of chromosomes is restored after fertilization. *Compare* mitosis. —**meiotic** *adj.*

Meissner's plexus (submucous plexus) (my-snerz) *n.* a fine network of parasympathetic nerve fibres in the wall of the alimentary canal, supplying the muscles and mucous membrane. [G. Meissner (1829–1905), German physiologist]

melaena (mi-lee-nă) *n.* black tarry faeces due to the presence of partly digested blood from higher up the digestive tract. It often occurs after vomiting blood (*see* haematemesis) and the causes are the same.

melan- (melano-) *prefix denoting* 1. black coloration. 2. melanin.

melancholia (mel-ăn-**koh**-liă) *n. see* depression, involutional melancholia.

melanin (mel-ăn-in) *n.* a dark-brown to black pigment occurring in the hair, the skin, and in the iris and choroid layer of the eyes.

melanism (melanosis) (mel-ăn-izm) *n.* an unusually pronounced darkening of body tissues caused by excessive production of the pigment melanin. Melanism may affect the skin after sunburn, during pregnancy, or in Addison's disease.

melanocyte (melanophore) (mel-ă-noh-syt) *n.* a cell within the epidermis of skin that produces melanin.

melanocyte-stimulating hormone (MSH) *n.* a hormone synthesized and released by the pituitary gland. In amphibians MSH brings about colour changes in the skin but its physiological role in man is uncertain.

melanoderma (mel-ă-noh-**der**-mă) *n.* an abnormal increase in the skin pigment melanin.

melanoma (mel-ă-**noh**-mă) *n.* a highly malignant tumour of melanocytes. Such tumours usually occur in the skin but are also found in the eye and the mucous membranes.

melanophore (mel-ă-noh-for) *n. see* melanocyte.

melanoplakia (mel-ă-nă-play-kiă) *n.* pigmented areas of melanin in the mucous membrane lining the inside of the cheeks.

melanosis (mel-ă-noh-sis) *n.* **1.** *see* melanism. **2.** a disorder in the body's production of the pigment melanin. **3.** cachexia associated with the spread of the skin cancer melanoma. —**melanotic** *adj.*

melanuria (mel-ăn-yoor-iă) *n.* the presence of dark pigment in the urine. This may occur in some cases of melanoma; it may alternatively be caused by metabolic disease, such as porphyria.

melasma (mi-laz-mă) *n. see* chloasma.

melioidosis (mee-li-oi-doh-sis) *n.* a disease of wild rodents caused by the bacterium *Pseudomonas pseudomallei*. It can be transmitted to man, causing pneumonia, multiple abscesses, and septicaemia.

melphalan (mel-fă-lan) *n.* a drug administered by mouth or injection to treat various types of cancer, including malignant melanoma, tumours of the breast and ovaries, and Hodgkin's disease. Trade name: **Alkeran**.

membrane (mem-brayn) *n.* **1.** a thin layer of tissue surrounding an organ or tissue, lining a cavity, or separating adjacent structures or cavities. *See also* basement membrane, mucous membrane, serous membrane. **2.** the lipoprotein envelope surrounding a cell (*cell m.*). —**membranous** (mem-brăn-ŭs) *adj.*

membranous labyrinth *n. see* labyrinth.

men- (meno-) *prefix denoting* menstruation.

menarche (men-ar-ki) *n.* the start of the menstrual periods. This may happen at any age between about 10 and 17 years.

Mendel's laws (men-d'lz) *pl. n.* rules of inheritance based on the breeding experiments of Gregor Mendel, which showed that the inheritance of characteristics is controlled by particles now known as genes. In modern terms they are as follows. (1) Each somatic cell of an individual carries two factors (genes) for every characteristic and each gamete carries only one. (2) Each pair of factors segregates independently of all other pairs at meiosis, so that the gametes show all possible combinations of factors. *See also* dominant, recessive. [G. J. Mendel (1822–84), Austrian monk]

Mendelson's syndrome (men-d'l-sŏnz) *n.* the condition resulting when the acid contents of the stomach are regurgitated and inhaled into the lungs, characterized by lung damage, pulmonary oedema, and bronchospasm. [C. L. Mendelson (1913–), US obstetrician]

menidrosis (menhidrosis) (men-id-roh-sis) *n.* the production of sweat, sometimes containing blood, instead of the normal menstrual flow.

Ménière's disease (Ménière's syndrome) (mayn-yairz) *n.* a disease affecting the inner ear in which deafness is associated with buzzing in the ears (tinnitus) and vertigo; its cause is not known. Between attacks there may be months without symptoms, but as the disease progresses the deafness becomes more marked. [P. Ménière (1799–1862), French physician]

mening- (meningo-) *prefix denoting* the meninges.

meninges (min-in-jeez) *pl. n.* (*sing.* **meninx**) the three connective tissue membranes that line the skull and vertebral canal and enclose the brain and spinal cord: the dura mater, arachnoid mater, and pia mater. —**meningeal** *adj.*

meningioma (min-in-ji-**oh**-mă) *n.* a tumour arising from the meninges. It is usually slow-growing and produces symptoms by pressure on the underlying nervous tissue. Some meningiomas (known as *meningeal sarcomas*) are malignant and invade neighbouring tissues. Treatment of the majority of cases is by surgical removal if the tumour is accessible.

meningism (**men**-in-jizm) *n.* stiffness of the neck mimicking that found in meningitis. It is usually a symptom of chest infection or inflammation in the upper respiratory tract.

meningitis (men-in-**jy**-tis) *n.* an inflammation of the meninges due to viral or bacterial infection. Meningitis causes an intense headache, fever, loss of appetite, intolerance to light and sound, rigidity of muscles, especially those in the neck (*see also* Kernig's sign), and in severe cases convulsions, vomiting, and delirium leading to death. Bacterial meningitis can be effectively treated with antibiotics or sulphonamides. *See also* cerebrospinal fever, leptomeningitis, pachymeningitis.

meningocele (min-**ing**-oh-seel) *n.* protrusion of the meninges through a gap in the spine. *See* neural tube defects.

meningococcus (min-ing-oh-**kok**-ŭs) *n.* (*pl.* **meningococci**) one of the bacteria causing meningitis: *Neisseria meningitidis.* —**meningococcal** *adj.*

meningoencephalitis (min-ing-oh-en-sef-ă-**ly**-tis) *n.* inflammation of the brain and the meninges caused by infection, as with the mumps virus or *Brucella* (the bacterium causing brucellosis).

meningoencephalocele (min-ing-oh-en-**sef**-ă-loh-seel) *n.* protrusion of the meninges and brain through a defect in the skull. *See* neural tube defects.

meningomyelocele (**myelocele, myelomeningocele**) (min-ing-oh-my-ĕ-loh-seel) *n.* protrusion of the meninges, spinal cord, and nerve roots through a gap in the spine, accompanied by paralysis of the legs and urinary incontinence. *See* neural tube defects.

meningovascular (min-ing-oh-**vas**-kew-ler) *adj.* relating to or affecting the meninges and the blood vessels that penetrate them to supply the underlying neural tissues.

meniscectomy (men-i-**sek**-tŏmi) *n.* surgical removal of a cartilage (meniscus) in the knee. This is carried out when the meniscus has been torn or is diseased.

meniscus (min-**isk**-ŭs) *n.* (in anatomy) a crescent-shaped structure, such as the fibrocartilaginous disc that divides the cavity of a synovial joint.

menopause (climacteric) (**men**-ŏ-pawz) *n.* the time in a woman's life when ovulation and menstruation cease and the woman is no longer able to bear children. The menopause can occur at any age between the middle thirties and the late fifties; it is associated with a change in the balance of sex hormones in the body, which sometimes leads to hot flushes,

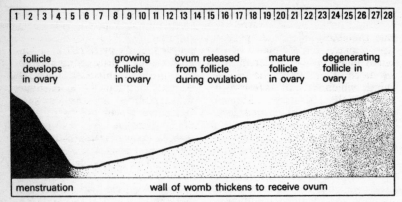

| 1 | 2 | 3 | 4 | 5 | 6 | 7 | 8 | 9 | 10 | 11 | 12 | 13 | 14 | 15 | 16 | 17 | 18 | 19 | 20 | 21 | 22 | 23 | 24 | 25 | 26 | 27 | 28 |

follicle develops in ovary

growing follicle in ovary

ovum released from follicle during ovulation

mature follicle in ovary

degenerating follicle in ovary

menstruation   wall of womb thickens to receive ovum

The menstrual cycle

palpitations, and emotional disturbances. —**menopausal** *adj.*

menorrhagia (epimenorrhagia) (men-ŏ-**ray**-jiă) *n.* abnormally heavy bleeding at menstruation. Menorrhagia may be associated with high blood pressure, hormonal disturbances, and many other conditions.

menses (men-seez) *n.* the blood and other materials discharged from the womb at menstruation.

menstrual cycle (men-stroo-ăl) *n.* the periodic sequence of events in sexually mature nonpregnant women by which an egg cell (ovum) is released from a follicle in the ovary at four-weekly intervals until the menopause (see illustration). The secretion of progesterone in the ruptured follicle causes the lining of the womb to become thicker and richly supplied with blood in preparation for pregnancy. If the ovum is not fertilized the womb lining is shed at menstruation.

menstruation (catamenia) (men-stroo-ay-shŏn) *n.* the discharge of blood and fragments of womb lining from the vagina at inter-

vals of about four weeks in women of child-bearing age (*see* menarche, menopause). The normal duration of discharge varies from three to seven days. *anovular m.* discharge that takes place without previous release of an egg cell from the ovary. *vicarious m.* bleeding from a mucous membrane other than the womb lining when normal menstruation is due. *See also* amenorrhoea, dysmenorrhoea, epimenorrhoea, hypomenorrhoea, menorrhagia, oligomenorrhoea.

mental¹ (men-t'l) *adj.* relating to or affecting the mind.

mental² *adj.* relating to the chin.

mental age *n.* a measure of an individual's level of intellectual functioning; for example, someone described as having a mental age of 6 years would be functioning at the level of an average 6-year-old child. *See also* intelligence quotient, intelligence test.

mental deficiency *n. see* subnormality.

Mental Health Act *n.* the Act of Parliament governing the care of the mentally disordered. It provides for compulsory admission when the mentally disordered put themselves or other people into danger.

mental illness *n.* a disorder of one or more of the functions of the mind, which causes suffering to the patient or others. Mental illness is broadly divided into psychosis, in which the capacity for appreciating reality is lost, and neurosis, in which insight is retained.

mental welfare officer *n.* (in Britain) an employee of a local authority with special training in and responsibility for people with mental illness. He obtains court orders for compulsory admission where necessary and provides surveillance and support for those being treated at home or in designated hostel accommodation.

menthol (men-thol) *n.* a compound extracted from peppermint oil, used in inhalants to relieve cold symptoms, in ointments and liniments, and to relieve itching. Formula: $C_{10}H_{20}O$.

mento- *prefix denoting* the chin.

mentum (men-tŭm) *n.* the chin.

mepacrine (mep-ă-kreen) *n.* a drug administered by mouth to treat various infections and infestations, particularly malaria, giardiasis, and taeniasis. Trade names: **Atebrin, Quinacrine**.

mephenesin (mi-fen-i-sin) *n.* a muscle-relaxant drug administered by mouth or injection to relieve muscular spasm and abnormal movements in such diseases as parkinsonism, chorea, and athetosis. Trade name: **Myanesin**.

meprobamate (mi-proh-bă-mayt) *n.* a mild tranquillizer administered by mouth or injection to relieve anxiety and nervous tension. Trade names: **Equanil, Mepavlon, Miltown**.

mepyramine (mi-py-ră-meen) *n.* an antihistamine drug administered by mouth or injection to treat allergies and sensitivity reactions and applied as a cream to treat skin allergies and itching. Trade name: **Anthisan**.

meralgia paraesthetica (mi-ral-jiă pa-ris-thet-ik-ă) *n.* painful tingling and numbness felt over the outer surface of the thigh when the lateral cutaneous nerve is trapped as it passes through the muscular tissues.

mercaptopurine (mer-kap-tŏ-pewr-een) *n.* a drug that prevents the growth of cancer cells and is administered by mouth, chiefly in the treatment of some types of leukaemia (*see* antimetabolite). Trade name: **Puri-Nethol**.

mercurialism (hydrargyria) (mer-kewr-iă-lizm) *n.* mercury poisoning. Acute poisoning causes vomiting, diarrhoea, and kidney damage. Treatment is with dimercaprol. Chronic poisoning causes mouth ulceration, loose teeth, and intestinal and renal disturbances. Treatment is removing the patient from further exposure.

mercury (mer-kewr-i) *n.* a silvery metallic element that is liquid at room temperature. Its toxicity has caused a decline in the use of its compounds in medicine. The main uses of mercury salts today are in antiseptics, fungicides, and antiparasitic agents. Symbol: Hg. *See also* mercurialism.

mes- (meso-) *prefix denoting* middle or medial.

mesaortitis (mes-ay-or-ty-tis) *n.* inflammation of the middle layer (media) of the wall of the aorta, generally the result of late syphilis.

mesarteritis (mes-ar-ter-I-tis) *n.* inflammation of the middle layer (media) of an artery, which is often combined with inflammation in all layers of the artery wall.

mescaline (mesk-ă-leen) *n.* an alkaloid present in the dried tops of the cactus *Lophophora williamsii* that produces inebriation and hallucinations when ingested.

mesencephalon (mes-en-sef-ă-lon) *n. see* midbrain.

mesentery (mes-ĕn-ter-i) *n.* a double layer of peritoneum attaching the stomach, small intestine, pancreas, spleen, and other abdominal organs to the posterior wall of the abdomen. —**mesenteric** (mes-ĕn-te-rik) *adj.*

mesial (mee-zi-ăl) *adj.* **1.** medial. **2.** relating to or situated in the median line or plane.

mesmerism (mez-mer-izm) *n.* hypnosis based on the ideas of Franz Mesmer, sometimes employing magnets and a variety of other equipment. [F. A. Mesmer (1734–1815), Austrian physician]

mesoappendix (mes-oh-ă-pen-diks) *n.* the mesentery of the appendix.

mesocolon (mes-oh-koh-lon) *n.* the fold of peritoneum by which the colon is fixed to the posterior abdominal wall.

mesoderm (mes-oh-derm) *n.* the middle germ layer of the early embryo. It gives rise to cartilage, muscle, bone, blood, kidneys, gonads and their ducts, and connective tissue. —**mesodermal** *adj.*

mesometrium (mes-oh-mee-tri-ŭm) *n.* the broad ligament of the uterus: a sheet of connective tissue that carries blood vessels to the uterus and attaches it to the abdominal wall.

mesomorphic (mes-oh-mor-fik) *adj.* describing a body type that has a well developed skeletal and muscular structure and a sturdy upright posture. —**mesomorph** *n.* —**mesomorphy** *n.*

mesonephros (Wolffian body) (mes-oh-nef-ross) *n.* kidney tissue that is functional only in the embryo. Its duct – the *mesonephric* (or *Wolffian*) *duct* – persists in males as the epididymis and vas deferens. —**mesonephric** *adj.*

mesosalpinx (mes-oh-sal-pinks) *n.* a fold of peritoneum that surrounds the Fallopian tubes. It is the upper part of the broad ligament, which surrounds the womb.

mesotendon (mes-oh-ten-dŏn) *n.* the delicate connective tissue membrane that surrounds a tendon.

mesothelioma (mes-oh-th'ee-li-oh-mă) *n.* a tumour of the epithelium making up the pleura, peritoneum, or pericardium. The occurrence of pleural mesothelioma has a strong association with exposure to asbestos dust (*see* asbestosis).

mesothelium (mes-oh-th'ee-liŭm) *n.* the single layer of cells that lines serous membranes. It is derived from embryonic mesoderm. *Compare* epithelium.

mesovarium (mes-oh-vair-iŭm) *n.* the mesentery of the ovaries.

messenger RNA (mes-in-jer) *n.* a type of RNA that carries the information of the genetic code of the DNA from the cell nucleus to the ribosomes, where the code is translated into protein. *See* transcription, translation.

mestranol (mes-tră-nol) *n.* a synthetic female sex hormone that is one of the most commonly used oestrogens in oral contraceptive pills.

met- (meta-) *prefix denoting* **1.** distal to; beyond; behind. **2.** change; transformation.

metabolism (mi-**tab**-ŏl-izm) *n.* **1.** the sum of all the chemical and physical changes that take place within the body and enable its continued growth and functioning. Metabolism involves the breakdown of complex organic constituents of the body (*see* catabolism) and the building up of complex substances from simple ones (*see* anabolism). *See also* basal metabolism. **2.** the sum of the biochemical changes undergone by a particular constituent of the body. —**metabolic** (met-ă-**bol**-ik) *adj.*

metabolite (mi-**tab**-ŏ-lyt) *n.* a substance that takes part in the process of metabolism.

metacarpal (met-ă-**kar**-păl) **1.** *adj.* relating to the metacarpus. **2.** *n.* any of the bones forming the metacarpus.

metacarpophalangeal (met-ă-kar-poh-fal-ăn-**jee**-ăl) *adj.* relating to the metacarpal bones and the phalanges, especially to the joints between these bones.

metacarpus (met-ă-**kar**-pŭs) *n.* the five bones of the hand that connect the carpus (wrist) to the phalanges (digits).

metamorphopsia (met-ă-mor-**fop**-siă) *n.* a condition in which objects appear distorted. It is usually due to a disorder of the retina affecting the macula.

metamorphosis (met-ă-**mor**-fŏ-sis) *n.* a structural change, especially the change from one developmental stage to another that occurs in certain animals (e.g. in amphibians from larval to adult form).

metaphase (met-ă-**fayz**) *n.* the second stage of mitosis and of each division of meiosis, in which the chromosomes line up at the centre of the spindle, with their centromeres attached to the spindle fibres.

metaphysis (mi-**taf**-i-sis) *n.* the growing portion of a long bone that lies between the epiphyses and the diaphysis.

metaplasia (met-ă-**play**-ziă) *n.* an abnormal change in the nature of a tissue. *myeloid m.* the development of bone marrow elements in organs such as the spleen and liver. This may occur after bone marrow failure.

metastasis (mi-**tas**-tă-sis) *n.* the distant spread of disease, especially a malignant tumour, from its site of origin. This occurs by three main routes: (1) through the bloodstream; (2) through the lymphatic system; (3) across body cavities. —**metastatic** (met-ă-**stat**-ik) *adj.*

metastasize (mi-**tas**-tă-syz) *vb.* (of a malignant tumour) to spread by metastasis.

metatarsal (met-ă-**tar**-săl) **1.** *adj.* relating to the metatarsus. **2.** *n.* any of the bones forming the metatarsus.

metatarsalgia (met-ă-tar-**sal**-jiă) *n.* aching pain in the metatarsal bones of the foot. Repeated injury and deformities of the foot are common causes, and corrective footwear may be prescribed.

metatarsus (met-ă-**tar**-sŭs) *n.* the five bones of the foot that connect the tarsus (ankle) to the phalanges (toes).

meteorism (meet-i-er-izm) *n. see* tympanites.

-meter *suffix denoting* an instrument for measuring.

metformin (met-for-min) *n.* a drug that reduces blood sugar levels and is administered by mouth to treat diabetes. Trade name: **Glucophage**.

methadone (meth-ă-dohn) *n.* a potent narcotic analgesic drug administered by mouth or injection to relieve severe pain and as a linctus to suppress coughs. Trade name: **Physopeptone**.

methaemalbumin (met-heem-al-bew-min) *n.* a chemical complex of the pigment portion of haemoglobin (haem) with the plasma protein albumin. It is formed in the blood in anaemias in which red blood cells are destroyed and free haemoglobin is released into the plasma.

methaemoglobin (met-hee-mŏ-gloh-bin) *n.* a substance formed when the iron atoms of haemoglobin have been oxidized from the ferrous to the ferric form (*compare* oxyhaemoglobin). Methaemoglobin cannot bind molecular oxygen and therefore cannot transport oxygen round the body.

methaemoglobinaemia (met-hee-mŏ-gloh-bin-ee-miă) *n.* the presence of methaemoglobin in the blood, which may result from ingestion of oxidizing drugs. Symptoms are fatigue, headache, dizziness and cyanosis.

methandienone (meth-ăn-dy-i-nohn) *n.* a synthetic male sex hormone with anabolic properties, administered by mouth to build up tissues in wasting diseases, such as osteoporosis, and during convalescence. Trade name: **Dianabol**.

methandriol (meth-an-dri-ol) *n.* a synthetic male sex hormone (*see* androgen) with the same actions and uses as methandienone.

methanol (meth-ă-nol) *n. see* methyl alcohol.

methapyrilene (meth-ă-pi-ri-leen) *n.* an antihistamine administered by mouth to relieve hay fever and other allergic reactions.

methaqualone (meth-ak-wă-lohn) *n.* a hypnotic and sedative drug administered by mouth to treat insomnia. Trade name: **Revonal**.

methenamine (meth-en-ă-meen) *n. see* hexamine.

methenolone (meth-en-oh-lohn) *n.* a synthetic male sex hormone with body-building actions (*see* anabolic). It is administered by mouth or injection.

methicillin (meth-i-sil-in) *n.* a semisynthetic form of penicillin administered by injection to treat infections caused by bacteria that destroy natural penicillin. Trade name: **Celbenin**.

methimazole (meth-im-ă-zohl) *n.* a drug that reduces thyroid activity, administered by mouth or injection to treat thyrotoxicosis and to prepare patients for surgical removal of the thyroid gland.

methionine (meth-I-ŏ-ńeen) *n.* a sulphur-containing essential amino acid. *See also* amino acid.

methixene (meth-iks-een) *n.* a drug with effects similar to those of atropine, administered by mouth to control the tremors and other symptoms in parkinsonism and to relieve spasm of smooth muscle in digestive disorders. Trade name: **Tremonil**.

methoin (meth-oh-in) *n.* an anticonvulsant drug administered by mouth to prevent or reduce the severity of grand mal fits in epilepsy. Trade name: **Mesontoin**.

methoserpidine (meth-oh-**ser**-pi-deen) *n.* a drug that lowers the blood pressure. It is administered by mouth. Trade name: **Decaserpyl**.

methotrexate (meth-oh-**treks**-ayt) *n.* a drug that interferes with cell growth and is administered by mouth or injection to treat various types of cancer, including leukaemia (*see* antimetabolite).

methotrimeprazine (meth-oh-try-mep-ră-zeen) *n.* a tranquillizing, sedative, and analgesic drug administered by mouth or injection to treat anxiety, tension, and agitation and to relieve moderate or severe pain. Trade name: **Veractil**.

methoxamine (meth-**oks**-ă-meen) *n.* a sympathomimetic drug that causes blood vessels to be constricted and therefore raises blood pressure. It is administered by injection to maintain the blood pressure during surgical operations. Trade name: **Vasoxine**.

methoxyphenamine (meth-oks-i-fen-ă-meen) *n.* a sympathomimetic drug administered by mouth to treat asthma and other allergic conditions, such as rhinitis, and added to cough mixtures. Trade name: **Orthoxine**.

methyl alcohol (methanol) (**mee**-thyl) *n.* wood alcohol: an alcohol that is oxidized in the body much more slowly than ethyl alcohol and forms poisonous products. As little as 10 ml of pure methyl alcohol can produce permanent blindness, and 100 ml is likely to be fatal. *See also* methylated spirits.

methylamphetamine (mee-thyl-am-fet-ămin) *n.* a drug with actions and side-effects similar to those of amphetamine. It is administered by mouth to treat narcolepsy and parkinsonism and some depressive states. It is also administered by injection to restore the blood pressure in surgical procedures and to treat drug overdosage.

methylated spirits (meth-il-ayt-id) *n.* a mixture consisting mainly of ethyl alcohol with methyl alcohol and petroleum hydrocarbons. It is used as a solvent, cleaning fluid, and fuel.

methylcellulose (mee-thyl-**sel**-yoo-lohz) *n.* a compound that absorbs water and is administered by mouth as a bulk laxative to treat constipation, to control diarrhoea, and in patients with a colostomy. Trade names: **Celevac, Cellucon, Cologel**.

methyldopa (mee-thyl-**doh**-pă) *n.* a drug that reduces blood pressure (*see* sympatholytic). It is administered by mouth or injection. Trade names: **Aldomet, Dopamet, Hydromet, Medomet**.

methylene blue (meth-il-een) *n.* a blue antiseptic dye that has been used to treat infections of the urinaɪy system, methaemoglobinaemia, and in a test for kidney function.

methylergometrine (mee-thyl-er-goh-met-reen) *n.* a drug that stimulates contractions of the womb. It is administered by mouth or injection in childbirth to control bleeding following delivery and to help the womb return to normal.

methylphenidate (mee-thyl-**fen**-id-ayt) *n.* a sympathomimetic drug that also stimulates the central nervous system. It is administered by mouth or injection to improve mental activity in convalescence and some depressive states and to overcome lethargy associated with drug treatment. Trade name: **Ritalin**.

methyl salicylate *n.* oil of wintergreen: a liquid with counterirritant and analgesic properties, applied to the skin to relieve pain in lumbago, sciatica, and rheumatic conditions.

methyltestosterone (mee-thyl-test-ost-er-ohn) *n.* a synthetic male sex hormone (*see* androgen) administered by mouth to treat sexual underdevelopment in men. It is also used to suppress lactation, to treat menstrual and menopausal disorders, and to treat breast cancer in women.

methylthiouracil (mee-thyl-th'y-oh-yoor-ă-sil) *n.* a drug that inhibits thyroid activity, administered by mouth to treat overactivity of the thyroid gland (*see* thyrotoxicosis).

methyprylone (meth-i-pry-lohn) *n.* a hypnotic and sedative drug administered by mouth to treat insomnia and to relieve anxiety and tension. Trade name: **Noludar**.

methysergide (meth-i-ser-jyd) *n.* a drug administered by mouth to prevent severe migraine attacks and to control diarrhoea associated with tumours in the digestive system. Trade name: **Deseril**.

metoclopramide (met-oh-kloh-pră-myd) *n.* a drug that speeds up digestion. It is administered by mouth or injection to treat nausea, vomiting, indigestion, heartburn, and flatulence. Trade names: **Maxolon**, **Primperan**.

metolazone (met-oh-lă-zohn) *n.* a diuretic administered by mouth to treat fluid retention (oedema) and high blood pressure. Trade name: **Zoroxolyn**.

metoprolol (met-oh-proh-lol) *n.* a drug that controls the activity of the heart (*see* beta blocker) and is administered by mouth to treat high blood pressure and angina. Trade names: **Betaloc**, **Lopressor**.

metr- (**metro-**) *prefix denoting* the womb.

metralgia (mi-tral-jiă) *n.* pain in the womb.

metre (mee-ter) *n.* the SI unit of length that is equal to 39.37 inches. Symbol: m.

metritis (mi-try-tis) *n.* inflammation of the womb. *See also* endometritis, myometritis.

metrocolpocele (met-roh-kol-poh-seel) *n.* protrusion of the womb into the vagina, which consequently becomes displaced downwards.

metronidazole (met-roh-ny-dă-zohl) *n.* a drug administered by mouth or in suppositories to treat infections of the urinary, genital, and digestive systems, such as trichomoniasis, amoebiasis, and giardiasis. Trade name: **Flagyl**.

metropathia haemorrhagica (essential uterine haemorrhage) (met-roh-path-iă hem-ŏ-rah-jik-ă) *n.* abnormal loss of blood in the womb, resulting from disease. The lining membrane of the womb usually thickens and there may be fluid-filled sacs in the ovary.

metroptosis (uterine prolapse) (met-rop-toh-sis) *n.* the downward displacement of the womb. The womb usually drops because the supporting tissues are weak or damaged, especially in women who have given birth. *Compare* metrocolpocele.

metrorrhagia (met-roh-ray-jiă) *n.* bleeding from the womb when menstruation is not due. Metrorrhagia may indicate the presence of cancer of the cervix or some other disease of the womb.

metrostaxis (met-roh-**staks**-iss) *n.* a slight but incessant loss of blood from the womb.

-metry *suffix denoting* measuring or measurement.

mianserin (mi-**an**-ser-in) *n.* a drug administered by mouth to relieve moderate or severe depression and anxiety. Trade name: **Bolvidon.**

Michel's clips (mee-**shelz**) *pl. n.* small metal clips used for suturing surgical wounds. [G. Michel (1875–1937), French surgeon]

micr- (micro-) *prefix denoting* **1.** small size. **2.** one millionth part.

microaneurysm (my-kroh-**an**-yoor-izm) *n.* a minute localized swelling of a capillary wall, which is found in the retina of patients with diabetic retinopathy.

microangiopathy (my-kroh-an-ji-**op**-ă-thi) *n.* damage to the walls of the smallest blood vessels. It may result from a variety of diseases, including diabetes mellitus, collagen diseases, infections, and cancer.

microbe (**my**-krohb) *n. see* microorganism.

microbiology (my-kroh-by-**ol**-ŏji) *n.* the science of microorganisms. Microbiology in relation to medicine is concerned mainly with the isolation and identification of the microorganisms that cause disease. **−microbiological** *adj.* **−microbiologist** *n.*

microcephaly (my-kroh-**sef**-ăli) *n.* abnormal smallness of the head: a congenital condition in which the brain is not fully developed. *Compare* macrocephaly.

microcheilia (my-kroh-**ky**-liă) *n.* abnormally small size of the lips. *Compare* macrocheilia.

Micrococcus (my-kroh-**kok**-ŭs) *n.* a genus of spherical Gram-positive bacteria occurring in colonies. They are saprophytes or parasites. *M. tetragenus* a species that can cause arthritis, endocarditis, meningitis, or abscesses in tissues.

microcyte (**my**-kroh-syt) *n.* an abnormally small red blood cell (erythrocyte). *See also* microcytosis. **−microcytic** *adj.*

microcytosis (my-kroh-sy-**toh**-sis) *n.* the presence of microcytes in the blood. Microcytosis is a feature of certain anaemias (*microcytic anaemias*), including those due to iron deficiency.

microdactyly (my-kroh-**dak**-tili) *n.* abnormal smallness or shortness of the fingers.

microdissection (my-kroh-dis-**sek**-shŏn) *n.* the process of dissecting minute structures under the microscope. Using this technique it is possible to dissect the nuclei of cells and even to separate individual chromosomes. *See also* microsurgery.

microdontia (my-kroh-**don**-tiă) *n.* a condition in which the teeth are unusually small.

microfilaria (my-kroh-fil-**air**-iă) *n.* (*pl.* **microfilariae**) the slender motile embryo of certain nematodes (*see* filaria). Microfilariae are commonly found in the circulating blood or lymph of patients suffering an infection with any of the filarial worms.

microglossia (my-kroh-**glos**-iă) *n.* abnormally small size of the tongue.

micrognathia (my-kroh-**nay**-thiă) *n.* a condition in which one jaw is unusually small.

microgram (**my**-kroh-gram) *n.* one millionth of a gram. Symbol: μg.

micrograph (photomicrograph) (my-kroh-graf) *n.* a photograph of an object viewed through a microscope. *electron m.* a micrograph photographed through an electron microscope. *light m.* a micrograph photographed through a light microscope.

micromanipulation (my-kroh-mă-nip-yoo-**lay**-shŏn) *n.* the manipulation of extremely small structures under the microscope, as in microdissection or microsurgery.

micromastia (micromazia) (my-kroh-**mas**-tiă) *n.* the condition of having abnormally small breasts.

micromelia (my-kroh-**mee**-liă) *n.* abnormally small size of the arms or legs. *Compare* macromelia.

micrometer (my-**krom**-it-er) *n.* an instrument for making extremely fine measurements of thickness or length.

micrometre (my-kroh-mee-ter) *n.* one millionth of a metre (10^{-6} m). Symbol: μm.

microorganism (microbe) (my-kroh-**or**-găn-izm) *n.* any organism too small to be visible to the naked eye. Microorganisms include bacteria, some fungi, mycoplasmas, protozoa, rickettsiae, and viruses.

micropsia (my-**krop**-siă) *n.* a condition in which objects appear smaller than they really are. It is usually due to disease of the retina.

microscope (my-krŏ-skohp) *n.* an instrument for producing a greatly magnified image of an object, which may be so small as to be invisible to the naked eye. *See also* electron microscope, operating microscope. —**microscopical** *adj.* —**microscopy** (my-kros-kŏ-pi) *n.*

microscopic (my-krŏ-**skop**-ik) *adj.*
1. too small to be seen clearly without the use of a microscope. **2.** of, relating to, or using a microscope.

microsonation (my-kroh-sŏn-ay-shŏn) *n.* the use of ultrasound waves generated inside the body from an extremely small source. This technique is used to obtain a picture of the fine structure of the neighbouring tissues.

Microsporum (my-kroh-**spor**-ŭm) *n.* a genus of fungi causing ringworm of the skin, hair, and nails. *M. audouini* the cause of ringworm of the scalp (tinea capitis).

microsurgery (my-kroh-**ser**-jer-i) *n.* the branch of surgery in which extremely intricate operations are performed through highly refined operating microscopes using miniaturized precision instruments. The technique enables surgery of previously inaccessible parts of the eye, inner ear, spinal cord, and brain.

microtome (my-krŏ-tohm) *n.* an instrument for cutting extremely thin slices of material that can be examined under a microscope.

microwave therapy (my-kroh-wayv) *n.* a form of diathermy using electromagnetic waves of extremely short wavelength.

micturition (mik-tewr-**ish**-ŏn) *n. see* urination.

midbrain (mesencephalon) (**mid**-brayn) *n.* the small portion of the brainstem, excluding the pons and the medulla, that joins the hindbrain to the forebrain.

middle ear (tympanic cavity) (**mi**-d'l) *n.* the air-filled part of the ear that transmits vibrations from the eardrum to the inner ear via three small bones (*see* ossicle). It is connected to the pharynx by the Eustachian tube.

midgut (**mid**-gut) *n.* the middle portion of the embryonic gut, which gives rise to most of the small intestine and part of the large intestine.

midwifery (mid-**wif**-ri) *n.* the profession of providing assistance and medical care to women undergoing labour and childbirth. *See also* domiciliary midwife, obstetrics. —**midwife** (**mid**-wyf) *n.*

migraine (**mee**-grayn) *n.* a recurrent throbbing headache that characteristically affects one side of the head and is often accompanied by prostration and vomiting. There is sometimes a preceding aura, consisting of flickering bright lights or blurring of vision.

miliaria (mili-**air**-iǎ) *n. see* prickly heat.

miliary (**mil**-yer-i) *adj.* describing or characterized by very small nodules or lesions, resembling millet seed. *m. tuberculosis* see tuberculosis.

milium (**mil**-iǔm) *n.* (*pl.* **milia**) a white nodule in the skin, particularly on the face. Up to 4 mm in diameter, milia are round masses of keratin occurring just beneath the epidermis.

milk (milk) *n.* the liquid food secreted by female mammals from the mammary gland. Milk is a complete food in that it has most of the nutrients necessary for life: protein, carbohydrate, fat, minerals, and vitamins. Cows' milk is comparatively deficient in vitamins C and D. Human milk contains more sugar (lactose) and less protein than cows' milk.

milk leg *n. see* white leg.

milk sugar *n. see* lactose.

milk teeth *pl. n.* the deciduous teeth of young children. *See* dentition.

Miller-Abbott tube (mil-er ab-ŏt) *n.* a double-channel rubber tube used to relieve obstruction of the small intestine. One channel terminates in a balloon that is inflated when the tube reaches the duodenum; the other is used for suction of the obstructing material. [T. G. Miller (1896–) and W. O. Abbott (1902–43), US physicians]

milli- *prefix denoting* one thousandth part.

milliampere (mili-**am**-pair) *n.* one thousandth of an ampere (10^{-3} A). Symbol: mA.

milligram (**mil**-i-gram) *n.* one thousandth of a gram. Symbol: mg.

millilitre (**mil**-i-lee-ter) *n.* one thousandth of a litre. Symbol: ml.

millimetre (**mil**-i-mee-ter) *n.* one thousandth of a metre (10^{-3} m). Symbol: mm.

Milton (**mil**-tŏn) *n. Trademark.* a solution of sodium hypochlorite, used especially for sterilizing babies' feeding bottles.

Miltown (**mil**-town) *n. see* meprobamate.

mineralocorticoid (min-er-ǎl-oh-**kor**-ti-koid) *n.* any of a group of corticosteroids, such as aldosterone, that are necessary for the regulation of salt and water balance.

miner's elbow (**my**-nerz) *n.* inflammation of the bursa over the elbow, caused by pressure on the olecranon process.

minim (**min**-im) *n.* a unit of volume used in pharmacy, equivalent to one sixtieth part of a fluid drachm.

mio- *prefix denoting* **1.** reduction or diminution. **2.** rudimentary.

miosis (myosis) (my-**oh**-sis) *n.* constriction of the pupil. This occurs normally in bright light, but persistent miosis is most commonly due to drug therapy for glaucoma. *See also* miotic. *Compare* mydriasis.

miotic (myotic) (my-**ot**-ik) *n.* a drug, such as physostigmine or pilocarpine, that causes the pupil of the eye to contract.

miscarriage (mis-ka-rij) *n. see* abortion.

miso- *prefix denoting* hatred.

missed case *n.* a person suffering from an infection in whom the symptoms and signs are so minimal that either there is no request for medical assistance or the doctor fails to make the diagnosis.

Misuse of Drugs Act (1971) *n.* (in the UK) an Act of Parliament restricting the use of dangerous drugs. These controlled drugs include the natural opiates and their synthetic substitutes, many stimulants (including amphetamine, cocaine, and pemoline), hallucinogens such as LSD and cannabis, and the sedative methaqualone.

mite (myt) *n.* a free-living or parasitic arthropod belonging to a group (Acarina) that also includes the ticks. Medically important mites include the many species causing dermatitis (e.g. *Dermatophagoides*).

mithramycin (mith-ră-**my**-sin) *n.* an antibiotic that prevents the growth of cancer cells. It is used mainly to treat cancer of the testis and is administered by injection.

mitobronitol (my-toh-**bron**-it-ol) *n.* a drug that prevents growth of cancer cells, administered by mouth to treat leukaemia. Trade name: **Myelobromol**.

mitochondrion (my-toh-**kon**-dri-ŏn) *n. (pl.* **mitochondria**) a structure, occurring in varying numbers in the cytoplasm of every cell, that is the site of the cell's energy production. Mitochondria contain ATP and the enzymes involved in the cell's metabolic activities. —**mitochondrial** *adj.*

mitosis (my-**toh**-sis) *n.* a type of cell division in which a single cell produces two genetically identical daughter cells. It is the way in which new body cells are produced for both growth and repair. *Compare* meiosis. —**mitotic** *adj.*

mitral incompetence (my-**trăl**) *n.* failure of the mitral valve to close, allowing a reflux of blood from the left ventricle of the heart to the left atrium. Its manifestations include breathlessness, atrial fibrillation, embolism, enlargement of the left ventricle, and a systolic murmur.

mitral stenosis *n.* narrowing of the opening of the mitral valve: a result of chronic scarring that follows rheumatic fever. Mild cases need no treatment, but severe cases are treated surgically by reopening the stenosis (*mitral valvotomy*) or by inserting an artificial valve (*mitral prosthesis*).

mitral valve (bicuspid valve) *n.* a valve in the heart consisting of two cusps attached to the walls at the opening between the left atrium and left ventricle. It allows blood to pass from the atrium to the ventricle, but prevents any backward flow.

mittelschmerz (mit-ĕl-**shmairts**) *n.* pain in the lower abdomen experienced about midway between successive menstrual periods, i.e. at ovulation.

ml *abbrev. for* millilitre.

MLD *n.* minimal lethal dose: the smallest quantity of a toxic compound that is recorded as having caused death.

modality (moh-**dal**-iti) *n.* **1.** a form of sensation, such as smell, hearing, tasting, or detecting temperature. **2.** one form of therapy as opposed to another, such as the modality of physiotherapy contrasted with that of radiotherapy.

modelling (**mod**-ĕl-ing) *n.* a technique used in behaviour modification, whereby an individual learns a behaviour by observing someone else doing it.

modiolus (moh-dy-oh-lŭs) *n.* the conical central pillar of the cochlea in the inner ear.

Mogadon (**mog**-ă-don) *n. see* nitrazepam.

molar (**moh**-ler) *n.* any one of the two (in the deciduous dentition) or three (in the permanent dentition) posterior teeth on each side of each jaw. *See also* dentition.

molarity (mol-**a**-ri-ti) *n.* the strength of a solution, expressed as the weight of dissolved substance in grams per litre divided by its molecular weight, i.e. the number of moles per litre.

mole¹ (mohl) *n.* the SI unit of amount of substance. One mole of a compound has a mass equal to its molecular weight expressed in grams. Symbol: mol.

mole² *n.* an area of pigment, usually brown, in the skin. Some moles are flat; others are raised and occasionally have hairs growing from them.

molecular biology (mŏ-**lek**-yoo-ler) *n.* the study of the molecules that are associated with living organisms, especially proteins and nucleic acids.

molecule (**mol**-i-kewl) *n.* a particle consisting of two or more atoms held together by chemical bonds. It is the smallest unit of an element or compound capable of existing independently. —**molecular** *adj.*

molluscum (mol-**usk**-ŭm) *n.* any of several skin diseases typified by the development of soft rounded tumours. *m. contagiosum* a virus disease that produces small rounded pearl-like swellings with craters containing broken-down matter.

mon- (mono-) *prefix denoting* one, single, or alone.

Mönckeberg's arteriosclerosis (*or* **degeneration**) (**mernk**-i-bergz) *n. see* arteriosclerosis. [J. G. Mönckeberg (1877–1925), German pathologist]

mongolism (**mong**-ŏ-lizm) *n. see* Down's syndrome.

Monilia (moh-**nil**-iă) *n.* the former name of the genus of fungi now known as *Candida.*

moniliasis (mon-i-**ly**-ă-sis) *n. see* candidiasis.

monitoring (mon-i-ter-ing) *n.* the periodic observation of a patient's condition, which may be by visual, manual, or automatic means.

monoamine oxidase (MAO) (mon-oh-**ay**-meen) *n.* an enzyme that catalyses the oxidation of a large variety of monoamines, including adrenaline, noradrenaline, and serotonin. Monoamine oxidase is found in most tissues, particularly the liver and nervous system. *See also* MAO inhibitor.

monoblast (mon-oh-blast) *n.* the earliest identifiable cell that gives rise to a monocyte. It is normally found in the blood-forming tissue of the bone marrow but may appear in the blood in certain diseases, most notably in *acute monoblastic leukaemia*.

monochromat (mon-oh-**kroh**-mat) *n.* a person who is completely colour-blind. The condition is probably inherited.

monocular (mon-**ok**-yoo-ler) *adj.* relating to or used by one eye only. *Compare* binocular.

monocyte (**mon**-oh-syt) *n.* a variety of white blood cell with a kidney-shaped nucleus. Its function is the ingestion of foreign particles, such as bacteria and tissue debris. —**monocytic** *adj.*

monocytosis (mon-oh-sy-**toh**-sis) *n.* an increase in the number of monocytes in the blood. Monocytosis occurs in a variety of diseases, including certain leukaemias (*monocytic leukaemias*).

monodactylism (mon-oh-**dak**-til-izm) *n.* the congenital absence of all but one digit on each hand and foot.

monomania (mon-oh-**may**-niă) *n.* the state in which a particular delusion or set of delusions is present in an otherwise normally functioning person. *See also* paranoia.

mononeuritis (mon-oh-newr-**I**-tis) *n.* disease affecting a single peripheral nerve. Entrapment of the nerve or interference with its blood supply are the commonest causes. *Compare* polyneuropathy.

mononuclear (mon-oh-**new**-kli-er) *adj.* (of a cell) having one nucleus.

mononucleosis (mon-oh-new-kli-**oh**-sis) *n.* the condition in which the blood contains an abnormally high number of mononuclear leucocytes (monocytes). *See* glandular fever (infectious mononucleosis).

monoplegia (mon-oh-**plee**-jiă) *n.* paralysis of one limb. —**monoplegic** *adj.*

monoploid (**mon**-ŏ-ploid) *adj. see* haploid.

monorchism (**mon**-or-kizm) *n.* absence of one testis. This is usually due to failure of one testicle to descend into the scrotum before birth.

monosaccharide (mon-oh-**sak**-ă-ryd) *n.* a simple sugar having the general formula $(CH_2O)_n$. The most abundant monosaccharide is glucose.

monosomy (**mon**-ŏ-soh-mi) *n.* a condition in which there is one chromosome missing from the normal (diploid) set. *Compare* trisomy. —**monosomic** *adj.*

monozygotic twins (mon-oh-zy-got-ik) *pl. n. see* twins.

mons (monz) *n.* (in anatomy) a rounded eminence. *m. pubis* the mound of fatty tissue lying over the pubic symphysis.

monster (**mon**-ster) *n.* a fetus or infant grossly malformed because of developmental abnormalities.

Montgomery's glands (mŏnt-**gom**-er-iz) *pl. n.* sebaceous glands on the areola surrounding the nipple of a woman's breast. They enlarge during pregnancy and their secretions lubricate and protect the breast during breast feeding. [W. F. Montgomery (1797–1859), Irish obstetrician]

Mooren's ulcer (moor-ĕnz) *n.* a rare chronic progressive ulceration of the cornea, occurring in the elderly. [A. Mooren (1829–99), German ophthalmologist]

morbid (**mor**-bid) *adj.* diseased or abnormal; pathological.

morbidity (mor-**bid**-iti) *n.* the state of being diseased. *m. rate* the number of cases of a disease found to occur in a stated number of the population, usually given as cases per 100,000 or per million.

morbilli (mor-**bill**) *n. see* measles.

morbilliform (mor-**bil**-i-form) *adj.* describing a skin rash resembling that of measles.

morbus (mor-**bŭs**) *n.* disease. The term is usually used as part of the medical name of a specific disease.

moribund (mo-ri-bund) *adj.* dying.

morning sickness (mor-ning) *n.* nausea and vomiting during early pregnancy. *Compare* hyperemesis. Medical name: **nausea gravidarum**.

moron (mor-on) *n. Obsolete.* a person afflicted by a mild degree of mental subnormality. *See* feeblemindedness.

Moro reflex (startle reflex) (**moh**-roh) *n.* the normal reaction of a newborn baby to a sudden loud noise. The infant moves its head and limbs and may cry. [E. Moro (1874–1951), German paediatrician]

morphine (mor-feen) *n.* a potent analgesic and narcotic drug administered by mouth or injection to relieve severe and persistent pain. Morphine causes feelings of euphoria; tolerance develops rapidly and dependence may occur.

morpho- *prefix denoting* form or structure.

morphoea (mor-fee-ă) *n.* a localized form of scleroderma in which the skin and sometimes the underlying tissues are replaced with connective tissue, forming areas or bands of infiltrating tissue.

morphogenesis (mor-foh-**jen**-i-sis) *n.* the development of form and structure of the body and its parts.

morphology (mor-**fol**-ŏji) *n.* the study of differences in form between species.

-morphous *suffix denoting* form or structure (of a specified kind).

mortality (mortality rate) (mor-**tal**-iti) *n.* the incidence of death in the population in a given period. *annual m. rate* the number of registered deaths in a year, multiplied by 1000 and divided by the population at the middle of the year. *See also* infant (mortality rate), maternal mortality rate.

mortification (mor-ti-fi-**kay**-shŏn) *n. see* necrosis.

morula (mo-roo-lă) *n.* an early stage of embryonic development formed by cleavage of the fertilized ovum. It consists of a solid ball of cells and is an intermediate stage between the zygote and blastocyst.

mosaicism (mŏ-**zay**-i-sizm) *n.* a condition in which the cells of an individual do not all contain identical chromosomes; there may be two or more genetically different populations of cells. —**mosaic** *adj.*

mosquito (mos-**kee**-toh) *n.* a small winged bloodsucking insect belonging to a large group – the Diptera. Female mosquitoes transmit the parasites responsible for several major infectious diseases, such as malaria. *See* Anopheles, Aëdes.

motile (**moh**-tyl) *adj.* being able to move spontaneously, without external aid: usually applied to a microorganism or a cell.

motions (**moh**-shŏnz) *pl. n.* the products of bowel evacuation.

motion sickness (**moh**-shŏn) *n. see* travel sickness.

motor cortex (**moh**-ter) *n.* the region of the cerebral cortex that is responsible for initiating nerve impulses that bring about voluntary activity in the muscles of the body.

motor nerve *n. see* nerve.

motor neurone *n.* one of the units (neurones) that goes to make up the nerve pathway between the brain and an effector organ, such as a skeletal muscle. *lower m. n.* a motor neurone that has a cell body in the spinal cord or brainstem and an axon that extends outwards to reach an effector. *upper m. n.* a motor neurone that has a cell body in the brain and an axon that extends into the spinal cord, where it ends in synapses.

motor neurone disease *n.* a progressive degenerative disease of the motor system occurring in middle age and causing muscle weakness and wasting. It primarily affects the cells of the anterior horn of the spinal cord, the motor nuclei in the brainstem, and the corticospinal fibres.

mould (mohld) *n.* any multicellular filamentous fungus that commonly forms a rough furry coating on decaying matter.

moulding (**mohld**-ing) *n.* the changing of the shape of an infant's head during labour, brought about by the pressures to which it is subjected when passing through the birth passage.

mountain sickness (**mownt**-in) *n. see* altitude sickness.

mouthwash (**mowth**-wosh) *n.* an aqueous solution with antiseptic, astringent, or deodorizing properties used for daily rinsing of the mouth and teeth.

MSH *n. see* melanocyte-stimulating hormone.

mucilage (**mew**-si-lij) *n.* (in pharmacy) a thick aqueous solution of a gum used as a lubricant in skin preparations, for the production of pills, and for the suspension of insoluble substances.

mucin (**mew**-sin) *n.* the principal constituent of mucus. Mucin is a glycoprotein.

muco- *prefix denoting* 1. mucus. 2. mucous membrane.

mucocele (**mew**-koh-seel) *n.* a space or organ distended with mucus. It may occur in the gall bladder when the exit duct becomes obstructed.

mucocutaneous (mew-koh-kew-**tay**-niŭs) *adj.* relating to or affecting mucous membrane and skin.

mucoid (**mew**-koid) *adj.* resembling mucus.

mucolytic (mew-koh-**lit**-ik) *n.* an agent, such as carbocysteine or tyloxapol, that dissolves or breaks down mucus. Mucolytics are used to treat chest conditions involving excessive or thickened mucus secretions.

mucoprotein (mew-koh-**proh**-teen) *n.* one of a group of proteins found in the globulin fraction of blood plasma. Mucoproteins are globulins combined with a carbohydrate group (an amino sugar).

mucopurulent (mew-koh-**pewr**-oolĕnt) *adj.* containing mucus and pus. See mucopus.

mucopus (**mew**-koh-pus) *n.* a mixture of mucus and pus.

mucormycosis (mew-kor-my-**koh**-sis) *n.* a disease caused by a fungus of the genus *Mucor*, affecting the external ear, skin, and respiratory passages.

mucosa (mew-**koh**-să) *n. see* mucous membrane. —**mucosal** *adj.*

mucous membrane (mucosa) (mew-kŭs) *n.* the moist membrane lining many tubular structures and cavities, including the nasal sinuses, respiratory tract, gastrointestinal tract, biliary, and pancreatic systems. The surface layer of the membrane contains glands that secrete mucus.

mucoviscidosis (mew-koh-vis-i-**doh**-sis) *n. see* cystic fibrosis.

mucus (**mew**-kŭs) *n.* a viscous fluid secreted by mucous membranes. Mucus acts as a protective barrier over the surfaces of the membranes, as a lubricant, and as a carrier of enzymes. —**mucous** *adj.*

Müllerian duct (mew-**leer**-iăn) *n. see* paramesonephric duct. [J. P. Müller (1801–58), German physiologist]

multi- *prefix denoting* many; several.

multifactorial (multi-fak-**tor**-iăl) *adj.* describing a condition, such as spina bifida, that is believed to have resulted from the interaction of genetic factors with an environmental factor or factors.

multifocal lenses (multi-**foh**-kăl) *pl. n.* lenses in which the power (*see* dioptre) of the lower part gradually increases towards the lower edge. The wearer can see clearly at any distance by lowering or raising his eyes to look through an appropriate part of the lens.

multigravida (multi-**grav**-id-ă) *n.* a woman who has been pregnant at least twice.

multipara (mul-**tip**-er-ă) *n.* a woman who has given birth to a live child after each of at least two pregnancies.

multiple myeloma (mul-ti-pŭl) *n. see* myeloma.

multiple sclerosis (disseminated sclerosis) *n.* a chronic disease of the nervous system affecting young and middle-aged adults. The myelin sheaths surrounding nerves in the brain and spinal cord are damaged, which affects the function of the nerves involved. The course of the illness is characterized by recurrent relapses followed by remissions. Symptoms include ataxia, nystagmus, dysarthria, spastic weakness, and retrobulbar neuritis.

mummification (mum-i-fi-**kay**-shŏn) *n.* the conversion of dead tissue into a hard shrunken mass, chiefly by dehydration.

mumps (mumps) *n.* a common virus infection mainly affecting children. Symptoms appear 2–3 weeks after exposure: fever, headache, and vomiting may precede a typical swelling of the parotid salivary glands. The infection may spread to other salivary glands and to the pancreas, brain, and testicles (*see* orchitis). Medical name: **infectious parotitis**.

Munchhausen's syndrome (muunch-how-zĕnz) *n.* a mental disorder in which the patient persistently tries to obtain hospital treatment for an illness that is nonexistent: an extreme form of malingering. [Baron von Munchhausen, a fictional character who told exaggerated stories]

murmur (bruit) (**mer**-mer) *n.* a noise, heard with the aid of a stethoscope, that is generated by turbulent blood flow within the heart or blood vessels produced by damaged valves, septal de-

A voluntary muscle in transverse section (left) and in longitudinal section at its junction with a tendon (right)

fects, narrowed arteries, or arteriovenous communications. *continuous m.* murmur heard throughout systole and diastole. *diastolic m.* murmur heard during diastole. *innocent m.* heart murmur heard in normal individuals. *systolic m.* murmur heard during systole.

Murphy's sign (mer-fiz) *n.* an indication of an inflamed gall bladder: continuous pressure over the gall bladder will cause the patient to catch his breath just before the peak of inhalation. [J. B. Murphy (1857–1916), US surgeon]

muscae volitantes (mus-kee vol-i-tan-teez) *pl. n.* black spots seen floating before the eyes usually due to the presence of opaque specks in the vitreous humour.

muscarine (musk-er-in) *n.* a highly poisonous alkaloid occurring in certain mushrooms, such as fly agaric (*Amanita muscaria*).

muscle (mus-ŭl) *n.* a tissue whose cells have the ability to contract, producing movement or force. The major functions of muscles are to produce movements of the body and of structures within it and to alter pressures or tensions of internal organs. There are

three types of muscle (*see* cardiac muscle, smooth muscle, striated muscle). **–muscular** (**mus**-kew-ler) *adj.*

muscle relaxant *n.* an agent that reduces tension in muscles. Drugs such as diazepam and mephensin are used to relieve skeletal muscular spasms in conditions such as parkinsonism. Other drugs, e.g. gallamine and tubocurarine, are used to relax the muscles during surgical operations.

muscular dystrophy *n.* any one of a group of muscle diseases in which there is a recognizable pattern of inheritance. They are marked by weakness and wasting of selected muscles: the affected muscle fibres degenerate and are replaced by fatty tissue. The most common form (*Duchenne dystrophy*) is nearly always restricted to boys and usually begins before the age of four. The child has a waddling gait and lordosis of the lumbar spine. The calf muscles – and later the shoulders and upper limbs – often become firm and bulky. *See also* dystrophia myotonica.

muscularis (mus-kew-lar-is) *n.* a muscular layer of the wall of a hollow organ (such as the stomach) or a tubular structure (such as the intestine or ureter).

musculo- *prefix denoting* muscle.

musculocutaneous nerve (mus-kew-loh-kew-tay-niŭs) *n.* a nerve of the brachial plexus that supplies some muscles of the arm and the skin of the lateral part of the forearm.

musculoskeletal (mus-kew-loh-skel-i-t'l) *adj.* relating to both the muscles and the bones.

mushroom (mush-room) *n.* the spore-producing body of various fungi. Great care must be taken in identifying edible mushrooms, as many species are poisonous (*see* Amanita).

mustine (nitrogen mustard) (must-een) *n.* a drug administered by injection to treat various types of cancer, including Hodgkin's disease and some types of leukaemia.

mutant (mew-tănt) *n.* 1. an individual in which a mutation has occurred, especially when the effect of the mutation is visible. 2. a characteristic showing the effects of a mutation. —mutant *adj.*

mutation (mew-tay-shŏn) *n.* a change in the amount or structure of the genetic material (DNA) of a cell, or the change this causes in a characteristic of the individual. A mutation affecting developing sex cells can be inherited. Mutations may occur spontaneously or be caused by external agents (e.g. radiation or certain viruses).

mutism (mewt-izm) *n.* inability or refusal to speak; dumbness. Innate speechlessness most commonly occurs in those who have been totally deaf since birth (*d. mutism*). Mutism may also result from brain damage (*see* aphasia)

or be caused by depression or psychological trauma. —mute *adj.*, *n.*

my- (myo-) *prefix denoting* muscle.

myalgia (my-al-jiă) *n.* pain in the muscles.

myasthenia (my-ăs-th'ee-niă) *n.* weakness of the muscles. *m. gravis* a chronic disease marked by abnormal fatiguability and weakness of selected muscles. Other symptoms include drooping of the upper eyelid (ptosis), double vision, and dysarthria. The cause appears to be associated with impaired ability of the neurotransmitter acetylcholine to induce muscular contraction. Drug treatment and surgical removal of the thymus lessen the severity of the symptoms.

myc- (myco-, mycet(o)-) *prefix denoting* a fungus.

mycelium (my-see-liŭm) *n.* (*pl.* mycelia) the tangled mass of fine branching threads that make up the feeding and growing part of a fungus.

mycetoma (my-si-toh-mă) *n.* a chronic inflammation of tissues caused by a fungus. *See* Madura foot.

Mycobacterium (my-koh-bak-teer-iŭm) *n.* a genus of rodlike Gram-positive aerobic bacteria. *M. leprae* (*Hansen's bacillus*) the species that causes leprosy. *M. tuberculosis* (*Koch's bacillus*) the species that causes tuberculosis.

mycology (my-kol-ŏji) *n.* the science of fungi. *See also* microbiology. —mycologist *n.*

mycoplasma (my-koh-plaz-mă) *n.* one of a group of minute nonmotile microorganisms that lack a rigid cell wall and hence display a variety of forms. The species *Mycoplasma pneumoniae* causes a pneumonia-like disease in man. The group also includes the *pleuropneumonia-like organisms (PPLO)*.

mycosis (my-koh-sis) *n.* any disease caused by a fungus, including actinomycosis, aspergillosis, cryptococcosis, rhinosporidiosis, ringworm, and sporotrichosis.

mycosis fungoides (fung-oid-eez) *n.* a variety of reticulosis usually confined to the skin. Chronic irritating eruptions occur, followed by purplish tumours. The disease is fatal, though partial remission may be effected with anti-cancer drugs.

Mycota (my-koh-ta) *n. see* undecenoic acid.

mydriasis (mid-ry-ă-sis) *n.* widening of the pupil, which occurs normally in dim light. The commonest cause of prolonged mydriasis is drug therapy (*see* mydriatic) or injury to the eye. *See also* cycloplegia. *Compare* miosis.

mydriatic (mid-ri-at-ik) *n.* a drug, such as atropine or phenylephrine, that causes the pupil of the eye to dilate.

myectomy (my-ek-tŏmi) *n.* a surgical operation to remove part of a muscle.

myel- (myelo-) *prefix denoting* **1.** the spinal cord. **2.** bone marrow. **3.** myelin.

myelencephalon (my-ĕl-en-sef-ă-lon) *n. see* medulla (oblongata).

myelin (my-ĕ-lin) *n.* a complex material formed of protein and phospholipid that is laid down as a sheath around the axons of certain neurones, known as *myelinated* (or *medullated*) *nerve fibres*.

myelination (my-ĕ-lin-ay-shŏn) *n.* the process in which myelin is laid down as an insulating layer around the axons of certain nerves.

myelitis (my-ĕ-ly-tis) *n.* **1.** an inflammatory disease of the spinal cord. The most usual kind (*transverse m.*) most often occurs during the development of multiple sclerosis. The inflammation spreads across the tissue of the spinal cord, resulting in paralysis of the legs and lower trunk. **2.** inflammation of the bone marrow. *See* osteomyelitis.

myeloblast (my-ĕ-loh-blast) *n.* the earliest identifiable cell that gives rise to a granulocyte. It is normally found in the blood-forming tissue of the bone marrow, but may appear in the blood in a variety of diseases, most notably in *acute myeloblastic leukaemia. See also* granulopoiesis. —**myeloblastic** *adj.*

myelocele (my-ĕ-loh-seel) *n. see* meningomyelocele.

myelocyte (my-ĕ-loh-syt) *n.* an immature form of granulocyte. It is normally found in the blood-forming tissue of the bone marrow, but may appear in the blood in a variety of diseases, including infections, infiltrations of the bone marrow, and certain leukaemias. *See also* granulopoiesis.

myelofibrosis (my-ĕ-loh-fy-broh-sis) *n.* a chronic but progressive disease characterized by fibrosis of the bone marrow, which leads to anaemia; enlargement of the spleen; and the presence of myeloid tissue in abnormal sites, such as the spleen and liver. Its cause is unknown.

myelography (my-ĕ-log-răfi) *n.* a specialized method of X-ray examination to demonstrate the spinal canal that involves injection of a radio-opaque contrast medium into the subarachnoid space. The X-rays obtained are called *myelograms*.

myeloid (my-ĕ-loid) *adj.* **1.** like, derived from, or relating to bone marrow. *m. leukaemia* a variety of leukaemia in which the type of blood cell that proliferates abnormally originates in the blood-forming tissue of the bone marrow. *m. tissue* a tissue in the bone marrow in which the various classes of blood cells are produced. *See also* haemopoiesis. **2.** resembling a myelocyte. **3.** relating to the spinal cord.

myeloma (multiple myeloma, myelomatosis) (my-ĕ-loh-mă) *n.* a malignant disease of the bone marrow, characterized by the presence of an excess of abnormal malignant plasma cells in the bone marrow. The patient may complain of tiredness due to anaemia and of bone pain and may develop pathological fractures. Treatment is usually with drugs, such as melphalan or cyclophosphamide, and radiotherapy. *See also* plasmacytoma.

myelomalacia (my-ĕ-loh-mă-lay-shiă) *n.* softening of the tissues of the spinal cord, most often caused by an impaired blood supply.

myelomatosis (my-ĕ-loh-mă-toh-sis) *n.* see myeloma.

myelomeningocele (my-ĕ-loh-min-ing-oh-seel) *n.* see meningomyelocele.

myenteron (my-en-ter-on) *n.* the muscular layer of the intestine, consisting of a layer of circular muscle inside a layer of longitudinal muscle. These muscles are used in peristalsis. —**myenteric** (my-en-te-rik) *adj.*

myiasis (my-ă-sis) *n.* an infestation of a living organ or tissue by maggots. Treatment of external myiases involves the destruction and removal of maggots followed by the application of antibiotics to wounds and lesions.

myo- *prefix. see* my-.

myoblast (my-oh-blast) *n.* a cell that develops into a muscle fibre. —**myoblastic** *adj.*

myocardial infarction (my-oh-kar-di-ăl) *n.* death of a segment of heart muscle, which follows interruption of its blood supply (*see* coronary thrombosis). The patient experiences sudden severe chest pain, which may spread to the arms and throat. The main danger is that of ventricular fibrillation, which accounts for most of the fatalities. Other complications include heart failure, rupture of the heart, phlebothrombosis, pulmonary embolism, pericarditis, shock, mitral incompetence, and perforation of the septum between the ventricles.

myocarditis (my-oh-kar-dy-tis) *n.* acute or chronic inflammation of the heart muscle. It may be seen alone or as part of endomyocarditis.

myocardium (my-oh-kar-diŭm) *n.* the middle of the three layers forming the wall of the heart (*see also* endocardium, epicardium). It is composed of cardiac muscle and forms the greater part of the heart wall. —**myocardial** *adj.*

myocele (my-oh-seel) *n.* protrusion of a muscle through a rupture in its sheath.

myoclonus (my-oh-kloh-nŭs) *n.* a sudden spasm of the muscles typically lifting and flexing the arms. Myoclonus is a major feature of some progressive neurological illnesses with extensive degeneration of brain cells. **—my-oclonic** (my-oh-**klon**-ik) *adj.*

myocyte (**my**-oh-syt) *n.* a muscle cell.

myodynia (my-oh-**din**-iă) *n.* pain in the muscles.

myofibrosis (my-oh-fy-**broh**-sis) *n.* the replacement of muscle tissue by fibrous tissue, with consequent loss of muscle function.

myogenic (my-oh-**jen**-ik) *adj.* originating in muscle: applied to the inherent rhythmicity of contraction of some muscles (e.g. cardiac muscle), which does not depend on neural influences.

myoglobin (my-oh-**gloh**-bin) *n.* an iron-containing pigment, resembling haemoglobin, found in muscle cells. It acts as an oxygen reservoir within the muscle fibres.

myoglobinuria (my-oh-gloh-bin-**yoor**-iă) *n.* the presence in the urine of the pigment myoglobin.

myogram (**my**-ŏ-gram) *n.* a recording of the activity of a muscle. *See* electromyography.

myograph (**my**-ŏ-graf) *n.* an instrument for recording the activity of muscular tissues. *See* electromyography.

myokymia (my-oh-ky-miă) *n.* prominent quivering of a few muscle fibres. It is a benign condition. *See also* fasciculation.

myology (my-**ol**-ŏji) *n.* the study of the structure, function, and diseases of the muscles.

myoma (my-oh-mă) *n.* a benign tumour of muscle. It may originate in smooth muscle (*see* leiomyoma) or in striated muscle.

myomectomy (my-oh-**mek**-tŏmi) *n.* an operation in which benign tumours (fibromyomas or fibroids) are removed from the muscular wall of the womb.

myometritis (my-oh-mi-**try**-tis) *n.*

focusing point falls short of retina

Uncorrected

Corrected

concave lens diverges light rays falling on the eye

Myopia (short-sightedness)

inflammation of the myometrium.

myometrium (my-oh-**mee**-tri-ŭm) *n.* the muscular tissue of the uterus, which surrounds the endometrium. It is composed of smooth muscle that undergoes small regular spontaneous contractions.

myoneural junction (my-oh-**newr**-ăl) *n. see* neuromuscular junction.

myopathy (my-**op**-ă-thi) *n.* any disease of the muscles. The myopathies are usually subdivided into those that are inherited (*see* muscular dystrophy) and those that are acquired. All are typified by weakness and wasting of the muscles in the upper parts of the arms and legs.

myopia (short-sightedness) (my-oh-piă) *n.* the condition in which parallel light rays are brought to a focus in front of the retina. The condition is corrected by wearing spectacles with concave lenses. *Compare* emmetropia, hypermetropia. **−myopic (my-op-**ik) *adj.*

myoplasm (my-oh-plazm) *n. see* sarcoplasm.

myoplasty (my-oh-plasti) *n.* the plastic surgery of muscle, in which part of a muscle is used to repair tissue defects or deformities in the vicinity of the muscle.

myosarcoma (my-oh-sar-**koh-**mă) *n.* a malignant tumour of muscle. *See also* leiomyosarcoma, rhabdomyosarcoma.

myosin (my-oh-sin) *n.* the most abundant protein in muscle fibrils, having the important properties of elasticity and contractility. *See* striated muscle.

myosis (my-oh-sis) *n. see* miosis.

myositis (my-oh-**sy-**tis) *n.* any of a group of muscle diseases in which inflammation and degenerative changes occur. Polymyositis is the most commonly occurring example. *m. ossificans* a condition in which muscle tissue is replaced by bone. It may be a hereditary disease or result from injury.

myotactic (my-oh-**tak-**tik) *adj.* relating to the sense of touch in muscles. *m. reflex see* stretch reflex.

myotic (my-**ot-**ik) *n. see* miotic.

myotomy (my-**ot-**ŏmi) *n.* the dissection or surgical division of a muscle.

myotonia (my-oh-**toh-**niă) *n.* a disorder of the muscle fibres that results in abnormally prolonged contractions. It is a feature of a hereditary condition starting in infancy or early childhood (*m. congenita*) and of a form of muscular dystrophy (dystrophia myotonica).

myotonic (my-oh-**ton-**ik) *adj.* relating to muscle tone.

myotonus (my-oh-**toh-**nŭs) *n.* **1.** a tonic muscular spasm. **2.** muscle tone.

myringa (mi-**ring-**ă) *n.* the eardrum (*see* tympanic membrane).

myringitis (mi-rin-**jy-**tis) *n.* inflammation of the eardrum. *See* otitis (media).

myringoplasty (tympanoplasty) (mi-**ring-**oh-plasti) *n.* surgical reconstruction of an eardrum damaged by infection or injury.

myringotome (mi-**ring-**oh-tohm) *n.* a surgical knife used to pierce the eardrum in myringotomy.

myringotomy (tympanotomy) (mi-**ring-**ot-ŏmi) *n.* incision of the eardrum to create an artificial opening, which relieves pressure and allows drainage of fluid from an inflamed middle ear.

myx- (myxo-) *prefix denoting* mucus.

myxoedema (miks-i-**dee-**mă) *n.* **1.** a dry firm waxy swelling of the skin and subcutaneous tissues found in patients with underactive thyroid glands (*see* hypothyroidism). **2.** the clinical syndrome due to hypothyroidism in adult life, including coarsening of the skin, intolerance to cold, weight gain, and mental dullness.

myxofibroma (miks-oh-fy-**broh-**mă) *n.* a benign tumour of fibrous tissue that contains myxomatous elements or has undergone mucoid degeneration.

myxoma (miks-**oh-**mă) *n.* a benign gelatinous tumour of connective tissue. *atrial m.* a tumour of the heart, usually of the left side, arising from the septum dividing the two upper chambers. Symptoms may include fever, lassitude, joint pains, and sudden loss of consciousness. —**myxomatous** *adj.*

myxosarcoma (miks-oh-sar-koh-mă) *n.* a sarcoma containing mucoid material.

myxovirus (miks-oh-vy-rŭs) *n.* one of a group of RNA-containing viruses that includes those causing influenza in animals and man. The related *paramyxoviruses* include the respiratory syncytial virus (RSV) and the agents causing measles, mumps, and parainfluenza.

N

nabothian follicle (nabothian cyst, nabothian gland) (nă-boh-thi-ăn) *n.* one of a number of cysts on the cervix of the womb. The sacs, which contain a thick liquid, form when the ducts of the glands in the cervix are blocked by a new growth of epithelium over an area damaged through infection. [M. Naboth (1675–1721), German anatomist]

Naegele's obliquity (anterior asynclitism) (nay-gi-liz) *n.* the entry of the head of a baby at birth into the vagina at an oblique angle, with the anterior part of the parietal bone of the skull presenting to the vagina. [F. K. Naegele (1777–1851), German obstetrician]

naevus (nee-vŭs) *n.* (*pl.* **naevi**) a birthmark: a clearly defined malformation of the skin, present at birth. Some naevi are composed of small blood vessels (*see* haemangioma). These include the *strawberry mark*, which usually disappears in early life, and the *port-wine stain*, which does not

disappear. Another kind of naevus is the mole.

Naga sore (nah-gă) *n. see* tropical ulcer.

nail (nayl) *n.* a horny structure, composed of keratin, formed from the epidermis on the dorsal surface of each finger and toe. Growth of the nail occurs at the end of the nail root, behind the exposed nail, by division of the germinative layer of the underlying epidermis. Anatomical name: **unguis.**

nalidixic acid (nal-i-diks-ik) *n.* a drug active against various bacteria and administered by mouth to treat infections of the urinary and digestive systems. Trade name: **Negram.**

nalorphine (nal-or-feen) *n.* a drug that reduces the effects of morphine and similar narcotic drugs and is administered by injection to stimulate breathing and restore consciousness after an overdose of these drugs. Trade name: **Lethidrone.**

nandrolone (nan-droh-lohn) *n.* a synthetic male sex hormone with effects and uses similar to those of methandienone. It is administered by injection. Trade name: **Durabolin.**

nano- *prefix denoting* 1. extremely small size. 2. one thousand-millionth part (10^{-9}).

nanometre (nan-oh-mee-ter) *n.* one thousand-millionth of a metre (10^{-9} m). One nanometre is equal to 10 angstrom. Symbol: nm.

nape (nayp) *n. see* nucha.

naphazoline (naf-az-oh-leen) *n.* a drug that constricts small blood vessels and is administered as nasal drops to relieve congestion in rhinitis and sinusitis.

napkin rash (**nap**-kin) *n.* **1.** a painful raw area of skin around the anus and buttocks of a young baby due to contact with frequent irritant stools. **2.** reddening over the genitals and napkin area due to the formation of ammonia in urine-soaked napkins. A neglected rash will become ulcerated. **3.** red raised areas of skin in the napkin region due to candidiasis.

naproxen (nă-**proks**-ĕn) *n.* an analgesic drug that also reduces inflammation and fever. It is administered by mouth to treat rheumatoid arthritis, ankylosing spondylitis, and gout. Trade name: **Naprosyn**.

narcissism (nar-sis-izm) *n.* excessive self-regard, with or without some rational basis. In Freudian terms it is a state in which the ego has taken itself as a love object. An extreme degree of narcissism may be a symptom of schizophrenia or personality disorder. —**narcissistic** *adj.*

narco- *prefix denoting* narcosis; stupor.

narcoanalysis (nar-koh-ă-**nal**-i-sis) *n.* a type of psychotherapy during which the patient is in a relaxed or sleeplike state induced by drugs.

narcolepsy (nar-kŏ-lep-si) *n.* an extreme tendency to fall asleep in quiet surroundings or when engaged in monotonous activities. The patient can be woken easily and is immediately alert. It is often associated with cataplexy. —**narcoleptic** *adj., n.*

narcosis (nar-**koh**-sis) *n.* a state of diminished consciousness or complete unconsciousness caused by the use of narcotic drugs. The body's normal reactions to stimuli are diminished and the body may become sedated or completely anaesthetized.

narcotic (nar-**kot**-ik) *n.* a drug that induces stupor and insensibility and relieves pain. The term is used particularly for morphine and other derivatives of opium (*see* opiate) but is also applied to other drugs that depress brain function (e.g. general anaesthetics and hypnotics).

nares (**nair**-eez) *pl. n.* (*sing.* **naris**) openings of the nose. *external* (or *anterior*) *n.* the nostrils, which lead from the nasal cavity to the outside. *internal* (or *posterior*) *n.* (*choanae*) the openings leading from the nasal cavity into the pharynx.

nasal (**nay**-zăl) *adj.* relating to the nose. *n. bone* either of a pair of narrow oblong bones that together form the bridge and root of the nose. *n. cavity* the space inside the nose that lies between the floor of the cranium and the roof of the mouth. *n. concha* (*turbinate bone*) any of three thin scroll-like bones that form the sides of the nasal cavity.

naso- *prefix denoting* the nose.

nasogastric (nay-zoh-**gas**-trik) *adj.* relating to the nose and stomach. *n. tube* a tube inserted into the stomach through the nose (*see* intubation).

nasolacrimal (nay-zoh-**lak**-ri-măl) *adj.* relating to the nose and the lacrimal (tear-producing) apparatus. *n. duct* the duct that drains the tears away from the lacrimal apparatus into the inferior meatus of the nose.

nasopharynx (rhinopharynx) (nay-zoh-fa-rinks) *n.* the part of the pharynx that lies above the soft palate. —**nasopharyngeal** (nay-zoh-fă-**rin**-ji-ăl) *adj.*

nates (nay-teez) *pl. n.* the buttocks. —**natal** (nay-t'l) *adj.*

National Health Service *n.* (in Britain) a comprehensive service offering therapeutic and preventive medical and surgical care, including the prescription and dispensing of medicines, spectacles, and medical and dental appliances. Exchequer funds pay for the services of doctors, nurses, and other professionals and meet a substantial part of the cost of the medicines and appliances.

natriuretic (nay-tri-yoor-et-ik) *n.* an agent that promotes the excretion of sodium salts in the urine. Most diuretics are natriuretics.

natural childbirth *n.* labour and delivery that relies largely on the efforts of the mother alone, with the minimum of medical intervention.

naturopathy (nay-cher-op-ă-thi) *n.* a system of medicine that relies upon the use of only 'natural' substances for the treatment of disease, rather than drugs.

nausea (naw-ziă) *n.* the feeling that one is about to vomit, as experienced in seasickness. Actual vomiting often occurs subsequently.

navel (nay-věl) *n.* see umbilicus.

navicular bone (nă-vik-yoo-ler) *n.* a boat-shaped bone of the ankle (*see* tarsus) that articulates with the three cuneiform bones in front and with the talus behind.

nearthrosis (nee-arth-roh-sis) *n. see* pseudarthrosis.

nebula (neb-yoo-lă) *n.* a faint opacity of the cornea that remains after an ulcer has healed.

nebulizer (neb-yoo-ly-zer) *n.* an instrument used for applying a liquid in the form of a fine spray.

Necator (ni-kay-ter) *n.* a genus of parasitic nematodes that live in the small intestine (*see* hookworm). *N. americanus* the species that infests man.

necatoriasis (ni-kay-ter-I-ă-sis) *n.* an infestation of the small intestine by the parasitic hookworm *Necator americanus.* See hookworm (disease).

neck (nek) *n.* **1.** a narrowed region of the body connecting the head to the trunk. It contains the cervical vertebrae. **2.** any other constricted region of an organ or part, such as the narrow section of the femur between the head and shaft. *See* cervix.

necro- *prefix denoting* death or dissolution.

necrobiosis (nek-roh-by-oh-sis) *n.* a gradual process by which cells lose their function and die.

necrology (nek-rol-ŏji) *n.* the study of the phenomena of death, involving determination of the moment of death and the different changes that occur in the tissues of the body after death.

necrophilism (necrophilia) (nek-rof-il-izm) *n.* sexual attraction to corpses. *See also* perversion. —**necrophile** (nek-roh-fyl) *n.*

necropsy (nek-rop-si) *n. see* autopsy.

necrosis (mortification) (nek-roh-sis) *n.* the death of some or all of the cells in an organ or tissue, caused by disease, physical or chemical injury, or interference with the blood supply (*see* gangrene). —**necrotic** *adj.*

necrospermia (nek-roh-sper-miă) *n.* the presence of either dead or motionless spermatozoa in the semen. *See* infertility.

necrotomy (nek-rot-ŏmi) *n.* **1.** the removal of a dead piece of bone (*see* sequestrum). **2.** dissection of a dead body.

needle (nee-d'l) *n.* a slender sharp-pointed instrument. Needles used for sewing up tissue during surgical operation are equipped with an eye for threading suture material. Hollow needles are used to inject substances into the body, to obtain specimens of tissue, or to withdraw fluid from a cavity. *See also* stop needle.

needling (need-ling) *n.* a form of capsulotomy in which a sharp needle is used to make a hole in the capsule surrounding the lens of the eye.

needs deprivation *n.* an unhealthy state said to exist if an individual is unable to meet basic human needs.

negativism (neg-ă-tiv-izm) *n.* uncooperative or obstructive behaviour. *active n.* negativism in which the individual does the opposite of what he is asked. This is usually associated with other features of catatonia. *passive n.* negativism in which the person fails to cooperate, occurring in schizophrenia and depression.

Neisseria (ny-**seer**-iǎ) *n.* a genus of spherical Gram-negative aerobic nonmotile bacteria characteristically grouped in pairs. *N. gonorrhoeae* (the *gonococcus*) the species that causes gonorrhoea, found within pus cells of urethral and vaginal discharge. *N. meningitidis* (the *meningococcus*) the species that causes cerebrospinal fever and meningitis. Meningococci are found within pus cells of infected cerebrospinal fluid and blood or in the nasal passages of carriers.

nematode (roundworm) (nem-ǎ-tohd) *n.* any one of a large group of worms having an unsegmented cylindrical body, tapering at both ends. Some nematodes, such as hookworms, filariae, pinworms, and guinea worms, are parasites of man.

Nembutal (nem-bew-tal) *n. see* pentobarbitone.

neo- *prefix denoting* new or newly formed.

neocerebellum (nee-oh-se-ri-**bel**-ŭm) *n.* the middle lobe of the cerebellum, excluding the pyramid and uvula.

neologism (ni-**ol**-ŏ-jizm) *n.* (in psychiatry) the invention of words to which meanings are attached. It may be a symptom of a psychotic illness, such as schizophrenia.

neomycin (nee-oh-**my**-sin) *n.* an antibiotic used to treat infections caused by a wide range of bacteria, mainly those affecting the skin and eyes. It is usually applied in creams or drops with other antibiotics, but can also be given by mouth.

neonatal death rate (nee-oh-**nay**-t'l) *n. see* infant (mortality rate).

neonate (nee-oh-**nayt**) *n.* an infant at any time during the first four weeks of life. The word is particularly applied to infants just born or in the first week of life. —**neonatal** *adj.*

neoplasm (nee-oh-plazm) *n.* a new and abnormal growth: any benign or malignant tumour.

neostigmine (nee-oh-**stig**-meen) *n.* a parasympathomimetic drug that acts by inhibiting the enzyme cholinesterase. It is used to diagnose and treat myasthenia gravis, as an antidote to some muscle-relaxant drugs, and to treat some intestinal disorders and glaucoma. Neostigmine is administered by mouth, injection, or in eye-drops. Trade name: **Prostigmin**.

nephr- (nephro-) *prefix denoting* the kidney(s).

nephralgia (ni-**fral**-jiă) *n.* pain in the kidney, which is felt in the loin and can be caused by a variety of kidney complaints.

nephrectomy (ni-**frek**-tŏmi) *n.* surgical removal of a kidney. *radical n.* removal of the entire organ together with its surrounding fat and the adjacent adrenal gland, performed for cancer of the kidney.

nephritis (Bright's disease) (ni-**fry**-tis) *n.* inflammation of the kidney. Nephritis is a nonspecific term used to describe a condition resulting from a variety of causes. *See* glomerulonephritis.

nephroblastoma (Wilms' tumour) (nef-roh-blas-**toh**-mă) *n.* a malignant tumour of the kidney found in children. The most obvious symptom is an abdominal swelling. Treatment is by nephrectomy followed by radiotherapy and cytotoxic drugs.

nephrocalcinosis (nef-roh-kal-sin-**oh**-sis) *n.* the presence of calcium deposits in the kidneys. This can be caused by excess calcium in the blood, due to overactivity of the parathyroid glands, or it may result from an underlying abnormality of the kidney.

nephrocapsulectomy (nef-roh-kaps-yoo-**lek**-tŏmi) *n.* surgical removal of the fibrous capsule around a kidney.

nephrolithiasis (nef-roh-lith-**I**-ă-sis) *n.* the presence of stones in the kidney (*see* calculus). Such stones can cause pain and blood in the urine, but they may produce no symptoms.

nephrolithotomy (nef-roh-lith-

distal convoluted tubule
efferent arteriole
afferent arteriole
Bowman's capsule
glomerulus
proximal convoluted tubule
collecting duct
loop of Henle

A single nephron

ot-ŏmi) *n.* the surgical removal of a stone from the kidney by an incision into the kidney substance.

nephrology (ni-**frol**-ŏji) *n.* the branch of medicine concerned with the study, investigation, and management of diseases of the kidney. *See also* urology. —**nephrologist** *n.*

nephroma (ni-**froh**-mă) *n.* a tumour of the kidney.

nephron (**nef**-ron) *n.* the active unit of excretion in the kidney (see illustration). Blood is filtered through the glomerulus into the Bowman's capsule so that water, nitrogenous waste, and many other substances pass into the renal tubule. Here most of the substances are reabsorbed back into the blood, the remaining fluid (urine) passing into the collecting duct, which drains into the ureter.

nephropexy (**nef**-roh-peks-i) *n.* an operation to fix a mobile kidney. The kidney is fixed to the twelfth rib and adjacent posterior abdominal wall.

nephroptosis (nef-rop-**toh**-sis) *n.* abnormal descent of a kidney into the pelvis on standing. If this is accompanied by pain and obstruction to free drainage of urine by the kidney, nephropexy may be advised.

nephrosclerosis (nef-roh-skleer-**oh**-sis) *n.* hardening of the arteries and arterioles of the kidneys.

nephrosis (ni-**froh**-sis) *n.* (in pathology) degenerative changes in the epithelium of the kidney tubules. The term is sometimes used loosely for the nephrotic syndrome.

nephrostomy (ni-**frost**-ŏmi) *n.* drainage of urine from the kidney by a tube (catheter) passing through the kidney via the skin surface. This is commonly used as a temporary procedure after operations on the kidney.

nephrotic syndrome (ni-**frot**-ik) *n.* a condition in which there is great loss of protein in the urine, reduced levels of albumin in the blood, and generalized oedema. It can be caused by a variety of disorders, most usually glomerulonephritis.

nephrotomy (ni-**frot**-ŏmi) *n.* surgical incision into the substance of the kidney. This is usually un-

Transverse section through a nerve

dertaken to remove a kidney stone (*see* nephrolithotomy).

nephroureterectomy (**ureteronephrectomy**) (nef-roh-yoor-i-ter-ek-tŏmi) *n.* surgical removal of a kidney together with its ureter, performed for cancer of the kidney pelvis or ureter.

nerve (nerv) *n.* a bundle of nerve fibres enclosed in a connective tissue sheath (see illustration). *motor n.* a nerve that transmits impulses from the brain or spinal cord to the muscles and glands. *sensory n.* a nerve that transmits impulses inwards from the sense organs to the brain and spinal cord.

nerve block *n.* a method of producing anaesthesia in part of the body by blocking the passage of pain impulses in the sensory nerves supplying it. A local anaesthetic, such as lignocaine, is injected into the tissues in the region to be anaesthetized.

nerve cell *n. see* neurone.

nerve ending *n.* the final part (terminal) of one of the branches of a nerve fibre, where a neurone makes contact either with another neurone or with a muscle or gland cell.

nerve fibre *n.* the long fine process that extends from the cell body of a neurone and carries nerve impulses. Bundles of nerve fibres running together form a nerve.

nerve gas *n.* any gas that disrupts the normal functioning of nerves and thus of the muscles they supply.

nerve impulse *n.* the electrical activity in the membrane of a neurone that is the means by which information is transmitted within the nervous system along the axons of the neurones.

nervous system (ner-vŭs) *n.* the vast network of cells specialized to carry information (in the form of nerve impulses) to and from all parts of the body in order to bring about bodily activity. *See* autonomic nervous system, central nervous system, peripheral nervous system.

nettle rash (ne-t'l) *n. see* urticaria.

neur- (neuro-) *prefix denoting* nerves or the nervous system.

neural (newr-ăl) *adj.* relating to a nerve or nerves. *n. arch see* vertebra.

neuralgia (newr-al-jă) *n.* a severe burning or stabbing pain often following the course of a nerve. *trigeminal n.* (*tic douloureux*) neuralgia in which there are brief paroxysms of searing pain felt in the distribution of one or more branches of the trigeminal nerve in the face.

neural tube *n.* a hollow tube of tissue in the embryo from which the brain and spinal cord develop. It is formed when two edges of a groove in a plate of primitive neural tissue (*neural plate*) come together and fuse.

neural tube defects *pl. n.* a group of congenital abnormalities involving defects in the spine or skull caused by failure of the neural tube to close. They include spina bifida, in which the bony arches of the spine fail to close, and more severe defects of bone fusion involving herniation of neural tissue and consequent mental and physical disorders, such as meningocele, meningomyelocele, and meningoencephalocele.

neurapraxia (newr-ă-praks-iă) *n.* temporary loss of nerve function resulting in tingling, numbness, and weakness. It is usually caused by compression of the nerve.

neurasthenia (newr-ăs-th'ee-niă) *n.* a set of psychological and physical symptoms, including fatigue, irritability, headache, and dizziness. It can be caused by organic damage, such as a head injury, or it can be due to neurosis. —**neurasthenic** *adj., n.*

neurectasis (newr-ek-tă-sis) *n.* the surgical procedure for stretching a peripheral nerve.

neurectomy (newr-ek-tŏmi) *n.* the surgical removal of the whole or part of a nerve.

neurilemma (neurolemma) (newr-i-lem-ă) *n.* the sheath of the axon of a nerve fibre. The neurilemma of a medullated fibre contains myelin. —**neurilemmal** *adj.*

neurilemmoma (newr-i-lem-oh-mă) *n. see* neurofibroma.

neurinoma (newr-i-noh-mă) *n. see* neurofibroma.

neuritis (newr-I-tis) *n.* a disease of the peripheral nerves showing the pathological changes of inflammation. The term is also used in a less precise sense as an alternative to neuropathy. *See also* retrobulbar neuritis.

neuroanatomy (newr-oh-ă-**nat**-ŏmi) *n.* the study of the structure of the nervous system.

neuroblast (**newr**-oh-blast) *n.* any of the nerve cells of the embryo that give rise to neurones.

neuroblastoma (newr-oh-blas-**toh**-mă) *n.* a malignant tumour composed of embryonic nerve cells. It may originate in any part of the sympathetic nervous system, most commonly in the medulla of the adrenal gland.

neurocranium (newr-oh-**kray**-niŭm) *n.* the part of the skull that encloses the brain.

neurodermatitis (neurodermatosis) (newr-oh-der-mă-ty-tis) *n.* a skin disease in which localized areas itch persistently and, because of constant scratching, become thickened (*see* lichenification). Common sites are the back of the neck, forearm, upper inner thighs, inner side of knees, and outer side of ankle.

neuroendocrine system (newr-oh-**end**-ŏ-kryn) *n.* the system of dual control of certain activities of the body by means of both nerves and circulating hormones. *See* neurohormone, neurosecretion.

neuroepithelioma (newr-oh-epith'ee-li-**oh**-mă) *n.* a malignant tumour of the retina of the eye. It is a form of glioma and commonly spreads into the brain.

neuroepithelium (newr-oh-epith'ee-liŭm) *n.* a type of epithelium associated with organs of special sense. It contains sensory nerve endings and is found in the retina, the membranous labyrinth, and the taste buds. —**neuroepithelial** *adj.*

neurofibroma (**neurilemmoma,** **neurinoma, neuroma, Schwannoma)** (newr-oh-fy-**broh**-mă) *n.* a benign tumour growing from the fibrous coverings of a peripheral nerve.

neurofibromatosis (von Recklinghausen's disease) (newr-oh-fy-broh-mă-**toh**-sis) *n.* a congenital disease, typified by numerous neurofibromas. Tumours may occur in the spinal canal, where they may press on the spinal cord. The tumours sometimes become malignant, giving rise to *neurofibrosarcomas.*

neurogenesis (newr-oh-**jen**-i-sis) *n.* the growth and development of nerve cells.

neurogenic (newr-oh-**jen**-ik) *adj.* **1.** caused by disease or dysfunction of the nervous system. **2.** arising in nervous tissue. **3.** caused by nerve stimulation.

neuroglia (newr-**og**-liă) *n. see* glia.

neurohormone (newr-oh-**hor**-mohn) *n.* a hormone, such as vasopressin or noradrenaline, that is produced within specialized nerve cells and is secreted from the nerve endings into the circulation.

neurohypophysis (newr-oh-hy-**pof**-i-sis) *n. see* pituitary gland.

neurolemma (newr-oh-**lem**-ă) *n. see* neurilemma.

neuroleptic (newr-oh-**lep**-tik) *n.* any drug that induces an altered state of consciousness, such as a major tranquillizer.

neurology (newr-**ol**-ŏji) *n.* the study of the structure, functioning, and diseases of the nervous system (including the brain, spinal cord, and all the peripheral nerves). —**neurological** *adj.* —**neurologist** *n.*

neuroma (newr-oh-mă) *n. see* neurofibroma.

neuromuscular junction (myoneural

dendrite
cell body
Nissl granules
neurofibrils
axon
myelin sheath
axon
motor end plate
cell body
dendrite
nerve impulse
nerve ending

Types of neurone:
motor (left) and sensory (right)

and trunk below the inflamed spinal cord, and retrobulbar (optic) neuritis affecting both optic nerves.

neurone (nerve cell) (newr-ohn) *n.* one of the basic functional units of the nervous system: a cell specialized to transmit electrical nerve impulses and so carry information from one part of the body to another (*see* illustration). Impulses enter the neurone through branches of the dendrites and are carried away from the cell body through the axon (nerve fibre). They are transmitted to adjacent neurones or to effector organs through minute gaps (*see* synapse, neuromuscular junction). *See also* motor neurone.

neuropathy (newr-op-ă-thi) *n.* any disease of the peripheral nerves, usually causing weakness and numbness. —**neuropathic** *adj.*

neurophysiology (newr-oh-fiz-i-ol-ŏji) *n.* the study of the complex chemical and physical changes that are associated with the activity of the nervous system.

neuroplasty (newr-oh-plasti) *n.* reconstructive surgery for damaged or severed peripheral nerves.

neurorrhaphy (newr-o-răfi) *n.* the operation of suturing a cut nerve.

neurosecretion (newr-oh-si-kree-shŏn) *n.* any substance produced within, and secreted by, a nerve cell. Important examples are the hormone-releasing factors produced by the cells of the hypothalamus.

neurosis (newr-**oh**-sis) *n.* (*pl.* **neuroses**) a mental illness in which insight is retained but there is a maladaptive way of behaving or thinking that causes suffering

junction) (newr-oh-**mus**-kew-ler) *n.* the meeting point of a motor nerve fibre and the muscle fibre that it supplies. It consists of a minute gap across which a neurotransmitter must diffuse from the nerve to trigger contraction of the muscle.

neuromyelitis optica (Devic's disease) (newr-oh-my-ĕ-ly-tis op-tik-ă) *n.* a condition that is closely related to multiple sclerosis. Typically there is a transverse myelitis, producing paralysis and numbness of the limbs (*compare* psychosis). The symptoms may include a pathologically severe emotional state, as in anxiety state or depression; distressing behaviour and thoughts, as in phobias or obsessions; or physical complaints, as in hysteria or hypochondria. Treatment for neurosis can include chemotherapy (often with tranquillizers), psychotherapy, or behaviour therapy. —**neurotic** *adj.*

neurosurgery (newr-oh-**ser**-jer-i) *n.* the surgical or operative treatment of diseases of the brain and spinal cord.

neurosyphilis (newr-oh-**sif**-i-lis) *n.* syphilis affecting the nervous system.

neurotmesis (newr-ot-**mee**-sis) *n.* an injury in which a nerve is severed.

neurotomy (newr-ot-ŏmi) *n.* the surgical procedure of severing a nerve.

neurotoxic (newr-oh-**toks**-ik) *adj.* poisonous or harmful to nerve cells.

neurotransmitter (newr-oh-tranz-**mit**-er) *n.* a chemical substance, such as acetylcholine, released from nerve endings to transmit impulses across synapses to other nerves and across the minute gaps between the nerves and the muscles or glands that they supply.

neurotripsy (newr-oh-**trip**-si) *n.* crushing or bruising of a nerve.

neurotrophic (newr-oh-**trof**-ik) *adj.* relating to the growth and nutrition of neural tissue in the body.

neurotropic (newr-oh-**trop**-ik) *adj.* growing towards or having an affinity for neural tissue. The term may be applied to viruses, chemicals, or toxins.

neutropenia (new-troh-**pee**-niă) *n.*

a decrease in the number of neutrophils in the blood. Neutropenia may occur in a wide variety of diseases, including aplastic anaemias, agranulocytosis, and acute leukaemias. It results in an increased susceptibility to infections.

neutrophil (polymorph) (**new**-trŏ-fil) *n.* a variety of granulocyte distinguished by the presence in its cytoplasm of fine granules that stain purple with Romanowsky stains. It is capable of ingesting and killing bacteria and provides an important defence against infection.

newton (**new**-t'n) *n.* the SI unit of force, equal to the force required to impart to 1 kilogram an acceleration of 1 metre per second per second. Symbol: N.

nexus (**neks**-ŭs) *n.* (in anatomy) a connection or link.

niacin (ny-ă-sin) *n. see* nicotinic acid.

nialamide (ny-al-ă-myd) *n.* a drug with effects similar to phenelzine, administered by mouth to treat all types of depression. Trade name: **Niamid.**

nicotinamide (nik-ŏ-tin-ă-myd) *n.* a B vitamin: the amide of nicotinic acid.

nicotine (nik-ŏ-teen) *n.* a poisonous alkaloid derived from tobacco, responsible for the dependence of regular smokers on cigarettes. In small doses nicotine has a stimulating effect on the autonomic nervous system. Large doses cause paralysis of the autonomic ganglia.

nicotinic acid (niacin) (nik-ŏ-**tin**-ik) *n.* a B vitamin. Nicotinic acid is required in the diet but can also be formed in small amounts in the body from the essential amino acid tryptophan. A deficiency of the vitamin leads to pellagra. Good sources of nicotinic acid are meat, yeast extracts, and some cereals.

nictitation (nik-ti-**tay**-shŏn) *n.* exaggerated and frequent blinking or winking of the eyes.

nidation (ny-**day**-shŏn) *n. see* implantation.

nidus (**ny**-dŭs) *n.* a place in which bacteria have settled and multiplied because of particularly suitable conditions: a focus of infection.

Niemann-Pick disease (**nee**-man pik) *n.* a rare inherited disease of phospholipid metabolism in which sphingomyelin and lecithin accumulate in the bone marrow, spleen, and lymph nodes. It is characterized by enlargement of the liver and spleen and physical and mental retardation. [A. Niemann (1880–1921), German paediatrician; F. Pick (1868–1935), German physician]

nifuratel (ny-**fewr**-ă-tel) *n.* a drug active against various microorganisms, administered by mouth or in pessaries to treat fungus infections of the genital and urinary systems (such as candidiasis of the vagina). Trade name: **Magmilor**.

night blindness (nyt) *n.* the inability to see in dim light or at night. It is due to a disorder of the rods in the retina and can result from dietary deficiency of vitamin A. Night blindness may progress to xerophthalmia and keratomalacia. Medical name: **nyctalopia**. *Compare* day blindness.

night sweat *n.* copious sweating during sleep. Night sweats may be an early indication of tuberculosis or other disease.

night terror *n.* the condition in which a young child, soon after falling asleep, starts screaming and appears terrified. The attack ceases when the child wakes up fully and is never remembered.

nihilistic (ny-i-**lis**-tik) *adj.* (in psychiatry) describing or relating to the state of a patient who believes that he and things about him do not exist.

nipple (**mamilla, papilla**) (**nip**-ŭl) *n.* the protuberance at the centre of the breast. In females the milk ducts open at the nipple.

niridazole (ni-**rid**-ă-zohl) *n.* an anthelmintic drug administered by mouth in the treatment of schistosomiasis. Niridazole should not be used in patients with impaired liver function.

Nissl granules (**nis**-ŭl) *pl. n.* collections of dark-staining material, containing RNA, seen in the cell bodies of neurones on microscopic examination. [F. Nissl (1860–1919), German neuropathologist]

nit (nit) *n.* the egg of a louse. The eggs of head lice are firmly cemented to the hair; those of body lice are fixed to the clothing.

nitrazepam (ny-**traz**-ĕ-pam) *n.* a hypnotic drug administered by mouth to treat insomnia and sleep disturbances. Trade names: **Mogadon, Remnos**.

nitric acid (**ny**-trik) *n.* a strong corrosive mineral acid, the concentrated form of which is capable of producing severe burns of the skin. Swallowing the acid leads to intense burning pain and ulceration of the mouth and throat. Treatment is by immediate administration of alkaline solutions. Formula: HNO_3.

nitrofurantoin (ny-troh-fewr-**ant**-oh-in) *n.* a drug administered by mouth to treat bacterial infections of the urinary system. Trade names: **Berkfurin, Furadantin, Furan, Macrodantin.**

nitrogen (ny-trŏ-jĕn) *n.* a gaseous element and a major constituent of air (79 per cent). Nitrogen is an essential constituent of proteins and nucleic acids and is obtained by man in the form of protein-containing foods. Nitrogenous waste is excreted as urea. Symbol N.

nitrogen mustard *n. see* mustine.

nitroglycerin (ny-troh-**glis**-er-in) *n. see* glyceryl trinitrate.

nitrous oxide (ny-trŭs) *n.* a colourless gas used as an anaesthetic with good analgesic properties. A mixture of nitrous oxide and oxygen is administered by inhalation for some dental procedures and in childbirth. Because it tends to excite the patient when used alone, nitrous oxide was formerly known popularly as *laughing gas.* Formula: N$_2$O.

nm *abbrev. for* nanometre.

Nocardia (noh-**kar**-diă) *n.* a genus of rodlike or filamentous Gram-positive nonmotile bacteria found in the soil. *N. asteroides* the species that causes nocardiosis. *N. madurae* the species associated with the disease Madura foot.

nocardiosis (noh-kar-di-**oh**-sis) *n.* a disease caused by bacteria of the genus *Nocardia*, primarily affecting the lungs, skin, and brain, resulting in the formation of abscesses.

noci- *prefix denoting* pain or injury.

nociceptive (noh-si-**sep**-tiv) *adj.* describing nerve fibres, endings, or pathways that are concerned with the condition of pain.

noct- (nocti-) *prefix denoting* night.

noctambulation (nok-tam-bew-lay-shŏn) *n. see* somnambulism.

nocturia (nokt-yoor-iă) *n.* the passage of urine at night. Nocturia usually occurs in elderly men with enlarged prostate glands, and is a common reason for patients to request prostatectomy.

nocturnal enuresis (nok-ter-năl) *n. see* enuresis.

node (nohd) *n.* a small swelling or knot of tissue. *See* atrioventricular node, sinoatrial node. *n. of Ranvier* one of the gaps that occur at regular intervals in the myelin sheath of medullated nerve fibres, between adjacent Schwann cells. [L. A. Ranvier (1835–1922), French pathologist]

nodule (**nod**-yool) *n.* a small swelling or aggregation of cells.

noma (**noh**-mă) *n.* a gangrenous infection of the mouth that spreads to involve the face. It is a severe form of ulcerative gingivitis that is usually found in debilitated or undernourished individuals.

non compos mentis (non **kom**-pŏs **men**-tis) *adj.* Latin: mentally incapable of managing one's own affairs.

noradrenaline (norepinephrine) (nor-ă-**dren**-ă-lin) *n.* a hormone, closely related to adrenaline, secreted by the medulla of the adrenal gland and also released as a neurotransmitter by sympathetic nerve endings. Among its many actions is constriction of small blood vessels leading to an increase in blood pressure, increase in the rate and depth of breathing, and relaxation of the smooth muscle in intestinal walls.

norepinephrine (nor-epi-**nef**-rin) *n.*
see noradrenaline.

norethandrolone (nor-eth-**an**-droh-
lohn) *n.* a synthetic male sex
hormone with body-building action. It has the same effects and
uses as methandienone and is
administered by mouth or injection.

norethisterone (nor-eth-**ist**-er-ohn)
n. a synthetic female sex hormone (*see* progestogen) administered by mouth to treat menstrual disorders, including amenorrhoea. It is also used in oral
contraceptives.

norma (**nor**-mă) *n.* a view of the
skull from one of several positions, from which it can be described or measured.

normo- *prefix denoting* normality.

normoblast (**nor**-moh-blast) *n.* a
nucleated cell that forms part of
the series giving rise to the red
blood cells and is normally
found in the blood-forming tissue of the bone marrow. *See
also* erythroblast, erythropoiesis.

normocyte (**nor**-moh-syt) *n.* a red
blood cell of normal size.
—**normocytic** *adj.*

normotensive (nor-moh-**ten**-siv)
adj. describing the state in which
the arterial blood pressure is
within the normal range. *Compare* hypertension, hypotension.

nortriptyline (nor-**trip**-ti-leen) *n.* a
tricyclic antidepressant drug administered by mouth to relieve
all types of depression. Trade
names: **Allegron, Aventyl**.

nose (nohz) *n.* the organ of olfaction, which also acts as an air
passage that warms, moistens,
and filters the air on its way to
the lungs. It consists of a triangular cartilaginous projection in
the front of the face that contains the nostrils (*see* nares). It

leads to the nasal cavity, which
is lined with mucous membrane
containing olfactory cells.

nosebleed (**nohz**-bleed) *n.* bleeding
from the nose, which may be
caused by physical injury or may
be associated with fever, high
blood pressure, or blood disorders. Medical name: **epistaxis**.

noso- *prefix denoting* disease.

nosocomial infection (nos-oh-
koh-mi-ăl) *n.* an infection that
originates in a hospital, such as
one acquired by a patient during
a hospital visit or one developing
among hospital staff.

nosology (nos-**ol**-ŏji) *n.* the naming
and classification of diseases.

nostrils (**nos**-trilz) *pl. n. see* nares.

notch (noch) *n.* (in anatomy) an
indentation, especially one in a
bone.

notifiable disease (noh-ti-**fy**-ăbŭl)
n. a disease that must be re-
ported to the health authorities
in order that speedy control and
preventive action may be undertaken if necessary. In Great
Britain such diseases include
cholera, diphtheria, dysentery,
food poisoning, infective jaundice, malaria, measles, poliomyelitis, smallpox, tuberculosis, typhoid, and whooping cough.

novobiocin (noh-voh-**by**-oh-sin) *n.*
an antibiotic administered by
mouth or injection to treat certain infections resistant to other
antibiotics.

noxious (**nok**-shŭs) *adj.* harmful:
applied particularly to drugs with
harmful effects.

nucha (**new**-kă) *n.* the nape of the
neck. —**nuchal** *adj.*

nucle- (nucleo-) *prefix denoting* a
cell nucleus.

**nuclear magnetic resonance
(NMR)** (new-**kli**-er) *n.* a technique used in chemical analysis

that has been applied in medicine for the diagnosis of brain abnormalities and cancer. Imaging of parts of the body can be performed in any plane and the procedure is without risk to the patient.

nuclease (new-kli-ayz) *n.* an enzyme that catalyses the breakdown of nucleic acids by cleaving the bonds between adjacent nucleotides.

nucleic acid (new-klee-ik) *n.* either of two organic acids, DNA or RNA, present in the nucleus and in some cases the cytoplasm of all living cells.

nucleolus (new-kli-oh-lŭs) *n.* (*pl.* **nucleoli**) a dense spherical structure within the cell nucleus that disappears during cell division. The nucleolus contains RNA for the synthesis of ribosomes.

nucleoprotein (new-kli-oh-proh-teen) *n.* a compound that occurs in cells and consists of nucleic acid and protein tightly bound together.

nucleoside (new-kli-ŏ-syd) *n.* a compound consisting of a nitrogen-containing base (a purine or pyrimidine) linked to a sugar. *See also* nucleotide.

nucleotide (new-kli-ŏ-tyd) *n.* a compound consisting of a nitrogen-containing base (a purine or pyrimidine) linked to a sugar and a phosphate group. Nucleic acids are long chains of linked nucleotides.

nucleus (new-kli-ŭs) *n.* (*pl.* **nuclei**) **1.** the part of a cell that contains the genetic material, DNA. The nucleus also contains RNA, most of which is located in the nucleolus. **2.** an anatomically and functionally distinct mass of nerve cells within the brain or spinal cord.

nucleus pulposus (pul-poh-sŭs) *n.* the central part of an intervertebral disc, which consists of a soft pulpy material.

nuclide (new-klyd) *n.* an artificially produced isotope that emits radioactive waves and may be used in radiotherapy for the treatment of tumours. *See* caesium-137, cobalt, yttrium-90.

nullipara (nul-ip-er-ă) *n.* a woman who has never given birth to an infant capable of survival.

nurse (ners) *n.* a person trained to care for the sick and carry out medical and surgical routines under the supervision of a doctor. In Britain nurses qualify for the State Roll of Assistant Nurses (*state enrolled n.*) or the State Register of Nurses (*state registered n.*). *See also* domiciliary midwife, health visitor, home nurse, nursing officer, school nurse.

nurse practitioner *n.* a nurse working in primary health care, to whom the patient has direct access for advice and help with health problems.

nursing officer (ners-ing) *n.* a higher grade of nurse concerned with administration and management in either tier of the British National Health Service (*regional* or *district n. o.*). *senior n. o.* a nurse responsible for a group of nurses in a particular specialty (e.g. surgical).

nursing process *n.* a method of organizing nursing work, usually using a problem-solving approach involving assessment, problem identification, planning, implementation, and evaluation as a continuous cycle. This produces individualized care for a patient rather than routine care for a disease.

nutation (new-**tay**-shŏn) *n.* the act of nodding the head.

nutrient (**new**-tri-ĕnt) *n.* a substance that must be consumed as part of the diet to provide a source of energy, material for growth, or substances to regulate growth or energy production.

nutrition (new-**trish**-ŏn) *n.* the study of food in relation to the physiological processes that depend on its absorption by the body. The science of nutrition includes the study of diets and deficiency diseases.

nux vomica (nuks **vom**-ik-ă) *n.* the seed of the tree *Strychnos nux-vomica*, which contains the poisonous alkaloid strychnine.

nyct- (**nycto-**) *prefix denoting* night or darkness.

nyctalopia (nik-tă-**loh**-piă) *n. see* night blindness.

nyctophobia (nik-toh-**foh**-biă) *n.* extreme fear of the dark. It is common in children and not unusual in normal adults.

nymphae (**nim**-fee) *pl. n.* the labia minora. *See* labium.

nympho- *prefix denoting* **1.** the labia minora. **2.** female sexuality.

nymphomania (nim-fŏ-**may**-niă) *n.* an extreme degree of sexual promiscuity in a woman. —**nymphomaniac** *adj., n.*

nystagmus (nis-**tag**-mŭs) *n.* rapid involuntary movements of the eyes that may be from side to side, up and down, or rotatory. Nystagmus may be congenital and associated with poor sight; it also occurs in disorders of the part of the brain responsible for eye movements and in disorders of the organ of balance in the ear.

nystatin (nis-tă-tin) *n.* an antibiotic active against fungi. It is applied as a cream for skin infections, by mouth for intestinal infections, as pessaries or suppositories for vaginal or anal infections, or as eye-drops for eye infections. Trade name: **Nystan**.

O

obesity (oh-**beess**-iti) *n.* the condition in which excess fat has accumulated in the body, mostly in the subcutaneous tissues. The accumulation of fat is caused by the consumption of more food than is required for producing enough energy for daily activities. —**obese** *adj.*

objective (ŏb-**jek**-tiv) *n.* **1.** (in microscopy) the arrangement of lenses in a light microscope that is nearest to the object under examination and furthest from the eyepiece. **2.** *see* behavioural objective.

objective signs *pl. n.* the signs of a disease apparent to the examiner, as opposed to the symptoms experienced by the patient.

obligate (**ob**-lig-ayt) *adj.* describing an organism that is restricted to one particular way of life. *Compare* facultative.

oblique muscles (ŏ-**bleek**) *pl. n.* **1.** two of the extrinsic muscles that control movement of the eyeball. *See* eye. **2.** two muscles in the wall of the abdomen.

obsession (ŏb-**sesh**-ŏn) *n.* a recurrent thought, feeling, or action that is unpleasant and provokes anxiety but cannot be got rid of. Although an obsession dominates the person, he (or she) realizes its senselessness and struggles to expel it. Obsessions can be treated with behaviour therapy and also with psychotherapy and tranquillizers. —**obsessional** *adj.*

obstetrics (ŏb-**stet**-riks) *n.* the branch of medical science concerned with the care of women during pregnancy, childbirth, and the period of about six weeks following the birth. *Compare* gynaecology. —**obstetrical** *adj.* —**obstetrician** (ob-stit-**rish**-ăn) *n.*

obturator (ob-tewr-ay-ter) *n.* **1.** a wire or rod within a cannula or hollow needle for piercing tissues or fitting aspirating needles. **2.** a removable form of denture that both closes a defect in the palate and also bears artificial teeth for cosmetic purposes. **3.** (*o. muscle*) either of two muscles that cover the outer surface of the anterior wall of the pelvis and are responsible for lateral rotation of the thigh and movements of the hip. *o. foramen* a large opening in the hip bone, below and slightly in front of the acetabulum. *See also* pelvis.

obtusion (ŏb-**tew**-zhŏn) *n.* the weakening or blunting of normal sensations. This may be associated with disease.

occipital bone (ok-**sip**-i-t'l) *n.* a saucer-shaped bone of the skull that forms the back and part of the base of the cranium. At the base of the occipital are two condyles that articulate with the first (atlas) vertebra of the backbone. Between the condyles is the foramen magnum.

occipito-anterior (ok-sip-i-toh-an-**teer**-i-er) *adj.* describing the position of a baby at the time of delivery in which the back of the head is towards the front of the mother's pelvis.

occipito-posterior (ok-sip-i-toh-pos-**teer**-i-er) *adj.* describing the position of a baby at the time of delivery in which the back of the head is towards the mother's backbone.

occiput (oks-ip-ut) *n.* the back of the head. —**occipital** *adj.*

occlusion (ŏ-kloo-*zh*ŏn) *n.* **1.** the closing or obstruction of a hollow organ or part. **2.** (in dentistry) the relation of the upper and lower teeth when they are in contact. *See also* malocclusion.

occlusive therapy (ŏ-**kloo**-siv) *n.* a method of correcting strabismus (squint) in which the normal eye is covered to encourage use of the affected one.

occult (ŏ-**kult**) *adj.* not apparent to the naked eye; not easily detected. *o. blood* blood present in such small quantities, for example in the faeces, that it can only be detected microscopically or by chemical testing.

occupational disease (ok-yoo-pay-shŏn-ăl) *n.* any one of various specific diseases to which workers in certain occupations are particularly prone. Examples include the various forms of pneumoconiosis, cataracts in glassblowers, decompression sickness in divers, and infectious diseases contracted from animals by farm workers. *See also* industrial disease, prescribed disease.

occupational therapy *n.* the treatment of physical and psychiatric conditions through specific activities in order to help people reach their maximum level of function and independence in all aspects of daily life.

oct- (**octa-, octi-, octo-**) *prefix denoting* eight.

ocular (ok-yoo-ler) *adj.* of or concerned with the eye or vision.

oculist (ok-yoo-list) *n.* a North American term for an ophthalmologist.

oculo- *prefix denoting* the eye(s).

oculogyric (ok-yoo-loh-**jy**-rik) *adj.* causing or concerned with movements of the eye.

oculomotor (ok-yoo-loh-**moh**-ter) *adj.* concerned with eye movements. *o. nerve* the third cranial nerve (III), which supplies muscles in and around the eye, including those responsible for altering the size of the pupil and those that turn the eyeball in different directions.

oculonasal (ok-yoo-loh-**nay**-zăl) *adj.* concerned with the eye and nose.

odont- (odonto-) *prefix denoting* a tooth.

odontalgia (od-on-**tal**-jiă) *n.* toothache.

odontoid process (od-**ont**-oid) *n.* a toothlike process from the upper surface of the axis vertebra.

odontology (od-on-**tol**-ŏji) *n.* the study of the teeth.

odontoma (od-on-**toh**-mă) *n.* any tumour of tissues that give rise to teeth. *See* ameloblastoma.

odontome (oh-**don**-tohm) *n.* an abnormal mass of calcified dental tissue.

-odynia *suffix denoting* pain in (a specified part).

odynophagia (od-i-noh-**fay**-jiă) *n.* discomfort, a burning sensation, or pain felt below the breastbone when food or fluid is swallowed. It is a symptom of reflux oesophagitis.

oedema (ee-**dee**-mă) *n.* excessive accumulation of fluid in the body tissues: popularly known as *dropsy.* The resultant swelling may be local, as with an injury or inflammation, or more general. In generalized oedema there may be collections of fluid within the chest cavity, abdomen

(*see* ascites), or within the air spaces of the lung (*pulmonary o.*). It may result from heart or kidney failure, cirrhosis of the liver, acute nephritis, the nephrotic syndrome, starvation, allergy, or certain drugs. Diuretics are administered to get rid of the excess fluid. *subcutaneous o.* oedema that commonly occurs in the legs and ankles; the swelling subsides with rest and elevation of the legs. *See also* angioneurotic oedema. —**oedematous** *adj.*

Oedipus complex (ee-dip-ŭs) *n.* repressed sexual feelings of a child for its opposite-sexed parent, combined with rivalry towards the same-sexed parent: a normal stage of development. Arrest of development at the Oedipal stage is said to be responsible for sexual deviations and other neurotic behaviour.

oesophag- (oesophago-) *prefix denoting* the oesophagus.

oesophageal ulcer (ee-sof-ă-**jee**-ăl) *n.* a peptic ulcer in the oesophagus, associated with reflux oesophagitis.

oesophagectomy (ee-sof-ă-**jek**-tŏmi) *n.* surgical removal of part or the whole of the oesophagus.

oesophagitis (ee-sof-ă-**jy**-tis) *n.* inflammation of the oesophagus. *reflux o.* the commonest form of oesophagitis, caused by frequent regurgitation of acid and peptic juices from the stomach. It may be associated with a hiatus hernia. The main symptoms are heartburn, regurgitation of bitter fluid, and sometimes difficulty in swallowing; complications include bleeding, narrowing (stricture) of the oesophageal canal, and ulceration.

oesophagocele (ee-sof-ă-goh-seel) *n.* protrusion of the lining (mucosa) of the oesophagus through a tear in its muscular wall.

oesophagoscope (ee-sof-ă-goh-skohp) *n.* an illuminated optical instrument used to inspect the interior of the oesophagus, dilate its canal, obtain material for biopsy, or remove a foreign body. —**oesophagoscopy** (ee-sof-ă-gos-kŏ-pi) *n.*

oesophagostomy (ee-sof-ă-gost-ŏmi) *n.* a surgical operation in which the oesophagus is opened onto the neck. It is usually performed after operations on the throat as a temporary measure to allow feeding.

oesophagotomy (ee-sof-ă-got-ŏmi) *n.* surgical opening of the oesophagus in order to inspect its interior or to remove or insert something.

oesophagus (ee-sof-ă-gŭs) *n.* the gullet: a muscular tube, about 23 cm long, that extends from the pharynx to the stomach. It is lined with mucous membrane, whose secretions lubricate food as it passes from the mouth to the stomach.

oestradiol (ees-tră-dy-ol) *n.* the major female sex hormone produced by the ovary. *See* oestrogen.

oestriol (ees-tri-ol) *n.* one of the female sex hormones produced by the ovary. *See* oestrogen.

oestrogen (ees-trŏ-jĕn) *n.* one of a group of steroid hormones (including oestriol, oestrone, and oestradiol) that control female sexual development. Oestrogens are synthesized mainly by the ovary; small amounts are also produced by the adrenal cortex, testes, and placenta. Naturally occurring and synthetic oestrogens, given by mouth or injection, are used to treat amenorrhoea, menopausal disorders, androgen-dependent cancers, and to inhibit lactation. Synthetic oestrogens are a major constituent of oral contraceptives. —**oestrogenic** *adj.*

oestrone (ees-trohn) *n.* one of the female sex hormones produced by the ovary. *See* oestrogen.

ohm (ohm) *n.* the SI unit of electrical resistance, equal to the resistance between two points on a conductor when a constant potential difference of 1 volt applied between these points produces a current of 1 ampere. Symbol: Ω.

-oid *suffix denoting* like; resembling.

ointment (oint-mĕnt) *n.* a greasy material, usually containing a medicament, applied to the skin or mucous membranes.

oleandomycin (oh-li-an-doh-my-sin) *n.* an antibiotic administered by mouth or injection to treat infections caused by a wide range of bacteria.

olecranon process (oh-lek-ră-non) *n.* the large process of the ulna that projects behind the elbow joint.

oleic acid (oh-lee-ik) *n. see* fatty acid.

oleo- *prefix denoting* oil.

oleum (oh-li-ŭm) *n.* (in pharmacy) an oil. *o. morrhuae* cod-liver oil. *o. olivae* olive oil. *o. ricini* castor oil.

olfaction (ol-fak-shŏn) *n.* **1.** the sense of smell. **2.** the process of smelling. Sensory cells in the mucous membrane that lines the nasal cavity are stimulated by the presence of chemical particles dissolved in the mucus. —**olfactory** (ol-fak-ter-i) *adj.*

olfactory nerve *n.* the first cranial nerve (I): the special sensory nerve of smell. Fibres of the nerve run upwards from smell receptors in the nasal mucosa and join to form the olfactory tract to the brain.

olig- (oligo-) *prefix denoting* **1.** few. **2.** a deficiency.

oligaemia (ol-ig-ee-miă) *n. see* hypovolaemia.

oligodactylism (ol-i-goh-**dak**-til-izm) *n.* the congenital absence of some of the fingers and toes.

oligodipsia (ol-i-goh-**dip**-siă) *n.* a condition in which thirst is diminished or absent.

oligodontia (ol-i-goh-**don**-shiă) *n.* the congenital absence of some of the teeth.

oligohydramnios (ol-i-goh-hy-**dram**-ni-os) *n.* a condition in which the amount of amniotic fluid bathing a fetus during pregnancy is abnormally small.

oligomenorrhoea (ol-i-goh-men-ŏ-**ree**-ă) *n.* sparse or infrequent menstruation.

oligophrenia (ol-i-goh-**free**-niă) *n. Obsolete.* mental subnormality.

oligospermia (ol-i-goh-**sper**-miă) *n.* the presence of less than the normal number of spermatozoa in the semen. The sperm usually have poor motility and often include many bizarre and immature forms. *See also* infertility.

oliguria (ol-ig-**yoor**-iă) *n.* the production of an abnormally small volume of urine. This may be a result of copious sweating, kidney disease, oedema, loss of blood, diarrhoea, or poisoning.

olive (**ol**-iv) *n.* a smooth oval swelling in the upper part of the medulla oblongata on each side. It contains a mass of nerve cells, mainly grey matter (*olivary nucleus*). —**olivary** *adj.*

olive oil *n.* an oil extracted from olives and used as a demulcent, faecal softener, and intestinal lubricant.

-ology *suffix. see* -logy.

om- (omo-) *prefix denoting* the shoulder.

-oma *suffix denoting* a tumour.

omentectomy (oh-men-**tek**-tŏmi) *n.* the removal of all or part of the omentum.

omentopexy (oh-men-toh-**peks**-i) *n.* an operation in which the omentum is attached to some other tissue, usually the abdominal wall in order to improve blood flow through the liver.

omentum (epiploon) (oh-**men**-tŭm) *n.* a double layer of peritoneum attached to the stomach and linking it with other abdominal organs. *great o.* a highly folded portion of the omentum that covers the intestines in an apronlike fashion. It acts as a heat insulator and prevents friction between abdominal organs. *lesser o.* a portion of the omentum that links the stomach with the liver. —**omental** *adj.*

omphal- (omphalo-) *prefix denoting* the navel or umbilical cord.

omphalitis (om-fă-**ly**-tis) *n.* inflammation of the navel, especially in newborn infants.

omphalocele (**om**-fă-loh-seel) *n.* an umbilical hernia.

omphalus (**om**-fă-lŭs) *n. see* umbilicus.

Onchocerca (onk-oh-**ser**-kă) *n.* a genus of parasitic worms (*see* filaria) occurring in central Africa and central America. *O. volvulus* the cause of onchocerciasis.

onchocerciasis (onk-oh-ser-**ky**-ă-sis) *n.* a tropical disease of the skin and underlying connective tissue caused by the parasitic worm *Onchocerca volvulus*. Fibrous nodular tumours grow around the adult worms in the skin; the migration of the larvae into the eye can cause total or partial blindness (*river blindness*). The drugs suramin and diethylcarbamazine are used in treatment.

onco- *prefix denoting* **1.** a tumour. **2.** volume.

oncogenesis (onk-oh-**jen**-i-sis) *n.* the development of a new abnormal growth (a benign or malignant tumour).

oncogenic (onk-oh-**jen**-ik) *adj.* describing a substance, organism, or environment that is known to be a causal factor in the production of a tumour. Some viruses are oncogenic. *See also* carcinogen.

oncology (onk-**ol**-ŏji) *n.* the study and practice of treating tumours.

oncolysis (onk-**ol**-i-sis) *n.* the destruction of tumours and tumour cells. This may occur spontaneously or, more usually, in response to treatment with drugs or radiotherapy.

oncometer (onk-**om**-it-er) *n. see* plethysmography.

oncotic (onk-**ot**-ik) *adj.* **1.** characterized by a tumour or swelling. **2.** relating to an increase in volume or pressure.

onomatomania (on-oh-mat-oh-**may**-niă) *n.* the repeated intrusion of a specific word or a name into a person's thoughts: a form of obsession.

ontogeny (on-**toj**-ĕ-ni) *n.* the history of the development of an individual from the fertilized egg to maturity.

onych- (onycho-) *prefix denoting* the nail(s).

onychauxis (on-i-**kawk**-sis) *n.* thickening or overgrowth of the nails.

onychia (on-**nik**-iă) *n.* inflammation of the matrix of the nail, which results in loss of the nail.

onychogryphosis (on-i-koh-grif-**oh**-sis) *n.* gross thickening and hardening of the nail, which becomes elongated and deformed.

onycholysis (on-i-**kol**-i-sis) *n.* separation or loosening of part or all of a nail from its bed. The condition may occur in psoriasis and in fungus infection of the skin and nail bed.

onychomadesis (on-i-koh-mă-**dee**-sis) *n.* loss of the nails.

onychomycosis (on-i-koh-my-**koh**-sis) *n.* fungus infection of the nails, usually caused by *Epidermophyton* or *Candida*. The nails become white, opaque, thickened, and brittle. *See also* tinea.

onychosis (on-i-**koh**-sis) *n.* any disease or deformity of the nails.

O'nyong nyong fever (joint-breaker fever) (oh-**n'yong**-n'yong) *n.* an East African disease caused by an arbovirus and transmitted to man by mosquitoes of the genus *Anopheles*. Symptoms include rigor, severe headache, an irritating rash, fever, and pains in the joints.

oo- *prefix denoting* an egg; ovum.

oocyesis (ovariocyesis) (oh-ŏ-sy-ee-sis) *n.* the development of an embryo in the ovary: ovarian pregnancy. *See also* ectopic pregnancy.

oocyte (**oh**-ŏ-syt) *n.* a cell in the ovary that undergoes meiosis to form an ovum. *See* oogenesis.

oogenesis (oh-ŏ-**jen**-i-sis) *n.* the process by which mature ova are produced in the ovary (see illustration). Primordial germ cells multiply to form oogonia, which start their first meiotic division to become oocytes in the fetus

Oogenesis

and complete it at ovulation. Fertilization stimulates the completion of the second meiotic division, which produces a mature ovum.

oogonium (oh-ŏ-**goh**-niŭm) *n.* (*pl.* **oogonia**) a cell produced at an early stage in the formation of an ovum. *See* oogenesis.

oophor- (oophoro-) *prefix denoting* the ovary.

oophoralgia (ovarialgia, ovaralgia) (oh-ŏ-fŏ-**ral**-jiă) *n.* pain in the ovary.

oophorectomy (ovariectomy) (oh-ŏ-fŏ-**rek**-tŏmi) *n.* surgical removal of an ovary.

oophoritis (ovaritis) (oh-ŏ-fŏ-**ry**-tis) *n.* inflammation of an ovary, either on the surface or within the organ. Oophoritis sometimes results from infection of the Fallopian tubes (*see* salpingitis) or the lower part of the abdominal cavity.

oophoroma (oh-off-ŏ-**roh**-mă) *n.* a rapidly developing cancerous growth in the ovary. *Compare* ovarian cyst.

oophoron (oh-off-ŏ-ron) *n.* the ovary.

oophoropexy (oophoropeliopexy, oophorrhaphy) (oh-off-ŏ-roh-peks-i) *n.* the stitching of a displaced ovary to the wall of the pelvic cavity.

oophorosalpingectomy (oh-off-ŏ-roh-sal-pin-**jek**-tŏmi) *n.* surgical removal of an ovary and its associated Fallopian tube.

opacity (ŏ-**pas**-iti) *n.* **1.** lack of transparency. **2.** an opaque area, as occurs in the lens of the eye in cataract.

operating microscope (op-er-ayt-ing) *n.* a binocular microscope used in surgery, e.g. in endarterectomy. The field of operation is illuminated through the objective lens by a light source within the microscope.

operculum (oh-per-kew-lŭm) *n.* (*pl.* **opercula**) a plug of mucus that blocks the cervical canal of the womb in a pregnant woman.

operon (op-er-on) *n.* a group of closely linked genes that regulate the production of enzymes.

ophthalm- (ophthalmo-) *prefix denoting* the eye.

ophthalmectomy (off-thal-mek-tŏmi) *n.* an operation in which the eye is removed. *See* enucleation.

ophthalmia (off-**thal**-miă) *n. Obsolete.* inflammation of the eye, particularly the conjunctiva (*see* conjunctivitis). *o. neonatorum* a form of conjunctivitis occurring in newborn infants, who contract the disease as they pass through an infected birth canal. If the mother has a gonorrhoeal infection, blindness will result unless antibiotic treatment or silver ni-disc for changing lenses

An ophthalmoscope

trate eyedrops are given promptly.

ophthalmic (off-**thal**-mik) *adj.* concerned with the eye.

ophthalmitis (off-thal-**my**-tis) *n.* inflammation of the eye. *See* conjunctivitis, uveitis.

ophthalmologist (off-thal-**mol**-ŏ-jist) *n.* a doctor who specializes in the diagnosis and treatment of eye diseases.

ophthalmology (off-thal-**mol**-ŏji) *n.* the branch of medicine that is devoted to the study and treatment of eye diseases. −**ophthalmological** *adj.*

ophthalmometer (off-thal-**mom**-it-er) *n.* *see* keratometer.

ophthalmoplegia (off-thal-moh-**plee**-jiă) *n.* paralysis of the muscles of the eye. *external o.* ophthalmoplegia affecting the muscles that move the eye. *internal o.* ophthalmoplegia affecting the iris and ciliary muscle.

ophthalmorrhexis (off-thal-moh-**rek**-sis) *n.* rupture of the eyeball.

This is usually due to a severe blow to the eye.

ophthalmoscope (off-**thal**-mŏ-skohp) *n.* an instrument for examining the interior of the eye (see illustration). −**ophthalmoscopy** (off-thal-**mos**-kŏ-pi) *n.*

ophthalmotomy (off-thal-**mot**-ŏmi) *n.* the operation of making an incision in the eyeball.

ophthalmotonometer (tonometer) (off-thal-moh-toh-**nom**-it-er) *n.* a small instrument for measuring the pressure inside the eye by applying pressure to the cornea.

-opia *suffix denoting* a defect of the eye or of vision.

opiate (**oh**-piăt) *n.* one of a group of drugs derived from opium, including apomorphine, codeine, morphine, and papaverine. Opiates depress the central nervous system: they relieve pain, suppress coughing, and stimulate vomiting. *See also* narcotic.

opisth- (opistho-) *prefix denoting* **1.** dorsal; posterior. **2.** backwards.

opisthorchiasis (op-iss-thor-ky-ă-sis) *n.* a condition caused by the presence of the parasitic fluke *Opisthorchis* in the bile ducts. Heavy infections can damage the tissues of the bile duct and liver and may progress to cirrhosis. The disease is treated with chloroquine.

Opisthorchis (op-iss-**thor**-kis) *n.* a genus of parasitic flukes occurring in E Europe and parts of SE Asia. The adult flukes, which live in the bile ducts, can cause opisthorchiasis.

opisthotonos (op-iss-**thot**-oh-nŏs) *n.* the position of the body in which the head, neck, and spine are arched backwards. It is assumed involuntarily by patients with tetanus and strychnine poisoning.

eyeball

optic nerve — — optic chiasma

optic tract

optic radiation

visual cortex

The optic chiasma

opium (oh-piŭm) *n.* an extract from the poppy *Papaver somniferum*, which has analgesic and narcotic action due to its content of morphine. It has the same uses and side-effects as morphine and prolonged use may lead to dependence. *See also* opiate.

opponens (oh-poh-nenz) *n.* one of a group of muscles in the hand that bring the digits opposite to other digits. *o. pollicis* the principal muscle causing opposition of the thumb.

-opsia *suffix denoting* a condition of vision.

opsonic index (op-son-ik) *n.* a numerical measurement of the power of a person's serum to attack invading bacteria and prepare them for destruction by phagocytes.

opsonin (op-sŏn-in) *n.* a serum component that attaches itself to invading bacteria and apparently makes them more susceptible to phagocytosis.

opt- (opto-) *prefix denoting* vision or the eye.

optic (op-tik) *adj.* concerned with the eye or vision. *o. atrophy* degeneration of the optic nerve. *o. chiasma* (*o. commissure*) the X-shaped structure formed by the two optic nerves as nerve fibres from the nasal side of the retina of each eye cross over to join fibres from the lateral side of the retina of the opposite eye (see illustration). *o. disc* (*o. papilla*) the start of the optic nerve, where nerve fibres from the rods and cones leave the eyeball. *See* blind spot. *o. nerve* the second cranial nerve (II), which is responsible for vision. It passes into the skull behind the eyeball to reach the optic chiasma, after which the visual pathway continues to the occipital lobe. *o. neuritis see* retrobulbar neuritis.

optician (op-tish-ăn) *n.* a person who either makes and fits glasses (*dispensing o.*) or who both tests people for glasses and also makes and fits them (*ophthalmic o.* or *optometrist*).

optometer (refractometer) (op-tom-it-er) *n.* an instrument for measuring the refraction of the eye.

optometrist (op-tom-i-trist) *n. see* optician.

optometry (op-tom-itri) *n.* the practice of testing the visual acuity of eyes and prescribing lenses to correct defects of vision.

oral (or-ăl) *adj.* **1.** relating to the mouth. **2.** taken by mouth: applied to medicines, etc.

oral contraceptive *n.* the Pill: a preparation, consisting of one or more synthetic female sex hormones, taken by women to prevent conception. Most oral contraceptives are combined pills, consisting of an oestrogen, which blocks the normal process of ovulation, and a progestogen, which acts on the pituitary gland to block the normal control of the menstrual cycle.

Orbenin (or-ben-in) *n.* *see* cloxacillin sodium.

orbicularis (or-bik-yoo-lar-iss) *n.* either of two circular muscles of the face. *o. oculi* the muscle around each orbit that is responsible for closing the eye. *o. oris* the muscle around the mouth that closes and compresses the lips.

orbit (or-bit) *n.* the cavity in the skull that contains the eye. It is formed from parts of the frontal, sphenoid, zygomatic, lacrimal, ethmoid, palatine, and maxillary bones. —**orbital** *adj.*

orchi- (orchido-, orchio-) *prefix denoting* the testis or testicle.

orchidalgia (or-kid-al-jiă) *n.* pain in the testicle. It may be caused by a hernia in the groin, a stone in the lower ureter, or a varicocele.

orchidectomy (or-kid-ek-tŏmi) *n.* surgical removal of a testis, usually to treat such diseases as seminoma (a malignant tumour of the testis).

orchidopexy (or-kid-oh-peks-i) *n.* the operation of mobilizing an undescended testis in the groin and fixing it in the scrotum.

orchidotomy (or-kid-ot-ŏmi) *n.* an incision into the testis, usually done to obtain biopsy material for histological examination.

orchis (or-kis) *n.* the testis or testicle.

orchitis (or-ky-tis) *n.* inflammation of the testis. This causes pain, redness, and swelling of the scrotum, and may be associated with inflammation of the epididymis (*epididymo-orchitis*). The condition is usually caused by infection spreading down the vas deferens but can develop in mumps (*mumps o.*).

orciprenaline (or-si-pren-ă-leen) *n.* a drug used to relieve bronchitis and asthma. It has the same actions and side-effects as isoprenaline. Trade name: **Alupent.**

orf (orf) *n.* a virus infection of sheep and goats that can be transmitted to man, causing a mild skin eruption on the fingers, hands, and forearms.

organ (or-găn) *n.* a part of the body, composed of more than one tissue, that forms a structural unit responsible for a particular function (or functions). *o. of Corti* (*spiral o.*) the sense organ of the cochlea, which converts sound signals into nerve impulses that are transmitted to the brain via the cochlear nerve. [A. Corti (1822–88), Italian anatomist]

organelle (or-gă-nel) *n.* a structure within a cell that is specialized for a particular function.

organic (or-gan-ik) *adj.* **1.** relating to any or all of the organs of the body. *o. disorder* a disorder associated with changes in the structure of an organ or tissue. *Compare* functional disorder. **2.** describing chemical compounds containing carbon, found in all living systems.

organism (or-găn-izm) *n.* any living thing, which may consist of a single cell (*see* microorganism) or a group of differentiated but interdependent cells.

organo- *prefix denoting* organ or organic.

orgasm (**or**-gazm) *n.* the climax of sexual excitement.

oriental sore (Baghdad boil, Delhi boil, Aleppo boil) (or-i-**en**-t'l) *n.* a skin disease, occurring in tropical and subtropical Africa and Asia, caused by the parasitic protozoan *Leishmania tropica.* The disease takes the form of a slow-healing open sore or ulcer, which sometimes becomes secondarily infected with bacteria.

orientation (or-i-en-**tay**-shŏn) *n.* (in psychology) awareness of oneself in time, space, and place. Orientation may be disturbed in such conditions as organic brain disease, toxic drug states, and concussion.

orifice (**o**-ri-fis) *n.* an opening in an anatomical part. *See* ostium.

origin (**o**-ri-jin) *n.* (in anatomy) **1.** the point of attachment of a muscle that remains relatively fixed during contraction of the muscle. *Compare* insertion. **2.** the point at which a nerve or blood vessel branches from a main nerve or blood vessel.

ornithine (**or**-ni-theen) *n.* an amino acid produced in the liver as a by-product during the conversion of ammonia to urea.

ornithosis (or-ni-**thoh**-sis) *n.* an infectious disease of birds, primarily pigeons; it can be transmitted to man and causes symptoms resembling those of pneumonia. *Compare* parrot disease.

oro- *prefix denoting* the mouth.

oropharynx (o-roh-**fa**-rinks) *n.* the part of the pharynx that lies between the soft palate and the hyoid bone.

orphenadrine (or-**fen**-ă-dreen) *n.* a drug that relieves spasm in muscle, administered by mouth or injection to treat all types of parkinsonism. Trade name: **Disipal**.

ortho- *prefix denoting* **1.** straight. **2.** normal.

orthodiagraph (orthŏ-**dy**-ă-grahf) *n.* an X-ray photograph designed to give an undistorted picture of part of the body so that accurate measurements may be made from it.

orthodontics (orthŏ-**don**-tiks) *n.* the branch of dentistry concerned with the growth and development of the teeth and the treatment of irregularities by means of various appliances.

orthopaedics (orthŏ-**pee**-diks) *n.* the science or practice of correcting deformities caused by disease of or damage to the bones and joints of the skeleton. —**orthopaedic** *adj.*

orthopnoea (or-thop-**nee**-ă) *n.* breathlessness that prevents the patient from lying down, so that he has to sleep propped up in bed or sitting in a chair. —**orthopnoeic** *adj.*

orthoptics (or-**thop**-tiks) *n.* the practice of using nonsurgical methods, particularly eye exercises, to treat abnormalities of vision and of coordination of eye movements (most commonly strabismus and amblyopia). —**orthoptist** *n.*

orthoptoscope (or-**thop**-toh-skohp) *n. see* amblyoscope.

orthostatic (orthŏ-**stat**-ik) *adj.* relating to the upright position of the body: used when describing this posture or a condition caused by it.

Ortolani's sign (or-toh-**lah**-niz) *n.* a sign used in a test for congenital dislocation of the hip. The baby's knees are flexed and rotation of the hip joint is attempted. A click is felt if the joint is unstable. [M. Ortolani, Italian orthopaedic surgeon]

os¹ (oss) *n.* (*pl.* **ossa**) a bone.

os² *n.* (*pl.* **ora**) the mouth or a mouthlike part.

osche- (oscheo-) *prefix denoting* the scrotum.

oscillation (oss-i-**lay**-shŏn) *n.* a regular side-to-side movement; vibration.

oscilloscope (oss-**il**-ŏ-skohp) *n.* a cathode-ray tube designed to display electronically a wave form corresponding to the electrical data fed into it. Oscilloscopes are used to provide a continuous record of many different measurements, such as the activity of the heart and brain. *See* electrocardiography, electroencephalography.

osculum (**osk**-yoo-lŭm) *n.* (in anatomy) a small aperture.

-osis *suffix denoting* **1.** a diseased condition. **2.** any condition. **3.** an increase or excess.

Osler's nodes (**ohss**-lerz) *pl. n.* small tender swellings in or beneath the skin at the ends of the fingers and toes, seen in subacute bacterial endocarditis. [Sir W. Osler (1849–1919), Canadian physician]

osm- (osmo-) *prefix denoting* **1.** smell or odour. **2.** osmosis or osmotic pressure.

osmolality (ǫz-moh-**lal**-iti) *n.* the osmotic pressure of a substance expressed in terms of osmoles of substance per kg of water. *Compare* osmolarity.

osmolarity (oz-moh-**la**-riti) *n.* the osmotic pressure of a substance expressed in terms of osmoles of substance per kg of solution.

osmole (**oz**-mohl) *n.* a unit of osmotic pressure equal to the molecular weight of a solute in grams divided by the number of ions or other particles into which it dissociates in solution.

osmoreceptor (oz-moh-ri-**sep**-ter) *n.* a group of cells in the hypothalamus that monitor blood concentration.

osmosis (oz-**moh**-sis) *n.* the passage of a solvent from a less concentrated to a more concentrated solution through a semipermeable membrane. In living organisms, the process of osmosis plays an important role in controlling the distribution of water. —**osmotic** (oz-**mot**-ik) *adj.*

osmotic pressure *n.* the pressure by which water is drawn into a solution through a semipermeable membrane; the more concentrated the solution, the greater its osmotic pressure.

osseous (**oss**-iŭs) *adj.* bony: applied to the bony parts of the inner ear.

ossicle (**oss**-i-kŭl) *n.* a small bone. *auditory o.* any of the three small bones (the incus, malleus, and stapes) in the middle ear.

ossification (osteogenesis) (oss-i-fi-**kay**-shŏn) *n.* the formation of bone, which takes place in three stages by the action of osteoblasts. A meshwork of collagen fibres is deposited in connective tissue, followed by the production of a cementing polysaccharide. Finally the cement is impregnated with minute crystals of calcium salts. The osteoblasts become enclosed within the matrix as osteocytes.

ost- (oste-, osteo-) *prefix denoting* bone.

ostectomy (oss-tek-tŏmi) *n.* the surgical removal of a bone or a piece of bone. *See also* osteotomy.

osteitis (osti-I-tis) *n.* inflammation of bone, due to infection, damage, or metabolic disorder. *o. deformans see* Paget's disease. *o. fibrosa cystica* the characteristic cystic changes that occur in bones during long-standing hyperparathyroidism.

osteo- *prefix. see* ost-.

osteoarthritis (osteoarthrosis) (osti-oh-arth-ry-tis) *n.* a disease of joint cartilage, associated with secondary changes in the underlying bone, which may ultimately cause pain and impair the function of the affected joint (usually the hip, knee, and thumb joints). The condition may result from overuse and is most common in those past middle life. Treatment consists of aspirin and other analgesics, reduction of pressure across the joint, and corrective and prosthetic surgery.

osteoarthropathy (osti-oh-arth-rop-ă-thi) *n.* any disease of the bone and cartilage adjoining a joint.

osteoarthrosis (osti-oh-arth-roh-sis) *n. see* osteoarthritis.

osteoarthrotomy (osti-oh-arth-rot-ŏmi) *n.* surgical excision of the bone adjoining a joint.

osteoblast (oss-ti-oh-blast) *n.* a cell, originating in the mesoderm of the embryo, that is responsible for the formation of bone. *See also* ossification.

osteochondritis (osti-oh-kon-dry-tis) *n.* inflammation of a bone associated with pain: the deposition of abnormal bony tissue (*see* os-

teosclerosis). The condition was formerly known as *osteochondrosis. See also* Köhler's disease, Legg-Calvé-Perthes disease. *o. dissecans* release of a small fragment (or fragments) of bone and cartilage into a joint, most frequently the knee, with resulting pain, swelling, and limitation of movement.

osteochondroma (osti-oh-kon-droh-mă) *n.* (*pl.* **osteochondromata**) a bone tumour composed of cartilage-forming cells. It appears as a painless mass, usually at the end of a long bone. As a small proportion of these tumours become malignant if untreated, they are excised.

osteochondrosis (osti-oh-kon-droh-sis) *n. see* osteochondritis.

osteoclasia (osteoclasis) (osti-oh-klay-ziă) *n.* 1. the deliberate breaking of a malformed or malunited bone, carried out by a surgeon to correct deformity. Also called: **osteoclasty.** 2. *see* osteolysis.

osteoclasis (osti-ok-lă-sis) *n.* 1. remodelling of bone by osteoclasts, during growth or the healing of a fracture. 2. *see* osteoclasia.

osteoclast (oss-ti-oh-klast) *n.* 1. a large multinucleate cell that resorbs calcified bone. 2. a device for fracturing bone for therapeutic purposes.

osteoclastoma (osti-oh-klas-toh-mă) *n.* a rare tumour of bone, caused by proliferation of osteoclast cells.

osteocyte (oss-ti-oh-syt) *n.* a bone cell. *See also* ossification.

osteodystrophy (osti-oh-dis-trŏ-fi) *n.* any generalized bone disease resulting from a metabolic disorder.

osteogenesis (osti-oh-**jen**-i-sis) *n.* *see* ossification. *o. imperfecta* (*fragilitas ossium*) a congenital disorder in which the bones are unusually brittle and fragile.

osteogenic (osti-oh-**jen**-ik) *adj.* originating in or composed of bone tissue. *o. sarcoma* a malignant tumour of bone (*see* osteosarcoma).

osteology (osti-**ol**-ŏji) *n.* the study of the structure and function of bones and related structures.

osteolysis (**osteoclasia**) (osti-**ol**-i-sis) *n.* dissolution of bone through disease, commonly by infection or loss of the blood supply (ischaemia) to the bone. —**osteolytic** *adj.*

osteoma (osti-**oh**-mă) *n.* a benign bone tumour. *cancellous o.* (*exostosis*) an outgrowth from the end of a long bone, usually rising to a point. *compact o.* (*ivory tumour*) an osteoma that is usually harmless but may rarely compress surrounding structures, as within the skull. *osteoid o.* an overgrowth of bone-forming cells, usually causing pain in the middle of a long bone.

osteomalacia (osti-oh-mă-**lay**-shiă) *n.* softening of the bones caused by a deficiency of vitamin D, which leads to progressive decalcification of bony tissues, often causing bone pain. The condition may become irreversible if treatment with vitamin D is not given.

osteomyelitis (osti-oh-my-ĕ-ly-tis) *n.* inflammation of the bone marrow due to infection. This may follow a compound fracture or be caused by blood-borne microorganisms. *acute o.* osteomyelitis occurring most commonly in children, in which there is severe pain, swelling, and redness at the site, often in the shaft of a long bone, accompanied by general illness and high fever. *chronic o.* osteomyelitis that may follow the acute form or develop insidiously.

osteopathy (osti-**op**-ă-thi) *n.* a system of healing based on the theory that most diseases are caused by displacement of bones from their correct positions. Treatment – manipulation and massage – provides relief for many disorders of bones and joints. —**osteopath** (ost-i-ŏ-path) *n.* —**osteopathic** (osti-ŏ-**path**-ik) *adj.*

osteopetrosis (**Albers-Schönberg disease, marble-bone disease**) (osti-oh-pi-**troh**-sis) *n.* a congenital abnormality in which bones become abnormally dense and brittle and tend to fracture. *See also* osteosclerosis.

osteophony (osti-**off**-ŏni) *n.* the conduction of sound by bone, such as occurs in the ossicles of the middle ear.

osteophyte (**oss**-ti-ŏ-fyt) *n.* a projection of bone, usually shaped like a rose thorn, that occurs at sites of cartilage degeneration or destruction near joints and intervertebral discs.

osteoplasty (**oss**-ti-ŏ-plasti) *n.* plastic surgery of bones.

osteoporosis (osti-oh-por-**oh**-sis) *n.* loss of bony tissue, resulting in bones that are brittle and liable to fracture. Infection, injury, and synovitis can cause localized osteoporosis. Generalized osteoporosis is common in the elderly, and in women often follows menopause.

osteosarcoma (osti-oh-sar-**koh**-mă) *n.* a malignant bone tumour. In children the usual site for the tumour is the leg, particularly the femur. Secondary growths (me-

An osteotome

tastases) are common, most frequently in the lungs (though other sites, such as the liver, may also be involved). Treatment of disease localized to the primary site is by amputation of the limb.

osteosclerosis (osti-oh-skleer-**oh**-sis) *n.* an abnormal increase in the density of bone, as a result of poor blood supply, chronic infection, or tumour. *See also* osteopetrosis.

osteotome (**oss**-ti-ŏ-tohm) *n.* a surgical chisel designed to cut bone.

osteotomy (osti-**ot**-ŏmi) *n.* a surgical operation to cut a bone into two parts, followed by realignment of the ends to allow healing. The operation may be performed to reduce pain and disability in an arthritic joint.

ostium (**oss**-tiŭm) *n.* (*pl.* **ostia**) (in anatomy) an opening. *o. abdominale* the opening of the Fallopian tube into the abdominal cavity.

-ostomy *suffix. see* -stomy.

ot- (**oto-**) *prefix denoting* the ear.

otalgia (oh-**tal**-jiă) *n.* pain in the ear.

otic (**oh**-tik) *adj.* relating to the ear.

otitis (oh-**ty**-tis) *n.* inflammation of the ear. *o. externa* inflammation of the canal between the eardrum and the external opening of the ear, often found in swimmers. *o. interna* (*labyrinthitis*) inflammation of the inner ear, causing the sudden onset of vomiting, vertigo, and loss of balance. *o. media* (*tympanitis*) inflammation, usually due to viral or bacterial infection, of the middle ear. Symptoms include severe pain and a high fever; unless treated (with antibiotics), it may lead to conductive deafness.

otoconium (oh-toh-**koh**-niŭm) *n. see* otolith.

otolaryngology (oh-toh-la-ring-ol-**ŏ**ji) *n.* the study of diseases of the ears and larynx. −**otolaryngologist** *n.*

otolith (**otoconium**) (**oh**-toh-lith) *n.* one of the small particles of calcium carbonate associated with a macula in the saccule or utricle of the inner ear.

otology (oh-**tol**-ŏji) *n.* the study of diseases of the ear. −**otologist** *n.*

-otomy *suffix. see* -tomy.

otomycosis (oh-toh-my-**koh**-sis) *n.* a fungus infection of the ear, causing irritation and inflammation of the canal between the eardrum and the external opening of the ear.

otoplasty (**oh**-toh-plasti) *n.* surgical repair or reconstruction of the ears after injury or in the correction of a congenital defect.

otorhinolaryngology (oh-toh-ry-noh-la-ring-ol-**ŏ**ji) *n.* the study of ear, nose, and throat diseases (i.e. ENT disorders). −**otorhinolaryngologist** *n.*

otorrhagia (oh-toh-**ray**-jiă) *n.* bleeding from the ear.

otorrhoea (oh-toh-**ree**-ă) *n.* any discharge from the ear, commonly a purulent discharge in chronic middle ear infection (otitis media).

otosclerosis (oh-toh-skleer-**oh**-sis) *n.* a hereditary disorder causing deafness in adult life. An overgrowth of the bone of the inner ear leads to the stapes becoming fixed to the fenestra ovalis, so that sounds cannot be conducted to the inner ear.

otoscope (oh-toh-skohp) *n. see* auriscope.

ouabain (wah-bah-in) *n.* a drug that stimulates the heart and is used to treat heart failure and other heart conditions. It is administered by mouth or injection and has the same actions and side-effects as digitalis.

outbreeding (owt-breed-ing) *n.* the production of offspring by parents who are not closely related. *Compare* inbreeding.

outer ear (owt-er) *n.* the pinna and the external auditory meatus of the ear.

out-patient (owt-pay-shěnt) *n.* a patient who receives treatment at a hospital but is not admitted to a bed in a hospital ward. Large hospitals have clinics at which out-patients can be given specialist treatment. *Compare* in-patient.

oval window (oh-văl) *n. see* fenestra (ovalis).

ovari- (ovario-) *prefix denoting* the ovary.

ovarian cyst (oh-vair-iăn) *n.* a fluid-filled sac, one or more of which may develop in the ovary. Although most ovarian cysts are not malignant, they may cause pain and vomiting; in such cases the cysts are usually surgically removed.

ovariectomy (oh-vair-i-ek-tŏmi) *n. see* oophorectomy.

ovariocele (oh-vair-i-oh-seel) *n.* hernia of an ovary.

ovariocyesis (oh-vair-i-oh-sy-ee-sis) *n. see* oocyesis.

ovariotomy (oh-vair-i-ot-ŏmi) *n.* **1.** incision into or surgical removal of an ovary. **2.** surgical removal of a tumour of the ovary.

ovaritis (oh-vă-ry-tis) *n. see* oophoritis.

ovary (oh-ver-i) *n.* the main female reproductive organ, which

perivitelline space
centrosome with two centrioles
nucleus
corona radiata
zona pellucida
ooplasm

A mature ovum
(magnification about × 600)

contains follicles that produce ova and steroid hormones in a regular cycle (*see* menstrual cycle). There are two ovaries, situated in the lower abdomen, one on each side of the womb (*see* reproductive system). **—ovarian** *adj.*

overcompensation (oh-ver-kom-pen-say-shŏn) *n.* (in psychology) the situation in which a person tries to overcome a disability by making greater efforts than are required.

overt (oh-vert) *adj.* plainly to be seen or detected: applied to diseases with observable signs and symptoms.

ovi (ovo-) *prefix denoting* an ovum.

oviduct (oh-vi-dukt) *n. see* Fallopian tube.

ovulation (ov-yoo-lay-shŏn) *n.* the process by which an ovum is released from a mature Graafian follicle. The fluid-filled follicle distends the surface of the ovary until a thin spot breaks down and the ovum floats out and starts to travel down the Fallopian tube to the womb.

ovum (egg cell, vitellus) (oh-vŭm) *n.* (*pl.* **ova**) the mature female sex cell (*see* gamete).

oxacillin (oks-ă-sil-in) *n.* an antibiotic administered by mouth or injection to treat infections caused by a wide variety of bacteria.

oxalate (oks-ă-layt) *n.* a salt of oxalic acid. *balanced o.* a mixture of ammonium and potassium oxalates (an anticoagulant) in which blood specimens are stored before laboratory examination.

oxalic acid (oks-**al**-ik) *n.* an extremely poisonous acid found in many plants, including sorrel and the leaves of rhubarb, and in some bleaching powders. When swallowed it produces burning sensations in the mouth and throat, vomiting of blood, breathing difficulties, and circulatory collapse. Treatment is with calcium lactate or other calcium salts, lime water, or milk. Formula: $C_2H_2O_4$.

oxaluria (oks-ăl-**yoor**-iă) *n.* the presence in the urine of oxalic acid or oxalates, especially calcium oxalate.

oxazepam (oks-**az**-ĕ-pam) *n.* a tranquillizing drug administered by mouth to relieve anxiety and tension and for the treatment of alcoholism. Trade name: **Serenid**.

oxidase (oks-i-dayz) *n. see* oxidoreductase.

oxidation (oks-i-**day**-shŏn) *n.* a reaction in which an atom or molecule loses electrons. Many biological oxidations are effected by the removal of hydrogen atoms, which combine with an *oxidizing agent*. For example, glucose is oxidized during cellular respiration: $C_6H_{12}O_6 + 6O_2 \rightarrow 6CO_2 + 6H_2O$.

oxidoreductase (oks-i-doh-ri-**duk**-tayz) *n.* one of a group of enzymes that catalyse oxidation-reduction reactions. This class includes the enzymes formerly known either as *dehydrogenases* or as *oxidases*.

oximeter (oks-**im**-it-er) *n.* an instrument for measuring the proportion of oxyhaemoglobin in the blood.

oxolinic acid (oks-oh-**lin**-ik) *n.* an antibacterial drug administered by mouth to treat infections of the urinary system. Trade name: **Prodoxol**.

oxprenolol (oks-**pren**-ŏ-lol) *n.* a drug that controls the activity of the heart (*see* beta blocker), administered by mouth or injection to treat angina, high blood pressure, and abnormal heart rhythm. Trade name: **Trasicor**.

oxycephaly (turricephaly) (oksi-**sef**-ăli) *n.* a deformity of the bones of the skull giving the head a pointed appearance. —**oxycephalic** (oksi-si-**fal**-ik) *adj.*

oxygen (**oks**-i-jĕn) *n.* an odourless colourless gas that makes up one-fifth of the atmosphere. Oxygen is essential to most forms of life; in man, it is absorbed into the blood from air breathed into the lungs. Oxygen is administered therapeutically in various conditions in which the tissues are unable to obtain an adequate supply through the lungs. Symbol: O. *o. deficit* a physiological condition that exists in cells during periods of temporary oxygen shortage. *o. tent see* tent.

oxygenation (oksi-ji-**nay**-shŏn) *n.* the process of becoming saturated with oxygen, such as occurs in the lungs during inhalation of air.

oxygenator (**oks**-i-ji-nay-ter) *n.* a machine that oxygenates blood outside the body. *See also* heartlung machine.

oxyhaemoglobin (oksi-hee-moh-**gloh**-bin) *n.* the bright-red substance formed when the pigment haemoglobin in red blood cells combines reversibly with oxygen. Oxyhaemoglobin is the form in which oxygen is transported from the lungs to the tissues. *Compare* methaemoglobin.

oxyntic cells (parietal cells) (oks-**in**-tik) *pl. n.* cells of the gastric glands that secrete hydrochloric acid in the fundic region of the stomach.

oxypertine (oksi-**per**-teen) *n.* a major tranquillizer administered by mouth to treat anxiety and tension in mental illnesses such as schizophrenia. Trade name: **Integrin.**

oxyphenbutazone (oksi-fen-**bew**-tă-zohn) *n.* an analgesic that also reduces inflammation and fever. It is administered by mouth or in suppositories to relieve pain in rheumatoid arthritis, gout, and similar conditions. Trade name: **Tanderil.**

oxyphencyclimine (oksi-fen-sy-kli-meen) *n.* a drug with actions similar to atropine. Since it slows down the digestive processes, it is used to treat stomach and duodenal ulcers and other digestive disorders. It is administered by mouth. Trade name: **Daricon.**

oxytetracycline (oksi-tet-ră-sy-kleen) *n.* an antibiotic used to treat infections caused by a wide variety of bacteria. It is administered by mouth or injection or applied to the skin in a cream. Trade names: **Clinimycin, Oxydon, Oxymycin, Terramycin,** etc.

oxytocic (oksi-**toh**-sik) *n.* a drug that induces or accelerates labour by stimulating the muscles of the womb to contract. *See also* oxytocin.

oxytocin (oksi-**toh**-sin) *n.* a hormone, released by the pituitary gland, that causes increased contraction of the womb during labour and stimulates the ejection of milk from the breasts. Oxytocin may be given by mouth or injection to assist labour.

oxyuriasis (oksi-yoor-I-ă-sis) *n. see* enterobiasis.

Oxyuris (oksi-**yoor**-iss) *n. see* pinworm.

ozaena (oh-**zee**-nă) *n.* a disorder of the nose in which the bones forming the sides of the nasal cavity become atrophied, with the production of an offensive discharge and crusts.

ozone (**oh**-zohn) *n.* a poisonous gas containing three oxygen atoms per molecule. Ozone is a very powerful oxidizing agent. It is found in the atmosphere at very high altitudes and is responsible for destroying a large proportion of the sun's ultraviolet radiation.

P

Pacchionian body (pak-i-**oh**-ni-ăn) *n. see* arachnoid. [A. Pacchioni (1665–1726), Italian anatomist]

pacemaker (**payss**-mayk-er) *n.* **1.** a device used to produce and maintain a normal heart rate in patients who have heart block. It consists of a battery that stimulates the heart through an insulated electrode wire attached to the surface of the ventricle (*epicardial p.*) or lying in contact with the lining of the heart (*endocardial p.*). A pacemaker may be temporary, with an external battery, or it may be permanent, when the whole apparatus is surgically implanted under the skin. **2.** the part of the heart that regulates the rate at which it beats: the sinoatrial node.

pachy- *prefix denoting* **1.** thickening of a part or parts. **2.** the dura mater.

pachydactyly (pak-i-**dak**-tili) *n.* abnormal enlargement of the fingers and toes, occurring either as a congenital abnormality or as part of an acquired disease (such as acromegaly).

pachydermia (pak-i-**der**-miă) *n.* any abnormal thickening of the skin.

pachymeningitis (pak-i-men-in-jy-tis) *n.* inflammation of the dura mater (*see* meningitis).

pachymeninx (pak-i-**mee**-ninks) *n.* the dura mater, outermost of the three meninges.

pachysomia (pak-i-**soh**-miă) *n.* thickening of parts of the body, which occurs in certain diseases.

Pacinian corpuscles (pă-**sin**-iăn) *pl. n.* sensory receptors for touch in the skin, consisting of sensory nerve endings surrounded by capsules of membrane. They are especially sensitive to changes in pressure and so detect vibration particularly well. [F. Pacini (1812–83), Italian anatomist]

pack (pak) *n.* a pad of folded moistened material, such as cotton-wool, applied to the body or inserted into a cavity.

packed cell volume (haematocrit) *n.* the volume of the red cells (erythrocytes) in blood, expressed as a fraction of the total volume of the blood.

pad (pad) *n.* cotton-wool, foam rubber, or other material used to protect a part of the body from friction, bruising, or other unwanted contact.

paed- (paedo-) *prefix denoting* children.

paediatrics (peed-i-**at**-riks) *n.* the general medicine of childhood. Handling the sick child requires detailed knowledge of genetics, obstetrics, psychological development, management of handicaps at home and in school, and effects of social conditions on child health. *See also* child health clinic. **—paediatrician** (peed-i-ă-**trish**-ăn) *n.*

Paget's disease (**paj**-its) *n.* **1.** a chronic disease of bones, occurring in the elderly and most frequently affecting the skull, backbone, pelvis, and long bones. Affected bones become thickened and severe continuous pain may result, which is relieved by a prolonged course of calcitonin injections. Medical name: **osteitis deformans**. **2.** an inflammatory condition of the nipple, resembling eczema in appearance, associated with underlying cancer of the milk ducts of the breast. *See also* breast cancer. [J. Paget (1814–99), British surgeon]

paint (paynt) *n.* (in pharmacy) a liquid preparation that is applied to the skin or mucous membranes. Paints usually contain antiseptics, astringents, caustics, or analgesics.

palaeo- *prefix denoting* **1.** ancient. **2.** primitive.

palate (**pal**-ăt) *n.* the roof of the mouth, which separates the mouth from the nasal cavity. *hard p.* the front part of the palate. It is formed by processes of the maxillae and palatine bones and is covered by mucous membrane. *soft p.* the posterior part of the palate: a movable fold of mucous membrane that tapers at the back of the mouth to form the uvula. *See also* cleft palate.

palatine bone (pal-ă-tyn) *n.* either of a pair of approximately L-shaped bones of the face that contribute to the hard palate, the nasal cavity, and the orbits.

palato- *prefix denoting* 1. the palate. 2. the palatine bone.

palatoplasty (pal-a-toh-plasti) *n.* plastic surgery of the roof of the mouth, usually to correct cleft palate or other congenital defects.

palatoplegia (pal-ă-toh-plee-jiă) *n.* paralysis of the soft palate.

palatorrhaphy (pal-ăt-o-răfi) *n. see* staphylorrhaphy.

pali- (**palin-**) *prefix denoting* repetition or recurrence.

palilalia (pal-i-lay-liă) *n.* a disorder of speech in which a word spoken by the individual is rapidly and involuntarily repeated.

palindromic (pal-in-drom-ik) *adj.* relapsing: describing diseases or symptoms that recur or get worse.

palliative (pal-i-ătiv) *n.* a medicine that gives temporary relief from the symptoms of a disease but does not actually cure the disease.

pallidectomy (pal-i-dek-tŏmi) *n.* a neurosurgical operation to destroy or modify the effects of the globus pallidus (*see* basal ganglia). This operation was used for the relief of parkinsonism and other conditions in which involuntary movements are prominent.

pallor (pal-er) *n.* abnormal paleness of the skin, due to reduced blood flow or lack of normal pigments. Pallor may indicate shock, anaemia, cancer, or other diseases.

palmar (pal-mer) *adj.* relating to the palm of the hand. *p. arches* two arterial arches (deep and superficial) in the palm of the hand, formed by anastomosis of the ulnar and radial arteries.

palmitic acid (pal-mit-ik) *n. see* fatty acid.

palpation (pal-pay-shŏn) *n.* the process of examining part of the body by careful feeling with the hands and fingertips.

palpebral (pal-pi-brăl) *adj.* relating to the eyelid (*palpebra*).

palpitation (pal-pi-tay-shŏn) *n.* an awareness of the heart beat. This is normal with fear, emotion, or exertion. It may also be a symptom of neurosis, arrhythmias, heart disease, and overactivity of the circulation.

palsy (pawl-zi) *n.* paralysis. *See* Bell's palsy, cerebral palsy.

paludism (pal-yoo-dizm) *n. see* malaria.

pan- (**pant(o)-**) *prefix denoting* all; every: hence (in medicine) affecting all parts of an organ or the body; generalized.

panacea (pan-ă-see-ă) *n.* a medicine said to be a cure for all diseases and disorders. Unfortunately panaceas do not exist, despite the claims of many patent medicine manufacturers.

Panadol (pan-ă-dol) *n. see* paracetamol.

panarthritis (pan-arth-ry-tis) *n.* inflammation of all the structures involved in a joint. *See* arthritis.

pancarditis (pan-kar-dy-tis) *n.* an inflammatory disorder affecting the pericardium, endocardium, and heart muscle.

pancreas (pank-ri-ăs) *n.* a compound gland, about 15 cm long, that lies behind the stomach. One end lies in the curve of the duodenum; the other end touches the spleen. It is composed of clusters (acini) of cells that secrete pancreatic juice into the duodenum via the *pancreatic duct*, which unites with the common bile duct. Interspersed among the acini are the islets of Langerhans, which secrete the hormones insulin and glucagon into the bloodstream. —**pancreatic** (pank-ri-at-ik) *adj.*

pancreatectomy (pank-ri-ă-tek-tŏmi) *n.* surgical removal of the pancreas, performed for tumours in the gland or because of chronic or relapsing pancreatitis. *partial p.* removal of a portion of the gland. *subtotal p.* removal of most of the gland. *total p.* (*Whipple's operation*) removal of the entire gland and part of the duodenum.

pancreatic juice *n.* the mixture of digestive enzymes secreted by the pancreas. Its production is stimulated by hormones secreted by the duodenum (*see* cholecystokinin-pancreozymin, secretin).

pancreatin (pank-ri-ă-tin) *n.* an extract obtained from the pancreas, containing the pancreatic enzymes. Pancreatin is administered for conditions in which pancreatic secretion is deficient; for example, in pancreatitis.

pancreatitis (pank-ri-ă-ty-tis) *n.* inflammation of the pancreas. *acute p.* a sudden illness in which the patient experiences severe pain in upper abdomen and back, with shock. Treatment consists of intravenous feeding and anticholinergic drugs. *chronic p.* pancreatitis that may produce symptoms similar to relapsing pancreatitis or may be painless; it leads to pancreatic failure causing malabsorption and diabetes mellitus. *relapsing p.* pancreatitis in which the symptoms

of acute pancreatitis are recurrent and less severe. It may be associated with gallstones or with alcoholism.

pancreatotomy (pank-ri-ă-tot-ŏmi) *n.* surgical opening of the duct of the pancreas in order to inspect the duct, to join the duct to the intestine, or to inject a contrast medium.

pancreozymin (pank-ri-oh-zy-min) *n. see* cholecystokinin-pancreozymin.

pancytopenia (pan-sy-toh-pee-niă) *n.* a simultaneous decrease in the numbers of red cells, white cells, and platelets in the blood. It occurs in a variety of disorders, including aplastic anaemias, hypersplenism, and tumours of the bone marrow.

pandemic (pan-dem-ik) *n.* an epidemic so widely spread that vast numbers of people in different countries are affected. —**pandemic** *adj.*

panhysterectomy (pan-hiss-ter-ek-tŏmi) *n.* the surgical removal of the entire womb, including its neck (cervix). *See* hysterectomy.

panhysterosalpingo-oophorectomy (pan-hiss-ter-oh-sal-ping-oh-oh-ŏ-fŏ-rek-tŏmi) *n.* surgical removal of the entire womb, the ovaries, and the Fallopian tubes.

panniculitis (pă-nik-yoo-ly-tis) *n.* inflammation of the panniculus adiposus, leading to multiple tender nodules in the thighs, trunk, and breasts. *See also* Weber-Christian disease.

panniculus (pă-nik-yoo-lŭs) *n.* a membranous sheet of tissue. *p. adiposus* the fatty layer of tissue underlying the skin.

pannus (pan-ŭs) *n.* invasion of the outer layers of the cornea of the eye by tissue containing many blood vessels, which grows in from the conjunctiva.

panophthalmitis (pan-off-thal-my-tis) *n.* inflammation involving the whole of the interior of the eye.

panosteitis (pan-osti-I-tis) *n.* inflammation of all the structures of a bone.

panotitis (pan-ŏ-ty-tis) *n.* inflammation of both the middle and the inner ears.

pant- (panto-) *prefix. see* pan-.

pantothenic acid (pan-tŏ-theen-ik) *n.* a B vitamin that is a constituent of coenzyme A. It plays an important role in the transfer of acetyl groups in the body.

pantropic (pan-trop-ik) *adj.* describing a virus that can invade and affect many different tissues of the body without showing a special affinity for any one of them.

Papanicolaou test (Pap test) (pap-ă-nik-oh-lay-oo) *n.* a test to detect cancer of the cervix or lining of the womb. A specimen of tissue taken from the womb is stained and examined under the microscope for the presence of abnormal cells. [G. N. Papanicolaou (1883–1962), Greek physician, anatomist, and cytologist]

papaveretum (pă-pav-er-ee-tŭm) *n.* a preparation of opium used for the relief of pain. It also contains several opium alkaloids, including papaverine.

papaverine (pă-pav-er-een) *n.* an alkaloid, derived from opium, that relaxes smooth muscle. It is administered by mouth or injection to treat muscle spasm in such conditions as colic and in sprays for the relief of asthma.

papilla (pă-pil-ă) *n.* (*pl.* **papillae**) any small nipple-shaped protuberance. Several different kinds of papillae occur on the tongue, in association with the taste buds. *optic p. see* optic (disc). —**papillary** *adj.*

papillitis (pap-i-ly-tis) *n.* inflammation of the optic disc.

papilloedema (pap-il-ee-dee-mă) *n.* swelling of the optic disc.

papilloma (pap-i-loh-mă) *n.* a benign growth on the surface of skin or mucous membrane. Warts are a type of papilloma.

papillomatosis (pap-i-loh-mă-toh-sis) *n.* a condition in which many papillomas grow on an area of skin or mucous membrane.

papovavirus (pap-oh-vă-vy-rŭs) *n.* one of a group of small DNA-containing viruses producing tumours in animals and man.

papule (pap-yool) *n.* a small superficial raised abnormality or spot on the skin. It usually forms part of a rash, such as appears with chickenpox. —**papular** *adj.*

papulo- *prefix denoting* a papule or pimple.

papulopustular (pap-yoo-loh-pus-tew-ler) *adj.* describing a rash that contains both papules and pustules.

papulosquamous (pap-yoo-loh-skway-mŭs) *adj.* **1.** describing a rash that is both papular and scaly. **2.** denoting a group of skin diseases that have this characteristic, including lichen planus and psoriasis.

para- *prefix denoting* **1.** beside or near. **2.** resembling. **3.** abnormal.

para-aminobenzoic acid (pa-ră-ă-mee-no-ben-zoh-ik) *n.* a naturally occurring drug used in lotions and creams to prevent sunburn. It was formerly administered by mouth to treat certain infections now treated with antibiotics.

para-aminosalicylic acid (PAS) (pa-ră-ă-mee-noh-sal-i-**sil**-ik) *n.* a drug administered by mouth, in conjunction with isoniazid or streptomycin, to treat tuberculosis. It is chemically related to aspirin.

paracentesis (pa-ră-sen-**tee**-sis) *n.* tapping: the process of drawing off excess fluid from a part of the body through a hollow needle or cannula.

paracetamol (pa-ră-**see**-tă-mol) *n.* an analgesic drug that also reduces fever. It is administered by mouth to treat mild or moderate pain, such as headache, toothache, and rheumatism. Trade names: **Panadol, Panasorb, Salzone.**

paracusis (pa-ră-**kew**-sis) *n.* any abnormality of hearing.

paradoxical breathing (pa-ră-**doks**-ikăl) *n.* breathing movements seen in patients with broken ribs: on inhalation the chest wall moves in instead of out, and vice versa on exhalation.

paraesthesiae (pa-ris-**theez**-i-ee) *pl. n.* spontaneously occurring abnormal tingling sensations, sometimes described as *pins and needles. Compare* dysaesthesiae.

paraffin (pa-ră-fin) *n.* one of a series of hydrocarbons derived from petroleum. *liquid p.* a mineral oil, which has been used as a laxative. *p. wax* (*hard p.*) a whitish mixture of solid hydrocarbons, used in medicine mainly as a base for ointments.

paraformaldehyde (pa-ră-for-**mal**-di-hyd) *n.* a white crystalline polymer of formaldehyde, used as a disinfectant fumigant and in the treatment of certain skin disorders.

parageusia (parageusis) (pa-ră-gew-siă) *n.* abnormality of the sense of taste.

paragonimiasis (endemic haemoptysis) (pa-ră-gon-i-**my**-ă-sis) *n.* a tropical disease, occurring principally in the Far East, caused by the presence of the fluke *Paragonimus westermani* in the lungs. Symptoms include the coughing up of blood and dyspnoea.

para-influenza viruses (pa-ră-in-floo-**en**-ză) *pl. n.* a group of large RNA-containing viruses that cause infections of the respiratory tract producing mild influenza-like symptoms. They are included in the paramyxovirus group (*see* myxovirus).

paraldehyde (pă-**ral**-di-hyd) *n.* a hypnotic and anticonvulsant drug administered by mouth, injection, or in suppositories to induce sleep in mental patients and to control convulsions in tetanus.

paralysis (pă-**ral**-i-sis) *n.* muscle weakness that varies in its extent, its severity, and the degree of spasticity or flaccidity according to the nature of the underlying disease and its distribution in the brain, spinal cord, peripheral nerves, or muscles. *See also* diplegia, hemiplegia, paraplegia, poliomyelitis. —**paralytic** (pa-ră-**lit**-ik) *adj.*

paramedian (pa-ră-**mee**-di-ăn) *adj.* situated close to or beside the median plane.

paramedical (pa-ră-**med**-ikăl) *adj.* describing or relating to the professions closely linked to the medical profession and working in conjunction with them. Paramedical personnel in a hospital include nurses, radiographers, physiotherapists, occupational therapists, and dietitians.

paramesonephric duct (Müllerian duct) (pa-ră-mes-oh-**nef**-rik) *n.* either of a pair of ducts in the embryo that develop into the Fallopian tubes, womb, and part of the vagina.

parameter (pă-**ram**-it-er) *n.* (in medicine) a measurement of some factor, such as blood pressure, pulse rate, or haemoglobin level, that may have a bearing on the condition being investigated.

paramethadione (pa-ră-meth-ă-**dy**-ohn) *n.* an anticonvulsant drug administered by mouth to prevent or reduce petit mal fits in epilepsy. Trade name: **Paradione**.

parametritis (pelvic cellulitis) (pa-ră-mi-**try**-tis) *n.* inflammation of the parametrium. The condition may be associated with puerperal fever.

parametrium (pa-ră-**mee**-triŭm) *n.* the layer of connective tissue surrounding the womb.

paramnesia (pa-ram-**nee**-ziă) *n.* a distorted memory, such as confabulation or déjà vu.

paramyotonia congenita (pa-ră-my-ŏ-**toh**-nia kŏn-**jen**-it-ă) *n.* a rare constitutional disorder in which myotonia develops when the patient is exposed to cold. This may be due to a disorder of potassium metabolism.

paranasal sinuses (pa-ră-**nay**-zăl) *pl. n.* the air-filled spaces, lined with mucous membrane, that occur in some bones of the skull and open into the nasal cavity. They comprise the *frontal sinuses* and the *maxillary sinuses* (one pair of each), the *ethmoid sinuses* (consisting of many spaces inside the ethmoid bone), and the two *sphenoid sinuses*.

paranoia (pa-ră-**noi**-ă) *n.* a mental disorder characterized by delusions organized into a system, without hallucinations or other marked symptoms of mental illness. The same term is sometimes used more loosely for a state of mind in which the individual has a strong belief that he is persecuted by others.

paranoid (pa-ră-noid) *adj.* **1.** describing a mental state characterized by fixed and logically elaborated delusions. There are many causes, including paranoid schizophrenia, manic-depressive psychosis, and severe emotional stress. **2.** describing a personality distinguished by such traits as excessive sensitivity to rejection by others, suspiciousness, hostility, and self-importance.

paraparesis (pa-ră-pă-**ree**-sis) *n.* weakness of both legs, resulting from disease of the nervous system.

paraphasia (pa-ră-**fay**-ziă) *n.* a disorder of language in which unintended syllables, words, or phrases are interpolated in the patient's speech.

paraphimosis (pa-ră-fi-**moh**-sis) *n.* retraction and constriction of the foreskin behind the glans penis. The tight foreskin cannot be drawn back over the glans and becomes painful and swollen.

paraphrenia (pa-ră-**free**-niă) *n.* a mental disorder, typically seen in the elderly and deaf, that is characterized by systematic delusions and prominent hallucinations but without any other marked symptoms of mental illness. Some sufferers eventually show other symtoms of schizophrenia.

paraplegia (pa-ră-**plee**-jiă) *n.* paralysis of both legs, usually due to disease or injury of the spinal cord. It is often accompanied by loss of sensation below the level of the injury and disturbed bladder function. —**paraplegic** *adj.*, *n.*

parapsoriasis (pa-ră-sŏ-**ry**-ă-sis) *n.* any one of a group of skin diseases (erythrodermas) that develop slowly and are typified by chronic red scaly patches that resemble psoriasis.

parapsychology (pa-ră-sy-**kol**-ŏji) *n.* the study of mental abilities that appear to defy natural law.

paraquat (**pa**-ră-kwot) *n.* the chemical compound dimethyl dipyridilium, widely used as a weed-killer. When swallowed it exerts its most serious effects upon the lungs, the tissues of which it destroys after a few days.

parasite (**pa**-ră-syt) *n.* any living thing that lives in or on another living organism (*see* host). Some parasites cause irritation and interfere with bodily functions; others destroy host tissues and release toxins into the body. Human parasites include fungi, bacteria, viruses, protozoa, and worms. *See also* commensal, symbiosis. —**parasitic** (pa-ră-**sit**-ik) *adj.*

parasiticide (pa-ră-**sit**-i-syd) *n.* an agent, such as gamma benzene hexachloride, that destroys parasites (excluding bacteria and fungi). *See also* acaricide, anthelmintic, trypanocide.

parasitology (pa-ră-sit-**ol**-ŏji) *n.* the study and science of parasites.

parasuicide (pa-ră-**soo**-i-syd) *n.* a self-injuring act (such as an overdose of sleeping pills) that is not motivated by a genuine wish to die. *Compare* (attempted) suicide.

parasympathetic nervous system (pa-ră-sim-pă-**thet**-ik) *n.* one of the two divisions of the autonomic nervous system, having fibres that leave the central nervous system from the brain and the lower portion of the spinal cord and are distributed to blood vessels, glands, and internal organs. The nerve endings release acetylcholine as a neurotransmitter.

parasympatholytic (pa-ră-sim-pă-thoh-**lit**-ik) *n.* a drug, such as atropine, that opposes the effects of the parasympathetic nervous system. The actions of parasympatholytic drugs include relaxation of smooth muscle, decreased secretion of saliva, sweat, and digestive juices, and dilation of the pupil of the eye.

parasympathomimetic (pa-ră-sim-pă-thoh-mi-**met**-ik) *n.* a drug that has the effect of stimulating the parasympathetic nervous system. The actions of the parasympathomimetic drugs include stimulation of skeletal muscle, vasodilatation, depression of heart rate, increasing the tension of smooth muscle, increasing secretions (such as saliva), and constricting the pupil of the eye.

parathion (pa-ră-**th'y**-on) *n.* an organic phosphorus compound, used as a pesticide, that causes poisoning when inhaled, ingested, or absorbed through the skin. The symptoms are headache, sweating, salivation, lacrimation, vomiting, diarrhoea, and muscular spasms. Treatment is by administration of atropine.

parathormone (pa-ră-**thor**-mohn) *n.* see parathyroid hormone.

parathyroidectomy (pa-ră-th'y-roid-ek-tŏmi) *n.* surgical removal of the parathyroid glands, usually as part of the treatment of hyperparathyroidism.

parathyroid glands (pa-ră-**th'y**-roid) *pl. n.* two pairs of yellowish-brown endocrine glands that are situated behind, or sometimes embedded within, the thyroid gland. They are stimulated to produce parathyroid hormone by a decrease in the amount of calcium in the blood.

parathyroid hormone (parathormone) *n.* a hormone, synthesized and released by the parathyroid glands, that controls the distribution of calcium and phosphate in the body. A deficiency of the hormone lowers blood calcium levels, causing tetany. *Compare* thyrocalcitonin.

paratyphoid fever (pa-ră-**ty**-foid) *n.* an infectious disease caused by the bacterium *Salmonella paratyphi* A, B, or C. Symptoms include diarrhoea, mild fever, and a pink rash on the chest. Treatment with chloramphenicol is effective. Vaccination with TAB provides temporary immunity against paratyphoid A and B.

paravertebral (pa-ră-ver-tib-răl) *adj.* close to or at the side of the backbone.

parenchyma (pă-**renk**-im-ă) *n.* the functional part of an organ, as opposed to the supporting tissue (stroma).

parenteral (pa-**rent**-er-ăl) *adj.* administered by any way other than through the mouth: applied, for example, to the introduction of drugs into the body by injection.

paresis (pă-**ree**-sis) *n.* muscular weakness caused by disease of the nervous system. It implies a lesser degree of weakness than paralysis, although the two

words are often used interchangeably.

paries (**pair**-i-eez) *n.* (*pl.* **parietes**) 1. the enveloping or surrounding part of an organ or other structure. 2. the wall of a cavity.

parietal (pă-**ry**-ĕ-t'l) *adj.* of or relating to the inner walls of a body cavity, as opposed to the contents. *p. bone* either of a pair of bones forming the top and sides of the cranium. *See* skull. *p. cells see* oxyntic cells. *p. lobe* one of the major divisions of each cerebral hemisphere (*see* cerebrum), lying beneath the crown of the skull. It contains the sensory cortex and association areas. *p. pleura see* pleura.

parity (**pa**-riti) *n.* the condition of a woman with regard to the number of pregnancies she has had that have each resulted in the birth of an infant capable of survival.

parkinsonism (par-kin-sŏn-izm) *n.* a disorder of middle-aged and elderly people characterized by tremor, rigidity and a poverty of spontaneous movements. The patient has an expressionless face, an unmodulated voice, and an increasing tendency to stoop. Parkinsonism is a disease affecting the basal ganglia of the brain; it can be induced by such drugs as chlorpromazine. Relief of the symptoms may be obtained with anticholinergic drugs and levodopa. [J. Parkinson (1755–1824), British physician]

paromomycin (pa-roh-moh-**my**-sin) *n.* an antibiotic, active against intestinal bacteria and amoebae, administered by mouth to treat dysentery and gastroenteritis.

paronychia (pa-roh-**nik**-iă) *n.* inflammation and swelling of the skin folds and tissues surrounding a fingernail or toenail. *See also* whitlow.

parosmia (pa-**roz**-miă) *n.* any disorder of the sense of smell.

parotid gland (pă-**rot**-id) *n.* one of a pair of salivary glands situated in front of each ear.

parotitis (pa-rŏ-**ty**-tis) *n.* inflammation of the parotid salivary glands. *See* mumps (infectious parotitis).

parous (**pa**-rŭs) *adj.* having given birth to one or more children.

paroxysm (**pa**-rŏk-sizm) *n.* **1.** a sudden violent attack, especially a spasm or convulsion. **2.** the abrupt worsening of symptoms or recurrence of disease. —**paroxysmal** (pa-rŏk-**siz**-măl) *adj.*

paroxysmal dyspnoea *n.* attacks of breathlessness occurring at night due to left ventricular heart failure.

paroxysmal tachycardia *n.* abnormally increased heart rate due to impulses generated anywhere in the heart outside the natural pacemaker (sinoatrial node).

parrot disease (**pa**-rŏt) *n.* an infectious disease of parrots and budgerigars; it can be transmitted to man and causes headache, bleeding from the nose, shivering, fever, and complications involving the lungs. The disease responds to tetracyclines or penicillin. Medical name: **psittacosis**. *Compare* ornithosis.

pars (parz) *n.* a specific part of an organ or other structure, such as any of parts of the pituitary gland.

parthenogenesis (par-thin-oh-**jen**-i-sis) *n.* reproduction in which an organism develops from an unfertilized ovum. It is common in plants and occurs in some lower animals (e.g. aphids).

parturition (par-tewr-**ish**-ŏn) *n.*

childbirth. *See* labour. —**parturient** (par-**tewr**-i-ĕnt) *adj.*

parvi- *prefix denoting* small size.

PAS *n. see* para-aminosalicylic acid.

pascal (**pas**-kăl) *n.* the SI unit of pressure, equal to 1 newton per square metre. Symbol: Pa.

Paschen bodies (**pah**-skĕn) *pl. n.* particles that occur in the cells of skin rashes in patients with cowpox or smallpox; they are thought to be the virus particles. [E. Paschen (1860–1936), German pathologist]

passive movement (**pas**-iv) *n.* movement not brought about by a patient's own efforts. Passive movements are induced by manipulation of the joints by a physiotherapist. *Compare* active movement.

Pasteurella (pas-cher-**el**-ă) a genus of small rodlike Gram-negative bacteria that are parasites of animals and man. *P. pestis* the species that causes plague in man.

pasteurization (pas-cher-I-**zay**-shŏn) *n.* the treatment of milk by heating it to 65°C for 30 minutes, or to 72°C for 15 minutes, followed by rapid cooling, to kill such bacteria as those of tuberculosis and typhoid.

pastille (**pas**-t'l) *n.* a medicinal preparation containing gelatine and glycerine that is dissolved in the mouth so that the medication is applied to the mouth or throat.

patch test (pach) *n.* a test to discover which of a number of possible substances is responsible for a patient's allergy. Small quantities of different allergens are applied to the skin; a positive reaction is typically a patch of swelling with a red flare.

patella (pă-tel-ă) *n.* the lens-shaped bone that forms the kneecap. It is situated in front of the knee in the tendon of the quadriceps muscle of the thigh. *See also* sesamoid bone. —**patellar** (pă-tel-er) *adj.*

patellar reflex *n.* the knee jerk, in which stretching the muscle at the front of the thigh by tapping its tendon below the kneecap causes a reflex contraction of the muscle, so that the leg kicks.

patellectomy (pat-ĕ-lek-tŏmi) *n.* surgical excision of the patella.

patent (pay-tĕnt) *adj.* open; unblocked. *p. ductus arteriosus see* ductus arteriosus.

path- (patho-) *prefix denoting* disease.

pathogen (pa-thŏ-jen) *n.* a microorganism, such as a bacterium, that parasitizes an animal (or plant) or man and produces a disease.

pathogenesis (pa-thŏ-jen-i-sis) *n.* the origin and development of a disease. —**pathogenetic** (pa-thoh-ji-net-ik) *adj.*

pathogenic (pa-thŏ-jen-ik) *adj.* capable of causing disease. The term is applied to a parasitic microorganism (especially a bacterium) in relation to its host. —**pathogenicity** *n.*

pathognomonic (pa-thŏg-noh-mon-ik) *adj.* describing a symptom or sign that is characteristic of or unique to a particular disease.

pathological (pa-thŏ-loj-ikăl) *adj.* relating to or arising from disease.

pathology (pă-thol-ŏji) *n.* the study of disease processes with the aim of understanding their nature and causes. *clinical p.* the application of the knowledge of disease processes to the treatment of patients. —**pathologist** *n.*

-pathy *suffix denoting* 1. disease. 2. therapy.

Paul's tube (pawlz) *n.* a glass tube with a projecting rim, used to drain the bowel after it has been brought to the surface of the abdomen and opened. [F. T. Paul (1851–1941), British surgeon]

Pearson bed (peer-sŏn) *n.* a special type of hospital bed for nursing patients with fractures.

peau d'orange (poh daw-rahnj) *n.* a dimpled appearance of the skin over a breast tumour, resembling the surface of an orange. The skin is thickened and the openings of hair follicles and sweat glands are enlarged.

pecten (pek-tin) *n.* 1. the middle section of the anal canal. 2. a sharp ridge on the upper branch of the pubis (part of the hip bone). —**pectineal** (pek-tin-iăl) *adj.*

pectoral (pek-ter-ăl) *adj.* relating to the chest or breast. *p. girdle see* shoulder girdle. *p. muscles* the chest muscles: the pectoralis major, which draws the arm forward across the chest, and the pectoralis minor, which depresses the shoulder.

pectoriloquy (pek-ter-il-ŏ-kwi) *n.* abnormal transmission of the patient's voice sounds through the chest wall so that they can be clearly heard through a stethoscope.

pectus (pek-tŭs) *n.* the chest or breast.

pedicle (ped-ikŭl) *n.* 1. the narrow neck of tissue connecting some tumours to the normal tissue from which they have developed. 2. (in plastic surgery) a narrow folded tube of skin by means of which a piece of skin used for grafting remains attached to its original site. **3.** (in anatomy) any slender stemlike process.

pediculicide (pi-**dik**-yoo-li-syd) *n.* an agent that kills lice; for example benzyl benzoate and gamma benzene hexachloride.

pediculosis (pi-dik-yoo-**loh**-sis) *n.* an infestation of the body and/or scalp with lice of the genus *Pediculus*, which causes intense itching. Body lice are destroyed by dusting the body and clothes with DDT powder; head lice are eliminated with gamma benzene hexachloride.

Pediculus (pi-**dik**-yoo-lŭs) *n.* a widely distributed genus of lice. *P. humanus capitis* the head louse. *P. humanus corporis* the body louse, which in some parts of the world transmits relapsing fever and typhus. *See also* pediculosis.

peduncle (pi-**dunk**-ŭl) *n.* a narrow process or stalklike structure, serving as a connection or support.

Pel–Ebstein fever (pel-eb-styn) *n.* a recurrent fever characteristic of patients with lymphoma or Hodgkin's disease. [P. K. Pel (1852–1919), Dutch physician; W. Ebstein (1836–1912), German physician]

pellagra (pil-**ag**-ră) *n.* a nutritional disease due to a deficiency of nicotinic acid (a B vitamin). It is common in maize-eating communities. The symptoms of pellagra are scaly dermatitis on exposed surfaces, diarrhoea, and depression.

pellet (**pel**-it) *n.* a small pill, especially one used as an implant.

pellicle (**pel**-ikŭl) *n.* a thin layer of skin, membrane, or any other substance.

pelvic girdle (**hip girdle**) (**pel**-vik)

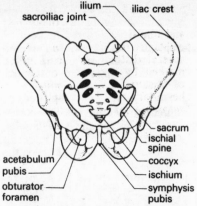

The male pelvis (ventral view)

n. the bony structure to which the bones of the lower limbs are attached. It consists of the right and left hip bones.

pelvimetry (pel-**vim**-itri) *n.* the measurement of the four internal diameters of the pelvis, using an instrument called a *pelvimeter*. Pelvimetry helps in determining whether it will be possible for a fetus to be delivered in the normal way.

pelvis (**pel**-vis) *n.* (*pl.* **pelves**) **1.** the bony structure formed by the hip bones, sacrum, and coccyx (see illustration). The hip bones are fused at the back to the sacrum to form a rigid structure that protects the organs of the lower abdomen and provides attachment for the bones and muscles of the lower limbs. **2.** the cavity within the bony pelvis. **3.** any structure shaped like a basin. *renal p.* the expanded part of the ureter in the kidney. —**pelvic** *adj.*

pemphigoid (**pem**-fig-oid) *n.* any of a group of skin disorders that resemble pemphigus but are distinct from it. A common type affects the elderly, with large blisters occurring on the trunk and limbs.

pemphigus (pem-fig-ŭs) *n.* any of several distinctive skin diseases marked by successive outbreaks of blisters. *benign familial p.* a hereditary type of pemphigus. *p. vulgaris* a rare serious disease occurring in middle age and initially affecting the mucous membranes.

-penia *suffix denoting* lack or deficiency.

penicillamine (pen-i-sil-ă-meen) *n.* a drug that binds metals and therefore aids their excretion (*see* chelating agent). It is administered by mouth to treat Wilson's disease, metal poisoning, and severe rheumatoid arthritis. Trade names: **Cuprimine, Distamine**.

penicillin (benzylpenicillin, penicillin G) (pen-i-sil-in) *n.* an antibiotic derived from the mould *Penicillium chrysogenum* and used to treat infections caused by a wide variety of bacteria. It is usually administered by injection. Some patients are allergic to penicillin and develop such reactions as skin rashes, swelling of the throat, and fever. Trade names: **Crystapen, Falapen, Icipen, Stabillin**.

penicillinase (pen-i-sil-in-ayz) *n.* an enzyme-like substance, produced by some bacteria, that is capable of antagonizing the antibacterial action of penicillin. Purified penicillinase may be used to treat reactions to penicillin.

Penicillium (pen-i-sil-iŭm) *n.* a genus of mouldlike fungi that commonly grow on decaying fruit, bread, or cheese. Some species are pathogenic to man, causing diseases of the skin and respiratory tract. *P. chrysogenum* the

The penis (median section)

major natural source of the antibiotic penicillin.

penis (pee-nis) *n.* the male organ that carries the urethra, through which urine and semen are discharged. Most of the organ is composed of erectile tissue (corpus cavernosum and corpus spongiosum), which becomes filled with blood under conditions of sexual excitement so that the penis is erected. *See also* glans, prepuce.

pent- (penta-) *prefix denoting* five.

pentaerythritol (pen-tă-i-rith-ri-tol) *n.* a drug that dilates blood vessels and is administered by mouth in the treatment of angina and other heart conditions. Trade names: **Cardiacap, Mycardol, Pentral, Peritrate**.

pentagastrin (pen-tă-gas-trin) *n.* a synthetic hormone that has the same effects as gastrin. It is injected to test for gastric secretion in the diagnosis of digestive disorders. Trade name: **Peptavlon**.

pentazocine (pen-taz-oh-seen) *n.* a potent analgesic drug administered by mouth, injection, or in suppositories to relieve moderate or severe pain. Trade name: **Fortral.**

pentobarbitone (pen-tŏ-**bar**-bi-tohn) *n.* a barbiturate drug used to relieve insomnia and agitation and also as an anticonvulsant. It is administered by mouth, injection, or in suppositories. Trade name: **Nembutal.**

pentose (**pen**-tohz) *n.* a simple sugar with five carbon atoms: for example, ribose and xylose.

pentosuria (pen-tohs-**yoor**-iă) *n.* an inborn defect of sugar metabolism causing abnormal excretion of pentose in the urine.

Pentothal (**pen**-tŏ-thal) *n. see* thiopentone.

peppermint (**pep**-er-mint) *n.* an oil extracted from a species of mint (*Mentha piperita*), used as a carminative and flavouring agent.

pepsin (**pep**-sin) *n.* an enzyme in the stomach that begins the digestion of proteins by splitting them into peptones (*see* peptidase). It is produced by the action of hydrochloric acid on *pepsinogen*, which is secreted by the gastric glands.

pepsinogen (pep-**sin**-ŏ-jĕn) *n. see* pepsin.

peptic (**pep**-tik) *adj.* **1.** relating to pepsin. **2.** relating to digestion. *p. ulcer* a breach in the lining (mucosa) of the digestive tract produced by digestion of the mucosa by pepsin and acid. This may occur when pepsin and acid are present in abnormally high concentrations. *See* duodenal ulcer, gastric (ulcer), oesophageal ulcer.

peptidase (**pep**-tid-ayz) *n.* one of a group of digestive enzymes that split proteins in the stomach and intestine into their constituent amino acids.

peptide (**pep**-tyd) *n.* a molecule consisting of two or more amino acids linked by bonds between the amino group and the carboxyl group. *See also* polypeptide.

peptone (**pep**-tohn) *n.* a large protein fragment produced by the action of enzymes on proteins in the first stages of protein digestion.

peptonuria (pep-tohn-**yoor**-iă) *n.* the presence in the urine of peptones.

perception (per-**sep**-shŏn) *n.* (in psychology) the process by which information about the world, received by the senses, is analysed and made meaningful.

percussion (per-**kush**-ŏn) *n.* the technique of examining part of the body by tapping it with the fingers or an instrument (plessor) and sensing the resultant vibrations. It is used to detect the presence of fluid or abnormal solidification or enlargement in different organs.

percutaneous (per-kew-**tay**-niŭs) *adj.* through the skin: often applied to the route of administration of drugs in ointments, etc., which are absorbed through the skin.

perforation (per-fer-**ay**-shŏn) *n.* the creation of a hole in an organ, tissue, or tube. This may occur in the course of a disease, such as duodenal ulcer, colonic diverticulitis, or stomach cancer. Treatment is usually by surgical repair of the perforation, but conservative treatment with antibiotics may result in spontaneous healing. Perforation may also be caused accidentally by instruments (for example a curette may perforate the womb) or by injury (for example to the eardrum).

perfusion (per-few-*zh*ŏn) *n.* **1.** the passage of fluid thorough a tissue, especially the passage of blood through the lung tissue to pick up oxygen in the alveoli and release carbon dioxide. **2.** the deliberate introduction of fluid into a tissue, usually by injection into the blood vessels supplying the tissue.

peri- *prefix denoting* near, around, or enclosing.

periadenitis (pe-ri-ad-in-I-tis) *n.* inflammation of tissues surrounding a gland.

perianal haematoma (external haemorrhoid) (pe-ri-ay-năl) *n.* a small painful swelling beside the anus, occurring after a bout of straining to pass faeces or coughing. Perianal haematomas are caused by the rupture of a small vein in the anus.

periarteritis nodosa (pe-ri-ar-ter-I-tis) *n. see* polyarteritis nodosa.

periarthritis (pe-ri-arth-ry-tis) *n.* inflammation of tissues around a joint capsule, including tendons and bursae. *chronic p.* a common cause of pain and stiffness of the shoulder; it usually responds to local steroid injections or physiotherapy.

pericard- (pericardio-) *prefix denoting* the pericardium.

pericardectomy (pe-ri-kar-dek-tŏmi) *n.* surgical removal of the pericardium. It is used in the treatment of chronic constrictive pericarditis and chronic pericardial effusion (*see* pericarditis).

pericardiocentesis (pe-ri-kar-di-oh-sen-tee-sis) *n.* removal of excess fluid from within the pericardium by means of needle aspiration

pericardiorrhaphy (pe-ri-kar-di-o-răfi) *n.* the repair of wounds in the pericardium, such as those due to injury or surgery.

pericardiostomy (pe-ri-kar-di-ost-ŏmi) *n.* an operation in which the pericardium is opened and the fluid within drained via a tube. It is sometimes used in the treatment of septic pericarditis.

pericarditis (pe-ri-kar-dy-tis) *n.* acute or chronic inflammation of the pericardium. Pericarditis may be seen alone or as part of pancarditis. It has numerous causes, including virus infections, uraemia, and cancer. *acute p.* pericarditis characterized by fever, chest pain, and a pericardial friction rub. Fluid may accumulate within the pericardial sac (*pericardial effusion*). *chronic constrictive p.* chronic thickening of the pericardium, which interferes with activity of the heart and has many features in common with heart failure.

pericardium (pe-ri-kar-diŭm) *n.* the membrane surrounding the heart. *fibrous p.* the outer portion of the pericardium, which completely encloses the heart and is attached to the large blood vessels emerging from the heart. *serous p.* the internal portion of the pericardium: a closed sac of serous membrane containing a very small amount of fluid, which prevents friction between the two surfaces as the heart beats. —**pericardial** *adj.*

pericardotomy (pe-ri-kar-dot-ŏmi) *n.* surgical opening or puncture of the pericardium. It is required to gain access to the heart in heart surgery and to remove excess fluid from within the pericardium.

perichondritis (pe-ri-kon-dry-tis) *n.* inflammation of cartilage and surrounding soft tissues, usually due to chronic infection. A common site is the external ear.

perichondrium (pe-ri-**kon**-driŭm) *n.* the dense layer of fibrous connective tissue that covers the surface of cartilage.

pericolpitis (paracolpitis) (pe-ri-kol-**py**-tis) *n.* inflammation of the connective tissues around the vagina.

pericranium (pe-ri-**kray**-niŭm) *n.* the periosteum of the skull.

pericystitis (pe-ri-sis-**ty**-tis) *n.* inflammation in the tissues around the bladder, causing pain in the pelvis, fever, and symptoms of cystitis. It usually results from infection in the Fallopian tubes or womb.

perifolliculitis (pe-ri-fŏ-lik-yoo-**ly**-tis) *n.* inflammation around the hair follicles.

perihepatitis (pe-ri-hep-ă-**ty**-tis) *n.* inflammation of the membrane covering the liver. It is usually associated with abnormalities of the liver or chronic peritonitis.

perilymph (**pe**-ri-limf) *n.* the fluid between the bony and membranous labyrinths of the ear.

perimeter (per-**im**-it-er) *n.* an instrument for mapping the absolute extent of the visual field and detecting any gaps or defects. —**perimetry** *n.*

perimetritis (pe-ri-mi-**try**-tis) *n.* inflammation of the membrane on the outer surface of the womb. The condition may be associated with parametritis.

perimetrium (pe-ri-**mee**-triŭm) *n.* the peritoneum of the womb.

perimysium (pe-ri-**mis**-iŭm) *n.* the fibrous sheath that surrounds each bundle of muscle fibres.

perinatal (pe-ri-**nay**-t'l) *adj.* relating to the period from about three months before to one month af-

ter birth. *p. mortality rate* the number of stillbirths and first-week or neonatal deaths per 1000 live births.

perineoplasty (pe-ri-nee-oh-plasti) *n.* a tissue-grafting operation to repair the perineum.

perineorrhaphy (pe-ri-ni-o-răfi) *n.* the stitching of a tear, possibly sustained during childbirth, in the perineum.

perinephric (pe-ri-**nef**-rik) *adj.* around the kidney.

perinephritis (pe-ri-ni-**fry**-tis) *n.* inflammation of the tissues around the kidney, usually due to spread of infection from the kidney itself. The patient has pain in the loins, fever, and fits of shivering.

perineum (pe-ri-**nee**-ŭm) *n.* the region of the body between the anus and the urethral opening, including both skin and underlying muscle. —**perineal** *adj.*

perineurium (pe-ri-**newr**-iŭm) *n.* the sheath of connective tissue that surrounds individual bundles of nerve fibres within a large nerve.

periodic fever (peer-i-**od**-ik) *n. see* malaria.

periodontal (pe-ri-ŏ-**don**-t'l) *adj.* denoting or relating to the tissues surrounding the teeth. *p. disease* disease of the gums and other structures supporting the teeth: the most common cause of tooth loss in older people. *p. membrane* (*p. ligament*) the ligament around a tooth, by which it is attached to the bone.

periodontium (pe-ri-ŏ-**don**-tiŭm) *n.* the tissues, collectively, surrounding the teeth: the gums (gingiva), periodontal membrane, and alveolar bone.

periosteotome (pe-ri-**ost**-i-ŏ-tohm) *n.* an instrument used for cutting the periosteum and separating it from the underlying bone.

periosteum (pe-ri-**ost**-iŭm) *n.* a layer of dense connective tissue that covers the surface of a bone and provides attachment for muscles, tendons, and ligaments. The outer layer of the periosteum contains a large number of blood vessels; the inner layer contains osteoblasts and fewer blood vessels. —**periosteal** *adj.*

periostitis (pe-ri-ost-**I**-tis) *n.* inflammation of the periosteum. *acute p.* periostitis that results from direct injury to the bone and is associated with a haematoma, which may later become infected. *chronic p.* periostitis that is often due to an inflammatory disease, such as tuberculosis or syphilis, or to a chronic ulcer overlying the bone involved.

peripheral nervous system (per-if-er-ăl) *n.* all parts of the nervous system lying outside the central nervous system. It includes the cranial nerves and spinal nerves and their branches and the autonomic nervous system.

periphlebitis (pe-ri-fli-**by**-tis) *n.* inflammation of the tissues around a vein: seen as an extension of phlebitis.

periproctitis (pe-ri-prok-**ty**-tis) *n.* inflammation of the tissues around the rectum and anus.

perisalpingitis (pe-ri-sal-pin-**jy**-tis) *n.* inflammation of the membrane on the outer surface of a Fallopian tube.

perisplenitis (pe-ri-spli-**ny**-tis) *n.* inflammation of the external coverings of the spleen.

peristalsis (pe-ri-**stal**-sis) *n.* a wavelike movement that progresses along some of the hollow muscular tubes of the body, such as the intestines. It occurs involuntarily, induced by distension of the walls of the tube. Alternate contraction and relaxation of the circular and longitudinal muscles tends to push the contents of the tube forward. —**peristaltic** *adj.*

peritendinitis (pe-ri-ten-di-**ny**-tis) *n.* *see* tenosynovitis.

peritomy (per-**it**-ŏmi) *n.* an eye operation in which an incision of the conjunctiva is made in a complete circle around the cornea. It is performed for the relief of pannus.

peritoneoscope (pe-ri-tŏn-**ee**-ŏ-skohp) *n.* *see* laparoscope.

peritoneum (pe-ri-tŏn-**ee**-ŭm) *n.* the serous membrane of the abdominal cavity. *parietal p.* the part of the peritoneum that lines the walls of the abdomen. *visceral p.* the part of the peritoneum that covers the abdominal organs. *See also* mesentery, omentum. —**peritoneal** *adj.*

peritonitis (pe-ri-tŏn-**I**-tis) *n.* inflammation of the peritoneum. *primary p.* peritonitis caused by bacteria spread via the bloodstream. Symptoms are diffuse abdominal pain and swelling, with fever and weight loss. *secondary p.* peritonitis due to perforation or rupture of an abdominal organ, such as the vermiform appendix, allowing access of bacteria and irritant digestive juices to the peritoneum. This produces sudden severe abdominal pain and shock. Treatment is usually by surgical repair of the perforation.

peritonsillar abscess (pe-ri-**ton**-sil-er) *n.* *see* quinsy.

liver
kidney
pancreas
stomach
duodenum
transverse colon
peritoneal cavity
mesentery
jejunum
ileum
bladder
pubic
symphysis
rectum

Sagittal section of the abdomen to show arrangement of the peritoneum

peritrichous (pe-ri-**try**-kŭs) *adj.* describing bacteria in which the flagella cover the entire cell surface.

perityphlitis (pe-ri-tif-**ly**-tis) *n.* *Archaic.* inflammation of the tissues around the caecum. *See* typhlitis.

periureteritis (pe-ri-yoor-i-ter-**I**-tis) *n.* inflammation of the tissues around a ureter. This is usually associated with inflammation of the ureter itself (ureteritis) often behind an obstruction caused by a stone or stricture.

perle (perl) *n.* a soft capsule containing medicine.

perleche (per-**lesh**) *n.* dryness and cracking of the corners of the mouth, sometimes with infection. Perleche may be caused by persistent lip licking or by a vitamin-deficient diet.

permeability (per-mi-ă-**bil**-iti) *n.*

the ability of membranes to allow soluble substances to pass through them. *See also* semipermeable membrane. —**permeable** (**per**-mi-ăbŭl) *adj.*

pernicious (per-**nish**-ŭs) *adj.* describing diseases that are highly dangerous or likely to result in death if untreated. *p. anaemia* a form of anaemia resulting from deficiency of vitamin B_{12}, due either to failure to produce intrinsic factor or to dietary deficiency of the vitamin. It is characterized by defective production of red blood cells and the presence of megaloblasts in the bone marrow.

pernio (**per**-ni-oh) *n. see* chilblain.

perniosis (per-ni-**oh**-sis) *n.* any one of a group of conditions caused by the effect of persistent cold on sensitive skin blood vessels. The small arteries constrict and the capillaries dilate slowing the blood flow: the affected area becomes blue, swollen, and cold. Perniosis includes chilblains, acrocyanosis, erythrocyanosis, and Raynaud's disease.

pero- *prefix denoting* deformity; defect.

peromelia (pe-roh-**mee**-liă) *n.* congenital deformity of one or more limbs.

peroneal (pe-rŏ-**nee**-ăl) *adj.* relating to or supplying the outer (fibular) side of the leg.

peroneus (pe-rŏ-**nee**-ŭs) *n.* one of the muscles of the leg that arises from the fibula and helps to turn the foot outwards.

peroral (per-**or**-ăl) *adj.* through the mouth.

perphenazine (per-**fen**-ă-zeen) *n.* a major tranquillizer administered by mouth or injection to relieve anxiety, tension, and agitation and to prevent nausea and vomiting. Trade name: **Fentazin**.

perseveration (per-sev-er-ay-shŏn) *n.* excessive persistence at a task that prevents the individual from turning his attention to new situations. It is a symptom of organic disease of the brain and sometimes of obsessional neurosis.

personality (per-sŏn-**al**-iti) *n.* (in psychology) an enduring disposition to act and feel in particular ways that differentiate one individual from another.

personality disorder *n.* a deeply ingrained and maladjusted pattern of behaviour, which persists through many years and causes suffering, either to the patient or to other people (or to both). *See* asthenic, hysterical, paranoid, psychopath, schizoid personality.

perspiration (per-sper-ay-shŏn) *n.* sweat or the process of sweating.

insensible p. sweat that evaporates immediately from the skin and is therefore not visible. *sensible p.* sweat that is visible on the skin in the form of drops.

Perthes' disease (**per**-tiz) *n. see* Legg-Calvé-Perthes disease.

pertussis (per-**tus**-iss) *n. see* whooping cough.

perversion (per-**ver**-shŏn) *n.* any abnormal sexual behaviour. The abnormality may be in the sexual object (as in homosexuality and fetishism) or in the activity engaged in (for example, sadism and exhibitionism).

pes (payz) *n.* (in anatomy) the foot or a part resembling a foot. *p. clavus see* claw-foot. *p. planus see* flat-foot.

pessary (**pess**-er-i) *n.* **1.** a plastic or metal instrument, often ring-shaped, that fits into the vagina and keeps the womb in position: used to treat prolapse. **2.** a plug or cylinder of soft material containing a drug that is fitted into the vagina for the treatment of such disorders as vaginitis. Also called: **vaginal suppository**.

pesticide (**pest**-i-syd) *n.* a chemical agent, such as parathion, used to kill insects or other organisms harmful to crops and other cultivated plants.

petechia (pi-**tee**-kiă) *n.* (*pl.* **petechiae**) a small round flat dark-red spot caused by bleeding into the skin or beneath the mucous membrane.

pethidine (**peth**-i-deen) *n.* a potent analgesic drug with mild sedative action, administered by mouth or injection to relieve moderate or severe pain.

petit mal (**pe**-tee mal) *n.* a form of idiopathic epilepsy in which there are brief spells of unconsciousness, lasting for a few seconds, during which posture and balance are maintained and the eyes stare blankly. Petit mal seldom appears before the age of three or after adolescence and often subsides spontaneously in adult life. It may be accompanied or followed by grand mal. Drug treatment (with sodium valproate or ethosuximide) is usually effective.

Petri dish (pet-ri) *n.* a flat shallow circular glass or plastic dish with a pillbox-like lid, used to hold solid agar or gelatin media for culturing bacteria. [J. R. Petri (1852–1921), German bacteriologist]

petrissage (pay-tri-**sah***zh*) *n.* kneading: a form of massage in which the skin is lifted up, pressed down and squeezed, and pinched and rolled.

petrositis (pet-roh-**sy**-tis) *n.* inflammation of the petrous part of the temporal bone, usually due to an extension of mastoiditis.

petrous bone (pet-rŭs) *n. see* temporal bone.

-pexy *suffix denoting* surgical fixation.

Peyer's patches (py-erz) *pl. n.* oval masses of lymphoid tissue on the mucous membrane lining the small intestine. [J. C. Peyer (1653–1712), Swiss anatomist]

Peyronie's disease (pay-roh-**neez**) *n.* a dense fibrous plaque in the penis. The penis curves or angulates at this point on erection and pain often results. [F. de la Peyronie (1678–1747), French surgeon]

pH *n.* a measure of the concentration of hydrogen ions in a solution, and therefore of its acidity or alkalinity. A pH of 7 indicates a neutral solution, a pH below 7 indicates acidity, and a pH in excess of 7 indicates alkalinity.

phaco- *prefix. see* phako-.

phaeochromocytoma (fi-oh-kroh-moh-sy-**toh**-mă) *n.* a small vascular tumour of the medulla of the adrenal gland. By its uncontrolled and irregular secretion of the hormones adrenaline and noradrenaline, the tumour causes attacks of raised blood pressure, increased heart rate, palpitations, and headache.

phag- **(phago-)** *prefix denoting* **1.** eating. **2.** phagocytes.

phage (fayj) *n. see* bacteriophage.

-phagia *suffix denoting* a condition involving eating.

phagocyte (**fag**-ŏ-syt) *n.* a cell that is able to engulf and digest bacteria, protozoa, cells and cell debris, and other small particles. Phagocytes include many white blood cells and macrophages, which play a major role in the body's defence mechanism. —**phagocytic** *adj.*

phagocytosis (fag-ŏ-sy-**toh**-sis) *n.* the engulfment and digestion of bacteria and other foreign particles by a phagocyte. *Compare* pinocytosis.

phako- **(phaco-)** *prefix denoting* the lens of the eye.

phalanges (fă-**lan**-jeez) *n.* (*sing.* **phalanx**) the bones of the fingers and toes (digits). The first digit (thumb/big toe) has two phalanges. Each of the remaining digits has three phalanges. —**phalangeal** *adj.*

phalangitis (fal-ăn-**jy**-tis) *n.* inflammation of a finger or toe, caused by infection of the soft tissues, bone, or joints or by rheumatic diseases. *See also* dactylitis.

phalanx (fal-anks) *n. see* phalanges.

phalloplasty (fal-oh-plasti) *n.* surgical reconstruction or repair of the penis, performed to correct a congenital deformity or following injury to the penis.

phallus (fal-ŭs) *n.* the embryonic penis, before the urethral duct has reached its final state of development.

phantasy (fant-ăsi) *n. see* fantasy.

phantom limb (fan-tŏm) *n.* the sensation that an arm or leg, or part of an arm or leg, is still attached to the body after it has been amputated.

phantom tumour *n.* a swelling, in the abdomen or elsewhere, caused by local muscular contraction or the accumulation of gases, that mimics a swelling caused by a tumour. The condition is usually associated with emotional disorder.

pharmaceutical (farm-ă-sewt-ikăl) *adj.* relating to pharmacy.

pharmacist (farm-ă-sist) *n.* a person who is qualified by examination and registered and authorized to dispense medicines.

pharmaco- *prefix denoting* drugs.

pharmacology (farm-ă-kol-ŏji) *n.* the science of the properties of drugs and their effects on the body. **—pharmacological** *adj.* **—pharmacologist** *n.*

pharmacopoeia (farm-ă-kŏ-pee-ă) *n.* a book containing a list of the drugs used in medicine, with details of their formulae, methods of preparation, dosages, standards of purity, etc.

pharmacy (farm-ăsi) *n.* **1.** the preparation and dispensing of drugs. **2.** premises registered to dispense medicines and sell poisons.

pharyng- (pharyngo-) *prefix denoting* the pharynx.

pharyngeal pouch (branchial or **visceral pouch) (fa-rin-jee-**ăl) *n.* any of the paired segmented pouches in the side of the throat of the early embryo. They give rise to the tympanic cavity, the parathyroid glands, the thymus, and probably the thyroid gland.

pharyngectomy (fa-rin-jek-tŏmi) *n.* surgical removal of part of the pharynx.

pharyngismus (fa-rin-jiz-mŭs) *n.* spasmodic contraction of the muscles of the pharynx.

pharyngitis (fa-rin-jy-tis) *n.* inflammation of the pharynx. It produces sore throat and is usually associated with tonsillitis.

pharyngocele (fă-ring-oh-seel) *n.* a pouch or cyst opening off the pharynx (*see* branchial cyst).

pharyngolaryngeal (fă-ring-oh-la-rin-jee-ăl) *adj.* relating to both the pharynx and the larynx.

pharyngoscope (fă-ring-ŏ-skohp) *n.* an endoscope for the examination of the pharynx.

pharyngotympanic tube (fă-ring-oh-tim-pan-ik) *n. see* Eustachian tube.

pharynx (fa-rinks) *n.* a muscular tube, lined with mucous membrane, that extends from the beginning of the oesophagus (gullet) up to the base of the skull. It communicates with the posterior nares, Eustachian tube, mouth, larynx, and oesophagus. The pharynx acts as a passageway for food, as an air passage from the nasal cavity and mouth to the larynx, and as a resonating chamber for the sounds produced in the larynx. **—pharyngeal** *adj.*

phenacemide (fin-ass-i-myd) *n.* an anticonvulsant drug administered by mouth in the treatment of epilepsy.

phenacetin (fin-**ass**-i-tin) *n.* an analgesic drug that also reduces fever, administered by mouth to relieve mild or moderate pain. Because prolonged high doses may cause kidney damage, its use in Britain was restricted by law in 1974.

phenazocine (fin-az-oh-seen) *n.* an analgesic drug administered by mouth or injection for rapid relief of moderate or severe pain. Trade name: **Narphen**.

phenazopyridine (fen-ă-zoh-pi-ri-deen) *n.* an analgesic drug administered by mouth to relieve pain in inflammatory conditions of the bladder and urinary tract, such as cystitis and urethritis. Trade name: **Pyridium**.

phenelzine (fen-ĕl-zeen) *n.* a drug administered by mouth to relieve depression and anxiety (*see* MAO inhibitor). Trade name: **Nardil**.

pheneturide (fen-et-yoor-ryd) *n.* an anticonvulsant drug administered by mouth in the treatment of major types of epilepsy. Trade name: **Benuride**.

phenformin (fen-for-min) *n.* a drug that reduces blood sugar levels and is administered by mouth to treat diabetes. Trade names: **Dibotin, Dipar, Meltrol**.

phenindione (fen-in-di-ohn) *n.* an anticoagulant drug administered by mouth or injection to treat thrombosis in the blood vessels of the heart and limbs. Trade name: **Dindevan**.

pheniodol (fin-I-ŏ-dol) *n.* an iodine-containing compound used as a contrast medium during X-ray examination of the gall bladder (*see* cholecystography).

pheniramine (fen-eer-ă-meen) *n.* an antihistamine used to treat allergic reactions such as hay fever and hives. It is administered by mouth or is applied to the skin in an ointment. Trade name: **Daneral**.

phenobarbitone (fee-noh-**bar**-bit-ohn) *n.* a barbiturate drug administered by mouth or injection to treat insomnia and anxiety and as an anticonvulsant in the treatment of epilepsy.

phenol (carbolic acid) (fee-nol) *n.* a strong disinfectant used for cleansing wounds, treating inflammations of the mouth, throat, and ear, and as a preservative in injections. It is administered as solution, ointments, and lotions and is highly toxic if taken by mouth.

phenolphthalein (fee-nol-**thal**-i-in) *n.* an irritant laxative administered by mouth, usually given at night to act the following morning.

phenolsulphonphthalein (fee-nol-sul-fohn-**thal**-i-in) *n.* a red dye administered by injection in a test for kidney function.

phenothiazines (fee-noh-**th'y**-ă-zeenz) *pl. n.* a group of chemically related compounds with various pharmacological actions. Some (e.g. chlorpromazine) are major tranquillizers; others (e.g. piperazine) are anthelmintics.

phenotype (fee-noh-typ) *n.* the observable characteristics of an individual, which result from interaction between his genotype and the environment.

phenoxybenzamine (fin-oks-i-ben-ză-meen) *n.* a drug that dilates blood vessels (*see* vasodilator). It is administered by mouth or injection to reduce blood pressure and to treat conditions involving poor circulation, such as Raynaud's disease and chilblains. Trade name: **Dibenyline**.

phenoxymethylpenicillin (fin-oks-i-meth-il-pen-i-**sil**-in) *n.* an antibiotic, similar to penicillin, administered by mouth to treat infections caused by a wide variety of microorganisms.

phensuximide (fen-**suks**-i-myd) *n.* an anticonvulsant drug administered by mouth to prevent or reduce petit mal fits in epilepsy.

phentermine (**fen**-ter-meen) *n.* a sympathomimetic drug that suppresses the appetite and is administered by mouth in the treatment of obesity. Trade names: **Duromine**, **Ionamin**.

phentolamine (fen-**tol**-ă-meen) *n.* a drug that dilates blood vessels (*see* vasodilator) and is administered by mouth or injection to reduce blood pressure in phaeochromocytoma and to treat conditions of poor circulation, such as Raynaud's disease and chilblains. Trade name: **Rogitine**.

phenylalanine (fee-nyl-**al**-ă-neen) *n.* ,an essential amino acid that is readily converted to tyrosine. Blockade of this metabolic pathway gives rise to phenylketonuria.

phenylbutazone (fee-nyl-**bew**-tă-zohn) *n.* an analgesic drug that reduces fever and inflammation and is administered by mouth or injection to relieve pain in rheumatic and related diseases. Trade names: **Butazolidin**, **Butazone**, **Flexazone**.

phenylephrine (fee-nyl-**ef**-reen) *n.* a drug that constricts blood vessels (*see* sympathomimetic). It is given by injection to increase blood pressure, in a nasal spray to relieve nasal congestion, and

in eye-drops to dilate the pupils. Trade name: **Neophryn**.

phenylketonuria (fee-nyl-kee-tŏn-**yoor**-iă) *n.* an inborn defect of protein metabolism causing an excess of the amino acid phenylalanine in the blood, which damages the nervous system and leads to severe mental retardation. The gene responsible for phenylketonuria is recessive, so that a child is affected only if both parents are carriers of the defective gene.

phenytoin (fen-i-**toh**-in) *n.* an anticonvulsant drug administered by mouth or injection to control major (grand mal) and focal fits in epilepsy. Trade name: **Epanutin**.

phial (**fy**-ăl) *n.* a small glass bottle for storing medicines or poisons.

-philia *suffix denoting* morbid craving or attraction.

phimosis (fy-**moh**-sis) *n.* narrowing of the opening of the foreskin, which cannot therefore be drawn back over the underlying glans penis.

phleb- (**phlebo-**) *prefix denoting* a vein or veins.

phlebectomy (fli-**bek**-tŏmi) *n.* the surgical removal of a vein (or part of a vein), sometimes performed for the treatment of varicose veins in the legs (*varicectomy*).

phlebitis (fli-**by**-tis) *n.* inflammation of the wall of a vein, which is most commonly seen in the legs as a complication of varicose veins. A segment of vein becomes painful and tender and the surrounding skin feels hot and appears red. Thrombosis (*thrombophlebitis*) commonly develops. Treatment consists of elastic support together with drugs, such as phenylbutazone.

phlebography (fli-**bog**-răfi) *n. see* venography.

phlebolith (**flee**-boh-lith) *n.* a stone-like structure that results from deposition of calcium in a venous blood clot.

phlebothrombosis (flee-boh-throm-**boh**-sis) *n.* obstruction of a vein by a blood clot, without preceding inflammation of its wall. It is most common within the deep veins of the calf of the leg. The affected leg may become swollen and tender and the clot may become detached and give rise to pulmonary embolism. Prolonged bed rest, heart failure, pregnancy, injury, and surgery predispose to thrombosis by encouraging sluggish blood flow. Anticoagulant drugs (such as warfarin and heparin) are used in prevention and treatment.

phlebotomy (**venesection**) (fli-**bot**-ŏmi) *n.* the surgical opening or puncture of a vein in order to remove blood (in the treatment of polycythaemia) or to infuse fluids, blood, or drugs in the treatment of many conditions.

phlegm (flem) *n.* a nonmedical term for sputum.

phlegmasia (fleg-**may**-ziă) *n.* inflammation. *p. alba dolens see* white leg.

phlycten (**flik**-těn) *n.* a small pinkish-yellow nodule surrounded by a zone of dilated blood vessels that occurs in the conjunctiva or in the cornea. Phlyctens are thought to be due to a type of allergy to the tubercle bacillus.

phobia (**foh**-biă) *n.* a pathologically strong fear of a particular event or thing. Avoiding the feared situation may severely restrict one's life and cause much suffering. Treatment is with behaviour therapy, especially desensitization and flooding. Psychotherapy and drug therapy are also useful.

-phobia *suffix denoting* morbid fear or dread.

phocomelia (foh-koh-**mee**-liă) *n.* congenital absence of the upper arm and/or upper leg, the hands or feet or both being attached to the trunk by a short stump.

pholcodine (**fol**-kŏ-deen) *n.* a drug that suppresses coughs and reduces irritation in the respiratory system (*see* antitussive). It is administered by mouth in cough mixtures.

phon- (phono-) *prefix denoting* sound or voice.

phonation (foh-**nay**-shŏn) *n.* the production of vocal sounds, particularly speech.

phonocardiogram (foh-noh-**kar**-di-ŏ-gram) *n. see* electrocardiophonography. —**phonocardiography** (foh-noh-**kar**-di-ŏ-gram) *n.*

-phoria *suffix denoting* (in ophthalmology) an abnormal deviation of the eyes or turning of the visual axis.

phosgene (**fos**-jeen) *n.* a poisonous gas developed during World War I. It is a choking agent, acting on the lungs to produce oedema, with consequent respiratory and cardiac failure.

phosphagen (**fos**-fă-jěn) *n.* creatine phosphate (*see* creatine).

phosphataemia (fos-fă-**tee**-miă) *n.* the presence of phosphates in the blood. Sodium, calcium, potassium, and magnesium phosphates are normal constituents.

phosphatase (**fos**-fă-tayz) *n.* one of a group of enzymes capable of catalysing hydrolysis of phosphoric acid esters. Phosphatases are important in the absorption and metabolism of carbohydrates, nucleotides, and phospholipids and are essential in the calcification of bone. *acid p.* a phosphatase present in kidney, semen, serum, and the prostate gland. *alkaline p.* a phosphatase that occurs in teeth, developing bone, plasma, kidney, and intestine.

phosphate (**fos**-fayt) *n.* any salt or ester of phosphoric acid.

phosphatidylcholine (fos-fat-i-dil-**koh**-leen) *n. see* lecithin.

phosphaturia (phosphuria) (fos-făt-**yoor**-iă) *n.* the presence of an abnormally high concentration of phosphates in the urine, making it cloudy. The condition may be associated with the formation of calculi in the kidneys or bladder.

phosphocreatine (fos-foh-**kree**-ă-teen) *n.* creatine phosphate (*see* creatine).

phospholipid (fos-foh-**lip**-id) *n.* a lipid containing a phosphate group as part of the molecule. Phospholipids are constituents of all tissues and organs, especially the brain. They are involved in many of the body's metabolic processes. Examples are cephalins, lecithins, and plasmalogens.

phosphonecrosis (fos-foh-nek-**roh**-sis) *n.* the destruction of tissues caused by excessive amounts of phosphorus in the system. The tissues likely to suffer are the liver, kidneys, muscles, bones, and the cardiovascular system.

phosphorus (**fos**-fer-us) *n.* a nonmetallic element that' is toxic in its pure state. Phosphorus compounds are major constituents in the tissues of both plants and animals. In man, phosphorus is mostly concentrated in bone. Symbol: P.

phot- (photo-) *prefix denoting* light.

photalgia (foh-**tal**-jiă) *n.* pain in the eye caused by very bright light.

photocoagulation (foh-toh-koh-ag-yoo-**lay**-shŏn) *n.* the destruction of tissue by heat released from the absorption of light shone on it. In eye disorders the technique is used to destroy diseased retinal tissue and to produce scarring between the retina and choroid, thus binding them together, in cases of detached retina.

photodermatitis (foh-toh-der-mă-ty-tis) *n.* a condition in which the skin becomes sensitized to a substance but only those parts of the skin subsequently exposed to light react by developing dermatitis.

photomicrograph (foh-toh-**my**-krŏ-grahf) *n. see* micrograph.

photophobia (foh-toh-**foh**-biă) *n.* an abnormal intolerance of light, in which exposure to light produces intense discomfort of the eyes with tight contraction of the eyelids. Photophobia may be associated with migraine, measles, German measles, or meningitis.

photophthalmia (foh-tof-**thal**-miă) *n.* inflammation of the eye due to exposure to light. It is usually caused by the damaging effect of ultraviolet light on the cornea, for example in snow blindness.

photoretinitis (foh-toh-ret-in-**I**-tis) *n.* damage to the retina of the eye caused by looking at the sun without adequate protection for the eyes. The central part of the visual field may be permanently lost (*sun blindness*).

photosensitivity (foh-toh-sen-si-tiv-iti) *n.* abnormal and severe reaction of the skin to sunlight. —**photosensitive** *adj.*

phototherapy (foh-toh-**th'e**-ră-pi) *n.* the treatment of disorders by exposing the patient to light. Phototherapy using fluorescent light is used to treat jaundice in the newborn, as the blue range of the light decomposes bilirubin.

photuria (foht-**yoor**-iă) *n.* the excretion of phosphorescent urine, due to the presence of certain phosphorus-containing compounds.

phren- (**phreno-**) *prefix denoting* 1. the mind or brain. 2. the diaphragm. 3. the phrenic nerve.

phrenemphraxis (phreniclasia) (fren-em-**fraks**-iss) *n.* surgical crushing of a portion of the phrenic nerve. This paralyses the diaphragm on the side operated upon, which is then pushed up by the abdominal contents, so pressing on the lung and partially collapsing it.

-phrenia *suffix denoting* a condition of the mind.

phrenic (**fren**-ik) *adj.* 1. relating to the mind. 2. relating to the diaphragm. *p. avulsion* the surgical removal of a section of the phrenic nerve, which paralyses the diaphragm. The procedure was used as a means of resting a lung infected with tuberculosis. *p. nerve* the nerve that supplies the muscles of the diaphragm. On each side it arises in the neck and passes downwards between the lungs and the heart.

phrenicectomy (fren-i-**sek**-tŏmi) *n.* surgical division or removal of part of the phrenic nerve. Partial removal of the nerve produces the same results as phrenemphraxis and division (*phrenicotomy*); it is done because the nerve sometimes regenerates after the other procedures.

phreniclasia (fren-i-**klay**-ziă) *n. see* phrenemphraxis.

phrenicotomy (fren-i-**kot**-ŏmi) *n. see* phrenicectomy.

phthalylsulphathiazole (thal-il-sul-fă-**th'y**-ă-zohl) *n.* a drug (*see* sulphonamide) that is slowly broken down in the gut and is therefore administered by mouth to treat bowel infections.

phthiriasis (thi-**ry**-ă-sis) *n.* infestation of the crab louse, *Phthirus pubis*, which causes intense itching; continued scratching by the patient may result in bacterial infection of the skin.

Phthirus (**thi**-rŭs) *n.* a widely distributed genus of lice. *P. pubis* the crab (or pubic) louse, a common parasite of man that lives permanently attached to the body hair, particularly that of the pubic or perianal regions. *See also* phthiriasis.

phthisis (**th'y**-sis) *n.* a former name for: 1. any disease resulting in wasting of tissues; 2. pulmonary tuberculosis.

phycomycosis (fy-koh-my-**koh**-sis) *n.* a disease caused by parasitic fungi of the genera *Rhizopus*, *Absidia*, and *Mucor*. The fungi grow within the blood vessels of the lungs and nervous tissue, causing blood clots that cut off the blood supply (*see* infarction). Treatment with the antibiotic amphotericin has proved effective.

physi- (**physio-**) *prefix denoting* 1. physiology. 2. physical.

physical (**fiz**-ikăl) *adj.* (in medicine) relating to the body rather than to the mind. *p. sign* a sign that a doctor can detect when examining a patient, such as abnormal dilation of the pupils or the absence of a knee-jerk reflex.

physical medicine *n.* the medical specialty concerned with the diagnosis and management of rheumatic diseases and the rehabilitation of patients with physical disabilities. *See also* rheumatology.

physician (fiz-ish-ăn) *n.* a registered medical practitioner who specializes in the diagnosis and treatment of disease by other than surgical means. *See also* Doctor.

physiological saline (fiz-i-ŏ-loj-ikăl) *n.* a 0.9% solution of sodium chloride in water, used for maintaining living cells.

physiological solution *n.* one of a group of solutions, including Ringer's solution, used to maintain tissues in a viable state. These solutions contain specific concentrations of substances that are vital for normal tissue function.

physiology (fiz-i-ol-ŏji) *n.* the science of the functioning of living organisms and of their component parts. —**physiological** *adj.* —**physiologist** *n.*

physiotherapy (fiz-i-oh-th'e-ră-pi) *n.* the branch of treatment that employs physical methods to promote healing, including the use of light, heat, electric current, massage, manipulation, and remedial exercise.

physo- *prefix denoting* air or gas.

physostigmine (eserine) (fy-soh-stig-meen) *n.* a parasympathomimetic drug used mainly to constrict the pupil of the eye and to reduce pressure inside the eye in glaucoma. It is administered by injection, in eyedrops, or in an ointment.

phyt- (phyto-) *prefix denoting* plants; of plant origin.

phytomenadione (fy-toh-men-ă-dy-ohn) *n.* a form of vitamin K that is used as an antidote to overdosage with anticoagulant drugs. It promotes the production of prothrombin, essential for the normal coagulation of blood.

pia (pia mater) (pee-ă) *n.* the innermost of the three meninges surrounding the brain and spinal cord. It contains numerous finely branching blood vessels that supply the nerve tissue within.

pian (pi-ahn) *n. see* yaws.

pica (py-kă) *n.* the indiscriminate eating of non-nutritious or harmful substances, such as grass, stones, or clothing. It is common in early childhood but may also be found in mentally handicapped and psychotic patients.

Pick's disease (piks) *n.* **1.** a rare cause of dementia in middle-aged people. The damage is mainly in the frontal and temporal lobes of the brain. [A. Pick (1851–1924), Czech psychiatrist] **2.** a syndrome in constrictive pericarditis, in which there is hepatic enlargement, ascites, and pleural effusion. [F. Pick (1867–1926), Czech physician]

picornavirus (pi-kor-nă-vy-rŭs) *n.* one of a group of small RNA-containing viruses. The group includes Coxsackie viruses, echoviruses, polioviruses, and rhinoviruses.

picric acid (trinitrophenol) (pik-rik) *n.* a yellow crystalline solid used as a dye and as a tissue fixative.

pigeon chest (pij-ŏn) *n.* forward protrusion of the breastbone resulting in deformity of the chest. The condition is painless and harmless.

pigeon toes *n*. an abnormal posture in which the toes are turned inwards. It is often associated with knock-knee.

pigment (**pig**-měnt) *n*. a substance giving colour. Physiologically important pigments include the blood pigments (especially haemoglobin), bile pigments, and retinal pigment (*see* rhodopsin).

pigmentation (pig-měn-**tay**-shŏn) *n*. coloration produced in the body by the deposition of one pigment, especially in excessive amounts. Pigmentation may be produced by natural pigments, such as melanin, or by foreign material, such as lead or arsenic in chronic poisoning.

piles (pylz) *pl. n. see* haemorrhoids.

pill (pil) *n*. **1.** a small round ball, sometimes coated with sugar, that contains one or more medicinal substances in solid form. It is taken by mouth. **2. the Pill** *see* oral contraceptive.

pillar (**pil**-er) *n*. (in anatomy) an elongated apparently supportive structure.

pilo- *prefix denoting* hair.

pilocarpine (py-loh-**kar**-peen) *n*. a drug with actions and uses similar to those of physostigmine. It is administered as eye-drops.

pilomotor nerves (py-loh-**moh**-ter) *pl. n.* sympathetic nerves that supply muscle fibres in the skin, around the roots of hairs. Activity of the sympathetic nervous system causes the muscles to contract, resulting in goose flesh.

pilonidal sinus (py-loh-**ny**-d'l) *n*. a short tract leading from an opening in the skin in the cleft at the top of the buttocks and containing hairs. The sinus may be recurrently infected, leading to pain and the discharge of pus.

pilosebaceous (py-loh-si-**bay**-shŭs) *adj*. relating to the hair follicles and their associated sebaceous glands.

pilosis (py-**loh**-sis) *n*. the abnormal growth of hair.

pilus (py-lŭs) *n*. a hair.

pimel- (**pimelo-**) *prefix denoting* fat; fatty.

pimozide (**pim**-oh-zyd) *n*. a major tranquillizer administered by mouth to relieve hallucinations and delusions occurring in schizophrenia. Trade name: **Orap**.

pimple (**pim**-pŭl) *n*. a small inflamed swelling on the skin that contains pus. It may be the result of bacterial infection of a skin pore that has become obstructed with fatty secretions from the sebaceous glands. *See also* acne.

pineal body (**pineal gland**) (**pin**-i-ăl) *n*. a pea-sized mass of tissue attached by a stalk to the posterior wall of the third ventricle of the brain. It may play a part in initiating the development of the gonads, but this is uncertain. Anatomical name: **epiphysis**.

pinguecula (ping-**wek**-yoo-lă) *n*. a degenerative change in the conjunctiva of the eye, seen most commonly in the elderly. Thickened yellow triangles develop on the conjunctiva at the inner and outer margins of the cornea.

pink disease *n*. a severe illness of children of the teething age, marked by pink cold clammy hands and feet, heavy sweating, raised blood pressure, rapid pulse, and photophobia. The condition may be an allergic reaction to mercury; it has virtually disappeared since all mercury-containing paediatric preparations have been banned. Medical names: **acrodynia, er-ythroedema, erythromelalgia.**

pink eye *n. see* conjunctivitis.

pinna (auricle) (pin-ă**)** *n.* the flap of skin and cartilage that projects from the head at the exterior opening of the external auditory meatus of the ear.

pinocytosis (pee-noh-sy-**toh**-sis) *n.* the intake of small droplets of fluid by a cell by cytoplasmic engulfment. *Compare* phagocytosis.

pinta (pin-tă**)** *n.* a skin disease, prevalent in tropical America, that seems to affect only the dark-skinned races. It is caused by the spirochaete *Treponema carateum.* Symptoms include thickening and eventual loss of pigment of the skin, particularly on the hands, wrists, feet, and ankles.

pinworm (threadworm) (pin-werm**)** *n.* a parasitic nematode worm of the genus *Enterobius* (*Oxyuris*), which lives in the upper part of the large intestine of man. Pinworms cause enterobiasis, a disease common in children throughout the world.

piperazine (pi-pe-**ră**-zeen) *n.* a drug administered by mouth to treat infestations by roundworms and threadworms. Trade names: **Antepar, Pripsen.**

piperidolate (pi-**pe**-ri-doh-layt) *n.* a drug, similar to atropine, administered by mouth to treat colic and other conditions involving spasm of the stomach and intestine. Trade name: **Dactil.**

piriform fossae (pi-ri-form) *pl. n.* two pear-shaped depressions that lie on either side of the opening to the larynx.

pisiform bone (py-si-form) *n.* the smallest bone of the wrist (*see* carpus): a pea-shaped bone that articulates with the triquetral bone and, indirectly by cartilage, with the ulna.

pit (pit) *n.* (in anatomy) a hollow or depression.

pithiatism (pith-I-ă-tizm) *n.* the treatment of certain disorders by persuading the patient that all is well.

pitting (pit-ing**)** *n.* the formation of depressed scars, as occurs on the skin following smallpox or acne. *p. oedema* oedema in which fingertip pressure leaves temporary indentations in the skin.

pituitary gland (hypophysis) (pit-**yoo**-it-eri) *n.* the master endocrine gland: a pea-sized body attached to the hypothalamus at the base of the skull. The anterior lobe (*adenohypophysis*) secretes thyroid-stimulating hormone, ACTH, gonadotrophins, growth hormone, prolactin, lipotrophin, and melanocyte-stimulating hormone. The posterior lobe (*neurohypophysis*) secretes vasopressin and oxytocin.

pityriasis (pit-i-**ry**-ă-sis) *n.* (originally) any of a group of skin diseases typified by the development of fine branlike scales. *p. alba* a common condition in children and adolescents in which uneven round pale macules appear on the face. *p. capitis see* dandruff. *p. rosea* a common skin complaint in which flat pink oval macules develop on the trunk and upper parts of the limbs. It occurs mainly in young people in spring and autumn.

pivot joint (piv-ŏt**)** *n. see* trochoid joint.

placebo (plă-**see**-boh) *n.* a medicine that is ineffective but may help to relieve a condition because the patient has faith in its powers. New drugs are tested against placebos in clinical trials.

placenta (plă-**sent**-ă) *n.* an organ within the uterus by means of which the embryo is attached to the wall of the uterus. Its primary function is to provide the embryo with nourishment, eliminate its wastes, and exchange respiratory gases. It also functions as a gland, secreting chorionic gonadotrophin, progesterone, and oestrogens. *See also* afterbirth. *p. praevia* the attachment of the placenta to the lower part of the womb (instead of to the upper part, as is normal). As it grows, the placenta may partially or completely cover the outlet from the womb to the vagina and delivery by Caesarean section may be necessary. —**placental** *adj.*

placentography (plas-en-**tog**-răfi) *n.* radiography of the pregnant womb in order to determine the position of the placenta.

plagiocephaly (play-ji-oh-**sef**-ăli) *n.* any distortion or lack of symmetry in the shape of the head, usually due to irregularity in the closure of the sutures between the bones of the skull.

plague (playg) *n.* **1.** any epidemic disease with a high death rate. **2.** an acute epidemic disease of rats and other wild rodents caused by the bacterium *Pasteurella pestis*, which is transmitted to man by rat fleas. *bubonic p.* the most common form of the disease, characterized by acute painful swellings of the lymph nodes (*see* bubo). In favourable cases the buboes burst and then heal; in other cases bleeding under the skin can lead to ulcers, which may prove fatal. *pneumonic p.* a

serious form of plague in which the lungs are affected. *septicaemic p.* a serious form of plague in which bacteria enter the bloodstream.

plane (playn) *n.* a level or smooth surface, especially any of the hypothetical flat surfaces used to divide the body (*see* coronal, sagittal).

planning (**plan**-ing) *n.* the stage of the nursing process in which an individual *care plan* is produced, stating the patient's problem(s), the objective, the goal or expected outcome, the nursing intervention, and the time or date by which the objective is expected to be achieved or by which the problem should be reviewed.

plantar (**plan**-ter) *adj.* relating to the sole of the foot (*planta*). *p. arch* the arch in the sole of the foot formed by anastomosing branches of the plantar arteries. *p. reflex* a reflex obtained by drawing a bluntly pointed object along the outer border of the sole of the foot. The normal response is a bunching and downward movement of the toes. *Compare* Babinski reflex. *p. wart see* wart.

plaque (plak) *n.* **1.** a layer composed of bacteria in an organic matrix that forms on the surface of a tooth, principally at its neck. It may cause caries or periodontal disease. **2.** a raised circular patch of skin or mucous membrane resulting from local damage, usually due to infection.

-plasia *suffix denoting* formation; development.

plasm- (plasmo-) *prefix denoting* **1.** blood plasma. **2.** protoplasm or cytoplasm.

plasma (blood plasma) (plaz-mă) *n.* the straw-coloured fluid in which the blood cells are suspended. It consists of a solution of various inorganic salts of sodium, potassium, calcium, etc., with a high concentration of protein and a variety of trace substances.

plasmacytoma (plaz-mă-sy-toh-mă) *n.* a malignant tumour of plasma cells, very closely allied to myeloma. It usually occurs as a solitary tumour of bone, but may be multiple; less frequently it affects soft tissues.

plasmapheresis (plaz-mă-fer-ee-sis) *n.* a method of removing a quantity of plasma from the blood. Blood is withdrawn from the patient and allowed to settle. The plasma is then drawn off and the blood cells transfused back into the patient.

plasmin (fibrinolysin) (plaz-min) *n.* an enzyme that digests the protein fibrin. Its function is the dissolution of blood clots (*see* fibrinolysis).

plasminogen (plaz-min-ŏ-jĕn) *n.* a substance normally present in the blood plasma that may be activated to form plasmin. *See* fibrinolysis.

Plasmodium (plaz-moh-diŭm) *n.* a genus of protozoans (*see* Sporozoa) that live as parasites within the red blood cells and liver cells of man. Four species cause malaria in man: *P. vivax*, *P. ovale*, *P. falciparum*, and *P. malariae*.

plaster (plah-ster) *n.* adhesive tape used in shaped pieces or as a bandage to keep a dressing in place.

plaster of Paris *n.* a preparation of gypsum (calcium sulphate) that sets hard when water is added. It is used in dentistry and orthopaedics for preparing plaster casts.

plastic lymph (plast-ik) *n.* a transparent yellowish liquid produced in a wound or other site of inflammation, in which connective tissue cells and blood vessels develop during healing.

plastic surgery *n.* a branch of surgery dealing with the reconstruction of deformed or damaged parts of the body. It also includes the replacement of parts of the body that have been lost.

plastron (plas-tron) *n.* the breastbone (sternum) together with the costal cartilages attached to it.

-plasty *suffix denoting* plastic surgery.

platelet (thrombocyte) (playt-lit) *n.* a disc-shaped structure, 1–2 μm in diameter, present in the blood. Platelets have several functions, all relating to the arrest of bleeding (*see* blood coagulation). *See also* thrombopoiesis.

platy- *prefix denoting* broad or flat.

platyhelminth (plat-i-hel-minth) *n.* *see* flatworm.

platysma (plă-tiz-mă) *n.* a broad thin sheet of muscle that extends from below the collar bone to the angle of the jaw. It depresses the corner of the mouth.

pledget (plej-it) *n.* a small wad of dressing material, such as lint, used either to cover a wound or sore or as a plug.

-plegia *suffix denoting* paralysis.

pleio- (pleo-) *prefix denoting* 1. multiple. 2. excessive.

pleocytosis (plee-oh-sy-toh-sis) *n.* the presence of an abnormally large number of lymphocytes in the cerebrospinal fluid.

parietal pleura
pleural cavity
chest wall
visceral pleura
diaphragm

The pleura

pleomorphism (plee-oh-**mor**-fizm) *n.* the condition in which an individual assumes a number of different forms during its life cycle. The malarial parasite (*Plasmodium*) displays pleomorphism.

pleoptics (plee-**op**-tiks) *n.* special techniques practised by orthoptists for developing normal function of the macula, in people whose macular function has previously been disturbed because of strabismus (squint).

plessor (plexor) (**ples**-er) *n.* a small hammer used to investigate nervous reflexes and in the technique of percussion.

plethora (**pleth**-er-ă) *n.* any excess of any bodily fluid, especially blood (*see* hyperaemia). —**plethoric** (pleth-o-rik) *adj.*

plethysmography (pleth-iz-**mog**-răfi) *n.* the process of recording the changes in the volume of a limb caused by alterations in blood pressure. The limb is inserted into a fluid-filled watertight casing (*oncometer*) and the pressure variations in the fluid are recorded.

pleur- (pleuro-) *prefix denoting* **1.** the pleura. **2.** the side of the body.

pleura (**ploor**-ă) *n.* the covering of the lungs (*visceral p.*) and of the inner surface of the chest wall (*parietal p.*), consisting of a closed sac of serous membrane. Fluid secreted by the membrane lubricates the opposing surfaces so that they can slide painlessly over each other during breathing. —**pleural** *adj.*

pleuracentesis (ploor-ă-sen-**tee**-sis) *n. see* pleurocentesis.

pleural cavity (**ploor**-ăl) *n.* the space between the visceral and parietal pleura, which is normally very small as the pleural membranes are in close contact.

pleurectomy (ploor-**ek**-tŏmi) *n.* surgical removal of part of the pleura, which is sometimes done to overcome recurrent pneumothorax or to remove diseased areas of pleura.

pleurisy (**ploor**-i-si) *n.* inflammation of the pleura, usually due to pneumonia in the underlying lung. The pleural surfaces become slightly sticky, so that there is pain on deep breathing. Pleurisy is always associated with some other disease in the lung, chest wall, diaphragm, or abdomen.

pleurocele (**ploor**-oh-seel) *n.* herniation of the pleura.

pleurocentesis (pleuracentesis, thoracentesis, thoracocentesis) (ploor-oh-sen-**tee**-sis) *n.* insertion of a hollow needle into the pleural cavity through the chest wall in order to withdraw fluid, blood, pus, or air.

pleurodesis (ploor-oh-**dee**-sis) *n.* a treatment for pneumothorax in which adhesions between the parietal and visceral pleura are induced by injecting a substance (e.g. silver nitrate) into the pleural cavity.

pleurodynia (ploor-oh-**din**-iă) *n.* severe paroxysmal pain arising from the muscles between the ribs. It is often thought to be of rheumatic origin.

pleurolysis (pneumolysis) (ploor-ol-i-sis) *n.* surgical stripping of the parietal pleura from the chest wall to allow the lung to collapse. The procedure was formerly used to help tuberculosis to heal.

pleuropneumonia (ploor-oh-new-moh-niă) *n.* inflammation involving both the lung and pleura. *See* pleurisy, pneumonia.

pleuropneumonia-like organisms (PPLO) *pl. n. see* mycoplasma.

plexor (pleks-er) *n. see* plessor.

plexus (pleks-ŭs) *n.* a network of nerves or blood vessels. *See* brachial plexus.

plica (plik-ă) *n.* a fold of tissue. —**plicate** *adj.*

plication (pli-kay-shŏn) *n.* a surgical technique in which the size of a hollow organ is reduced by taking tucks or folds in the walls.

plombage (plom-bahᴢh) *n.* a surgical technique used to correct a detached retina. A small piece of silicone plastic is sewn on the outside of the eyeball to produce an indentation over the region where a retinal hole has been found.

plumbism (plum-bizm) *n.* lead poisoning. *See* lead.

Plummer-Vinson syndrome (plum-er vin-sŏn) *n.* a disorder characterized by difficulty in swallowing associated with severe iron-deficiency anaemia. [H. S. Plummer (1874–1936) and P. P. Vinson (1890–), US physicians]

pluri- *prefix denoting* more than one; several.

pneo- *prefix denoting* breathing; respiration.

pneum- (pneumo-) *prefix denoting* 1. the presence of air or gas. 2. the lung(s). 3. respiration.

pneumat- (pneumato-) *prefix denoting* 1. the presence of air or gas. 2. respiration.

pneumatocele (new-mat-oh-seel) *n.* herniation of lung tissue.

pneumaturia (new-măt-yoor-iă) *n.* the presence in the urine of bubbles of air or other gas, due to the formation of gas by bacteria infecting the urinary tract or to a fistula between the urinary tract and bowel.

pneumocephalus (pneumocele) (new-moh-sef-ă-lŭs) *n.* the presence of air within the skull, usually resulting from a fracture passing through one of the air sinuses.

pneumococcus (new-moh-kok-ŭs) *n.* (*pl.* **pneumococci**) the bacterium associated with pneumonia: *Streptococcus pneumoniae*. —**pneumococcal** *adj.*

pneumoconiosis (new-moh-koh-ni-oh-sis) *n.* a lung disease caused by inhaling dust. In practice industrial exposure to coal dust (*see* anthracosis), silica (*see* silicosis), and asbestos (*see* asbestosis) produces most of the cases of pneumoconiosis.

pneumocyte (new-moh-syt) *n.* a type of cell that lines the walls separating the air sacs (*see* alveolus) in the lungs.

pneumoencephalography (new-moh-en-sef-ă-log-răfi) *n.* a technique used in the X-ray diagnosis of disease within the skull. Air is introduced into the ventricles of the brain to displace the cerebrospinal fluid, thus acting as a contrast medium. X-ray photographs show the size and disposition of the ventricles and the subarachnoid spaces.

pneumogastric (new-moh-**gas**-trik) *adj*. relating to the lungs and stomach. *p. nerve* the vagus nerve.

pneumograph (**new**-moh-grahf) *n*. an instrument used to record the movements made during respiration.

pneumohaemothorax (new-moh-hee-moh-**thor**-aks) *n*. *see* haemopneumothorax.

pneumohydrothorax (new-moh-hy-droh-**thor**-aks) *n*. *see* hydropneumothorax.

pneumolysis (new-**mol**-i-sis) *n*. *see* pleurolysis.

pneumomycosis (new-moh-my-**koh**-sis) *n*. any infection of the lungs caused by fungi, such as aspergillosis.

pneumon- (**pneumono-**) *prefix denoting* the lung(s).

pneumonectomy (new-mŏ-**nek**-tŏmi) *n*. surgical removal of a lung, usually for cancer.

pneumonia (new-**moh**-niă) *n*. inflammation of the lung caused by bacteria, in which the alveoli fill up with pus so that air is excluded and the lung becomes solid (*see* consolidation). The symptoms generally include cough and chest pain, with shadows on the chest X-ray. Treatment with antibiotics is usually effective. *bronchopneumonia* the most common type of pneumonia, which starts around the bronchi and bronchioles. *hypostatic p.* pneumonia that develops in dependant parts of the lung in people who are otherwise ill, chilled, or immobilized. *lobar p.* pneumonia that affects whole lobes of either or both lungs. *Compare* pneumonitis.

pneumonitis (new-mŏ-ny-tis) *n*. inflammation of the lung that is confined to the walls of the alveoli and often caused by viruses or unknown agents. It may be acute and transient or chronic, leading to increasing respiratory disability. It does not respond to antibiotics but corticosteroids may be helpful. *Compare* pneumonia.

pneumoperitoneum (new-moh-pe-ri-tŏn-ee-ŭm) *n*. air or gas in the peritoneal or abdominal cavity, usually due to a perforation of the stomach or bowel.

pneumoradiography (new-moh-ray-di-**og**-răfi) *n*. X-ray examination of part of the body using a gas, such as air or carbon dioxide, as a contrast medium.

pneumothorax (new-moh-**thor**-aks) *n*. air in the pleural cavity, which results from breach of the lung surface or chest wall and causes the lung to collapse. *artificial p.* the deliberate injection of air into the pleural cavity to collapse the lung: a former treatment for pulmonary tuberculosis. *spontaneous p.* pneumothorax that occurs without apparent cause, in otherwise healthy people. *tension p.* pneumothorax in which a breach in the lung surface acts as a valve, admitting air into the pleural cavity when the patient breathes in but preventing its escape when he breathes out. *traumatic p.* pneumothorax that results from injuries to the chest.

-pnoea *suffix denoting* a condition of breathing.

pock (pok) *n*. a small pus-filled eruption on the skin characteristic of chickenpox and smallpox rashes. *See also* pustule.

pod- *prefix denoting* the foot.

podagra (pŏ-**dag**-ră) *n*. gout of the foot, especially the big toe.

podalic version (pŏ-**dal**-ik) *n.* altering the position of a fetus in the womb so that its feet will emerge first at birth. *See also* version.

-poiesis *suffix denoting* formation; production.

poikilo- *prefix denoting* variation; irregularity.

poikilocyte (poi-kil-oh-syt) *n.* an abnormally shaped erythrocyte. *See also* poikilocytosis.

poikilocytosis (poi-kil-oh-sy-**toh**-sis) *n.* the presence of poikilocytes in the blood. Poikilocytosis is particularly marked in myelofibrosis but can occur to some extent in almost any blood disease.

poikilothermic (poi-kil-oh-**therm**-ik) *adj.* cold-blooded: being unable to regulate the body temperature, which fluctuates according to that of the surroundings. *Compare* homoiothermic. —**poikilothermy** *n.*

poison (poi-zŏn) *n.* any substance that irritates, damages, or impairs the activity of the body's tissues. The term is usually reserved for substances, such as arsenic, cyanide, and strychnine, that are harmful in relatively small amounts.

polar body (**poh**-ler) *n.* one of the small cells produced by division of an oocyte that does not develop into a functional egg cell. *See* oogenesis.

poldine (**pol**-deen) *n.* a drug, similar to atropine, that inhibits gastric secretion and is administered by mouth to treat such disorders as gastric and duodenal ulcers. Trade name: **Nacton**.

pole (pohl) *n.* (in anatomy) the extremity of the axis of the body, an organ, or a cell.

poli- (polio-) *prefix denoting* the grey matter of the nervous system.

polioencephalitis (viral encephalitis) (poh-li-oh-en-sef-ă-ly-tis) *n.* a virus infection of the brain, causing particular damage to the grey matter of the cerebral hemispheres and the brainstem. The infection is usually transmitted to man by the bite of a mosquito or tick. *See also* encephalitis.

polioencephalomyelitis (poh-li-oh-en-sef-ă-loh-my-ĕ-ly-tis) *n.* any virus infection of the central nervous system affecting the grey matter of the brain and spinal cord. Rabies is the outstanding example.

poliomyelitis (infantile paralysis, polio) (poh-li-oh-my-ĕ-ly-tis) *n.* an infectious virus disease affecting the central nervous system. Immunization, using the Sabin vaccine or the Salk vaccine, is highly effective. *abortive p.* poliomyelitis in which only the throat and intestines are infected and the symptoms are those of a stomach upset or influenza. *bulbar p.* paralytic poliomyelitis in which the muscles of the respiratory system are affected. *nonparalytic p.* a form of the disease in which the symptoms of abortive poliomyelitis are accompanied by muscle stiffness. *paralytic p.* a less common form of poliomyelitis in which the symptoms of the milder forms of the disease are followed by weakness and eventual paralysis of the muscles.

poliovirus (poh-li-oh-vy-rŭs) *n.* one of a small group of RNA-containing viruses causing poliomyelitis. They are included within the picornavirus group.

Politzer's bag (**pol**-it-zerz) *n.* a flexible rubber bag for inflating the middle ear through the Eustachian tube. [A. Politzer (1835–1920), Austrian otologist]

pollex (**pol**-eks) *n.* (*pl.* **pollices**) the thumb.

pollinosis (poli-**noh**-sis) *n.* a more precise term than hay fever for an allergy due to the pollen of grasses, trees, or shrubs.

poly- *prefix denoting* **1.** many; multiple. **2.** excessive. **3.** generalized; affecting many parts.

polyarteritis nodosa (periarteritis nodosa) (poli-ar-ter-**I**-tis noh-**doh**-să) *n.* a disease of unknown cause in which there is patchy inflammation of the walls of the arteries. It is one of the collagen diseases. Common manifestations include arthritis, asthma, hypertension, and kidney failure.

polyarthritis (poli-arth-ry-tis) *n.* rheumatic disease involving several joints, either together or in sequence, causing pain, stiffness, swelling, tenderness, and loss of function. Rheumatoid arthritis is the most common cause.

polycystic disease of the kidneys (poli-**sis**-tik) *n.* an inherited disorder in which the substance of both kidneys is largely replaced by numerous cysts. Symptoms, including haematuria, urinary tract infection, and hypertension, are associated with chronic kidney failure.

polycythaemia (poli-sy-**theem**-iă) *n.* an increase in the haemoglobin concentration of the blood. This may be due either to a decrease in the total volume of the plasma (*relative p.*) or to an increase in the total volume of the red cells (*absolute p.*). The latter may occur as a primary disease or as a secondary condition in association with various respiratory or circulatory disorders and with certain tumours. *p. vera* (*erythraemia, Vaques-Osler disease*) a disease in which absolute polycythaemia is often accompanied by an increase in the numbers of white blood cells and platelets. Symptoms include headache, thromboses, cyanosis, and plethora.

polydactylism (poli-**dak**-til-izm) *n.* *see* hyperdactylism.

polydipsia (poli-**dip**-siă) *n.* abnormally intense thirst: a symptom of diabetes mellitus and diabetes insipidus.

polymer (**pol**-im-er) *n.* a substance formed by the linkage of a large number of smaller molecules known as *monomers*. An example of a monomer is glucose, whose molecules link together to form glycogen, a polymer.

polymorph (polymorphonuclear leucocyte) (**pol**-i-morf) *n.* *see* neutrophil.

polymyalgia rheumatica (poli-my-al-jiă roo-**mat**-ikă) *n.* a rheumatic disease causing aching and progressive stiffness of the muscles of the shoulders and hips. The condition is most common in the elderly and is often associated with temporal arteritis. The symptoms respond rapidly and effectively to corticosteroid treatment.

polymyositis (poli-my-oh-sy-tis) *n.* a generalized disease of the muscles that may be acute or chronic. It particularly affects the muscles of the shoulder and hip girdles, which are weak and tender to the touch. Relief of the symptoms is obtained with corticosteroid drugs. *See also* dermatomyositis.

polymyxin B (poli-**miks**-in) *n.* an antibiotic used to treat infections caused by Gram-negative bacteria, especially *Pseudomonas*. It is usually administered by injection but is also taken by mouth or applied externally for ear and eye infections. Trade name: **Aerosporin**.

polyneuritis (poli-newr-**I**-tis) *n.* any disorder involving all the peripheral nerves. The term is often used interchangeably with polyneuropathy although its specific use implies inflammation of the nerves.

polyneuropathy (poli-newr-**op**-ă-thi) *n.* any disease involving all of the peripheral nerves. The symptoms first affect the tips of the fingers and toes and subsequently spread towards the trunk. *See* neuropathy.

polyopia (poli-**oh**-piă) *n.* the sensation of multiple images of one object. It is sometimes experienced by people with early cataract. *See also* diplopia.

polyp (polypus) (**pol**-ip) *n.* a growth, usually benign, protruding from a mucous membrane. Polyps are commonly found in the nose and sinuses, giving rise to obstruction, chronic infection, and discharge. Other sites include the ear, the stomach, and the bowel. Polyps are usually removed by cauterization.

polypeptide (poli-**pep**-tyd) *n.* a molecule consisting of three or more amino acids linked together by peptide bonds. Protein molecules are polypeptides.

polyphagia (poli-**fay**-jiă) *n.* gluttonous excessive eating.

polypharmacy (poli-**farm**-ă-si) *n.* treatment of a patient with more than one type of medicine.

polyploid (**pol**-i-ploid) *adj.* describ-ing cells, tissues, or individuals in which there are three or more complete sets of chromosomes. *Compare* diploid, haploid. —**polyploidy** *n.*

polypoid (**pol**-i-poid) *adj.* having the appearance of a polyp.

polyposis (poli-**poh**-sis) *n.* a condition in which numerous polyps form in an organ or tissue. *familial p. coli* a hereditary disease in which multiple polyps develop in the colon at puberty. As these polyps often become malignant, total colectomy is usually performed. *Compare* pseudopolyposis.

polypus (**pol**-i-pŭs) *n. see* polyp.

polyradiculitis (polyradiculopathy) (poli-ră-dik-yoo-**ly**-tis) *n.* any disorder of the peripheral nerves (*see* neuropathy) in which the brunt of the disease falls on the nerve roots where they emerge from the spinal cord.

polysaccharide (poli-**sak**-eryd) *n.* a carbohydrate formed from many monosaccharides joined together in long linear or branched chains. Examples are glycogen and cellulose.

polyserositis (poli-seer-oh-**sy**-tis) *n.* inflammation of the membranes that line the chest, abdomen, and joints, with accumulation of fluid in the cavities.

polyspermia (poli-**sper**-miă) *n.* **1.** excessive formation of semen. **2.** *see* polyspermy.

polyspermy (polyspermia) (poli-**sper**-mi) *n.* fertilization of a single ovum by more than one spermatozoon: the development is abnormal and the embryo dies.

polyuria (poli-**yoor**-iă) *n.* the production of large volumes of dilute urine. The phenomenon may be due simply to excessive liquid intake or to disease, particularly diabetes mellitus, diabetes insipidus, and kidney disorders.

pompholyx (pom-foh-liks) *n.* eczema of the hands and feet. Because the horny layer of the skin in these parts is so thick the vesicles typical of eczema cannot rupture. There is intense itching until the skin eventually peels. Pompholyx is commonest in early adulthood.

pons (ponz) *n.* any portion of tissue that joins two parts of an organ. *p. Varolii* the part of the brainstem that links the medulla oblongata and the thalamus. It contains numerous nerve tracts between the cerebral cortex and the spinal cord. [C. Varolius (1543–75), Italian anatomist] —**pontine** (pon-teen) *adj.*

popliteus (pop-lit-iŭs) *n.* a flat triangular muscle at the back of the knee joint, between the femur and tibia, that helps to flex the knee. —**popliteal** *adj.*

pore (por) *n.* a small opening. *sweat p.* the opening of a sweat gland on the surface of the skin.

porencephaly (por-en-sef-ăli) *n.* an abnormal communication between the lateral ventricle and the surface of the brain. This is usually a consequence of brain injury or cerebrovascular disease.

porphin (por-fin) *n.* a complex nitrogen-containing ring structure and parent compound of the porphyrins.

porphyria (por-fi-riă) *n.* one of a group of rare inherited disorders due to disturbance of the metabolism of the breakdown products (porphyrins) of haemoglobin, which are excreted in the urine. The prominent features include sensitivity of the skin to sunlight, neuritis, mental disturbances, and attacks of abdominal pain.

porphyrin (por-fi-rin) *n.* one of a number of pigments derived from porphin, which are widely distributed in living things. All porphyrins form chelates with iron, magnesium, zinc, nickel, copper, and cobalt. These chelates are constituents of haemoglobin, myoglobin, the cytochromes, and chlorophyll. *See also* protoporphyrin IX.

porphyrinuria (por-fi-rin-yoor-iă) *n.* the presence in the urine of porphyrins, sometimes causing discoloration. *See* porphyria.

porta (por-tă) *n.* the aperture in an organ through which its associated vessels pass. Such an opening occurs in the liver (*p. hepatis*). —**portal** *adj.*

portacaval anastomosis (portacaval shunt) (por-tă-kay-văl) *n.* **1.** a surgical technique in which the hepatic portal vein is joined to the inferior vena cava, thus bypassing the liver. It is used in the treatment of portal hypertension. **2.** any of the natural communications between the branches of the hepatic portal vein in the liver and the inferior vena cava.

portal hypertension (por-t'l) *n.* a state in which the pressure within the hepatic portal vein is increased, causing enlargement of the spleen and ascites. The commonest cause is cirrhosis. Treatment is by diuretic drugs or surgery (*see* portacaval anastomosis).

portal system *n.* a vein or group of veins that terminates at both ends in a capillary bed. *hepatic p. s.* the best known portal system, consisting of the portal vein and its tributaries.

genupectoral position

lithotomy position

Trendelenburg's position

semi-prone position

Types of position

portal vein *n.* a vein that conveys blood from the stomach, intestines, spleen, and pancreas to the liver.

position (pŏ-**zish**-ŏn) *n.* a posture or attitude assumed by a patient in order to facilitate nursing, diagnostic, or surgical procedures (see illustration).

positive pressure ventilation (**poz**-it-iv) *n.* the forcible passage of air into the lungs to stimulate breathing movements. *See also* respirator.

posology (pŏ-**sol**-ŏji) *n.* the science of the dosage of medicines.

posseting (**poss**-it-ing) *n.* the regurgitation of food by an infant.

Possum (**poss**-ŭm) *n.* a device that enables severely paralysed patients to use typewriters, telephones, and other machines. Modern Possums are operated by micro-switches that require only the slightest movement in any limb. The name derives from *Patient-Operated Selector Mechanism (POSM)*.

post- *prefix denoting* 1. following; after. 2. (in anatomy) behind.

postcibal (pohst-**sy**-băl) *adj.* occurring after eating.

postconcussional syndrome (pohst-kŏn-**kush**-ŏn-ăl) *n.* persistent headaches, giddiness, and lack of concentration that may follow a head injury.

postepileptic (pohst-epi-**lep**-tik) *adj.* occurring after an epileptic fit.

posterior (poss-**teer**-i-er) *adj.* situated at or near the back of the body or an organ.

postero- *prefix denoting* posterior.

postganglionic (pohst-gang-li-**on**-ik) *adj.* describing a neurone in a nerve pathway that starts at a ganglion and ends at the muscle or gland that it supplies. *Compare* preganglionic.

posthitis (poss-**th'y**-tis) *n.* inflammation of the foreskin. This usually occurs in association with balanitis (*see* balanoposthitis).

posthumous birth (**poss**-tew-mŭs) *n.* 1. delivery of a child by Caesarean section after the mother's death. 2. birth of a child after the father's death.

postmature (pohst-mă-**tewr**) *adj.* describing a baby that has remained in the womb for longer than 280 days. —**postmaturity** *n.*

post mortem (pohst **mor**-tĕm) Latin: after death. *See* autopsy.

postnatal (pohst-**nay**-t'l) *adj.* following childbirth.

postoperative (pohst-**op**-er-ă-tiv) *adj.* following operation: referring to the condition of a patient or to the treatment given at this time.

postpartum (pohst-**par**-tŭm) *adj.* relating to the period of a few days immediately after birth.

postprandial (pohst-**pran**-di-ăl) *adj.* occurring after eating.

potassium chloride (pŏ-**tas**-iŭm) *n.* a salt of potassium administered by mouth or injection to prevent and treat potassium deficiency, especially during treatment with certain diuretics. Trade names: **Kalium, Kay-Cee-L, K-Contin, Slow-K.**

potassium hydroxyquinoline (hy-droks-i-**kwin**-ŏ-leen) *n.* a salt of potassium that has antifungal, antibacterial, and deodorant activities.

potassium perchlorate (per-**klor**-ayt) *n.* a salt of potassium that is administered by mouth to treat overactivity of the thyroid gland (thyrotoxicosis). Trade name: **Peroidin.**

potassium permanganate (per-**mang**-ă-nayt) *n.* a salt of potassium used for disinfecting and cleansing wounds and as a general skin antiseptic. It irritates mucous membranes and is poisonous if taken into the body.

Pott's disease (pots) *n.* tuberculosis of the backbone, usually transmitted by infected cows' milk. Untreated, it can lead to a hunchback deformity. [P. Pott (1714–88), British surgeon]

Pott's fracture *n. see* fracture.

pouch (powch) *n.* (in anatomy) a small sac-like structure, especially occurring as an outgrowth of a larger structure.

poultice (fomentation) (**pohl**-tis) *n.* a preparation of hot moist material applied to any part of the body to increase local circulation, alleviate pain, or soften the skin.

Poupart's ligament (poo-**parz**) *n. see* inguinal (ligament). [F. Poupart (1661–1708) French anatomist]

powder (**pow**-der) *n.* (in pharmacy) a medicinal preparation consisting of a mixture of two or more drugs in the form of fine particles.

pox (poks) *n.* **1.** an infectious disease causing a skin rash. **2.** a rash of pimples that become pus-filled, as in chickenpox and smallpox.

poxvirus (**poks**-vy-rŭs) *n.* one of a group of large DNA-containing viruses including those that cause smallpox (variola) and cowpox (vaccinia).

PPLO *pl. n. see* mycoplasma.

pre- *prefix denoting* **1.** before; preceding. **2.** (in anatomy) in front of; anterior to.

precancerous (pree-**kan**-ser-ŭs) *adj.* describing a growth that is not yet malignant but that is known to become so if left untreated.

precipitin (pri-**sip**-it-in) *n.* any antibody that combines with its antigen to form a complex that is seen as a precipitate. The precipitin reaction is a useful means of confirming the identity of an unknown antigen or establishing that a serum contains antibodies to a known disease. *See also* agglutination.

precocity (pri-**kos**-iti) *n.* an acceleration of normal development. The intellectually precocious child has a high IQ and may become isolated from his contemporaries or frustrated at school. —**precocious** (pri-**koh**-shŭs) *adj.*

precordium (pree-**kor**-diŭm) *n.* the region of the thorax immediately over the heart. —**precordial** *adj.*

precursor (pri-**ker**-ser) *n.* a substance from which another, usually more biologically active, substance is formed. For example, trypsinogen is the precursor of the enzyme trypsin.

predigestion (pree-dy-**jes**-chŏn) *n.* the partial digestion of foods by artificial means before they are taken into the body.

predisposition (pree-dis-pŏ-**zish**-ŏn) *n.* a tendency to be affected by a particular disease or kind of disease. *See also* diathesis.

prednisolone (pred-**nis**-ŏ-lohn) *n.* a synthetic corticosteroid used to treat rheumatic diseases and inflammatory and allergic conditions. It is administered by mouth, injected into joints, or applied in creams, lotions, and ointments. Trade names: **Codelcortone**, **Delta-Cortef**, **Deltacortril**, **Deltastab**, **Precortisyl**, **Prednesol**.

prednisone (**pred**-ni-sohn) *n.* a synthetic corticosteroid administered by mouth to treat rheumatic diseases, severe allergic conditions, inflammatory conditions, and leukaemia. Trade names: **Deltacortone**, **Di-Adreson**.

pre-eclampsia (pree-i-**klamp**-siă) *n.* a condition that affects women at an advanced stage of pregnancy and is marked by high blood pressure, swelling of the ankles, and the presence of protein in the urine. *See also* eclampsia, toxaemia (of pregnancy).

prefrontal leucotomy (pree-**frun**-t'l) *n. see* leucotomy.

prefrontal lobe *n.* the region of the brain at the very front of each cerebral hemisphere. The functions of the lobe are concerned with emotions, memory, learning, and social behaviour.

preganglionic (pree-gang-li-**on**-ik) *adj.* describing fibres in a nerve pathway that end in a ganglion, where they form synapses with postganglionic fibres.

pregnancy (**preg**-năn-si) *n.* the period during which a woman carries a developing fetus. Pregnancy lasts for approximately 266 days, from conception until the baby is born, and the fetus normally develops in the womb (*compare* ectopic pregnancy). *See also* pseudocyesis (phantom pregnancy). *p. test* any of several methods used to demonstrate whether or not a woman is pregnant. A commonly used laboratory test of early pregnancy is based on detection of a hormone, chorionic gonadotrophin, in the urine. —**pregnant** *adj.*

pregnanediol (preg-nayn-**dy**-ol) *n.* a steroid that is formed during the metabolism of the female sex hormone progesterone. It occurs in the urine during pregnancy and certain phases of the menstrual cycle.

pregnenolone (preg-**neen**-ŏ-lohn) *n.* a steroid synthesized in the adrenal glands, ovaries, and testes. Pregnenolone is an important intermediate product in steroid hormone synthesis.

premature beat (**prem**-ă-tewr) *n. see* ectopic beat.

premature birth *n.* birth of a baby before full term. Since the date of conception is often not precisely known, a premature baby is defined as one weighing less than 2500 g (5½ lb) at birth.

premedication (pree-med-i-kay-shŏn) *n.* drugs administered to a patient before an operation. Premedication usually comprises injection of a sedative together with a drug, such as atropine, to dry up the secretions of the lungs (which might otherwise be inhaled during anaesthesia).

premenstrual tension (pree-men-stroo-ăl) *n.* a condition of nervousness, irritability, emotional disturbance, headache, and/or depression affecting some women for up to 10 days before menstruation.

premolar (pree-moh-ler) *n.* either of the two teeth on each side of each jaw behind the canines and in front of the molars in the adult dentition.

prenatal diagnosis (antenatal diagnosis) (pree-nay-t'l) *n.* diagnostic procedures carried out on pregnant women in order to discover genetic or other abnormalities in the developing fetus. The investigations involve the use of X-rays, ultrasound scanning, thermography, and analysis of amniotic fluid (*see* amniocentesis).

prenylamine (pri-nil-ă-meen) *n.* a drug that dilates blood vessels (*see* vasodilator). It is administered by mouth to treat angina. Trade name: **Synadrin.**

preoperative (pree-op-er-ă-tiv) *adj.* before operation: referring to the condition of a patient or to treatment, such as sedation, given at this time.

prepubertal (pree-pew-ber-t'l) *adj.* relating to or occurring in the period before puberty.

prepuce (foreskin) (pree-pewss) *n.* the fold of skin that grows over the glans penis. On its inner surface modified sebaceous glands (*preputial glands*) secrete a lubricating fluid over the glans. —**preputial** (pree-pew-shăl) *adj.*

presby- (presbyo-) *prefix denoting* old age.

presbyacusis (prezbi-ă-kew-sis) *n.* the progressive perceptive deafness that occurs with age.

presbyopia (prezbi-oh-piă) *n.* difficulty in reading at the usual distance and in performing other close work, due to the decline with age in the ability of the eye to focus on close objects.

prescribed disease (pri-skrybd) *n.* one of a number of illnesses (currently 48) arising as a result of employment requiring close contact with a hazardous substance or circumstance. Examples include decompression sickness in divers and infections such as anthrax in those handling wool.

prescription (pri-skrip-shŏn) *n.* a written direction from a registered medical practitioner to a pharmacist for preparing and dispensing a drug.

presenility (pree-sin-il-iti) *n.* premature ageing of the mind and body, so that a person shows the reduction in mental and physical abilities normally found only in old age. *See also* dementia, progeria. —**presenile** (pree-see-nyl) *adj.*

presentation (prez-ĕn-tay-shŏn) *n.* the part of the infant's body that appears first at the opening from the neck of the womb during childbirth, as perceived on inserting the finger into the vagina. Normally the head appears first (*cephalic p.*). However, the infant's buttocks (*see* breech presentation), its side (*transverse p.*), its feet, or the placenta may be the first parts to appear.

pressor (**pres**-er) *n*. an agent that raises blood pressure. *See* vasoconstrictor.

pressure area (**presh**-er) *n*. any of the areas of the body where a bone is close to the skin surface, so that pressure on that area (e.g. by lying in bed) deprives the overlying tissues of their blood supply (*see* bedsore).

pressure point *n*. a point at which an artery lies over a bone on which it may be compressed by finger pressure, to arrest haemorrhage beyond.

pressure sore *n*. *see* bedsore.

presystole (pree-sis-tŏ-li) *n*. the period in the cardiac cycle just preceding systole.

preventive medicine (pri-ven-tiv) *n*. the branch of medicine whose main aim is the prevention of disease.

priapism (pry-ă-pizm) *n*. persistent erection of the penis. It is commonly due to a blood clot in the erectile tissue of the penis and is most often encountered in patients with kidney failure undergoing intermittent dialysis.

prickle cells (prik-ŭl) *pl. n.* cells with cytoplasmic processes that form intercellular bridges. The germinative layer of the epidermis is sometimes called the prickle cell layer.

prickly heat (**heat rash**) (prik-li) *n*. an itchy rash of small raised red spots. It occurs usually on the face, neck, back, chest, and thighs in hot moist weather. Medical name: **miliaria**.

prilocaine (**pril**-oh-kayn) *n*. a local anaesthetic used particularly in ear, nose, and throat surgery and in dentistry. It is applied in a solution to mucous membranes or injected. Trade name: **Citanest**.

primaquine (pry-mă-kween) *n*. a drug used to treat malaria. It is administered by mouth, usually in combination with other antimalarial drugs, such as chloroquine. Trade name: **Mysoline**.

primary nursing (pry-mer-i) *n*. a method of organizing nursing care in which one nurse (the *primary nurse*) is responsible for assessing the patient, planning his care, and evaluating his progress throughout his stay in hospital.

prime mover (prym **moov**-er) *n*. *see* agonist.

primidone (pry-mid-ohn) *n*. an anticonvulsant drug administered by mouth to treat major (grand mal) epilepsy. Trade name: **Mysoline**.

primigravida (**unigravida**) (pry-mi-**grav**-id-ă) *n*. a woman experiencing her first pregnancy.

primipara (**unipara**) (pry-**mip**-er-ă) *n*. a woman who has given birth to one infant capable of survival.

primordial (pry-**mor**-di-ăl) *adj*. (in embryology) describing cells or tissues that are formed in the early stages of embryonic development.

pro- *prefix denoting* **1.** before; preceding. **2.** a precursor. **3.** in front of.

probang (**proh**-bang) *n*. a long flexible rod with a small sponge, ball, or tuft at the end, used to remove obstructions from the larynx or oesophagus.

probe (prohb) *n*. a thin rod of pliable metal with a blunt swollen end. The instrument is used for exploring cavities, wounds, fistulas, or sinus channels.

probenecid (proh-**ben**-ĕ-sid) *n*. a drug that reduces the level of uric acid in the blood (*see* uricosuric drug), administered by mouth in the treatment of gout. Trade name: **Benemid**.

problem-solving approach *n.* a method of planning work involving assessment, problem identification, planning, implementation, and evaluation. *See* nursing process.

procainamide (proh-**kayn**-ă-myd) *n.* a drug that slows down the activity of the heart and is administered by mouth or injection to control abnormal heart rhythm. Trade name: **Pronestyl**.

procaine (**proh**-kayn) *n.* a local anaesthetic administered by injection for spinal anaesthesia. It was formerly used in dentistry. Trade name: **Novutex**.

procaine penicillin *n.* an antibiotic, consisting of penicillin and procaine, used to treat infections caused by organisms sensitive to penicillin. It is injected into muscle so that the penicillin is released slowly. Trade names: **Bicillin**, **Depocillin**.

procarbazine (proh-**kar**-bă-zeen) *n.* a drug that inhibits growth of cancer cells by preventing cell division and is administered by mouth to treat such cancers as Hodgkin's disease. Trade name: **Natulan**.

process (**proh**-ses) *n.* (in anatomy) a thin prominence or protuberance.

prochlorperazine (proh-klor-**per**-ă-zeen) *n.* a major tranquillizer used to treat schizophrenia and other mental disorders, migraine, vertigo, nausea, and vomiting. It is administered by mouth, injection, or in suppositories. Trade name: **Stemetil**.

procidentia (pros-i-**den**-shiă) *n.* the complete prolapse of an organ, especially the womb (*uterine p.*), which protrudes from the vaginal opening.

proct- (procto-) *prefix denoting* the anus and/or rectum.

proctalgia (proctodynia) (prok-**tal**-jiă) *n.* pain in the rectum or anus. *p. fugax* severe pain that suddenly affects the rectum and may last for minutes or hours. There is no structural disease and the pain is probably due to muscle spasm.

proctatresia (prok-tă-**tree**-ziă) *n.* see imperforate (anus).

proctectasia (prok-tek-**tay**-ziă) *n.* enlargement or widening of the rectum, usually due to long-standing constipation.

proctectomy (prok-**tek**-tŏmi) *n.* surgical removal of the rectum. It is usually performed for cancer of the rectum and requires the construction of a permanent opening in the colon (*see* colostomy).

proctitis (prok-**ty**-tis) *n.* inflammation of the rectum. Symptoms are tenesmus, diarrhoea, and often bleeding. Proctitis is invariably present in ulcerative colitis and sometimes in Crohn's disease, but may occur independently (*idiopathic p.*).

proctocele (rectocele) (**prok**-toh-seel) *n.* bulging or pouching of the rectum, usually a forward protrusion of the rectum into the vagina in association with prolapse of the womb.

proctoclysis (prok-**tok**-li-sis) *n.* an infusion of fluid into the rectum: formerly used to replace fluid but rarely employed now.

proctocolectomy (prok-toh-kŏ-**lek**-tŏmi) *n.* a surgical operation in which the rectum and colon are removed. Removal of the whole rectum and colon (*panproctocolectomy*) requires a permanent opening of the ileum (*see* ileostomy).

proctocolitis (prok-toh-kŏ-ly-tis) *n.* inflammation of the rectum and colon, usually due to ulcerative colitis. *See also* proctitis.

proctodynia (prok-toh-**din**-iă) *n. see* proctalgia.

proctology (prok-**tol**-ŏji) *n.* the study of disorders of the rectum and anus.

proctorrhaphy (prokt-o-răfi) *n.* a surgical operation to stitch tears of the rectum or anus.

proctoscope (**prok**-tŏ-skohp) *n.* an illuminated instrument through which the lower part of the rectum and the anus may be inspected. —**proctoscopy** *n.*

proctosigmoiditis (prok-toh-sig-moid-I-tis) *n.* inflammation of the rectum and the sigmoid colon. *See also* proctocolitis.

proctotomy (prok-tot-ŏmi) *n.* incision into the rectum or anus to relieve stricture of these canals or to open an imperforate anus.

procyclidine (proh-sy-kli-deen) *n.* a drug, similar in its effects to atropine, administered by mouth or injection to reduce muscle tremor and rigidity in parkinsonism. Trade name: **Kemadrin**.

prodromal (proh-**droh**-măl) *adj.* relating to the period of time between the appearance of the first symptoms of an infectious disease and the development of a rash or fever. *p. rash* a rash that precedes the full rash of an infectious disease.

prodrome (**proh**-drohm) *n.* a symptom indicating the onset of a disease.

proenzyme (zymogen) (proh-en-zym) *n.* the inactive form in which certain enzymes (e.g. digestive enzymes) are originally produced and secreted.

proflavine (proh-**flay**-vin) *n.* a dye used as an antiseptic in the form of skin applications and eyedrops.

profunda (proh-fun-dă) *adj.* describing blood vessels that are deeply embedded in the tissues they supply.

progeria (proh-**jeer**-iă) *n.* a very rare condition in which all the signs of old age appear and progress in a child, so that 'senility' is reached before puberty.

progesterone (proh-**jest**-er-ohn) *n.* a steroid hormone secreted by the corpus luteum of the ovary, the placenta, and also (in small amounts) by the adrenal cortex and testes. It is responsible for preparing the endometrium for pregnancy.

progestogen (proh-**jest**-oh-jĕn) *n.* one of a group of naturally occurring or synthetic steroid hormones, including progesterone, that maintain the normal course of pregnancy. Progestogens are used to treat threatened or habitual abortion, premenstrual tension, amenorrhoea, and abnormal bleeding from the womb. Because they prevent ovulation, progestogens are a major constituent of oral contraceptives.

proglottis (proh-**glot**-iss) *n.* (*pl.* **proglottids** or **proglottides**) one of the segments of a tapeworm. Mature segments, situated at the posterior end of the worm, each consist mainly of a branched uterus packed with eggs.

prognathism (**prog**-nă-thizm) *n.* the state of one jaw being markedly larger than the other and therefore in front of it. —**prognathic** (prog-**nath**-ik) *adj.*

prognosis (prog-**noh**-sis) *n.* an assessment of the future course and outcome of a patient's disease.

proguanil (proh-**gwan**-il) *n.* a drug that kills malaria parasites and is administered by mouth in the prevention and treatment of malaria. Trade name: **Paludrine**.

proinsulin (proh-**ins**-yoo-lin) *n.* a substance produced in the pancreas from which the hormone insulin is derived.

projection (prŏ-**jek**-shŏn) *n.* (in psychology) the attribution of one's own qualities to other people. In psychoanalytic psychology this is one of the defence mechanisms; people who cannot tolerate their own feelings may cope by imagining that other people have those feelings.

prolactin (lactogenic hormone, luteotrophic hormone, luteotrophin) (proh-**lak**-tin) *n.* a hormone, synthesized and stored in the anterior pituitary gland, that stimulates milk production after childbirth and also stimulates production of progesterone by the corpus luteum in the ovary.

prolapse (**proh**-laps) *n.* downward displacement of an organ or a part from its normal position. *See also* metroptosis (uterine prolapse).

prolapsed intervertebral disc (PID) *n.* a 'slipped disc': protrusion of the pulpy inner material of an intervertebral disc through the fibrous outer coat, causing pressure on adjoining nerve roots, ligaments, etc. Treatment is by complete bed rest on a firm surface, manipulation, traction, and analgesics; if these fail, a laminectomy may be performed.

proliferate (prŏ-**lif**-er-ayt) *vb.* to grow rapidly by cell division: applied particularly to malignant tumours. —**proliferation** *n.*

proline (**proh**-leen) *n.* an amino acid found in many proteins.

promazine (**proh**-mă-zeen) *n.* a major tranquillizer administered by mouth or injection to relieve agitation, confusion, severe pain, anxiety, nausea, and vomiting and in the treatment of alcoholism and drug withdrawal symptoms. Trade name: **Sparine**.

promethazine (proh-**meth**-ă-zeen) *n.* a powerful antihistamine drug administered by mouth or injection to treat allergic conditions and insomnia. It is also used as an antitussive in cough mixtures. Trade name: **Phenergan**.

promontory (**prom**-ŏn-ter-i) *n.* (in anatomy) a projecting part of an organ or other structure.

pronation (proh-**nay**-shŏn) *n.* the act of turning the hand so that the palm faces downwards. In this position the radius and ulna are crossed. *Compare* supination.

pronator (proh-**nay**-ter) *n.* any muscle that causes pronation of the forearm and hand.

prone (prohn) *adj.* **1.** lying with the face downwards. **2.** (of the forearm) in the position in which the palm of the hand faces downwards. *Compare* supine.

propanidid (proh-**pan**-i-did) *n.* an anaesthetic that is injected to give rapid complete anaesthesia for a short period of time, for use in minor surgical operations. Trade name: **Epontol**.

propantheline (proh-**panth**-ĕ-leen) *n.* a drug that decreases activity of smooth muscle (*see* parasympatholytic) and is administered by mouth or injection to treat disorders of the digestive system, including stomach and duodenal ulcers, and enuresis (bed wetting). Trade name: **Pro-Banthine**.

properdin (proh-per-din) *n.* a group of substances in blood plasma that, in combination with complement and magnesium ions, is capable of destroying certain bacteria and viruses.

prophase (proh-fayz) *n.* the first stage of mitosis and of each division of meiosis, in which the chromosomes become visible under the microscope.

prophylactic (pro-fil-ak-tik) *n.* an agent that prevents the development of a condition or disease.

prophylaxis (pro-fil-aks-iss) *n.* any means taken to prevent disease, such as immunization. —**prophylactic** *adj.*

propranolol (proh-pran-ŏ-lol) *n.* a drug (*see* beta blocker) administered by mouth or injection to treat abnormal heart rhythm, angina, and high blood pressure and to relieve anxiety. Trade name: **Inderal.**

proprietary name (prŏ-pry-ĕt-er-i) *n.* (in pharmacy) the trade name of a drug: the name assigned to it by the firm that manufactured it.

proprioceptor (proh-pri-ŏ-sep-ter) *n.* a specialized sensory nerve ending (*see* receptor) that monitors internal changes in the body brought about by movement and muscular activity. Proprioceptors in muscles and tendons assist in coordinating muscular activity.

proptosis (prop-toh-sis) *n.* forward displacement of an organ, especially the eye (*see* exophthalmos).

propylthiouracil (proh-pil-th'y-oh-yoor-ă-sil) *n.* a drug that reduces thyroid activity and is administered by mouth to treat thyrotoxicosis and to prepare patients for surgical removal of the thyroid gland.

prosop- (prosopo-) *prefix denoting* the face.

prostaglandin (pros-tă-gland-in) *n.* one of a group of hormone-like substances present in a wide variety of tissues and body fluids. Prostaglandins have many actions, one of which is to cause contraction of the womb: for this reason they have been used therapeutically to aid labour and induce abortion.

prostatectomy (pros-tă-tek-tŏmi) *n.* surgical removal of the prostate gland. The operation is necessary to relieve retention of urine or impaired urinary flow due to enlargement of the prostate. It can be performed through the bladder (*transvesical p.*), through the surrounding capsule of the prostate (*retropubic p.*), or through the urethra (*transurethral p.*).

prostate gland (pros-tayt) *n.* a male accessory sex gland that opens into the urethra just below the bladder and vas deferens. During ejaculation it secretes an alkaline fluid that forms part of the semen. The prostate may become enlarged in elderly men. This obstructs the neck of the bladder and requires surgical treatment (*see* prostatectomy).

The prostate gland and associated structures (median view)

prostatitis (pros-tă-**ty**-tis) *n.* inflammation of the prostate gland. This may be due to bacterial infection and can be either acute or chronic.

prostatocystitis (pros-tă-toh-sis-ty-tis) *n.* inflammation of the prostate gland associated with inflammation of the urinary bladder.

prostatorrhoea (pros-tă-tŏ-**ree**-ă) *n.* an abnormal discharge of thin watery fluid from the prostate gland. This occurs in some patients with acute prostatitis.

prosthesis (pros-**th'ee**-sis) *n.* (*pl.* **prostheses**) any artificial device that is attached to the body as a substitute for a missing or nonfunctional part. Prostheses include artificial limbs, hearing aids, dentures, and implanted pacemakers. —**prosthetic** (pros-**thet**-ik) *adj.*

prostration (pros-**tray**-shŏn) *n.* extreme exhaustion.

protamine (**proh**-tă-meen) *n.* one of a group of simple proteins that can be conjugated with nucleic acids to form nucleoproteins. *p. zinc insulin* a combination of protamine and insulin that is absorbed much more slowly than ordinary insulin and thus reduces the frequency of injections.

protanopia (proh-tă-**noh**-piă) *n. see* Daltonism.

protease (**proh**-ti-ayz) *n. see* proteolytic enzyme.

protein (**proh**-teen) *n.* one of a group of organic compounds made up of one or more chains of amino acids. Proteins are essential constituents of the body; they form the structural material of muscles, tissues, organs, etc., and are equally important as regulators of function, as enzymes and hormones. Proteins are synthesized in the body from their constituent amino acids, which are obtained from the digestion of protein in the diet.

proteinuria (proh-tin-**yoor**-iă) *n. see* albuminuria.

proteolysis (proh-ti-**ol**-i-sis) *n.* the process whereby protein molecules are broken down by proteolytic enzymes into their constituent amino acids, which are then absorbed into the bloodstream. —**proteolytic** (proh-ti-ŏ-**lit**-ik) *adj.*

proteolytic enzyme (protease) *n.* a digestive enzyme that causes the breakdown of protein.

proteose (**proh**-ti-ohz) *n.* a product of the hydrolytic decomposition of protein.

Proteus (**proh**-ti-ŭs) *n.* a genus of rodlike Gram-negative flagellate highly motile bacteria common in the intestines and in decaying organic material. *P. morganii* a species associated with acute enteritis in children. *P. vulgaris* a species that can cause urinary tract infections.

prothionamide (proh-th'y-on-ă-myd) *n.* a drug used in the treatment of tuberculosis. It is administered by mouth, usually together with other antituberculosis drugs. Trade name: **Trevintix**.

prothipendyl (proh-th'y-**pen**-dil) *n.* a tranquillizer and sedative drug administered by mouth or injection to relieve anxiety, agitation, restlessness, and excitement, to induce sleep, and to prevent nausea and vomiting. Trade name: **Tolnate**.

prothrombin (proh-**throm**-bin) *n.* a substance, present in blood plasma, that is the inactive precursor from which the enzyme thrombin is derived during the process of blood coagulation. *See also* coagulation factors.

proto- *prefix denoting* **1.** first. **2.** primitive; early. **3.** a precursor.

protopathic (proh-tŏ-**path**-ik) *adj.* describing the ability to perceive only strong stimuli of pain, heat, etc. *Compare* epicritic.

protoplasm (**proh**-tŏ-plazm) *n.* the material of which living cells are made, which includes the cytoplasm and nucleus. —**protoplasmic** *adj.*

protoporphyrin IX (proh-toh-**por**-firin) *n.* the most common type of porphyrin found in nature. It is a constituent of haemoglobin, myoglobin, and the commoner chlorophylls.

Protozoa (proh-tŏ-**zoh**-ă) *n.* a group of microscopic single-celled animals. Most Protozoa are free-living but some, such as *Plasmodium* and *Leishmania*, are important disease-causing parasites of man. *See also* amoeba. —**protozoan** *adj., n.*

protriptyline (proh-**trip**-ti-leen) *n.* a tricyclic antidepressant drug administered by mouth to treat moderate or severe depression, especially in apathetic and withdrawn patients. Trade name: **Concordin**.

protuberance (prŏ-**tew**-ber-ăns) *n.* (in anatomy) a rounded projecting part.

proud flesh (prowd) *n.* a large amount of soft granulation tissue that may develop during the healing of a wound of large surface area.

provitamin (proh-**vit**-ă-min) *n.* a substance that is not itself a vitamin but can be converted to a vitamin in the body. An example is β-carotene, which can be converted into vitamin A.

proximal (**proks**-i-măl) *adj.* (in anatomy) situated close to the origin or point of attachment or close to the median line of the body. *Compare* distal.

prurigo (proor-**I**-goh) *n.* a chronic itchy skin disease of unknown cause. It usually starts in childhood with small pale pimples arising deep in the skin. Prurigo may occur in association with hay fever or asthma or start in warm weather.

pruritus (proor-**I**-tŭs) *n.* itching, caused by local irritation of the skin or sometimes nervous disorders. Severe itching is a symptom of some forms of jaundice. Pruritus of the vulva in women may be due to vaginal infection. Pruritus of the anal region may be due to poor hygiene, haemorrhoids, or intestinal worms.

prussic acid (**prus**-ik) *n. see* hydrocyanic acid.

psammoma (sam-**oh**-mă) *n.* a tumour containing gritty sandlike particles (*p. bodies*). Such tumours may be found in the meninges, the ovary, etc.

pseud- (**pseudo-**) *prefix denoting* superficial resemblance to; false.

pseudarthrosis (**nearthrosis**) (s'yood-arth-**roh**-sis) *n.* a 'false' joint, formed around a displaced bone end after dislocation.

pseudoangina (s'yoo-doh-an-**jy**-nă) *n.* pain in the centre of the chest in the absence of heart disease. It is associated with anxiety and may be part of the effort syndrome.

pseudocholinesterase (s'yoo-doh-koh-lin-**est**-er-ayz) *n.* an enzyme found in the blood and other tissues that breaks down acetylcholine, but much more slowly than cholinesterase.

pseudocoxalgia (s'yoo-doh-koks-al-jiǎ) *n.* *see* Legg-Calvé-Perthes disease.

pseudocrisis (s'yoo-doh-kry-sis) *n.* a false crisis: a sudden but temporary fall of temperature in a patient with fever.

pseudocroup (s'yoo-doh-kroop) *n.* spasmodic contraction of the larynx that is not caused by inflammation of the glottis or associated with coughing. It occurs particularly in children with rickets.

pseudocyesis (phantom pregnancy) (s'yoo-doh-sy-ee-sis) *n.* a condition in which a nonpregnant woman exhibits symptoms of pregnancy, e.g. enlarged abdomen, morning sickness, and absence of menstruation. The condition usually has an emotional basis.

pseudocyst (s'yoo-doh-sist) *n.* a fluid-filled space without a proper wall or lining, within an organ. *pancreatic p.* a pseudocyst, filled with pancreatic juice, that may develop in cases of chronic pancreatitis or as a complication of acute pancreatitis. It may cause episodes of abdominal pain accompanied by a rise in the level of enzymes in the blood. Treatment is by surgical drainage, usually by marsupialization.

pseudohermaphroditism (s'yoo-doh-her-maf-rŏ-dyt-izm) *n.* a congenital abnormality in which the external genitalia of a male or a female resemble those of the opposite sex.

pseudohypertrophy (s'yoo-doh-hy-per-trŏ-fi) *n.* increase in the size of an organ or structure caused by excessive growth of cells that have a packing or supporting role. The result is usually a decline in the efficiency of the organ. —**pseudohypertrophic** (s'yoo-doh-hy-per-trof-ik) *adj.*

pseudohypoparathyroidism (s'yoo-doh-hy-poh-pa-rǎ-th'y-roid-izm) *n.* a syndrome of mental retardation, restricted growth, and bony abnormalities due to a genetic defect that causes lack of response to parathyroid hormone.

pseudologia fantastica (s'yoo-doh-loh-jiǎ fan-tas-tik-ǎ) *n.* the telling of elaborate and fictitious stories as if they were true. It is sometimes a feature of chronic mental illness and of personality disorders, particularly psychopathy.

Pseudomonas (s'yoo-doh-moh-nǎs) *n.* a genus of rodlike motile pigmented Gram-negative bacteria. Most live in soil and decomposing organic matter. *P aeruginosa* a species that occurs in pus from wounds; it is associated with urinary tract infections. *P. pseudomallei* the causative agent of melioidosis.

pseudomyxoma (s'yoo-doh-miks-oh-mǎ) *n.* a mucoid tumour of the peritoneum, often seen in association with myxomas of the ovary.

pseudoplegia (s'yoo-doh-plee-jiǎ) *n.* paralysis of the limbs not associated with organic abnormalities. It may be a hysterical symptom.

pseudopodium (s'yoo-doh-poh-diŭm) *n.* (*pl.* **pseudopodia**) a temporary and constantly changing extension of the body of an amoeba or an amoeboid cell. Pseudopodia engulf bacteria and other particles as food and are responsible for the movements of the cell.

pseudopolyposis (s'yoo-doh-pol-i-poh-sis) *n.* a condition in which the bowel lining (mucosa) is covered by elevated or protuberant plaques (*pseudopolyps*) that are not true polyps but abnormal growth of inflamed mucosa. It is usually found in chronic ulcerative colitis.

psilosis (sy-loh-sis) *n. see* sprue.

psittacosis (sit-ă-koh-sis) *n. see* parrot disease.

psoas (psoas major) (soh-ăs) *n.* a muscle in the groin that acts jointly with the iliacus muscle to flex the hip joint. A smaller muscle (*p. minor*) has the same action but is often absent.

psoriasis (sŏ-ry-ă-sis) *n.* a chronic skin disease in which itchy scaly red patches form on the elbows, forearms, knees, legs, scalp, and other parts of the body. Psoriasis is one of the commonest skin diseases in Britain, but its cause is not known. It sometimes occurs in association with arthritis (*psoriatic arthritis*). Occasionally the disease may be very severe, affecting much of the skin and causing considerable disability in the patient. —**psoriatic** (sor-i-at-ik) *adj.*

psych- (psycho-) *prefix denoting* **1.** the mind; psyche. **2.** psychology.

psyche (sy-ki) *n.* the mind or the soul; the mental (as opposed to the physical) functioning of the individual.

psychedelic (sy-ki-**del**-ik) *adj.* describing drugs, such as cannabis and LSD, that can induce changes in the level of consciousness of the mind.

psychiatrist (si-ky-ă-trist) *n.* a medically qualified physician who specializes in the study and treatment of mental disorders.

psychiatry (si-ky-ă-tri) *n.* the study of mental disorders and their diagnosis, management, and prevention. —**psychiatric** (sy-ki-at-rik) *adj.*

psychic (sy-kik) *adj.* **1.** of or relating to the psyche. **2.** relating to parapsychological phenomena.

psychoanalysis (sy-koh-ă-**nal**-i-sis) *n.* a school of psychology and a method of treating mental disorders based upon the teachings of Sigmund Freud (1856–1939). Psychoanalysis employs the technique of free association in the course of intensive psychotherapy in order to bring repressed fears and conflicts to the conscious mind, where they can be dealt with (*see* repression). —**psychoanalyst** (sy-koh-**an**-ă-list) *n.* —**psychoanalytic** (sy-koh-an-ă-**lit**-ik) *adj.*

psychodrama (sy-koh-drah-mă) *n.* a form of group psychotherapy in which individuals acquire insight into themselves by acting out situations from their past with other group members. *See* group therapy.

psychodynamics (sy-koh-dy-**nam**-iks) *n.* the study of the mind in action. —**psychodynamic** *adj.*

psychogenic (sy-koh-**jen**-ik) *adj.* having an origin in the mind rather than in the body. The term is applied particularly to symptoms and illnesses.

psychogeriatrics (sy-koh-je-ri-at-riks) *n.* the branch of psychiatry that deals with the mental disorders of old people. —**psychogeriatric** *adj.*

psychologist (sy-kol-ŏ-jist) *n.* a person who is engaged in the scientific study of the mind. *clinical p.* a psychologist trained in aspects of the assessment and treatment of the ill and handicapped. He usually works in a hospital. *educational p.* a psychologist trained in aspects of the cognitive and emotional development of children. He usually works in close association with schools.

psychology (sy-**kol**-ŏji) *n.* the science concerned with the behaviour of man and animals. The different schools of psychology include behaviourism, psychoanalysis, and gestaltism. —**psychological** (sy-kŏ-**loj**-ikăl) *adj.*

psychometrics (sy-koh-**met**-riks) *n.* the measurement of individual differences in psychological functions (such as intelligence and personality) by means of standardized tests. —**psychometric** *adj.*

psychomotor (sy-koh-**moh**-ter) *adj.* relating to muscular and mental activity. The term is applied to disorders in which muscular activities are affected by cerebral disturbance.

psychoneurosis (sy-koh-newr-**oh**-sis) *n.* a neurosis that is manifest in psychological rather than organic symptoms.

psychopath (sy-koh-path) *n.* a person who behaves in an antisocial way and shows little or no guilt for antisocial acts and little capacity for forming emotional relationships with others. *See also* personality disorder. —**psychopathic** *adj.* —**psychopathy** (sy-**kop**-ă-thi) *n.*

psychopathology (sy-koh-pă-**thol**-ŏji) *n.* **1.** the study of mental disorders, with the aim of explaining and describing aberrant behaviour. *Compare* psychiatry. **2.** the symptoms, collectively, of a mental disorder. —**psychopathological** *adj.*

psychopharmacology (sy-koh-farm-ă-**kol**-ŏji) *n.* the study of the effects of drugs on mental processes and behaviour, particularly psychotropic drugs.

psychophysiology (sy-koh-fiz-i-**ol**-ŏji) *n.* the branch of psychology that records physiological measurements, such as heart rate and size of the pupil, and relates them to psychological events. —**psychophysiological** *adj.*

psychosexual development (sy-koh-**seks**-yoo-ăl) *n.* the process by which an individual becomes more mature in his sexual feelings and behaviour. Gender identity, sex-role behaviour, and choice of sexual partner are the three major areas of development.

psychosis (sy-**koh**-sis) *n.* a severe mental illness in which the sufferer loses contact with reality. Delusions and hallucinations occur and thought processes may be altered. The major varieties are *organic* and *functional*; in the latter no physical cause has been demonstrated. The most important functional psychoses are schizophrenia and manic-depressive psychosis. —**psychotic** (sy-**kot**-ik) *adj.*

psychosomatic (sy-koh-sŏ-**mat**-ik) *adj.* relating to or involving both the mind and body: usually applied to illnesses, such as asthma and peptic ulcer, that are caused by the interaction of mental and physical factors.

psychosurgery (sy-koh-**ser**-jer-i) *n.* surgery of the brain to relieve psychological symptoms, such as severe chronic anxiety, depression, and untreatable pain. The operation most commonly performed is leucotomy, but cingulectomy and amygdalectomy are sometimes also used. —**psychosurgical** *adj.*

psychotherapy (sy-koh-**th'e**-răpi) *n.* psychological (as opposed to physical) methods for the treatment of mental disorders and psychological problems. There are many different approaches to psychotherapy, including psychoanalysis, client-centred therapy, and group therapy. *See also* behaviour therapy, counselling. —**psychotherapeutic** (sy-koh-th'e-rǎ-**pew**-tik) *adj.* —**psychotherapist** *n.*

psychoticism (sy-**kot**-i-sizm) *n.* a dimension of personality derived from psychometric tests, which appears to indicate a degree of emotional coldness and some cognitive impairment.

psychotropic (sy-koh-**trop**-ik) *adj.* describing drugs that affect mood. Antidepressants, sedatives, stimulants, and tranquillizers are psychotropic.

pterion (**teer**-i-ŏn) *n.* the point on the side of the skull at which the sutures between the parietal, temporal, and sphenoid bones meet.

pteroylglutamic acid (te-roh-il-gloo-**tam**-ik) *n. see* folic acid.

pterygium (tě-**rij**-iŭm) *n.* a triangular overgrowth of the cornea, usually the inner side, by thickened and degenerative conjunctiva.

pterygo- *prefix denoting* the pterygoid process.

pterygoid process (te-ri-goid) *n.* either of two large processes of the sphenoid bone.

ptomaine (**toh**-mayn) *n.* any of various substances, such as putrescine, cadaverine, and neurine, produced in decaying foodstuffs and responsible for the unpleasant taste and smell of such foods. Ptomaines themselves are harmless, but they are often associated with toxic bacteria.

ptosis (**toh**-sis) *n.* drooping of the upper eyelid. This may be due to a disorder of the oculomotor nerve, a disease of the eye muscles, or myasthenia gravis; it may also occur as part of Horner's syndrome or as an isolated congenital feature.

-ptosis *suffix denoting* a lowered position of an organ or part; prolapse.

ptyal- (ptyalo-) *prefix denoting* saliva.

ptyalin (**ty**-ǎ-lin) *n.* an enzyme (an amylase) found in saliva.

ptyalism (sialorrhoea) (ty-ǎ-lizm) *n.* the excessive production of saliva: a symptom of certain nervous disorders, poisoning, or infection (rabies). *Compare* xerostomia.

ptyalith (ty-ǎ-lith) *n.* a stone (calculus) in a salivary gland or duct.

ptyalography (ty-ǎ-**log**-rǎfi) *n. see* sialography.

puberty (**pew**-ber-ti) *n.* the time at which the onset of sexual maturity occurs and the reproductive organs become functional. This is manifested in both sexes by the appearance of secondary sexual characteristics and in girls by the start of menstruation. —**pubertal** *adj.*

pubes (**pew**-beez) *n.* **1.** the body surface that overlies the pubis, at the front of the pelvis. **2.** *see* pubis. —**pubic** *adj.*

pubiotomy (pew-bi-**ot**-ŏmi) *n.* an operation to divide the pubic bone near the symphysis, performed during childbirth to increase the size of an abnormally small pelvis.

pubis (**pew**-bis) *n.* (*pl.* **pubes**) a bone forming the lower and anterior part of each side of the hip bone (*see also* pelvis). The two pubes meet at the front of the pelvis at the *pubic symphysis*. *See also* pubes.

pudendal block (pew-**den**-d'l) *n*. anaesthesia of the pudendum and surrounding areas by injecting a local anaesthetic into the nerves that supply them. It is performed to relieve the pain of the expulsive stage of labour. *See also* nerve block.

pudendum (pew-**den**-dŭm) *n*. (*pl.* **pudenda**) the external genital organs, especially those of the female (*see* vulva). —**pudendal** *adj*.

puerpera (pew-**er**-per-ă) *n*. a woman who has recently given birth and whose womb has not yet returned to its normal non-pregnant dimensions.

puerperal (puerperous) (pew-er-per-ăl) *adj*. relating to childbirth or the period that immediately follows it. *p. fever* (*childbed fever*) blood poisoning (septicaemia) in a mother shortly after childbirth resulting from infection of the lining of the womb or the vagina.

puerperalism (pew-er-per-ăl-izm) *n*. illness of a mother or her baby associated with childbirth.

puerperium (childbed) (pew-er-**peer**-iŭm) *n*. the period of up to about six weeks after childbirth, during which the size of the womb decreases to normal.

Pulex (**pew**-leks) *n*. a genus of widely distributed fleas. *P. irritans* the human flea: a common parasite of man whose bite may give rise to intense irritation and bacterial infection.

pulicide (**pew**-li-syd) *n*. any chemical agent, for example DDT or malathion, used for killing fleas.

pulmo- (pulmon(o)-) *prefix denoting* the lung(s).

pulmonary (pul-**mŏn**-er-i) *adj*. relating to, associated with, or af-

The pulse points

fecting the lungs. *p. artery* the artery that conveys deoxygenated blood from the heart to the lungs for oxygenation. *p. circulation see* circulation. *p. embolism see* embolism. *p. hypertension* raised blood pressure within the blood vessels supplying the lungs. Pulmonary hypertension may complicate pulmonary embolism, septal defects, heart failure, diseases of the mitral valve, and chronic lung diseases. *p. stenosis* congenital narrowing of the outlet of the right ventricle of the heart. Severe pulmonary stenosis may produce angina pectoris, faintness, and heart failure. The defect is corrected by surgery. *p. tuberculosis see* tuberculosis. *p. valve see* semilunar valve. *p. vein* a vein carrying oxygenated blood from the lung to the left atrium.

pulp (pulp) *n.* **1.** a soft mass of tissue (for example, of the spleen). **2.** the mass of connective tissue containing blood vessels and nerve fibres at the centre of a tooth (*p. cavity*).

pulsation (pul-**say**-shŏn) *n.* a rhythmical throbbing or beating, as of the heart or arteries.

pulse (puls) *n.* a series of pressure waves within an artery caused by contractions of the left ventricle and corresponding with the heart rate. It is easily detected over certain superficial arteries (*p. points* – see illustration). The average adult pulse rate at rest is 60–80 per minute, but exercise, injury, illness, and emotion may produce much faster rates.

pulsus alternans (pul-sus awl-ter-nanz) *n.* a pulse in which there is a regular alternation of strong and weak beats without changes in the length of the cycle.

pulsus paradoxus (pa-ră-doks-ŭs) *n.* a large fall in systolic blood pressure and pulse volume when the patient breathes in. It is seen in constrictive pericarditis, pericardial effusion, and asthma.

pulvis (pul-vis) *n.* (in pharmaceutics) a powder.

punch-drunk syndrome *n.* a group of symptoms consisting of progressive dementia, tremor of the hands, and epilepsy. It is a consequence of repeated blows to the head that have been severe enough to cause concussion.

punctate (punk-tayt) *adj.* spotted or dotted.

punctum (punk-tŭm) *n* (*pl.* **puncta**) (in anatomy) a point or small area. *puncta lacrimalia* the two openings of the tear ducts in the inner corners of the upper and lower eyelids (*see* lacrimal (apparatus)).

puncture (punk-cher) **1.** *n.* a wound made accidentally or deliberately by a sharp object or instrument. Punctures are performed for diagnostic purposes, in order to withdraw tissue or fluid for examination. *See also* lumbar (puncture). **2.** *vb.* to pierce a tissue with a sharp instrument.

pupil (pew-pil) *n.* the circular opening in the centre of the iris, through which light passes into the lens of the eye. –**pupillary** (pew-pil-er-i) *adj.*

pupillary reflex (light reflex) *n.* the reflex change in the size of the pupil according to the amount of light entering the eye.

purgation (per-gay-shŏn) *n.* the use of drugs to stimulate intestinal activity and clear the bowels. *See* laxative.

purgative (per-gă-tiv) *n. see* laxative.

purine (pewr-reen) *n.* a nitrogen-containing compound with a two-ring molecular structure. Examples of purines are adenine and guanine, which occur in nucleic acids, and uric acid.

Purkinje cells (per-**kin**-ji) *pl. n.* nerve cells found in great numbers in the cortex of the cerebellum. [J. E. Purkinje (1787–1869), Bohemian physiologist]

Purkinje fibres *pl. n. see* atrioventricular bundle.

purpura (per-pew-ră) *n.* a skin rash resulting from bleeding into the skin from blood capillaries; the rash is made up of individual purple spots (petechiae). Purpura may be due either to defects in the capillaries (*nonthrombocytopenic p.*) or to a deficiency of blood platelets (*thrombocytopenic p.*). *acute idiopathic thrombocytopenic p.* a disease of children in which antibodies are produced that destroy the patient's platelets. *See also* thrombocytopenia, Schönlein-Henoch purpura.

purulent (**pewr**-uu-lĕnt) *adj.* forming, consisting of, or containing pus.

pus (pus) *n.* a thick yellowish or greenish liquid formed at the site of an established infection. Pus contains dead white blood cells, both living and dead bacteria, and fragments of dead tissue. *See also* mucopus, seropus.

pustule (**pus**-tewl) *n.* a small pus-containing blister on the skin.

putamen (pew-**tay**-men) *n.* a part of the lenticular nucleus (*see* basal ganglia).

putrefaction (pew-tri-**fak**-shŏn) *n.* the process whereby proteins are decomposed by bacteria. This is accompanied by the formation of amines (such as putrescine and cadaverine) having a strong and very unpleasant smell.

py- (**pyo-**) *prefix denoting* pus; a purulent condition.

pyaemia (py-ee-miă) *n.* blood poisoning by pus-forming bacteria released from an abscess. Widespread formation of abscesses may develop, with fatal results. *Compare* sapraemia, septicaemia, toxaemia.

pyarthrosis (py-arth-**roh**-sis) *n.* an infected joint filled with pus. Drainage, combined with antibiotic treatment, is necessary.

pyel- (**pyelo-**) *prefix denoting* the pelvis of the kidney.

pyelitis (py-ĕ-**ly**-tis) *n.* inflammation of the pelvis of the kidney, usually caused by a bacterial infection. The patient experiences pain in the loins, shivering, and a high temperature. Treatment is by the administration of a suitable antibiotic, together with analgesics and a high fluid intake.

pyelocystitis (py-ĕ-loh-sis-ty-tis) *n.* inflammation of the renal pelvis and urinary bladder (*see* pyelitis, cystitis).

pyelogram (py-ĕ-loh-gram) *n.* an X-ray picture obtained by pyelography.

pyelography (py-ĕ-**log**-răfi) *n.* X-ray examination of the kidneys using radio-opaque contrast material. *intravenous p.* (*excretion urography*) pyelography in which the contrast medium is injected into a vein and is concentrated and excreted by the kidneys. *retrograde p.* pyelography in which fine catheters are passed up the ureter to the kidneys at cystoscopy and contrast material is injected directly into the renal pelvis.

pyelolithotomy (py-ĕ-loh-lith-ot-ŏmi) *n.* surgical removal of a stone from the kidney through an incision made in the pelvis of the kidney.

pyelonephritis (py-ĕ-loh-ni-**fry**-tis) *n.* bacterial infection of the kidney substance. *acute p.* pyelonephritis in which the patient has pain in the loins, a high temperature, and shivering fits. Treatment is by the administration of an appropriate antibiotic. *chronic p.* pyelonephritis in which the kidneys become small and scarred and kidney failure ensues. Vesicoureteric reflux in childhood is one of the causes.

pyeloplasty (py-ĕ-loh-plasti) *n.* an operation to relieve obstruction at the junction of the pelvis kidney and the ureter. *See* hydronephrosis, Dietl's crisis.

pyelotomy (py-ĕ-**lot**-ŏmi) *n.* surgical incision into the pelvis of the kidney. This operation is usually undertaken to remove a stone (*see* pyelolithotomy).

pyg- (**pygo-**) *prefix denoting* the buttocks.

pykno- *prefix denoting* thickness or density.

pyknolepsy (pik-noh-lep-si) *n. Obsolete.* a very high frequency of petit mal attacks.

pyl- (**pyle-**) *prefix denoting* the portal vein.

pylephlebitis (**portal pyaemia**) (py-li-fli-**by**-tis) *n.* septic inflammation and thrombosis of the hepatic portal vein, resulting from the spread of infection within the abdomen. The condition causes fever, liver abscesses, and ascites. Treatment is by antibiotic drugs and surgical drainage of abscesses.

pylethrombosis (py-li-throm-**boh**-sis) *n.* obstruction of the portal vein by a blood clot (*see* thrombosis), resulting from such conditions as pylephlebitis and cirrhosis of the liver. Portal hypertension is a frequent result.

pylor- (**pyloro-**) *prefix denoting* the pylorus.

pylorectomy (py-lor-ek-tŏmi) *n.* a surgical operation in which the muscular outlet of the stomach (pylorus) is removed. *See* antrectomy, pyloroplasty.

pyloric stenosis (py-**lor**-ik) *n.* narrowing of the pylorus. This causes delay in passage of the stomach contents to the duodenum, which leads to repeated vomiting. Pyloric stenosis in adults is caused by a peptic ulcer close to the pylorus or by a cancerous growth obstructing it. *congenital hypertrophic p. s.* pyloric stenosis that occurs in babies about 10 to 14 days old (particularly boys) in which the thickened pyloric muscle can be felt as a nodule. Treatment is by pyloromyotomy.

pyloromyotomy (**Ramstedt's operation**) (py-lor-oh-my-ot-ŏmi) *n.* a surgical operation in which the muscle around the pylorus is divided down to the lining (mucosa) in order to relieve congenital pyloric stenosis.

pyloroplasty (py-**lor**-oh-plasti) *n.* a surgical operation in which the pylorus is widened by a form of reconstruction. It is done to allow the contents of the stomach to pass more easily into the duodenum.

pylorospasm (py-**lor**-oh-spazm) *n.* closure of the pylorus due to muscle spasm, leading to delay in the passage of stomach contents to the duodenum and vomiting. It is usually associated with duodenal or pyloric ulcers.

pylorus (py-**lor**-ŭs) *n.* the lower end of the stomach, which leads to the duodenum. It terminates at a ring of muscle (*pyloric sphincter*), which contracts to close the opening by which the stomach communicates with the duodenum. —**pyloric** *adj.*

pyo- *prefix. see* py-.

pyocele (py-oh-seel) *n.* a swelling caused by an accumulation of pus in a part of the body.

pyocolpos (py-oh-kol-pos) *n.* the presence of pus in the vagina.

pyocyanin (py-oh-sy-ă-nin) *n.* an antibiotic substance produced by the bacterium *Pseudomonas aeruginosa* and active principally against Gram-positive bacteria.

pyoderma (py-oh-**der**-mă) *n.* any infected skin disease in which pus is produced.

pyogenic (py-oh-**jen**-ik) *adj.* causing the formation of pus.

pyometra (py-oh-**mee**-tră) *n.* the presence of pus in the womb.

pyomyositis (py-oh-my-oh-sy-tis) *n.* bacterial or fungal infection of a muscle resulting in painful inflammation.

pyonephrosis (py-oh-ni-**froh**-sis) *n.* obstruction and infection of the kidney resulting in pus formation. A kidney stone is the usual cause of the obstruction, and the kidney becomes distended by pus and destroyed by the inflammation. Treatment is urgent nephrectomy under antibiotic cover.

pyopericarditis (py-oh-pe-ri-kar-dy-tis) *n.* inflammation of the pericardium, with the formation of pus.

pyopneumothorax (py-oh-new-moh-thor-aks) *n.* pus and gas or air in the pleural cavity. The condition can arise if air is introduced during attempts to drain the pus from an empyema. Alternatively a hydropneumothorax may become infected.

pyorrhoea (py-ŏ-ree-ă) *n.* a former name for periodontal disease.

pyosalpinx (py-oh-**sal**-pinks) *n.* the accumulation of pus in a Fallopian tube.

pyosis (py-**oh**-sis) *n.* the formation and discharge of pus.

pyothorax (py-oh-**thor**-aks) *n. see* empyema.

pyr- (**pyro-**) *prefix denoting* **1.** fire. **2.** a burning sensation. **3.** fever.

pyramid (pi-ră-mid) *n.* **1.** one of the conical masses that make up the medulla of the kidney. **2.** one of the elongated bulging areas on the anterior surface of the medulla oblongata in the brain. —**pyramidal** (pi-ram-i-d'l) *adj.*

pyramidal cell *n.* a type of neurone found in the cerebral cortex, with a pyramid-shaped cell body.

pyramidal system *n.* a collection of nerve tracts within the pyramid of the medulla oblongata, en route from the cerebral cortex to the spinal cord.

pyrazinamide (py-ră-zin-ă-myd) *n.* a drug administered by mouth, usually in combination with other drugs, to treat tuberculosis. Trade name: **Zinamide**.

pyret- (**pyreto-**) *prefix denoting* fever.

pyrexia (py-**reks**-iă) *n. see* fever.

pyridostigmine (pi-ri-doh-stig-meen) *n.* a drug that inhibits the enzyme cholinesterase and is used to treat myasthenia gravis. It has a more prolonged action and is less toxic than neostigmine.

pyridoxal phosphate (pi-ri-doks-ăl) *n.* a derivative of vitamin B_6 that is an important coenzyme in certain reactions of amino-acid metabolism. *See* transamination.

pyridoxine (vitamin B_6) (pi-ri-doks-een) *n. see* vitamin B.

pyrimidine (pi-**rim**-i-deen) *n.* a nitrogen-containing compound with a ring molecular structure. The commonest pyrimidines are cytosine, thymine, and uracil, which form the nucleotides of nucleic acids.

pyrogen (**py**-roh-jen) *n.* any substance or agent producing fever. —**pyrogenic** *adj.*

pyromania (py-roh-**may**-niă) *n.* an excessively strong impulse to set things on fire. —**pyromaniac** *adj.*, *n.*

pyrosis (py-**roh**-sis) *n.* another term (chiefly US) for heartburn.

pyruvic acid (**pyruvate**) (py-**roo**-vik) *n.* a compound, derived from carbohydrates, that may be oxidized in the Krebs cycle to yield carbon dioxide and energy in the form of ATP.

pyuria (py-**yoor**-iă) *n.* the presence of pus in the urine, making it cloudy. This is a sign of bacterial infection in the urinary tract.

Q

Q fever *n.* an acute infectious disease of cattle, sheep, and goats that is caused by a rickettsia, *Coxiella burnetti*, and can be transmitted to man primarily through contaminated unpasteurized milk. Symptoms include fever, severe headache, and respiratory problems. Treatment with tetracyclines or chloramphenicol is effective. *See also* typhus.

quadratus (kwod-**ray**-tŭs) *n.* any of various four-sided muscles. *q. femoris* a flat muscle at the head of the femur, responsible for lateral rotation of the thigh.

quadri- *prefix denoting* four.

quadriceps (**kwod**-ri-seps) *n.* one of the great extensor muscles of the legs. It is situated in the thigh and is subdivided into four distinct portions: the *rectus femoris*, *vastus lateralis*, *vastus medialis*, and *vastus intermedius*.

quadriplegia (**tetraplegia**) (kwod-ri-**plee**-jiă) *n.* paralysis affecting all four limbs. —**quadriplegic** *adj.*, *n.*

quadruple vaccine (kwod-roo-pŭl) *n.* a combined vaccine used to produce immunity against diphtheria, whooping cough, poliomyelitis, and tetanus.

quarantine (**kwo**-răn-teen) *n.* the period for which a person (or animal) is kept in isolation to prevent the spread of a contagious disease. Different diseases have different quarantine periods.

quartan fever (kwor-t'n) *n.* a type of malaria, caused by *Plasmodium malariae*, in which there is a three-day interval between fever attacks.

Queckenstedt test (kwek-ĕn-stet) *n.* a part of the routine lumbar puncture procedure. It is used to determine whether or not the flow of cerebrospinal fluid is blocked in the spinal cord. [H. H. G. Queckenstedt (1876–1918), German physician]

quickening (kwik-ĕn-ing) *n.* the first movement of a baby in the womb that is felt by the mother, usually after about four months of pregnancy.

quiescent (kwi-**es**-ĕnt) *adj.* describing a disease that is in an inactive or undetectable phase.

quinestradol (kwin-ee-strä-dol) *n.* a synthetic female sex hormone (*see* oestrogen) administered by mouth to treat inflammation of the vagina, particularly after the menopause. Trade name: **Pentovis**.

quinestrol (kwin-ee-strol) *n.* a synthetic female sex hormone (*see* oestrogen) administered by mouth to inhibit lactation in mothers not breast feeding. Trade name: **Estrovis.**

quinidine (kwin-i-deen) *n.* a drug that slows down the activity of the heart and is administered by mouth to control abnormal and increased heart rhythm. Trade names: **Kinidin, Natisedine, Quinicardine.**

quinine (kwin-een) *n.* a drug formerly used to prevent and treat malaria, now largely replaced by more effective less toxic drugs. It is administered by mouth or injection; large doses can cause severe poisoning (*see* cinchonism).

quinism (kwin-izm) *n.* the symptoms of overdosage or too prolonged treatment with quinine. *See* cinchonism.

quinsy (kwin-zi) *n.* a pus-filled swelling in the soft palate around the tonsil: a complication of tonsillitis. The patient has great difficulty in swallowing and surgical incision of the abscess may be necessary. Medical name: **peritonsillar abscess.**

quotidian fever (kwoh-tid-iăn) *n.* a severe type of malaria, caused by *Plasmodium falciparum*, in which the interval between fever attacks varies from a few hours to two days.

quotient (kwoh-shěnt) *n. see* intelligence quotient, respiratory quotient.

R

rabbit fever (rab-it) *n. see* tularaemia.

rabies (hydrophobia) (ray-beez) *n.* an acute virus disease of the central nervous system that may be transmitted to man by a bite from an infected dog. Symptoms include malaise, fever, difficulty in breathing, salivation, and painful muscle spasms of the throat induced by swallowing. In the later stages of the disease the mere sight of water induces convulsions and paralysis; death occurs within 4–5 days. Injections of rabies vaccine and antiserum may prevent the disease from developing in a person bitten by an infected animal. —**rabid** (rab-id) *adj.*

racemose (ras-i-mohs) *adj.* resembling a bunch of grapes. The term is applied particularly to a compound gland the secretory part of which consists of a number of small sacs.

rachi- (rachio-) *prefix denoting* the spine.

rachiotomy (ray-ki-ot-ŏmi) *n. see* laminectomy.

rachis (ray-kis) *n. see* backbone.

rachischisis (ray-kis-ki-sis) *n. see* spina bifida.

rachitic (ră-kit-ik) *adj.* afflicted with rickets.

rad (rad) *n.* a unit of absorbed dose of ionizing radiation equal to an absorbed energy of 0.01 joule per kilogram of irradiated material.

radial (ray-di-ăl) *adj.* relating to or associated with the radius. *r. artery* a branch of the brachial artery, beginning at the elbow and passing down the forearm, around the wrist, and into the palm of the hand. *r. nerve* an important mixed sensory and motor nerve of the arm, forming the largest branch of the brachial plexus. *r. reflex* flexion of the forearm (and sometimes also of the fingers) that occurs when the lower end of the radius is tapped.

radiation (ray-di-**ay**-shŏn) *n*. energy in the form of waves or particles, such as gamma rays, X-rays, ultraviolet rays, visible light, and infrared rays (radiant heat). *r. sickness* any acute illness caused by exposure to rays emitted by radioactive substances, e.g. X-rays or gamma rays. Very high doses cause death within hours. Lower doses cause immediate symptoms of nausea, vomiting, and diarrhoea followed by damage to the bone marrow, loss of hair, and bloody diarrhoea.

radical treatment (**rad**-ikăl) *n*. vigorous treatment that aims at the complete cure of a disease rather than the mere relief of symptoms. *Compare* conservative treatment.

radicle (**rad**-ikŭl) *n*. (in anatomy) 1. a small root. 2. the initial fibre of a nerve or the origin of a vein. —**radicular** (ră-**dik**-yoo-ler) *adj*.

radiculitis (ră-dik-yoo-**ly**-tis) *n*. inflammation of the root of a nerve. *See* polyradiculitis.

radio- *prefix denoting* 1. radiation. 2. radioactive substances.

radioactivity (ray-di-oh-ak-**tiv**-iti) *n*. disintegration of the nuclei of certain elements, with the emission of energy in the form of alpha, beta, or gamma rays. Naturally radioactive elements include radium and uranium. *See also* radioisotope. —**radioactive** *adj*.

radioautography (ray-di-oh-aw-**tog**-răfi) *n*. *see* autoradiography.

radiobiology (ray-di-oh-by-**ol**-ŏji) *n*. the study of the effects of radia-tion on living tissues. —**radiobiologist** *n*.

radiodermatitis (ray-di-oh-der-mă-ty-tis) *n*. inflammation of the skin after its exposure to ionizing radiation. The skin becomes dry, hairless, and atrophied, losing its colouring.

radiography (ray-di-**og**-răfi) *n*. the technique of examining the body by directing X-rays through it to produce images (*radiographs*) on photographic plates or fluorescent screens. Radiography is used in the diagnosis of such disorders as broken bones, gastric ulcers, and gallstones, when inspection from outside the body is insufficient for diagnosis. —**radiographer** *n*.

radioimmunoassay (ray-di-oh-im-yoo-noh-**ass**-ay) *n*. the technique of using radioactive tracers to determine the levels of particular antibodies in the blood.

radioisotope (ray-di-oh-**I**-sŏ-tohp) *n*. an isotope of an element that emits alpha, beta, or gamma radiation during its decay into another element. Artificial radioisotopes, such as iodine-131 and cobalt-60, are produced by bombarding elements with beams of neutrons. They are widely used in medicine as tracers and as sources of radiation for the different techniques of radiotherapy.

radiology (ray-di-**ol**-ŏji) *n*. the branch of medicine concerned with the use of radiation, including X-rays, and radioactive substances in the diagnosis and treatment of disease. *See also* radiotherapy. *Compare* radiography. —**radiologist** *n*.

radio-opaque (ray-di-oh-oh-**payk**) *adj*. having the property of absorbing, and therefore being opaque to, X-rays. Radio-opaque materials, many of them containing iodine, are used as contrast media in radiography.

radio pill (ray-di-oh) *n.* a capsule containing a miniature radio transmitter that can be swallowed by a patient. During its passage through the digestive tract it transmits information about internal conditions (acidity, etc.).

radioscopy (ray-di-osk-ŏ-pi) *n.* examination of an X-ray image on a fluorescent screen (*see* fluoroscope).

radiosensitive (ray-di-oh-sen-sit-iv) *adj.* describing certain forms of cancer cell that are particularly susceptible to radiation and are likely to be dealt with successfully by radiotherapy.

radiotherapy (ray-di-oh-th'e-răpi) *n.* the treatment of disease with penetrating radiation, such as X-rays, beta rays, or gamma rays. Beams of radiation may be directed at a diseased part from a distance (*see* telecurietherapy), or radioactive material, in the form of needles, wires, or pellets, may be implanted in the body.

radium (ray-diŭm) *n.* a radioactive metallic element that emits alpha and gamma rays during its decay into other elements. The gamma radiation is employed in radiotherapy for the treatment of cancer. Symbol: Ra. *See also* thorium-X.

radius (ray-di-ŭs) *n.* the outer and shorter bone of the forearm (*compare* ulna). It partially revolves about the ulna, permitting pronation and supination of the hand. —**radial** *adj.*

radix (ray-diks) *n. see* root.

radon (ray-don) *n.* a radioactive gaseous element that is produced during the decay of radium. It

A rib raspatory

emits alpha and gamma radiation. Symbol: Rn. *r. seeds* sealed capsules containing radon, used in radiotherapy for the treatment of cancer.

rale (rahl) *n. see* crepitation.

Ramstedt's operation (rahm-stets) *n. see* pyloromyotomy. [W. C. Ramstedt (1867–1963), German surgeon]

ramus (ray-mŭs) *n.* (*pl.* **rami**) 1. a branch, especially of a nerve fibre or blood vessel. 2. a thin process projecting from a bone.

ranula (ran-yoo-lă) *n.* a cyst found under the tongue, formed when the duct leading from a salivary or mucous gland is obstructed and distended.

raphe (ray-fi) *n.* a line, ridge, seam, or crease in a tissue or organ; for example, the furrow that passes down the centre of the dorsal surface of the tongue.

rarefaction (rair-i-fak-shŏn) *n.* thinning of bony tissue sufficient to cause decreased density of bone to X-rays, as in osteoarthritis.

rash (rash) *n.* a temporary eruption on the skin, usually typified by reddening and itching. A rash may be a local skin reaction or the outward sign of a disorder affecting the body.

raspatory (rah-spă-ter-i) *n.* a file-like surgical instrument used for scraping the surface of bone.

rat-bite fever (sodokosis) (rat-byt) *n.* a disease, contracted from the bite of a rat, due to infection by either the bacterium *Spirillum minus*, which causes ulceration of the skin and recurrent fever, or by the fungus *Strepto-bacillus moniliformis*, which causes inflammation of the skin, muscular pains, and vomiting. Both infections respond well to penicillin.

rationalization (rash-ŏn-ă-ly-zay-shŏn) *n.* (in psychiatry) the explanation of events or behaviour in terms that avoid giving the true reasons.

rauwolfia (raw-wuul-fiă) *n.* the dried root of the shrub *Rauwolfia serpentina*, which contains several alkaloids, including reserpine. Rauwolfia and its alkaloids lower blood pressure and depress activity of the central nervous system.

Raynaud's disease (ray-nohz) *n.* a condition of unknown cause in which the arteries of the fingers are unduly reactive and enter spasm when the hands are cold. This produces attacks of pallor, numbness, and discomfort in the fingers. Gangrene or ulceration of the finger tips may result. Warm gloves and antispasmodic drugs may relieve the condition. [M. Raynaud (1834–81), French physician]

reaction (ri-ak-shŏn) *n.* **1.** the response to a stimulus. **2.** the interaction of two or more substances that results in chemical changes in them. **3.** the effect produced by an allergen (*see* allergy).

reactive (ri-ak-tiv) *adj.* describing mental illnesses that are precipitated by events in the psychological environment.

reagent (ree-ay-jĕnt) *n.* a compound that reacts with another, especially one used to detect the presence of the other compound.

reagin (ree-ă-jin) *n.* a type of antibody, formed against an aller-gen, that remains fixed in various tissues. Subsequent contact with the allergen causes damage to the tissue and the release of histamine and serotonin, which are responsible for the allergic reaction (*see* anaphylaxis).

reality shock (ri-al-iti) *n.* the psychological condition said to result when a newly qualified nurse, trained in an academic setting and to idealistic standards, is confronted with the practical difficulties of working in a hospital ward.

recall (ri-kawl) **1.** *n.* the process of eliciting a representation (especially an image) of a past experience. **2.** *vb.* to elicit such a representation.

receptaculum (ree-sep-tak-yoo-lŭm) *n.* the dilated portion of a tubular anatomical part. *r.* (or *cis-terna*) *chyli* the dilated end of the thoracic duct, into which lymph vessels from the lower limbs and intestines drain.

receptor (ri-sep-ter) *n.* a cell or group of cells specialized to detect changes in the environment and trigger impulses in the sensory nervous system. All sensory nerve endings act as receptors. *See* exteroceptor, interoceptor, proprioceptor.

recess (ri-ses) *n.* (in anatomy) a hollow chamber or a depression in an organ or other part.

recessive (ri-ses-iv) *adj.* describing a gene (or its corresponding characteristic) whose effect is shown in the individual only when its allele is the same. *Compare* dominant. —**recessive** *n.*

recipient (ri-sip-iĕnt) *n.* a person who receives something from a donor, such as a blood transfusion or a kidney transplant.

recrudescence (ree-kroo-**des**-ĕns) *n.* a fresh outbreak of a disorder in a patient after a period during which its signs and symptoms had died down.

rect- (recto-) *prefix denoting* the rectum.

rectocele (rek-toh-seel) *n.* *see* proctocele.

rectopexy (rek-toh-peks-i) *n.* the surgical fixation of a prolapsed rectum.

rectosigmoid (rek-toh-sig-moid) *n.* the region of the large intestine around the junction of the sigmoid colon and the rectum.

rectovesical (rek-toh-ves-ikăl) *adj.* relating to the rectum and the urinary bladder.

rectum (rek-tŭm) *n.* the terminal part of the large intestine, which runs from the sigmoid colon to the anal canal. Faeces are stored in the rectum before defecation. —**rectal** (rek-t'l) *adj.*

rectus (rek-tŭs) *n.* any of several straight muscles. *r. abdominis* a long flat muscle that extends bilaterally along the entire length of the front of the abdomen. *r. femoris see* quadriceps. *r. muscles of the orbit* some of the extrinsic eye muscles.

recumbent (ri-kum-bĕnt) *adj.* lying down. —**recumbency** *n.*

recurrent (ri-ku-rĕnt) *adj.* (in anatomy) describing a structure, such as a nerve or blood vessel, that turns back on its course, forming a loop.

red blood cell *n.* *see* erythrocyte.

red lotion *n.* an astringent solution containing zinc sulphate.

reduction (ri-duk-shŏn) *n.* (in surgery) the restoration of a displaced part of the body, such as a hernia or a dislocated joint, to its normal position by manipulation or operation.

A reflex arc

reduction division *n.* the first division of meiosis, in which the chromosome number is halved.

referred pain (synalgia) (ri-ferd) *n.* pain felt in a part of the body other than where it might be expected. An abscess beneath the diaphragm, for example, may cause a referred pain in the shoulder area. The confusion arises because sensory nerves from different parts of the body share common pathways when they reach the spinal cord.

reflex (ree-fleks) *n.* an automatic or involuntary response to a stimulus, which is brought about by relatively simple nervous circuits without consciousness being necessarily involved. *See* conditioned reflex, patellar reflex, plantar (reflex). *r. arc* the nervous circuit involved in a reflex, being at its simplest a sensory nerve with a receptor, linked at a synapse in the brain or spinal cord with a motor nerve, which supplies a muscle or gland.

reflux (**ree**-fluks) *n*. a backflow of liquid, against its normal direction of movement. *See also* (reflux) oesophagitis, vesicoureteric reflux.

refraction (ri-**frak**-shŏn) *n*. **1.** the change in direction of light rays when they pass obliquely from one transparent medium to another, of a different density. Refraction occurs as light enters the eye and passes through the cornea, lens, etc., to come to a focus on the retina. Errors of refraction include astigmatism and long- and short-sightedness. **2.** determination of the power of refraction of the eye. This determines whether or not the patient needs glasses and, if so, how strong they should be.

refractometer (ree-frak-**tom**-it-er) *n*. *see* optometer.

refractory (ri-**frakt**-er-i) *adj*. unresponsive: applied to a condition that fails to respond satisfactorily to a given treatment.

refractory period *n*. (in neurology) the time of recovery needed for a nerve cell that has just transmitted a nerve impulse or for a muscle fibre that has just contracted. During the refractory period a normal stimulus will not bring about excitation of the cell.

refrigeration (ri-frij-er-**ay**-shŏn) *n*. lowering the temperature of a part of the body to reduce the metabolic activity of its tissues or to provide a local anaesthetic effect.

regeneration (ri-jen-er-**ay**-shŏn) *n*. the natural regrowth of a tissue or other part lost through injury.

regimen (**rej**-i-men) *n*. (in therapeutics) a prescribed systematic form of treatment, such as a diet or a course of drugs, for curing disease or improving health.

regional ileitis (ree-jŏn-**ăl**) *n*. *see* Crohn's disease.

registrar (rej-i-**strar**) *n*. (in a hospital) an experienced physician or surgeon responsible for the care of a number of patients with the assistance of junior doctors, whom he instructs.

regression (ri-**gresh**-ŏn) *n*. **1.** (in psychiatry) reversion to a more immature level of functioning. **2.** the stage of a disease during which the signs and symptoms disappear and the patient recovers.

regurgitation (ri-ger-ji-**tay**-shŏn) *n*. **1.** the bringing up of undigested material from the stomach to the mouth (*see* vomiting). **2.** the flowing back of a liquid in a direction opposite to the normal one.

rehabilitation (ree-ă-bil-i-**tay**-shŏn) *n*. **1.** (in physical medicine) the treatment of an ill, injured, or disabled patient by massage, electrotherapy, and graduated exercises to restore normal health and functions. **2.** any means for restoring the independence of a patient after disease or injury.

Reiter's syndrome (**ry**-terz) *n*. a disease of men involving diarrhoea, urethritis, conjunctivitis, and arthritis. The symptoms resemble those of gonorrhoea. No causative agent has been positively identified, although a virus may be implicated. [H. Reiter (1881–1969), German physician]

relapse (ri-**laps**) *n*. a return of disease symptoms after recovery had apparently been achieved or the worsening of an apparently recovering patient's condition.

relapsing fever (ri-**laps**-ing) *n*. an infectious disease caused by bacteria of the genus *Borrelia*, which is transmitted by ticks or lice and results in recurrent fever. The first episode of fever is accompanied by severe headache and aching muscles and joints. Subsequent attacks are milder and occur at intervals of 3–10 days. Treatment with antibiotics is effective.

relative density (rel-ă-tiv) *n.* the ratio of the density of a substance at a specified temperature to the density of a reference substance (for liquids, this is water at 4°C). It was formerly known as *specific gravity*.

relaxant (ri-laks-ănt) *n.* an agent that reduces tension and strain, particularly in muscles (*see* muscle relaxant).

relaxation (ree-laks-ay-shŏn) *n.* (in physiology) the diminution of tension in a muscle, which occurs when it ceases to contract. *r. therapy* treatment by teaching a patient to decrease his anxiety by reducing the tone in his muscles.

relaxin (ri-laks-in) *n.* a hormone, secreted by the placenta in the terminal stages of pregnancy, that causes the cervix of the womb to dilate and prepares the womb for the action of oxytocin during labour.

REM rapid eye movement: describing a stage of sleep during which the muscles of the eyeballs are in constant motion behind the eyelids. REM sleep usually coincides with dreaming.

remission (ri-mish-ŏn) *n.* a lessening in the severity of symptoms or their temporary disappearance during the course of an illness.

remittent fever (ri-mit-ĕnt) *n. see* fever.

renal (ree-năl) *adj.* relating to or affecting the kidneys. *r. artery* either of two large arteries arising from the abdominal aorta and supplying the kidneys. *r. cell carcinoma see* hypernephroma. *r. tubule* (*uriniferous tubule*) the fine tubular part of a nephron, through which water and certain dissolved substances are reabsorbed back into the blood.

reni- (**reno-**) *prefix denoting* the kidney.

renin (ree-nin) *n.* a substance released into the blood by the kidney in response to stress. It produces angiotensin, which causes constriction of blood vessels and thus an increase in blood pressure. Excessive production of renin results in renal hypertension.

rennin (ren-in) *n.* an enzyme produced in the stomach that coagulates milk. It converts caseinogen (milk protein) into insoluble casein in the presence of calcium ions. This ensures that the milk remains in the stomach, exposed to protein-digesting enzymes, for as long as possible.

renography (ri-nog-răfi) *n.* the radiological study of the kidneys by a gamma camera following the intravenous injection of a radioactive substance, which is concentrated and excreted by the kidneys. The resultant graph of each kidney gives information regarding function and rate of drainage.

reovirus (ree-oh-vy-rŭs) *n.* one of a group of small RNA-containing viruses that infect both respiratory and intestinal tracts without producing specific or serious diseases (and were therefore termed *r*espiratory *e*nteric *o*rphan viruses). *Compare* echovirus.

Male reproductive system

Female reproductive system

replication (rep-li-**kay**-shŏn) *n*. the process by which DNA makes copies of itself when the cell divides. The two strands of the DNA molecule unwind and each strand directs the synthesis of a new strand complementary to itself.

repolarization (ri-poh-ler-I-zay-shŏn) *n*. the process in which the membrane of a nerve cell returns to its normal electrically charged state after a nerve impulse has passed.

repositor (ri-**poz**-it-er) *n*. an instrument used to return a displaced part of the body to its normal position.

repression (ri-**presh**-ŏn) *n*. (in psychoanalysis) the process of excluding an unacceptable wish or an idea from conscious mental life. The repressed material continues to control behaviour and may give rise to symptoms.

reproductive system (ree-prŏ-**duk**-tiv) *n*. the combination of organs and tissues associated with the process of reproduction. In males it includes the testes, vasa deferentia, prostate gland, seminal vesicles, urethra, and penis; in females it includes the ovaries, Fallopian tubes, uterus, vagina, and vulva.

resection (ri-**sek**-shŏn) *n*. surgical removal of a portion of any part of the body. *submucous r*. removal of part of the cartilage septum of the nose that has become deviated, usually by injury. *transurethral r*. (*TUR, r. of the prostate*) an operation performed when the prostate gland becomes enlarged. It involves removal of the gland through the urethra using an instrument called a *resectoscope*.

resectoscope (ri-**sek**-tŏ-skohp) *n*. *see* (transurethral) resection.

reserpine (**res**-er-peen) *n*. a drug extracted from rauwolfia and administered by mouth or injection to lower high blood pressure and, occasionally, to relieve anxiety. Trade name: **Serpasil**.

residual urine (ri-**zid**-yoo-ăl) *n*. urine remaining in the bladder after micturition.

residual volume *n*. the volume of air that remains in the lungs after the individual has breathed out as much as he can. This volume is increased in emphysema.

resistance (ri-zist-ăns) n. 1. the degree of immunity that the body possesses. 2. the degree to which a disease or disease-causing organism remains unaffected by antibiotics or other drugs.

resolution (rez-ŏ-loo-shŏn) n. 1. the stage during which inflammation gradually disappears. 2. the degree to which individual details can be distinguished by the eye, as through a microscope.

resonance (rez-ŏn-ăns) n. the sound produced by percussion of a part of the body during a physical examination. *See also* vocal resonance.

resorcinol (ri-zor-sin-ol) n. a drug that causes the skin to peel. It is applied to the skin in ointments to treat such conditions as acne, and used in hair lotions for dandruff.

resorption (ri-sorp-shŏn) n. loss of substance through physiological or pathological means.

respiration (res-per-ay-shŏn) n. the process of gaseous exchange between an organism and its environment. *external r.* breathing: the stage of respiration in which oxygen is taken up by the capillaries of the lung alveoli and carbon dioxide is released from the blood. *internal r.* the stage of respiration in which oxygen is released to the tissues and carbon dioxide absorbed by the blood. *See also* lung. —**respiratory** (rĕs-pir-ă-ter-i) *adj.*

respirator (res-per-ayt-er) n. 1. a device used to maintain the breathing movements of paralysed patients. *cuirass r.* a respirator that works on a similar principle to the iron lung, but leaves the limbs free.

Drinker r. (*iron lung*) a type of respirator in which the patient is enclosed, except for the head, in an airtight container in which the air pressure is decreased and increased mechanically. This draws air into and out of the lungs, through the normal air passages. *positive-pressure r.* a respirator that blows air into the patient's lungs via a tube passed either through the mouth into the trachea or through a tracheostomy. 2. a face mask for administering oxygen or other gas or for filtering harmful fumes, dust, etc. *See also* artificial respiration.

respiratory distress syndrome (hyaline membrane disease) n. the condition of a newborn infant in which the lungs are imperfectly expanded. Breathing is rapid, laboured, and shallow. The condition is most common and serious among premature infants (especially between the 32nd and 37th weeks of gestation). It is treated by careful nursing, intravenous fluids, and oxygen, with or without positive pressure by a respirator.

respiratory quotient (RQ) n. the ratio of the volume of carbon dioxide transferred from the blood into the alveoli to the volume of oxygen absorbed into the alveoli. The RQ is usually about 0.8.

respiratory syncytial virus (RSV) n. a paramyxovirus (*see* myxovirus) that causes infections of the nose and throat. It is a major cause of bronchiolitis and pneumonia in young children.

respiratory system n. the combination of organs and tissues associated with breathing. It includes the nasal cavity, pharynx, larynx, trachea, bronchi, and lungs.

response (ri-**spons**) *n*. the way in which the body or part of the body reacts to a stimulus.

resuscitation (ri-sus-i-**tay**-shŏn) *n*. the process of reviving someone who appears to be dead; for example by cardiac massage or artificial respiration.

retardation (ree-tar-**day**-shŏn) *n*. the slowing up of a process. *mental r.* mental subnormality: the use of this term implies that the subnormality is a delay in development rather than a qualitative defect. *psychomotor r.* a marked slowing down of activity and speech. It is a symptom of severe depression.

retching (**rech**-ing) *n*. repeated unavailing attempts to vomit.

rete (**ree**-ti) *n*. a network of blood vessels, nerve fibres, or other strands of interlacing tissue in the structure of an organ.

retention (ri-**ten**-shŏn) *n*. inability to pass urine, which is retained in the bladder. The condition may be acute and painful or chronic and painless. The commonest cause is enlargement of the prostate gland in men.

retention cyst *n*. a cyst that arises when the outlet of a glandular duct is blocked.

retention defect *n*. (in psychology) a memory defect in which items that have been registered in the memory are lost from storage. It is a feature of dementia.

reticular (ri-**tik**-yoo-ler) *adj*. (of tissues) resembling a network; branching. *r. fibres* branching fibres of connective tissue that form a delicate supportive meshwork around blood vessels, muscle fibres, glands, nerves, etc. *r. formation* a network of nerve pathways and nuclei throughout the brainstem, connecting motor

and sensory nerves to and from the spinal cord, the cerebellum and the cerebrum, and the cranial nerves.

reticulin (ri-**tik**-yoo-lin) *n*. the collagen-like protein of reticular fibres.

reticulocyte (ri-**tik**-yoo-loh-syt) *n*. an immature red blood cell (erythrocyte). Reticulocytes normally comprise about 1% of the total red cells.

reticulocytosis (ri-tik-yoo-loh-sy-**toh**-sis) *n*. an increase in the proportion of reticulocytes in the bloodstream: a sign of increased output of new red cells from the bone marrow.

reticuloendothelial system (RES) (ri-tik-yoo-loh-en-doh-**theel**-iăl) *n*. a community of phagocytes that is spread throughout the body. The RES is concerned with defence against microbial infection and with the removal of worn-out blood cells from the bloodstream. *See also* spleen.

reticuloendotheliosis (histiocytosis X) (ri-tik-yoo-loh-en-doh-theel-i-**oh**-sis) *n*. overgrowth of cells of the reticuloendothelial system, causing either isolated swelling of the bone marrow (*eosinophilic granuloma*) or destruction of the bones of the skull (*Hand-Schüller-Christian disease*). The most acute form is associated with tumours containing histiocytes in the internal organs (*Letterer-Siwe disease*).

reticulosis (ri-tik-yoo-**loh**-sis) *n*. abnormal overgrowth, usually malignant, of any of the cells of the lymphatic glands or the immune system. *See* lymphoma, Hodgkin's disease, Burkitt's tumour.

reticulum (ri-**tik**-yoo-lŭm) *n*. a network of tubules or blood vessels. *See* endoplasmic reticulum.

retin- (retino-) *prefix denoting* the retina.

retina (ret-in-ă) *n.* the light-sensitive layer that lines the interior of the eye. The inner part of the retina, next to the cavity of the eyeball, contains rods and cones (light-sensitive cells) and their associated nerve fibres. The outer part is pigmented to prevent the passage of light. —**retinal** *adj.*

retinaculum (ret-in-ak-yoo-lŭm) *n.* (*pl.* **retinacula**) a thickened band of tissue that serves to hold various tissues in place.

retinal (retinene) (ret-in-al) *n.* the aldehyde of retinol (vitamin A). *See also* rhodopsin.

retinene (ret-in-een) *n. see* retinal.

retinitis (ret-i-ny-tis) *n.* inflammation of the retina. *r. pigmentosa* a noninflammatory hereditary condition involving progressive degeneration of the retina.

retinoblastoma (ret-in-oh-blas-toh-mă) *n.* a rare malignant tumour of the retina, occurring in infants.

retinol (ret-in-ol) *n. see* vitamin A.

retinopathy (ret-in-op-ă-thi) *n.* any disorder of the retina resulting in impairment or loss of vision. It may occur as a complication of diabetes (*diabetic r.*) or high blood pressure.

retinoscope (ret-in-oh-skohp) *n.* an instrument used to determine the power of refraction of the eye. —**retinoscopy** *n.*

retraction (ri-trak-shŏn) *n.* **1.** (in obstetrics) the permanent shortening of the muscle fibres of the womb wall that occurs each time they contract during labour. *r. ring* **a.** (or *Bandl's ring*) a depression on the surface of the womb that may be felt through the abdominal wall during labour. It

wound retractor

abdominal retractor

Retractors

indicates a constriction around the womb, which tends to prevent the infant from emerging into the cervical canal. **b.** the dividing line between the upper contracting part of the womb in labour and the lower dilating part. **2.** (in dentistry) the drawing back of one or more teeth into a better position by an orthodontic appliance.

retractor (ri-trak-ter) *n.* a surgical instrument used to expose the operation site by drawing aside the cut edges of skin, muscle, or other tissues.

retro- *prefix denoting* at the back or behind.

retrobulbar neuritis (optic neuritis) (ret-roh-bulb-er) *n.* inflammation of the optic nerve behind the eye, causing increasingly blurred vision. Retrobulbar neuritis is one of the symptoms of multiple sclerosis but it can also occur as an isolated lesion.

retroflexion (ret-roh-flek-shŏn) *n.* the bending backward of an organ or part of an organ, especially of the upper part of the womb (*uterine r.*).

retrograde (ret-roh-grayd) *adj.* going backwards, or moving in the opposite direction to the normal. *See also* (retrograde) amnesia, (retrograde) pyelography.

retrogression (ret-roh-**gresh**-ŏn) *n.* return to a less complex state or condition; regression.

retrolental fibroplasia (ret-roh-len-t'l) *n.* the abnormal proliferation of fibrous tissue immediately behind the lens of the eye, leading to blindness: formerly seen in premature infants due to overadministration of oxygen.

retro-ocular (ret-roh-**ok**-yoo-ler) *adj.* behind the eye.

retropharyngeal (ret-roh-fă-**rin**-ji-ăl) *adj.* behind the pharynx. *r. abscess* a collection of pus in the tissues behind the pharynx, resulting in difficulty in swallowing, pain, and fever.

retropubic (ret-roh-**pew**-bik) *adj.* behind the pubis. *r. prostatectomy see* prostatectomy.

retropulsion (ret-roh-**pul**-shŏn) *n.* a compulsive tendency to walk backwards. It is a symptom of parkinsonism.

retrospection (ret-roh-**spek**-shŏn) *n.* (in psychology) the systematic reviewing of past experiences.

retroversion (ret-roh-**ver**-shŏn) *n.* the backward inclination of an organ, especially of the womb (*uterine r.*), when it is tipped back so that the cervix points towards the pubic symphysis.

rhabdomyosarcoma (rab-doh-my-oh-sar-**koh**-mă) *n.* a malignant tumour originating in, or showing the characteristics of, striated muscle. *embryonal r.* a type of rhabdomyosarcoma that affects infants, children, and young adults. *pleomorphic r.* a type of rhabdomyosarcoma that occurs in late middle age, in the muscles of the limbs.

rhagades (**rag**-ă-deez) *pl. n.* cracks or long thin scars in the skin, particularly around the mouth. The fissures around the mouth and nose of babies with congenital syphilis eventually heal to form rhagades.

rheo- *prefix denoting* 1. a flow of liquid. 2. an electric current.

rhesus factor (Rh factor) (ree-sŭs) *n.* a group of antigens that may or may not be present on the surface of the red blood cells; it forms the basis of the rhesus blood group system. Most people have the rhesus factor, i.e. they are *Rh-positive*. People who lack the factor are termed *Rh-negative*. Incompatibility between Rh-positive and Rh-negative blood is an important cause of blood transfusion reactions and haemolytic disease of the newborn. *See also* blood group.

rheumatic fever (acute rheumatism) (roo-**mat**-ik) *n.* a disease affecting mainly children and young adults that arises as a delayed complication of infection of the upper respiratory tract with haemolytic streptococci. The main features are fever, arthritis, chorea, and inflammation of the membrane surrounding the heart. The infection is treated with antibiotics (e.g. penicillin) and bed rest. *chronic rheumatic heart disease* a complication of rheumatic fever, in which there is scarring and chronic inflammation of the heart and its valves leading to heart failure, murmurs, and damage to the valves.

rheumatism (**room**-ă-tizm) *n.* any disorder in which aches and pains affect the muscles and joints. *See* rheumatoid arthritis, rheumatic fever, osteoarthritis, gout.

rheumatoid arthritis (**room**-ă-toid) *n.* a form of arthritis that involves the joints of the fingers, wrists, feet, and ankles and often the hips and shoulders. The condition is diagnosed by a blood test and by X-rays revealing typical changes (*rheumatoid erosions*) around the affected joints. A wide variety of treatments, usually based on anti-inflammatory analgesics, provide relief of symptoms.

rheumatology (room-ă-**tol**-ŏji) *n.* the medical specialty concerned with the diagnosis and management of disease involving joints, tendons, muscles, ligaments, and associated structures. *See also* physical medicine. —**rheumatologist** *n.*

Rh factor *n. see* rhesus factor.

rhin- (rhino-) *prefix denoting* the nose.

rhinitis (ry-**ny**-tis) *n.* inflammation of the mucous membrane of the nose. *acute r. see* (common) cold. *allergic r. see* hay fever. *atrophic r.* rhinitis in which the mucous membrane becomes thinned and fragile. *chronic catarrhal r.* rhinitis in which there is overgrowth of, and increased secretion by, the membrane.

rhinology (ry-**nol**-ŏji) *n.* the branch of medicine concerned with disorders of the nose and nasal passages.

rhinomycosis (ry-noh-my-**koh**-sis) *n.* fungal infection of the lining of the nose.

rhinophyma (ry-noh-**fy**-mă) *n.* permanent redness and swelling of the nose. It commonly occurs with rosacea, in which the characteristic nodular swelling may produce grotesque deformity.

rhinoplasty (ry-noh-plasti) *n.* reparative or cosmetic surgery of the nose.

rhinorrhoea (ry-nŏ-ree-ă) *n.* a persistent watery mucous discharge from the nose, as in the common cold.

rhinoscopy (ry-**nosk**-ŏ-pi) *n.* examination of the interior of the nose.

rhinosporidiosis (ry-noh-sper-id-i-**oh**-sis) *n.* a fungal infection of the mucous membranes of the nose, larynx, eyes, and genitals that is characterized by the formation of polyps.

rhinovirus (ry-noh-vy-rŭs) *n.* any one of a group of RNA-containing viruses that cause respiratory infections in man resembling the common cold. They are included in the picornavirus group.

rhiz- (rhizo-) *prefix denoting* a root.

rhizotomy (ry-zot-ŏmi) *n.* a surgical procedure in which selected nerve roots are cut at the point where they emerge from the spinal cord. The posterior (sensory) nerve roots are cut for the relief of intractable pain; the anterior (motor) nerve roots are sometimes cut for the relief of severe muscle spasm.

rhodopsin (visual purple) (roh-**dop**-sin) *n.* a pigment in the retina of the eye consisting of retinal and a protein. The presence of rhodopsin is essential for vision in dim light. *See* rod.

rhombencephalon (rom-ben-sef-ă-lon) *n. see* hindbrain.

rhomboid (rom-boid) *n.* either of two muscles situated in the upper part of the back, between the backbone and shoulder blade. They help to move the shoulder blade backwards and upwards.

rhonchus (ronk-ŭs) *n.* (*pl.* **rhonchi**) an abnormal musical noise produced by air passing through narrowed bronchi. It is heard through a stethoscope, usually when the patient breathes out.

rhythm method (*rith*-ĕm) *n.* a contraceptive method in which sexual intercourse is restricted to the days at the beginning and end of the menstrual cycle when conception is least likely to occur (*safe period*). The method depends for its reliability on the woman having uniform regular periods and its failure rate is higher than with mechanical methods.

rib (rib) *n.* a curved strip of bone forming part of the skeleton of the thorax. There are 12 pairs of ribs. The head of each rib articulates with one of the 12 thoracic vertebrae of the backbone; the other end is attached to a costal cartilage. *false r.* any of the three pairs of ribs below the true ribs. Each is connected by its cartilage to the rib above it. *floating r.* any of the last two pairs of ribs, which end freely in the muscles of the body wall. *true r.* any of the first seven pairs of ribs, which are connected directly to the sternum by their costal cartilages. Anatomical name: **costa.**

riboflavin (vitamin B₂) (ry-boh-flay-vin) *n. see* vitamin B.

ribonuclease (ry-boh-new-kli-ayz) *n.* an enzyme, located in the lysosomes of cells, that splits RNA at specific places in the molecule.

ribonucleic acid (ry-boh-new-klee-ik) *n. see* RNA.

ribose (ry-bohz) *n.* a pentose sugar that is a component of RNA and several coenzymes. Ribose is also involved in intracellular metabolism.

ribosome (ry-bŏ-sohm) *n.* a particle, consisting of RNA and protein, that occurs in cells and is the site of protein synthesis in the cell (*see* translation). —**ribosomal** *adj.*

ricewater stools (rys-waw-ter) *pl. n. see* cholera.

ricin (ry-sin) *n.* a highly toxic albumin obtained from castor-oil seeds (*Ricinus communis*) that inhibits protein synthesis and becomes attached to the surface of cells, resulting in gastroenteritis, hepatic congestion and jaundice, and cardiovascular collapse.

rickets (rik-its) *n.* a disease of children in which the bones do not harden and are malformed due to a deficiency of vitamin D. *See also* osteomalacia. *renal r.* a type of rickets that is due to impaired kidney function: the bones are malformed as bone-forming minerals are excreted in the urine.

rickettsiae (ri-ket-si-ee) *pl. n.* (*sing.* **rickettsia**) a group of very small nonmotile spherical or rodlike parasitic organisms. They cause such illnesses as rickettsial pox, Rocky Mountain spotted fever, and typhus. Rickettsiae infect arthropods (ticks, mites, etc.), through whom they can be transmitted to mammals (including man). —**rickettsial** (ri-ket-si-ăl) *adj.*

rickettsial pox *n.* a disease of mice caused by the microorganism *Rickettsia akari* and transmitted to man by mites: it produces chills, fever, muscular pain, and a rash similar to that of chickenpox. *See also* typhus.

ridge (rij) *n.* **1.** (in anatomy) a crest or a long narrow protuberance, e.g. on a bone. **2.** (in dental anatomy) *see* alveolus.

rifampicin (rif-**am**-pi-sin) *n.* an antibiotic administered by mouth to treat various infections, particularly tuberculosis. Trade names: **Rifadin, Rimactane**.

rifamycin (rif-ă-**my**-sin) *n.* an antibiotic used to treat certain infections, particularly tuberculosis. It is administered by injection, inhalation, or in a solution applied to the infected area.

rigidity (ri-**jid**-iti) *n.* (in neurology) resistance to the passive movement of a limb that persists throughout its range. It is a symptom of parkinsonism. *Compare* spasticity.

rigor (**ry**-ger) *n.* an abrupt attack of shivering and a sensation of coldness, accompanied by a rapid rise in body temperature. This often marks the onset of a fever and may be followed by a feeling of heat, with copious sweating. *r. mortis* the stiffening of a body that occurs within some eight hours of death, due to chemical changes in muscle tissue. It starts to disappear after about 24 hours.

rima (**ry**-mă) *n.* (in anatomy) a cleft. *r. glottidis* the space between the vocal cords.

rimiterol (rim-i-**te**-rol) *n.* a drug, similar to isoprenaline, administered by inhalation as a bronchodilator to relieve asthma and chronic bronchitis. Trade name: **Pulmadil**.

ring (ring) *n.* (in anatomy) *see* annulus.

Ringer's solution (Ringer's mixture) (**ring**-erz) *n.* a clear colourless physiological solution of sodium chloride, potassium chloride, and calcium chloride prepared with recently boiled pure water. [S. Ringer (1835–1910), British physiologist]

ringworm (**ring**-werm) *n. see* tinea.

Rinne's test (**rin**-iz) *n.* a test to determine whether deafness is conductive or perceptive. A vibrating tuning fork is held first in the air, close to the ear, and then with its base placed on the mastoid process. If the sound conducted by air is heard for a longer time than the sound conducted by bone the test is positive and the deafness perceptive; a negative result indicates conductive deafness. [H. A. Rinne (1819–68), German otologist]

risus sardonicus (ry-sŭs sar-**don**-ik-ŭs) *n.* an abnormal grinning expression resulting from involuntary prolonged contraction of facial muscles, as seen in tetanus.

river blindness *n. see* onchocerciasis.

RNA (ribonucleic acid) *n.* a nucleic acid, occurring in the nucleus and cytoplasm of cells, that is concerned with synthesis of proteins (*see* messenger RNA, ribosome, transfer RNA, translation). In some viruses RNA is the genetic material.

Rocky Mountain spotted fever (spotted fever, tick fever) *n.* a disease of rodents and other small mammals in the USA caused by the microorganism *Rickettsia rickettsii* and transmitted to man by ticks. Symptoms include fever, muscle pains, and a profuse reddish rash like that of measles. Treatment with tetracycline or chloramphenicol is effective. *See also* typhus.

rod (rod) *n.* one of the two types of light-sensitive cells in the retina of the eye (*compare* cone). Rods are necessary for seeing in dim light. They contain the pigment rhodopsin, which is bleached in the light and regenerated in the dark. When all the pigment is bleached (i.e. in bright light) the rods no longer function. *See also* dark adaptation, light adaptation.

rodent ulcer (roh-děnt) *n.* a slow-growing malignant tumour of the face, usually at the edge of the eyelids, lips, or nostrils. Rodent ulcers can be treated by surgery or radiotherapy; if untreated, they destroy skin muscle and bone but they do not spread to other parts of the body. Medical name: **basal cell carcinoma**.

roentgen (ront-gěn) *n.* a unit of exposure dose of X- or gamma-radiation.

roentgenology (ront-gě-nol-ŏji) *n.* the study of the applications of X-rays (roentgen rays) in medicine.

role playing (rohl-play-ing) *n.* acting out another person's expected behaviour, usually in a contrived situation, in order to understand him better. It is used in family psychotherapy, in teaching social skills to patients, and also in the training of psychiatric (and other) staff.

Romanowsky stains (roh-mă-nof-ski) *pl. n.* a group of stains used for microscopical examination of blood cells, consisting of variable mixtures of thiazine dyes with eosin. [D. L. Romanowsky (1861–1921), Russian physician]

Romberg's sign (rom-bergz) *n.* evidence of a sensory disorder affecting those nerves that transmit information to the brain about the position of the limbs and joints and the tension in the muscles. The patient is unable to maintain an upright posture when his eyes are closed. [M.

Romberg (1795–1873), German neurologist]

rongeur (rawn-*zh*er) *n.* powerful biting forceps for cutting tissue, particularly bone.

root (root) *n.* **1.** (in neurology) a bundle of nerve fibres at its emergence from the spinal cord. **2.** (in dentistry) the part of a tooth that is buried in a socket in the jawbone. **3.** the origin of any structure, i.e. the point at which it diverges from another structure. Anatomical name: **radix**.

Rorschach test (ror-shahk) *n.* a test to measure aspects of personality, consisting of ten inkblots in colour and black and white. The responses to the different inkblots are used to derive hypotheses about the subject. [H. Rorschach (1884–1922), Swiss psychiatrist]

rosacea (roh-zay-shiă) *n.* a skin disease of the face in which the blood vessels enlarge, giving the cheeks and nose a flushed appearance. Rosacea usually occurs after the age of 30 and affects women more often than men, with the menopause sometimes acting as a trigger.

roseola (roh-zee-ŏ-lă) *n.* any rose-coloured rash, such as occurs in measles, the secondary stage of syphilis, or typhoid fever.

rostrum (ros-trŭm) *n.* (*pl.* **rostra**) (in anatomy) a beaklike projection, such as that on the sphenoid bone. —**rostral** *adj.*

rotator (roh-tay-ter) *n.* a muscle that brings about rotation of a part.

Rothera's test (ro*th*-er-ăz) *n.* a method of testing urine for the presence of acetone or acetoacetic acid: a sign of diabetes mellitus. [A. C. H. Rothera

(1880 – 1915), Australian bio-chemist]

Roth spot (roht) *n.* a pale area surrounded by haemorrhage sometimes seen in the retina of those who have bacterial endo-carditis, septicaemia, or leukae-mia. [M. Roth (1839 – 1915), Swiss physician]

roughage (**ruf**-ij) *n. see* dietary fibre.

rouleau (**roo**-loh) *n.* (*pl.* **rouleaux**) a cylindrical structure in the blood formed from several red blood cells piled one upon the other and adhering by their rims.

round ligaments (rownd) *pl. n.* the fibromuscular bands that pass from the uterus along the broad ligaments to terminate in the labia majora.

round window *n. see* fenestra (rotunda).

roundworm (**rownd**-werm) *n. see* nematode.

Rovsing's sign (**rov**-singz) *n.* pain in the right iliac fossa induced by pressure on the left iliac fossa: a sign of acute appendicitis. [N. T. Rovsing 1868 – 1927), Danish surgeon]

-rrhagia (**-rrhage**) *suffix denoting* excessive or abnormal flow or discharge from an organ or part.

-rrhaphy *suffix denoting* surgical sewing; suturing.

-rrhexis *suffix denoting* splitting or rupture of a part.

-rrhoea *suffix denoting* a flow or discharge from an organ or part.

RSV *n. see* respiratory syncytial virus.

rubefacient (roo-bi-**fay**-shĕnt) *n.* an agent that causes reddening and warming of the skin. Rubefacients are often used as counterirritants for the relief of muscular pain.

rubella (roo-**bel**-ă) *n. see* German measles.

rubeola (roo-**bee**-ŏ-lă) *n. see* measles.

rubor (**roo**-ber) *n.* redness: one of the four classical signs of inflam-mation in a tissue. *See also* calor, dolor, tumor.

ruga (**roo**-gă) *n.* (*pl.* **rugae**) a fold or crease, especially one of the folds of mucous membrane that line the stomach.

rumination (roo-mi-**nay**-shŏn) *n.* (in psychiatry) an obsessional type of thinking in which the same thoughts or themes are ex-perienced repetitively. The thoughts are irrational and re-sisted by the patient.

rupia (**roo**-piă) *n.* dark raised crusts on the skin, as occurs in secondary syphilis.

rupture (**rup**-cher) **1.** *n. see* hernia. **2.** *n.* the bursting apart or open of an organ or tissue; for exam-ple, the splitting of the mem-branes enclosing an infant during childbirth. **3.** *vb.* (of tissues, etc.) to burst apart or open.

Russell traction (**rus**-ĕl) *n.* a form of traction used to align a frac-tured femur. The lower leg is supported in a sling just below the knee and pulling forces are exerted upwards and longitudi-nally by means of pulleys and weights. [R. H. Russell (1860 – 1933), Australian surgeon]

Ryle's tube (rylz) *n.* a thin flexible tube of rubber or plastic, in-serted through the mouth or nose of a patient and used for withdrawing fluid from the stom-ach or giving a test meal. [J. A. Ryle (1889 – 1950), British physi-cian]

S

Sabin vaccine (say-bin) *n.* an oral vaccine against poliomyelitis. [A. B. Sabin 1906–), US bacteriologist]

sac (sak) *n.* a pouch or baglike structure. Sacs can enclose natural cavities in the body, e.g. in the lungs (*see* alveolus), or they can be pathological, as in a hernia.

sacchar- (saccharo-) *prefix denoting* sugar.

saccharide (sak-eryd) *n.* a carbohydrate. *See also* disaccharide, monosaccharide, polysaccharide.

saccharine (sak-er-een) *n.* a sweetening agent. Saccharine is 400 times as sweet as sugar and has no energy content. It is very useful as a sweetener in diabetic and low-calorie foods.

Saccharomyces (sak-er-oh-my-seez) *n. see* yeast.

sacculated (sak-yoo-layt-id) *adj.* pursed out with small pouches or sacs.

saccule (sacculus) (sak-yool) *n.* the smaller of the two membranous sacs within the vestibule of the ear. It contains a macula, which responds to gravity and relays information to the brain about the position of the head.

sacralization (say-kră-ly-zay-shŏn) *n.* abnormal fusion of the fifth lumbar vertebra with the sacrum.

sacral nerves (say-krăl) *pl. n.* the five pairs of spinal nerves that emerge from the spinal column in the sacrum. The nerves carry sensory and motor fibres from the upper and lower leg and from the anal and genital regions.

sacral vertebrae *pl. n. see* sacrum.

sacro- *prefix denoting* the sacrum.

sacrococcygeal (say-kroh-kok-sij-iăl) *adj.* relating to or between the sacrum and the coccyx.

sacroiliac (say-kroh-il-i-ak) *adj.* relating to the sacrum and the ilium.

sacroiliitis (say-kroh-il-i-I-tis) *n.* inflammation of the sacroiliac joint. Involvement of both joints is a common feature of ankylosing spondylitis and associated rheumatic diseases. The resultant low back pain and stiffness may be alleviated by rest and analgesics.

sacrum (say-krŭm) *n.* (*pl.* **sacra**) a curved triangular element of the backbone consisting of five fused vertebrae (*sacral vertebrae*). It articulates with the last lumbar vertebra above, the coccyx below, and the hip bones laterally. *See also* vertebra. —**sacral** *adj.*

saddle-nose (sa-d'l-nohz) *n.* flattening of the bridge of the nose, such as may occur in congenital syphilis.

sadism (say-dizm) *n.* sexual excitement in response to inflicting pain upon other people. *See also* masochism, perversion. —**sadist** *n.* —**sadistic** (să-**dis**-tik) *adj.*

safe period (sayf) *n. see* rhythm method.

sagittal (saj-it'l) *adj.* describing the dorsoventral plane that extends down the long axis of the body, dividing it into right and left halves. **s. suture** the immovable joint between the two parietal bones of the skull.

salbutamol (sal-bew-tă-mol) *n.* a drug, similar to isoprenaline, administered by mouth, injection, or inhalation as a bronchodilator to relieve asthma, chronic bronchitis, and emphysema. Trade name: **Ventolin**.

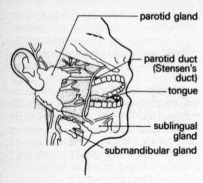

parotid gland

parotid duct (Stensen's duct)

tongue

sublingual gland

submandibular gland

Salivary glands

salicylamide (sal-i-**sil**-ă-myd) *n.* an analgesic drug with effects and uses similar to those of aspirin. It is administered by mouth. Trade name: **Salimed**.

salicylate (să-**lis**-i-layt) *n.* a salt of salicylic acid. *See* methyl salicylate, sodium salicylate.

salicylic acid (sal-i-**sil**-ik) *n.* a drug that causes the skin to peel and destroys bacteria and fungi. It is applied to the skin to treat ulcers, dandruff, eczema, psoriasis, warts, and corns.

salicylism (sal-i-**sil**-izm) *n.* poisoning due to an overdose of aspirin or other salicylate-containing compounds. The main symptoms are headache, dizziness, tinnitus, disturbances of vision, and vomiting.

saline (**say**-lyn) *n.* a solution containing 0.9% sodium chloride. Saline may be used clinically as a diluent for drugs administered by injection and as a plasma substitute.

saliva (să-**ly**-vă) *n.* the alkaline liquid secreted by the salivary glands and the mucous membrane of the mouth. Its principal constituents are water and mucus, which keep the mouth moist

and lubricate food, and enzymes that begin the digestion of starch. —**salivary** (să-**ly**-ver-i) *adj.*

salivary gland *n.* a gland that produces saliva. There are three pairs of salivary glands: the parotid glands, sublingual glands, and submandibular glands (see illustration).

salivation (sal-i-**vay**-shŏn) *n.* the secretion of saliva by the salivary glands of the mouth, increased in response to the chewing action of the jaws or to the thought, taste, smell, or sight of food. *See also* ptyalism.

Salk vaccine (sawlk) *n.* a vaccine against poliomyelitis. It is administered by injection. [J. E. Salk (1914–), US bacteriologist]

Salmonella (sal-mŏ-**nel**-ă) *n.* a genus of Gram-negative motile rodlike bacteria that inhabit the intestines of animals and man. Certain species cause such diseases as food poisoning, gastroenteritis, and septicaemia. *S. paratyphi* a species that causes paratyphoid fever. *S. typhi* a species that causes typhoid fever.

salmonellosis (sal-mŏ-nel-**oh**-sis) *n.* an infestation of the digestive system by bacteria of the genus *Salmonella. See also* food poisoning.

salping- (salpingo-) *prefix denoting* **1.** the Fallopian tube. **2.** the auditory tube (meatus).

salpingectomy (sal-pin-**jek**-tŏmi) *n.* the surgical removal or cutting of a Fallopian tube. The operation involving both tubes is a permanent and completely effective method of sterilization.

salpingitis (sal-pin-**jy**-tis) *n.* inflammation of a tube, most commonly of one or both of the Fallopian tubes caused by bacterial infection spreading from the vagina or womb or carried in the blood. *acute s.* salpingitis in which there is sharp pain in the lower abdomen. The infection may spread to the peritoneum (*see* peritonitis); in severe cases the tubes may become blocked with scar tissue.

salpingography (sal-ping-og-răfi) *n.* radiography of one or both Fallopian tubes after a radio-opaque substance has been introduced into them via an injection into the womb.

salpingo-oophorectomy (sal-pɪ.ɪg-oh-oh-ŏ-fŏ-**rek**-tŏmi) *n.* surgical removal of a Fallopian tube and the ovary associated with it.

salpingo-oophoritis (salpingo-oothecitis) (sal-ping-oh-oh-ŏ-fŏ-ry-tis) *n.* inflammation of a Fallopian tube and an ovary.

salpingo-oophorocele (salpingo-oothecocele) (sal-ping-oh-oh-**off**-ŏ-roh-seel) *n.* hernia involving a Fallopian tube and an ovary.

salpingostomy (sal-ping-ost-ŏmi) *n.* the surgical creation of an artificial opening in a blocked Fallopian tube in order to restore its patency.

salpinx (**sal**-pinks) *n.* (in anatomy) a tube, especially a Fallopian tube or the external auditory meatus.

salt (sawlt) *n.* (in chemistry) a compound formed when the hydrogen in an acid is replaced by a metal. An acid and a base react together to form a salt and water. *common s. see* sodium chloride. *s. depletion* excessive loss of sodium chloride from the body. This may result from sweating, persistent vomiting or diarrhoea, or loss of fluid in wounds. The main symptoms are muscular weakness and cramps.

sanatorium (san-ă-**tor**-iŭm) *n.* **1.** a hospital or institution for the rehabilitation and convalescence of patients of any kind. **2.** an institution for patients who have suffered from pulmonary tuberculosis.

sandfly fever (sand-fly) *n.* a viral influenza-like disease transmitted to man by the bite of the sandfly *Phlebotomus papatasii*. Sandfly fever occurs principally in countries surrounding the Persian Gulf and the tropical Mediterranean.

sangui- (sanguino-) *prefix denoting* blood.

sanguineous (sang-**win**-iŭs) *adj.* **1.** containing, stained, or covered with blood. **2.** (of tissues) containing more than the normal quantity of blood.

sanies (**say**-ni-eez) *n.* a foul-smelling watery discharge from a wound or ulcer, containing serum, blood, and pus.

saphena (să-**fee**-nă) *n. see* saphenous vein.

saphenous nerve (să-**fee**-nŭs) *n.* a large branch of the femoral nerve that supplies the skin from the knee to below the ankle with sensory nerves.

saphenous vein (saphena) *n.* either of two superficial veins of the leg, draining blood from the foot. *long s. v.* the longest vein in the body, running from the foot to the groin. *short s. v.* the vein that runs up the back of the calf.

sapiential authority (say-pi-**en**-shăl) *n.* authority vested in an individual by virtue of his (or her) special knowledge or expertise in a particular area or subject.

saponify (să-**pon**-i-fy) *vb.* (in chemistry) to hydrolyse an ester with a hydroxide, especially a fat with

a hydroxide to form a soap.
—**saponification** n.

sapr- (sapro-) prefix denoting **1.**
putrefaction. **2.** decaying matter.

sapraemia (sap-ree-miǎ) n. blood
poisoning by toxins of sapro-
phytic bacteria. Compare
pyaemia, septicaemia, toxaemia.

saprophyte (sap-roh-fyt) n. any
free-living organism that lives
and feeds on the dead and pu-
trefying tissues of animals or
plants. Compare parasite. —**sapro-
phytic** (sap-roh-**fit**-ik) adj.

sarc- (sarco-) prefix denoting **1.**
flesh or fleshy tissue. **2.** muscle.

sarcoid (**sar**-koid) **1.** adj. fleshy. **2.**
n. a fleshy tumour.

sarcoidosis (sar-koid-**oh**-sis) n. a
chronic disorder of unknown
cause in which the lymph nodes
in many parts of the body are
enlarged and granulomas develop
in the lungs, liver, and spleen.
The skin, nervous system, eyes,
and salivary glands are also
commonly affected, and the condition has features similar to tuberculosis.

sarcolemma (sar-koh-**lem**-ǎ) n. the
cell membrane that encloses a
muscle cell (muscle fibre).

sarcoma (sar-**koh**-mǎ) n. any cancer of connective tissue. These
tumours may occur in any part
of the body; they arise in fibrous tissue, muscle, fat, bone,
cartilage, synovium, blood and
lymphatic vessels, and various
other tissues. See also chondrosarcoma, fibrosarcoma, leiomyosarcoma, liposarcoma,
lymphangiosarcoma, osteo-
sarcoma, rhabdomyosarcoma.
—**sarcomatous** adj.

sarcomatosis (sar-koh-mǎ-**toh**-sis)
n. sarcoma that has spread
widely throughout the body,

most commonly through the
bloodstream.

sarcoplasm (myoplasm) (**sar**-koh-
plazm) n. the cytoplasm of muscle cells.

Sarcoptes (sar-**kop**-teez) n. a genus
of small oval mites. S. scabiei
the human itch mite. The female
tunnels into the skin, where it
lays its eggs. The presence of the
mites causes severe irritation,
which eventually leads to scabies.

sartorius (sar-**tor**-iǔs) n. a narrow
ribbon-like muscle at the front
of the thigh. The longest muscle
in the body, the sartorius flexes
the leg on the thigh and the
thigh on the abdomen.

saucerization (saw-ser-I-**zay**-shŏn)
n. **1.** an operation in which tissue is cut away from a wound to
form a saucer-like depression. It
is carried out to facilitate healing
of injuries or disorders in which
bone is infected. **2.** the concave
appearance of the upper surface
of a vertebra that has been fractured by compression.

Sayre's jacket (**say**-erz) n. a plaster of Paris cast used to support
the backbone when the vertebrae
have been severely damaged by
disease, such as tuberculosis. [L.
A. Sayre (1820–1900), US sur-
geon]

scab (skab) n. a hard crust of
dried blood, serum, or pus that
develops over a sore, cut, or
scratch.

scabicide (**skay**-bi-syd) n. a drug
that kills the mites causing scabies.

scabies (**skay**-beez) n. a skin infection caused by the itch mite,
Sarcoptes scabiei. Scabies is typified by severe itching, red papules, and often secondary infection. The mites pass easily from
person to person by contact.

Commonly infected areas are the groin, penis, nipples, and the skin between the fingers. Local treatment is with hexa-chlorophane or benzyl benzoate creams.

scala (skay-lă) *n.* one of the spiral canals of the cochlea.

scald (skawld) *n.* a burn produced by a hot liquid or vapour, such as boiling water or steam.

scale (skayl) 1. *n.* any of the flakes of dead epidermal cells shed from the skin. 2. *vb.* to scrape deposits of calculus from the teeth (*see* scaler).

scalenus (skay-leen-ŭs) *n.* one of four paired muscles of the neck (*s. anterior, medius, minimus,* and *posterior*). They are responsible for raising the first and second ribs in inspiration and for bending the neck forward and to either side.

scalenus syndrome (thoracic outlet syndrome) *n.* the group of symptoms caused by the scalenus anterior muscle compressing the lower roots of the brachial plexus against the outlet of the upper thoracic vertebrae. Loss of sensation and wasting may be found in the affected arm.

scaler (skayl-er) *n.* an instrument for removing calculus from the teeth, either by hand scraping or by employing rapid ultrasonic vibrations.

scalp (skalp) *n.* the skin that covers the cranium and is itself covered with hair.

scalpel (skal-pĕl) *n.* a small pointed surgical knife with a straight handle and detachable disposable blades of various shapes.

scanning speech (skan-ing) *n.* a disorder of articulation in which the syllables are inappropriately separated and equally stressed. It is caused by cerebellar disease.

scaphocephaly (skaf-oh-**sef**-ăli) *n.* an abnormally long and narrow skull due to premature closure of the sagittal suture. It is usually associated with mental retardation. −**scaphocephalic** (skaf-oh-si-**fal**-ik) *adj.*

scaphoid bone (skay-foid) *n.* a boat-shaped bone of the wrist (*see* carpus). It articulates with the trapezium and trapezoid bones in front and with the radius behind.

scapul- (scapulo-) *prefix denoting* the scapula.

scapula (**skap**-yoo-lă) *n.* (*pl.* **scapulas** *or* **scapulae**) the shoulder blade: a triangular bone, a pair of which form the back part of the shoulder girdle. −**scapular** *adj.*

scar (skar) *n. see* cicatrix.

scarification (ska-rifi-**kay**-shŏn) *n.* the process of making a series of shallow cuts or scratches in the skin to allow a substance, such as a droplet of smallpox vaccine, to penetrate the body.

scarlatina (skar-lă-**tee**-nă) *n. see* scarlet fever.

scarlet fever (**skar**-lit) *n.* a highly contagious disease, mainly of childhood, caused by bacteria of the genus *Streptococcus.* Symptoms include fever, sickness, sore throat, and a widespread scarlet rash that spreads from the armpits and groin to the neck, chest, back, limbs, and tongue. Treatment with antibiotics prevents such complications as ear and kidney infections and swollen neck glands. Medical name: **scarlatina**. *Compare* German measles.

Scarpa's triangle (skar-păz) *n. see* femoral (triangle). [A. Scarpa (1747–1832), Italian anatomist and surgeon]

scat- (scato-) *prefix denoting* faeces.

Scheuermann's disease (shoi-ermanz) *n.* a form of osteochondritis affecting the vertebrae. It develops in adolescents and results in outward curvature of the spine. [H. W. Scheuermann (1877–1960), Danish surgeon]

Schick test (shik) *n.* a test to determine whether a person is susceptible to diphtheria. A small quantity of diphtheria toxin is injected under the skin; a patch of reddening and swelling shows that the person has no immunity. [B. Schick (1877–1967), US paediatrician]

Schilling test (shil-ing) *n.* a test used to assess a patient's capacity to absorb vitamin B_{12} from the bowel. Radioactive vitamin B_{12} is given by mouth and urine collected. A patient with pernicious anaemia will excrete less than 5% of the original dose over a period of 24 hours.

schindylesis (skin-di-lee-sis) *n.* a form of synarthrosis (immovable joint) in which a crest of one bone fits into a groove of another.

-schisis *suffix denoting* a cleft or split.

schisto- *prefix denoting* a fissure; split.

Schistosoma (Bilharzia) (shist-ŏ-soh-mă) *n.* a genus of blood flukes, three species of which are important parasites of man causing the tropical disease schistosomiasis.

schistosomiasis (bilharziasis) (shist-ŏ-soh-my-ă-sis) *n.* a tropical disease caused by blood flukes of the genus *Schistosoma*. The disease is contracted when larvae penetrate the skin of anyone bathing in infected water. Adult flukes eventually settle in the blood vessels of the intestine (*S. mansoni* and *S. japonicum*) or bladder (*S. haematobium*); the release of their spiked eggs causes anaemia, inflammation, and the formation of scar tissue. Additional symptoms include diarrhoea, dysentery, cirrhosis of the liver, haematuria, and cystitis. The disease is treated with various drugs, including stibophen and niridazole.

schiz- (schizo-) *prefix denoting* a split or division.

schizoid personality (skits-oid) *n.* a personality characterized by solitariness, emotional coldness to others, excessive introspection, and eccentricity of behaviour. *See* personality disorder.

schizophrenia (skits-ŏ-freen-iă) *n.* a severe mental disorder (or group of disorders) characterized by a disintegration of the process of thinking, of contact with reality, and of emotional responsiveness. The patient suffers from hallucinations and delusions and feels that his thoughts, sensations, and actions are controlled by, or shared with, others. Treatment is with drugs such as phenothiazines and by vigorous psychological and social management and rehabilitation. *catatonic s.* schizophrenia in which there are marked motor disturbances (*see* catatonia). *hebephrenic s. see* hebephrenia. *paranoid s.* schizophrenia characterized by prominent delusions. *simple s.* schizophrenia in which increasing social withdrawal and personal ineffectiveness are the major changes.

–**schizophrenic** (skits-ŏ-**fren**-ik) *adj.*

Schlatter's disease (**shlat**-erz) *n.* a form of osteochondritis affecting the tuberosity at the top of the tibia. It is most common in adolescent boys. [C. Schlatter (1864–1934), Swiss surgeon]

Schlemm's canal (shlemz) *n.* a channel in the eye, at the junction of the cornea and the sclera, through which the aqueous humour drains. [F. Schlemm (1795–1858), German anatomist]

Schönlein-Henoch purpura (**shern**-lyn **hen**-ohk) *n.* a blood disease that affects young children; its cause is not known. It is characterized by a purple skin rash due to bleeding into the skin from defective capillaries; abdominal pain; and kidney disturbance. *See also* purpura. [J. L. Schönlein (1793–1864), German physician; E. H. Henoch (1820–1910), German paediatrician]

school health service (skool) *n.* (in Britain) a service concerned with the early detection of physical, mental, and emotional abnormalities in schoolchildren and their subsequent treatment and surveillance.

school nurse *n.* a member of the school health service who conducts routine examinations and/ or treats minor ailments. Health visitors may sometimes work in this capacity but state registered and state enrolled nurses may also perform these tasks.

Schwann cells (shwon) *pl. n.* the cells that lay down the myelin sheath around the axon of a medullated nerve fibre. [T. Schwann (1810–82), German anatomist and physiologist]

Schwannoma (shwon-**oh**-mă) *n. see* neurofibroma.

Schwartze's operation (**shvarts**-ĕz) *n.* an operation to open and drain the air cells in the mastoid in severe cases of mastoiditis. [H. H. R. Schwartze (1837–1910), German otologist]

sciatica (sy-**at**-ik-ă) *n.* pain felt down the back and outer side of the thigh, leg, and foot. It is usually caused by degeneration of an intervertebral disc, which protrudes laterally to compress a spinal nerve root. The onset may be sudden, brought on by an awkward lifting or twisting movement.

sciatic nerve (sy-**at**-ik) *n.* the major nerve of the leg and the nerve with the largest diameter. It runs down behind the thigh from the lower end of the spine.

scintigram (**sin**-ti-gram) *n.* a diagram showing the distribution of radioactive tracer in a part of the body, produced by recording the flashes of light given off by a scintillator as it is struck by radiation of different intensities. By scanning the body, section by section, a 'map' of the radioactivity in various regions is built up, aiding the diagnosis of cancer or other disorders. Such a record is known as a *scintiscan*.

scintillascope (sin-**til**-ă-skohp) *n.* the instrument used to produce a scintigram. It incorporates a scintillator, a device to magnify the fluorescence produced, and a means of recording the results, often aided by a computer. *See also* gamma camera.

scintillator (sin-ti-**lay**-ter) *n.* a substance that produces a fluorescent flash when struck by high-energy radiation, such as beta or gamma rays. *See also* scintigram.

scintiscan (sin-ti-skan) *n. see* scintigram.

scirrhous (si-rŭs) *adj.* describing carcinomas that are stony hard to the touch. Such a carcinoma is known as a *scirrhus*.

scissor leg (siz-er) *n.* a disability in which one leg becomes permanently crossed over the other as a result of spasticity of its adductor muscles. The condition occurs in children with brain damage and in adults after strokes.

scissura (scissure) (si-zhor-ă) *n.* a cleft or splitting, such as the splitting open of tissues when a hernia forms.

scler- (sclero-) *prefix denoting* 1. hardening or thickening. 2. the sclera. 3. sclerosis.

sclera (sclerotic coat) (skleer-ă) *n.* the white fibrous outer layer of the eyeball. At the front of the eye it becomes the cornea. *See* eye. —**scleral** *adj.*

scleritis (skleer-I-tis) *n.* inflammation of the sclera.

scleroderma (skleer-oh-der-mă) *n.* persistent hardening and contraction of the body's connective tissue. The skin is thickened and tough, often with pigmented patches. Scleroderma may be localized (*see* morphoea) or it can spread slowly throughout the body, eventually causing death.

scleroma (skleer-oh-mă) *n.* a hardened patch of skin or mucous membrane, consisting of granulation tissue.

scleromalacia (skleer-oh-mă-lay-shiă) *n.* thinning of the sclera (white of the eye) as a result of inflammation.

sclerosis (skleer-oh-sis) *n.* hardening of tissue, usually due to scarring (fibrosis) after inflammation. It can affect the lateral columns of the spinal cord and the medulla of the brain (*amyotrophic lateral s.*), causing progressive muscular paralysis (*see* motor neurone disease). *See also* arteriosclerosis, atherosclerosis, multiple sclerosis, tuberous sclerosis.

sclerotherapy (skleer-oh-th'e-ră-pi) *n.* treatment of varicose veins by the injection of an irritant solution. This causes thrombophlebitis, which encourages obliteration of the varicose vein by thrombosis and subsequent scarring.

sclerotic (skleer-ot-ik) 1. (*or* sclerotic coat) *n. see* sclera. 2. *adj.* affected with sclerosis.

sclerotome (skleer-ŏ-tohm) *n.* a surgical knife used in the operation of sclerotomy.

sclerotomy (skleer-ot-ŏmi) *n.* an operation in which an incision is made in the sclera.

scolex (skoh-leks) *n.* (*pl.* **scolices**) the head of a tapeworm. Suckers and/or hooks on the scolex enable the worm to attach itself to the wall of its host's gut.

scoliosis (skoh-li-oh-sis) *n.* lateral (sideways) deviation of the backbone, caused by congenital or acquired abnormalities of the vertebrae, muscles, and nerves. *See also* kyphosis, kyphoscoliosis.

-scope *suffix denoting* an instrument for observing or examining.

scopolamine (skŏ-pol-ă-meen) *n. see* hyoscine.

scorbutic (skor-bew-tik) *adj.* affected with scurvy.

scoto- *prefix denoting* darkness.

scotoma (skoh-toh-mă) *n.* (*pl.* **scotomata**) a small area of abnormally decreased or absent vision in the visual field, surrounded by normal sight.

scotometer (skoh-tom-it-er) *n.* an instrument used for mapping defects in the visual field. *See also* perimeter.

scotopic (skoh-**top**-ik) *adj.* relating to or describing conditions of poor illumination. *s. vision* vision in dim light in which the rods of the retina are involved (*see* dark adaptation).

screening test (**skreen**-ing) *n.* a simple test carried out on a large number of apparently healthy people to separate those who probably have a specified disease from those who do not. Examples are mass X-rays and cervical smears.

scrofula (**skrof**-yoo-lă) *n.* tuberculosis of lymph nodes, usually those in the neck, causing the formation of abscesses. Treatment with antituberculous drugs is effective. The disease, which is now rare, most commonly affects young children. —**scrofulous** *adj.*

scrofuloderma (skrof-yoo-loh-**der**-mă) *n.* tuberculosis of the skin in which the skin breaks down over suppurating tuberculous glands, with the formation of irregular-shaped ulcers with blue-tinged edges. Treatment is with antituberculous drugs.

scrotum (**skroh**-tŭm) *n.* the paired sac that holds the testes and epididymides outside the abdominal cavity. Its function is to allow the production and storage of spermatozoa to occur at a lower temperature than that of the abdomen. —**scrotal** *adj.*

scrub typhus (tsutsugamushi disease) (skrub) *n.* a disease, widely distributed in SE Asia, caused by the parasitic microorganism *Rickettsia tsutsugamushi* and transmitted to man through the bite of mites. Symptoms include headache, chills, high temperature, a red rash, a cough,

and delirium. A small ulcer forms at the site of the bite. Scrub typhus is treated with tetracycline antibiotics. *See also* rickettsiae, typhus.

scurf (skerf) *n. see* dandruff.

scurvy (**sker**-vi) *n.* a disease that is caused by a deficiency of vitamin C and results from the consumption of a diet devoid of fresh fruit and vegetables. The first sign of scurvy is swollen bleeding gums; this may be followed by subcutaneous bleeding. Treatment with vitamin C soon reverses the effects.

scybalum (**sib**-ă-lŭm) *n.* a lump or mass of hard faeces.

seasickness (**see**-sik-nis) *n. see* travel sickness.

sebaceous cyst (steatoma, wen) (si-**bay**-shŭs) *n.* a cyst arising in a sebaceous gland. It may be filled with yellowish cheesy sebum, which sometimes becomes infected. Sebaceous cysts are found most commonly on the scalp, scrotum, and vulva.

sebaceous gland *n.* any of the simple or branched glands in the skin that secrete an oily substance, sebum. They open into hair follicles and their secretion is produced by the disintegration of their cells.

seborrhoea (seb-ŏ-**ree**-ă) *n.* excessive secretion of sebum by the sebaceous glands. The glands are enlarged, especially beside the nose and in other parts of the face. The condition predisposes to acne and is common at puberty. Seborrhoea is sometimes associated with a kind of eczema (seborrhoeic dermatitis). —**seborrhoeic** *adj.*

sebum (**see**-bŭm) *n.* the oily substance secreted by the sebaceous glands. Sebum provides a thin film of fat over the skin, which slows the evaporation of water; it also has an antibacterial effect.

secondary medical care (sek-ŏnd-er-i) *n. see* general practitioner.

secondary prevention *n.* the avoidance or alleviation of the serious consequences of disease by early detection.

secondary sexual characteristics *pl. n.* the physical characteristics that develop after puberty. In boys they include the growth of facial and pubic hair and the breaking of the voice. In girls they include the growth of pubic hair and the development of the breasts.

secretagogue (si-**kree**-tă-gog) *n.* a substance that stimulates secretion.

secretin (si-**kree**-tin) *n.* a hormone secreted from the duodenum when acidified food leaves the stomach. It stimulates the secretion of relatively enzyme-free alkaline juice by the pancreas and of bile by the liver.

secretion (si-**kree**-shŏn) *n.* **1.** the process by which a gland isolates constituents of the blood or tissue fluid and chemically alters them to produce a substance that it discharges for use by the body or excretes. **2.** the substance that is produced by a gland.

section (**sek**-shŏn) *n.* **1.** (in surgery) the act of cutting (the cut or division made is also called a section). **2.** (in microscopy) a thin slice of the specimen to be examined under a microscope.

sedation (si-**day**-shŏn) *n.* the production of a restful state of mind, particularly by the use of drugs (*see* sedative).

sedative (**sed**-ă-tiv) *n.* a drug that

has a calming effect, relieving anxiety and tension. Barbiturates as sedatives have largely been replaced by tranquillizers, which are less likely to cause drowsiness or dependence.

sedimentation rate (sed-i-men-tay-shŏn) *n.* the rate at which solid particles sink in a liquid under the influence of gravity. *See also* ESR (erythrocyte sedimentation rate).

segment (**seg**-měnt) *n.* (in anatomy) a portion of a tissue or organ, usually distinguishable from other portions by lines of demarcation.

Seidlitz powder (**sed**-lits) *n.* a mixture of sodium bicarbonate, sodium potassium tartrate, and tartaric acid, taken as a laxative when dissolved in water.

self-actualization (self-ak-tew-ă-ly-zay-shŏn) *n.* the tendency to realize and fulfil one's maximum potential. *See* Maslow's hierarchy of human needs.

self-care (self-**kair**) *n.* the practice of activities that are necessary to sustain life and health, normally initiated and carried out by the individual for himself.

sella turcica (**sel**-ă **ter**-sik-ă) *n.* a depression in the body of the sphenoid bone that encloses the pituitary gland.

semeiology (see-mi-**ol**-ŏji) *n. see* symptomatology.

semen (seminal fluid) (**see**-men) *n.* the fluid ejaculated from the penis at sexual climax. Each ejaculate may contain 300–500 million sperms suspended in a fluid secreted by the prostate gland and seminal vesicles with a small contribution from Cowper's glands. **—seminal** (sem-in-ăl) *adj.*

semi- *prefix denoting* half.

semicircular canals (sem-i-ser-kew-ler) *pl. n.* three tubes that form part of the membranous labyrinth of the ear. They are concerned with balance and each canal registers movement in a different plane.

semilunar cartilage (sem-i-**loo**-ner) *n.* one of a pair of crescent-shaped cartilages in the knee joint situated between the femur and tibia.

semilunar valve *n.* either of the two valves in the heart situated at the origin of the aorta (*aortic valve*) and the pulmonary artery (*pulmonary valve*). Each consists of three flaps (cusps), which maintain the flow of blood in one direction.

seminal vesicle *n.* either of a pair of male accessory sex glands that open into the vas deferens. The seminal vesicles secrete most of the liquid component of semen.

seminiferous tubule (sem-in-**if**-er-ŭs) *n.* any of the long convoluted tubules that make up the bulk of the testis.

seminoma (sem-in-**oh**-mă) *n.* a malignant tumour of the testis, appearing as a swelling, often painless, in the scrotum. The best treatment for localized disease is orchidectomy. A similar tumour occurs in the ovary (*see* dysgerminoma).

semipermeable membrane (sem-i-per-mi-ăbŭl) *n.* a membrane that allows the passage of some molecules but not others. Semipermeable membranes are used clinically in haemodialysis.

semiprone (sem-i-**prohn**) *adj.* describing the position of a patient lying face downwards, but with one or both knees flexed to one side. *Compare* prone, supine.

senescence (si-**nes**-ĕns) *n.* the condition of ageing, which is often marked by a decrease in physical and mental abilities. —**senescent** *adj.*

Sengstaken tube (sengz-tay-kĕn) *n.* a tube containing a triple lumen and inflatable balloons that is passed down the oesophagus to the stomach to compress bleeding oesophageal varicose veins. [R. W. Sengstaken (1923–), US neurosurgeon]

senile dementia (see-nyl) *n.* loss of the intellectual faculties, beginning for the first time in old age. *See also* dementia.

senility (sin-il-iti) *n.* the state of physical and mental deterioration that is associated with the ageing process. —**senile** *adj.*

senna (sen-ă) *n.* the dried fruits of certain shrubs of the genus *Cassia*, administered by mouth as an irritant laxative to relieve constipation and to empty the bowels before X-ray examination.

sensation (sen-say-shŏn) *n.* a feeling: the result of messages from the body's sensory receptors registering in the brain as information about the environment.

sense (sens) *n.* one of the faculties by which the qualities of the external environment are appreciated – sight, hearing, smell, taste, or touch. *s. organ* a collection of specialized cells (receptors), connected to the nervous system, that is capable of responding to a particular stimulus from either outside or inside the body.

sensibility (sen-si-**bil**-iti) *n.* the ability to be affected by, and respond to, changes in the surroundings. Sensibility is a characteristic of cells of the nervous system.

sensible (sen-sibŭl) *adj*. **1**. perceptible to the senses. **2**. capable of sensibility.

sensitive (sen-sit-iv) *adj*. possessing the ability to respond to a stimulus.

sensitization (sen-si-ty-**zay**-shŏn) *n*. **1**. alteration of the responsiveness of the body to the presence of foreign substances. In the development of an allergy, an individual becomes sensitized to a particular allergen. The phenomena of sensitization are due to the production of antibodies. **2**. (in behaviour therapy) a form of aversion therapy in which anxiety-producing stimuli are associated with the unwanted behaviour.

sensory (sen-ser-i) *adj*. relating to the input division of the nervous system, which carries information from receptors throughout the body towards the brain and spinal cord. **s. cortex** the region of the cerebral cortex responsible for receiving incoming information relayed by sensory nerve pathways from all parts of the body. **s. deprivation** a condition resulting from partial or complete absence of sensory stimuli, leading to confusion and disorientation. **s. nerve** *see* nerve.

sepsis (sep-sis) *n*. the putrefactive destruction of tissues by disease-causing bacteria or their toxins.

sept- (**septi-**) *prefix denoting* **1**. seven. **2**. (*or* **septo-**) a septum, especially the nasal septum. **3**. sepsis.

septal defect (sep-t'l) *n*. a hole in the partition (septum) between the left and right halves of the heart. This congenital condition is due to an abnormality of heart development in the fetus. It may be found between the two atria (*atrial s. d.*) or between the ventricles (*ventricular s. d.*). A septal defect permits abnormal circulation of blood from the left side of the heart to the right, which results in excessive blood flow through the lungs. Pulmonary hypertension develops and heart failure may occur.

septic (**sep**-tik) *adj*. relating to or affected with sepsis.

septicaemia (septi-**seem**-iă) *n*. widespread destruction of tissues due to absorption of disease-causing bacteria or their toxins from the bloodstream. *Compare* pyaemia, sapraemia, toxaemia.

Septrin (sep-trin) *n. see* co-trimoxazole.

septum (sep-tŭm) *n*. (*pl.* **septa**) a partition or dividing wall within an anatomical structure. —**septal** *adj*. —**septate** (sep-tayt) *adj*.

sequela (si-kwee-lă) *n*. (*pl.* **sequelae**) any disorder or pathological condition that results from a preceding disease or accident.

sequestration (see-kwes-**tray**-shŏn) *n*. the formation of a sequestrum and its separation from the surrounding tissue.

sequestrectomy (see-kwes-trek-tŏmi) *n*. surgical removal of a sequestrum.

sequestrum (si-kwes-trŭm) *n*. (*pl.* **sequestra**) a portion of dead bone formed in an infected bone in chronic osteomyelitis. It can cause irritation and the formation of pus, which may discharge through a sinus, and is usually surgically removed.

ser- (**sero-**) *prefix denoting* **1**. serum. **2**. serous membrane.

serine (se-reen) *n. see* amino acid.

serology (si-**rol**-ŏji) *n*. the study of blood serum and its constituents, particularly their contribution to the protection of the body against disease. —**serological** adj.

seropus (seer-oh-pus) n. a mixture of serum and pus, which forms, for example, in infected blisters.

serosa (sı-**roh**-să) n. see serous membrane.

serositis (seer-oh-**sy**-tis) n. inflammation of a serous membrane. See polyserositis.

serotherapy (seer-oh-th'e-ră-pi) n. the use of serum containing known antibodies (see antiserum) to treat a patient with an infection or to confer temporary passive immunity upon a person at special risk.

serotonin (5-hydroxytryptamine) (se-rŏ-**toh**-nin) n. a compound widely distributed in the tissues, particularly in the blood platelets, intestinal wall, and central nervous system. It is thought to play a role in inflammation similar to that of histamine and it also possibly acts as a neurotransmitter.

serotype (seer-oh-typ) n. a category into which material is placed based on its serological activity, particularly in terms of the antigens it contains or the antibodies that may be produced against it.

serous (seer-ŭs) adj. **1.** relating to or containing serum. **2.** resembling serum or producing a fluid resembling serum.

serous membrane (serosa) n. a smooth transparent membrane lining certain large cavities of the body, such as the abdomen (see peritoneum) and chest (see pleura). The *parietal* portion of the membrane lines the walls of the cavity, and the *visceral* portion covers the organs concerned. The two form a closed sac, the inner surface of which is moistened by a thin fluid derived from blood serum, allowing frictionless movement of organs within their cavities. *Compare* mucous membrane.

serpiginous (ser-**pij**-in-ŭs) adj. having an indented or wavy margin: applied to certain skin lesions.

serrated (ser-**ayt**-id) adj. having a saw-toothed edge. —**serration** n.

serum (blood serum) (seer-ŭm) n. the fluid that separates from clotted blood or blood plasma that is allowed to stand. Serum is essentially similar in composition to plasma but lacks fibrinogen and other substances that are used in the coagulation process. *s. sickness* a reaction that sometimes occurs 7–12 days after injection of a quantity of foreign serum. The usual symptoms are rashes, fever, joint pains, and enlargement of the lymph nodes.

sesamoid bone (ses-ă-moid) n. an oval nodule of bone that lies within a tendon and slides over another bony surface. The patella (kneecap) is a sesamoid bone.

sessile (se-syl) adj. (of a tumour) having no stalk.

sex chromatin (seks) n. chromatin found only in female cells and believed to represent a single X chromosome in a nondividing cell. It can be used to discover the sex of a baby before birth by examination of cells obtained by amniocentesis.

sex chromosome n. a chromosome that is involved in the determination of the sex of the individual. Women have two X chromosomes; men have one X chromosome and one Y chromosome. *Compare* autosome.

sex hormone *n.* any steroid hormone, produced mainly by the ovaries or testes, that is responsible for controlling sexual development and reproductive function. Oestrogens and progesterone are the female sex hormones; androgens are the male sex hormones.

sex-linked (seks-linkt) *adj.* describing genes (or the characteristics controlled by them) that are carried on the sex chromosomes. The genes for certain disorders, e.g. haemophilia, are carried on the X chromosome.

sexology (seks-ol-ōji) *n.* the study of sexual matters, including anatomy, physiology, behaviour, and techniques.

sexual intercourse (seks-yoo-ăl **in-**ter-kors) *n. see* coitus.

SGOT *n.* serum glutamic oxaloacetic transaminase. *See* glutamic oxaloacetic transaminase.

SGPT *n.* serum glutamic pyruvic transaminase. *See* glutamic pyruvic transaminase.

sheath (sheeth) *n.* (in anatomy) the layer of connective tissue that envelops structures such as nerves, arteries, tendons, and muscles.

Sheehan's syndrome (shee-ănz) *n.* subnormal activity of the pituitary gland (*see* hypopituitarism) resulting from a reduction in its blood supply, due to postpartum haemorrhage. [H. L. Sheehan (1900–), British pathologist]

Shigella (shig-el-ă) *n.* a genus of nonmotile rodlike Gram-negative bacteria normally present in the intestinal tract of man. Some species are pathogenic. *S. dysenteriae* a species associated with bacillary dysentery.

shigellosis (shig-el-oh-sis) *n.* an infestation of the digestive system by bacteria of the genus *Shigella*, causing bacillary dysentery.

shin bone (shin) *n. see* tibia.

shingles (shing-ŭlz) *n. see* herpes (zoster).

Shirodkar's operation (shirod-karz) *n.* an operation in which the neck (cervix) of the womb is closed by means of a purse-string suture in order to prevent miscarriage. [N. V. Shirodkar (1900–71), Indian obstetrician]

shock (shok) *n.* the condition associated with circulatory collapse, when the arterial blood pressure is too low to maintain an adequate supply of blood to the tissues. The patient has a cold sweaty pallid skin, a weak rapid pulse, irregular breathing, dry mouth, dilated pupils, and a reduced flow of urine. Shock may be due to a decrease in the volume of blood, as occurs after haemorrhage, dehydration, burns, etc., or it may be caused by reduced activity of the heart, as in coronary thrombosis. It may also be due to widespread dilation of the veins so that there is insufficient blood to fill them. This may be caused by the presence of bacteria in the bloodstream (*bacteraemic s.*), a severe allergic reaction (*anaphylactic s.*: *see* anaphylaxis), drug overdosage, or emotional shock (*neurogenic s.*).

short circuit (short-**ser-**kit) *n. see* anastomosis.

short-sightedness (short-**syt-**id-nis) *n. see* myopia.

shoulder girdle (pectoral girdle) (shohl-der) *n.* the bony structure to which the bones of the upper limbs are attached. It consists of the right and left scapulas and clavicles.

show (shoh) *n. Informal.* a discharge of blood-stained mucus from the vagina that occurs at the start of labour.

shunt (shunt) *n.* (in medicine) a passage connecting two anatomical channels and diverting blood from one to the other. It may occur as a congenital abnormality or be surgically created. *See also* anastomosis.

sial- (**sialo-**) *prefix denoting* **1.** saliva. **2.** a salivary gland.

sialadenitis (sy-ăl-ad-i-ny-tis) *n.* inflammation of a salivary gland.

sialogogue (sy-al-ŏ-gog) *n.* a drug that promotes the secretion of saliva. Parasympathomimetic drugs have this action.

sialography (**ptyalography**) (sy-ă-log-răfi) *n.* X-ray examination of the salivary glands, after introducing a quantity of radio-opaque material into the ducts of the salivary glands in the mouth.

sialolith (sy-al-oh-lith) *n.* a stone (calculus) in a salivary gland or duct. The flow of saliva is obstructed, causing swelling and intense pain.

sialorrhoea (sy-ă-lŏ-ree-ă) *n. see* ptyalism.

Siamese twins (sy-ă-meez) *pl. n.* identical twins that are physically joined together at birth. The condition ranges from twins joined only by the umbilical blood vessels to those in whom conjoined heads or trunk are inseparable.

sib (sib) *n. see* sibling.

sibilant (sib-i-lănt) *adj.* whistling or hissing. The term is applied to certain abnormal sounds heard through a stethoscope.

sibling (sib) (sib-ling) *n.* one of a number of children of the same parents, i.e. a brother or sister.

sickle-cell disease (**drepanocytosis**) (sik-ŭl-sel) *n.* a hereditary blood disease that affects negroes. It is characterized by the production of an abnormal type of haemoglobin in the red blood cells. The cells are distorted into the characteristic sickle shape and are rapidly removed from the circulation, leading to anaemia.

side-effect (syd-i-fekt) *n.* an unwanted effect produced by a drug in addition to its desired therapeutic effects. Side-effects may be harmful.

sidero- *prefix denoting* iron.

sideropenia (sid-er-oh-pee-niă) *n.* iron deficiency. This may result from dietary inadequacy; increased requirement of iron by the body, as in pregnancy or childhood; or increased loss of iron from the body, usually due to chronic bleeding.

siderosis (sid-er-oh-sis) *n.* the deposition of iron oxide dust in the lungs, occurring in silver finishers, arc welders, and haematite miners. Pulmonary fibrosis may develop if fibrogenic dusts such as silica are also inhaled.

sigmoid- *prefix denoting* the sigmoid colon.

sigmoid colon (**sigmoid flexure**) (sig-moid) *n.* the S-shaped terminal part of the descending colon, which leads to the rectum.

sigmoidectomy (sig-moid-ek-tŏmi) *n.* removal of the sigmoid colon by surgery. It is performed for tumours, severe diverticular disease, or sigmoid volvulus.

sigmoidoscope (sig-moid-ŏ-skohp) *n.* an instrument inserted through the anus in order to inspect the interior of the rectum and sigmoid colon.

sigmoidoscopy (sig-moid-**osk**-ŏpi) *n.* examination of the rectum and sigmoid colon with a sigmoidoscope. It is used in the investigation of diarrhoea or rectal bleeding, particularly to detect colitis or cancer of the rectum.

sigmoidostomy (sig-moid-**ost**-ŏmi) *n.* an operation in which the sigmoid colon is brought through the abdominal wall and opened. *See* colostomy.

sign (syn) *n.* an indication of a particular disorder that is observed by a physician but is not apparent to the patient. *Compare* symptom.

silicone (**sil**-i-kohn) *n.* any of a group of synthetic organic compounds of silicon that are water-repellant and are used in medicine in prostheses and as lubricants and adhesives.

silicosis (sil-i-**koh**-sis) *n.* a lung disease – a form of pneumoconiosis – produced by inhaling silica dust particles. It affects workers in mineral mining, quarrying, stone dressing, and boiler scaling. Silica stimulates fibrosis of lung tissue, which produces progressive breathlessness and considerably increased susceptibility to tuberculosis.

silver nitrate (**sil**-ver **ny**-trayt) *n.* a salt of silver with caustic, astringent, and disinfectant properties. It is applied in solutions or creams to destroy warts and to treat skin injuries, including burns. Formula: $AgNO_3$.

Simmond's disease (**sim**-ŏnz) *n.* loss of sexual function, loss of weight, and other features of hypopituitarism occurring in women after childbirth complicated by bleeding (postpartum haemorrhage). [M. Simmonds (1855–1925), German physician]

sinew (**sin**-yoo) *n.* a tendon.

singultus (sing-**gul**-tŭs) *n. see* hiccup.

sinistr- (sinistro-) *prefix denoting* left or the left side.

sino- (sinu-) *prefix denoting* **1.** a sinus. **2.** the sinus venosus.

sinoatrial node (SA node) (sy-noh-ay-tri-ăl) *n.* the pacemaker of the heart: a microscopic area of specialized cardiac muscle located in the upper wall of the right atrium near the entry of the vena cava. Fibres of the SA node contract at around 70 times per minute. Following each contraction, the impulse spreads along connecting fibres to the atrioventricular node. Impulses arriving at the SA node accelerate or decrease the heart rate.

sinogram (**sy**-noh-gram) *n.* an X-ray photograph of a sinus that has been injected with a radio-opaque substance. —**sinography** (sy-**nog**-răfi) *n.*

sinus (**sy**-nŭs) *n.* **1.** an air cavity within a bone, especially any of the cavities within the bones of the face or skull (*see* paranasal sinuses). **2.** any wide channel containing blood, usually venous blood. *s. arrhythmia see* arrhythmia. *s. venosus* a chamber in the embryonic heart that becomes part of the right atrium after birth. **3.** a pocket or bulge in a tubular organ, especially a blood vessel. **4.** an infected tract leading from a focus of infection to the surface of the skin or a hollow organ. *See* pilonidal sinus.

sinusitis (sy-nŭs-**I**-tis) *n.* inflammation of one or more of the paranasal sinuses. It is often caused by infection spreading from the nose. Symptoms include headache and tenderness over

skull

mandible

cervical vertebrae

clavicle

scapula

ribs

sternum

humerus

thoracic vertebrae

lumbar vertebrae

ilium

ulna

sacrum

radius

metacarpals

carpals

phalanges

coccyx

femur

patella

tibia

fibula

tarsals

phalanges

metatarsals

The skeleton

the affected sinus, which may become filled with a purulent material. In persistent cases treatment may require the affected sinus to be washed out or drained by a surgical operation.

sinusoid (sy-new-soid) *n.* a small blood vessel found in certain organs, such as the adrenal gland and liver.

siphonage (sy-fŏn-ij) *n.* the transfer of liquid from one container to another by means of a bent tube. The procedure is used in gastric lavage.

sito- *prefix denoting* food.

sitz bath (sits) *n.* a fairly shallow hip bath in which the person is seated.

SI units (Système International d'Unités) *pl. n.* the internationally agreed system of units, based on the metre-kilogram-second system, now in use for all scientific purposes. *See* Appendix 9.

skatole (methyl indole) (skat-ohl) *n.* a derivative of the amino acid tryptophan, excreted in the urine and faeces.

skeletal muscle (skel-i-t'l) *n. see* striated muscle.

skeleton (skel-i-tŏn) *n.* the rigid framework of connected bones that gives form to the body, protects and supports its soft organs and tissues, and provides attachments for muscles and a system of levers essential for locomotion. (See illustration.) —**skeletal** *adj.*

skia- *prefix denoting* shadow.

skiagram (sky-ă-gram) *n.* a 'shadow-photograph', such as an X-ray photograph produced in radiography. —**skiagraphy** (sky-ag-răfi) *n.*

skin (skin) *n.* the outer covering of the body, consisting of an outer layer, the epidermis, and an inner layer, the dermis. The epidermis protects the body from injury and from invasion by parasites. It also helps to prevent the body from becoming dehydrated. The combination of erectile hairs, sweat glands, and blood capillaries in the skin form part of the temperature-regulating mechanism of the body. The skin also acts as an organ of excretion (by the secretion of sweat) and as a sense organ (it contains receptors that are sensitive to heat, cold, touch, and pain). Anatomical name: **cutis**. **s. graft** a portion of healthy skin cut from one area of the body and used to cover a part that has lost its skin, usually as a result of injury, burns, or operation.

skull (skul) *n.* the skeleton of the head and face, which is made up of 22 bones. It can be divided into the cranium, which encloses the brain, and the face, including the lower jaw (mandible). (See illustration.) All the bones of the skull except the mandible are connected to each other by immovable joints (*see* suture). The skull contains cavities for the eyes and nose and a large opening at its base (foramen magnum) through which the spinal cord passes.

sleeping sickness (African trypanosomiasis) (sleep-ing) *n.* a disease of tropical Africa caused by the presence in the blood of the parasitic protozoans *Trypanosoma gambiense* or *T. rhodesiense*, which are transmitted to man through the bite of tsetse flies. Initial symptoms include fever, headache, and chills, followed later by enlargement of the

Section through the skin

Side view of the skull

lymph nodes, anaemia, and pains in the limbs and joints. The parasites eventually invade the minute blood vessels supplying the central nervous system, causing drowsiness and lethargy.

sleep-walking (sleep-wawk-ing) *n.* *see* somnambulism.

sling (sling) *n.* a bandage arranged to support and rest an injured limb so that healing is not hindered by activity. The most common sling is a triangular bandage tied behind the neck to support the weight of a broken arm.

slipped disc (slipt) *n.* *see* prolapsed intervertebral disc.

slit lamp (slit) *n.* a device for providing a narrow beam of light, used in conjunction with a special microscope. It can be used to examine minutely the structures within the eye, one layer at a time.

slough (sluf) *n.* dead tissue, such as skin, that separates from healthy tissue after inflammation or infection.

smallpox (smawl-poks) *n.* an acute infectious virus disease causing high fever and a rash that scars the skin. The rash consists of red spots (macules) that appear on the face, spread to the trunk and extremities, and gradually develop into pustules. Most patients recover but serious complications such as nephritis or pneumonia may develop. Treatment with thiosemicarbazone is effective. Immunization against smallpox has now totally eradicated the disease. Medical name: **variola**. *See also* alastrim, cowpox.

smear (smeer) *n.* a specimen of tissue or other material taken from part of the body and smeared on a microscope slide

A nasal snare

for examination. *See* cervical (smear).

smegma (smeg-mă) *n.* the secretion of the glands of the foreskin (prepuce), which accumulates under the foreskin and has a white cheesy appearance.

Smith-Petersen nail (smith-**pee**-ter-sĕn) *n.* a stainless steel nail used to fix fragments of bone when the neck of the femur is fractured. [M. N. Smith-Petersen (1886–1953), US orthopaedic surgeon]

smooth muscle (involuntary muscle) (smoo*th*) *n.* muscle that produces slow long-term contractions of which the individual is unaware. Smooth muscle occurs in hollow organs, such as the stomach, intestine, blood vessels, and bladder. *Compare* striated muscle.

snare (snair) *n.* an instrument consisting of a wire loop designed to remove polyps, tumours, and other projections of tissue. *See also* diathermy.

sneeze (sneez) **1.** *n.* an involuntary violent reflex expulsion of air through the nose and mouth provoked by irritation of the mucous membrane lining the nasal cavity. **2.** *vb.* to produce a sneeze.

Snellen chart (snel-ĕn) *n.* the commonest chart used for testing sharpness of distant vision (*see* visual acuity). It consists of rows of capital letters, called *test types*, the letters of each row becoming smaller down the chart.

[H. Snellen (1834–1908), Dutch ophthalmologist]

snow blindness (snoh) *n.* a painful disorder of the cornea of the eye due to excessive exposure to ultraviolet light reflected from the snow.

snuffles (snuf-ĕlz) *n.* **1.** partial obstruction of breathing in infants, caused by the common cold. **2.** (formerly) discharge through the nostrils associated with necrosis of the nasal bones: seen in infants with congenital syphilis.

socket (sok-it) *n.* (in anatomy) a hollow or depression into which another part fits.

sodium (soh-diŭm) *n.* a mineral element and an important constituent of the human body. The amount of sodium in the body is controlled by the kidneys. An excess of sodium leads to the condition of hypernatraemia, which often results in oedema. Sodium is also implicated in hypertension: a high-sodium diet is thought to increase the risk of hypertension in later life. Symbol: Na.

sodium aminosalicylate (ă-mee-noh-să-**lis**-i-layt) *n.* a drug with effects and uses similar to those of para-aminosalicylic acid. Trade name: **Paramisan**.

sodium bicarbonate (by-**kar**-bŏn-ayt) *n.* a salt of sodium that neutralizes acid and is administered by mouth or injection to treat stomach and digestive disorders, acidosis, and sodium deficiency. *See also* antacid.

sodium chloride (**klor**-ryd) *n.* common salt: a salt of sodium that is an important constituent of the body and is used to replace lost fluids and electrolytes and to irrigate body cavities. Formula: NaCl.

sodium citrate (**sit**-rayt) *n.* a salt of sodium used to prevent the clotting of stored blood and as a mild diuretic and laxative.

sodium fusidate (**few**-si-dayt) *n.* an antibiotic used mainly to treat infections caused by *Staphylococcus.* It is administered by mouth or injection or applied in an ointment for skin infections. Trade name: **Fucidin**.

sodium nitrite (**ny**-tryt) *n.* a sodium salt administered by injection, with sodium thiosulphate, to treat cyanide poisoning. It also has effects similar to glyceryl trinitrate and has been used to treat angina.

sodium salicylate *n.* a drug with actions and side-effects similar to those of aspirin. It is used mainly to treat rheumatic fever. Trade name: **Entrosalyl**.

sodium thiosulphate (th'y-oh-**sul**-fayt) *n.* a salt of sodium administered by intravenous injection, with sodium nitrite, to treat cyanide poisoning.

sodium valproate (**val**-proh-ayt) *n.* an anticonvulsant drug administered by mouth to treat all types of epilepsy. Trade name: **Epilim**.

sodokosis (soh-doh-**koh**-sis) *n. see* rat-bite fever.

soft sore (chancroid) (soft) *n.* a venereal disease caused by the bacterium *Haemophilus ducreyi*, resulting in enlargement and ulceration of lymph nodes in the groin. Treatment with sulphonamides is effective.

solarium (sŏ-**lair**-iŭm) *n.* a room in which patients are exposed to either sunlight or artificial sunlight (a blend of visible light and infrared and ultraviolet radiation).

solar plexus (coeliac plexus) (soh-ler **pleks**-ŭs) *n.* a network of sympathetic nerves and ganglia high in the back of the abdomen.

soleus (soh-li-ŭs) *n.* a broad flat muscle in the calf of the leg. The soleus flexes the foot, so that the toes point downwards.

solution (sŏ-**loo**-shŏn) *n.* a homogeneous mixture of two or more dissimilar substances, usually of a liquid (the *solvent*) in which a solid (the *solute*) is dissolved.

solvent (**sol**-vĕnt) *n. see* solution.

soma (**soh**-mă) *n.* 1. the entire body excluding the germ cells. 2. the body as distinct from the mind.

somat- *prefix denoting* 1. the body. 2. somatic.

somatic (sŏ-**mat**-ik) *adj.* 1. relating to the nonreproductive parts of the body. 2. relating to the body wall (i.e. excluding the viscera). *Compare* splanchnic. 3. relating to the body rather than the mind.

somatotrophin (soh-mă-toh-**troh**-fin) *n. see* growth hormone.

somnambulism (noctambulation) (som-**nam**-bew-lizm) *n.* sleepwalking: walking about and performing other actions in a semiautomatic way during sleep without later memory of doing so. It is common during childhood and can also arise as the result of stress or hypnosis. —**somnambulistic** *adj.*

somnolism (**som**-noh-lizm) *n.* a hypnotic trance. *See* hypnosis.

Sonne dysentery (**son**-i) *n.* bacillary dysentery caused by the species *Shigella sonnei.* [C. Sonne (1882–1948), Danish bacteriologist]

sonoplacentography (soh-noh-plas-en-**tog**-răfi) *n.* the technique of using ultrasound waves to determine the position of the placenta during pregnancy.

sonotopography (soh-noh-tŏ-**pog**-răfi) *n.* the use of ultrasound waves to determine the position of structures within the body, such as the position of a fetus within the womb.

soporific (sop-er-if-ik) *n. see* hypnotic.

sorbitol (**sor**-bit-ol) *n.* a carbohydrate with a sweet taste, used by diabetics as a substitute for cane sugar. It is also administered by mouth or injection in disorders of carbohydrate metabolism and in drip feeding.

sordes (**sor**-deez) *pl. n.* the brownish encrustations that form around the mouth and teeth of patients suffering from fevers.

sore (sor) *n.* a lay term for any ulcer or other open wound of the skin or mucous membranes. *See also* bedsore, soft sore.

sore throat *n.* pain at the back of the mouth, commonly due to tonsillitis or pharyngitis. If infection persists the lymph nodes in the neck may become tender and enlarged (cervical adenitis).

sotalol (**soh**-tă-lol) *n.* a drug (*see* beta blocker) administered by mouth or injection to treat abnormal heart rhythm, angina, and high blood pressure and to relieve symptoms in thyrotoxicosis. Trade names: **Beta-Cardone**, **Sotacor**.

souffle (soo-fĕl) *n.* a soft blowing sound heard through the stethoscope, usually produced by blood flowing in vessels.

sound (sownd) (in surgery) 1. *n.* a long rodlike instrument, often with a curved end, used to explore body cavities or to dilate strictures in the urethra or other canals. 2. *vb.* to explore a cavity using a sound.

Southey's tubes (su*th*-iz) *pl. n.* fine-calibre tubes for insertion into subcutaneous tissue to drain excess fluid. They are rarely used in practice today. [R. Southey (1835–99), English physician]

Spanish fly (**span**-ish) *n.* the blister beetle, *Lytta vesicatoria*: source of the irritant and toxic chemical compound cantharidin.

spansule (**span**-sewl) *n.* a drug in the form of a capsule prepared in such a way that, when taken orally, its contents are released slowly.

spasm (spazm) *n.* a sustained involuntary muscular contraction, which may occur either as part of a generalized disorder or as a local response to an otherwise unconnected painful condition. *carpopedal s.* a spasm that affects the muscles of the hands and feet and is caused by a deficiency of available calcium in the body.

spasmo- *prefix denoting* spasm.

spasmodic (spaz-**mod**-ik) *adj.* occurring in spasms or resembling a spasm.

spasmolytic (spaz-moh-**lit**-ik) *n.* a drug that relieves spasm of smooth muscle, e.g. papaverine or piperidolate. Spasmolytics may be used as bronchodilators to stimulate the heart in the treatment of angina, or to relieve colic.

spasmus nutans (spaz-mŭs new-tanz) *n.* a combination of symptoms including a slow nodding movement of the head, nystagmus, and spasm of the neck muscles. It affects infants and it normally disappears within a year or two.

spastic (**spast**-ik) **1.** *adj.* characterized by spasms. *s. colon see* irri-

table bowel syndrome. *s. paralysis* weakness of a limb or limbs associated with increased reflex activity. This results in spasticity and is caused by disease affecting the nerve fibres of the corticospinal tract. *See* cerebral palsy. **2.** *n.* an individual suffering from spastic paralysis.

spasticity (spas-**tis**-iti) *n.* resistance to the passive movement of a limb that is maximal at the beginning of the movement and gives way as more pressure is applied. It is a symptom of damage to the corticospinal tracts in the brain or spinal cord. *Compare* rigidity.

spatula (**spat**-yoo-lă) *n.* an instrument with a flat blunt blade used to spread ointments or plasters.

special hospital (spesh-ăl) *n.* a hospital for the care of mentally ill patients who are also dangerous and must therefore be kept securely.

special school *n.* (in Britain) an education establishment for handicapped children.

species (**spee**-shiz) *n.* the smallest unit used in the classification of living organisms. Members of the same species are able to interbreed and produce fertile offspring. Similar species are grouped together within one genus.

specific (spi-**sif**-ik) **1.** *n.* a medicine that has properties especially useful for the treatment of a particular disease. **2.** *adj.* (of a disease) caused by a particular microorganism that causes no other disease. **3.** *adj.* of or relating to a species.

specific gravity (**grav**-iti) *n. see* relative density.

Cusco's

Fergusson's

Sims's

Vaginal specula

spectinomycin (spek-tin-oh-my-sin) *n.* an antibiotic administered by injection to treat various infections, particularly gonorrhoea. Trade name: **Trobicin**.

spectroscope (spek-trŏ-skohp) *n.* an instrument used to split up light or other radiation into components of different wavelengths. The simplest spectroscope uses a prism, which splits white light into the rainbow colours of the visible spectrum.

spectrum (spek-trŭm) *n.* (in pharmacology) the range of effective-ness of an antibiotic. *broad s.* effectiveness against a wide range of microorganisms.

speculum (spek-yoo-lŭm) *n.* (*pl.* **specula**) a metal instrument for inserting into and holding open a cavity of the body, such as the vagina, rectum, or nasal orifice, in order that the interior may be examined.

speech therapy (speech) *n.* the rehabilitation of patients who are unable to speak coherently because of congenital causes, accidents, or illness.

sperm (sperm) *n. see* spermatozoon.

sperm- (spermi(o)- spermo-) *prefix denoting* sperm or semen.

spermat- (spermato-) *prefix denot-*

Spermatogenesis

ing **1.** sperm. **2.** organs or ducts associated with sperm.

spermatic artery (sper-mat-ik) *n.* either of two arteries that originate from the abdominal aorta and travel downwards to supply the testes.

spermatic cord *n.* the cord, consisting of the vas deferens, nerves, and blood vessels, that runs from the abdominal cavity to the testicle in the scrotum.

spermatocele (**sperm**-ă-toh-seel) *n.* a cystic swelling in the scrotum containing sperm. The cyst arises from the epididymis and can be felt as a lump above the testis. Treatment is by surgical removal.

spermatogenesis (sperm-ă-toh-**jen**-i-sis) *n.* the process by which mature spermatozoa are produced in the testis. Spermatogonia, in the outermost layer of the seminiferous tubules, multiply throughout reproductive life. Some of them divide by meiosis into spermatocytes, which produce haploid spermatids. These are transformed into mature spermatozoa by the process of *spermiogenesis*. The whole process takes 70–80 days.

spermatorrhoea (sperm-ă-tŏ-**ree**-ă) *n.* the involuntary discharge of semen without orgasm.

spermatozoon (sperm) (sperm-ă-toh-**zoh**-ŏn) *n.* (*pl.* **spermatozoa**) a mature male sex cell (*see* gamete). The tail of a sperm enables it to swim, which is important as a means for reaching and fertilizing the ovum. *See also* acrosome, fertilization.

spermaturia (sperm-ăt-**yoor**-iă) *n.* the presence of spermatozoa in the urine. Abnormal ejaculation into the bladder on orgasm (retrograde ejaculation) may occur after prostatectomy or other sur-

A spermatozoon

gical procedures or in certain neurological conditions.

sperm count *n.* an estimate of the concentration of spermatozoa in ejaculated semen, which is used as a measure of male fertility.

spermicide (**sperm**-i-syd) *n.* an agent that kills spermatozoa. Contraceptive creams and jellies contain chemical spermicides. —**spermicidal** *adj.*

spermiogenesis (sperm-i-oh-**jen**-i-sis) *n.* *see* spermatogenesis.

spheno- *prefix denoting* the sphenoid bone.

sphenoid bone (sfee-noid) *n.* a bone forming the base of the cranium behind the eyes. *See* skull.

spherocyte (sfeer-oh-syt) *n.* an abnormal form of red blood cell (erythrocyte) that is spherical rather than disc-shaped. Spherocytes tend to be removed from the blood as they pass through the spleen, resulting in anaemia. *See also* spherocytosis.

spherocytosis (sfeer-oh-sy-toh-sis) *n.* the presence in the blood of spherocytes. Spherocytosis may occur as a hereditary disorder (*hereditary s.*) or in certain haemolytic anaemias.

sphincter (sfink-ter) *n.* a specialized ring of muscle that surrounds an orifice. Contractions of the sphincter partly or completely close the orifice. Sphincters are found, for example, around the anus (*anal s.*) and at the opening between the stomach and duodenum (*pyloric s.*).

sphincter- *prefix denoting* a sphincter.

sphincterectomy (sfink-ter-ek-tŏmi) *n.* **1.** the surgical removal of any sphincter muscle. **2.** surgical removal of part of the iris in the eye at the border of the pupil.

sphincterotomy (sfink-ter-ot-ŏmi) *n.* surgical division of any sphincter muscle.

sphygmo- *prefix denoting* the pulse.

sphygmocardiograph (sfig-moh-kar-di-ŏ-grahf) *n.* an apparatus for producing a continuous record of both the heart beat and the subsequent pulse in one of the blood vessels. The recording can be shown on a moving tape or on an electronic screen.

Types of spica

sphygmograph (sfig-moh-grahf) *n.* an apparatus for producing a continuous record of the pulse in one of the blood vessels, showing the strength and rate of the beats.

sphygmomanometer (sfig-moh-mă-nom-it-er) *n.* an instrument for measuring blood pressure in the arteries. It consists of an inflatable cuff connected via a rubber tube to a column of mercury with a graduated scale.

spica (spy-kă) *n.* a bandage wound repeatedly in a figure-of-eight around an injured limb, forming a series of V-shapes.

spicule (spik-yool) *n.* a small splinter of bone.

spigot (spig-ŏt) *n.* a glass or plastic peg used to close the opening of a tube, used in nasogastric tubes and catheters.

spina bifida (rachischisis) (spy-nă bif-id-ă) *n.* a developmental defect in which the newborn baby has part of the spinal cord and its coverings exposed through a gap in the backbone. The symptoms may include paralysis of the legs, incontinence, and mental retardation from the commonly associated brain defect, hydrocephalus. Spina bifida can be diagnosed at about the 16th week of pregnancy by a test on the amniotic fluid (*see* amniocentesis). *See also* neural tube defects.

spinal accessory nerve (spy-năl) *n. see* accessory nerve.

spinal anaesthesia *n.* 1. suppression of sensation in part of the body by the injection of a local anaesthetic into the space surrounding the spinal cord. Spinal anaesthesia is useful in patients whose condition makes them unsuitable for a general anaesthetic, for certain obstetric procedures, or in circumstances where a skilled anaesthetist is not available. *epidural s. a.* spinal anaesthesia in which the anaesthetic is injected into the outer lining of the spinal cord. 2. loss of sensation in part of the body as a result of injury or disease to the spinal cord.

spinal column *n. see* backbone.

spinal cord *n.* the portion of the central nervous system enclosed in the vertebral column, consisting of nerve cells and bundles of nerves connecting all parts of the body with the brain. It extends from the medulla oblongata in the skull to the level of the second lumbar vertebra.

spinal nerves *pl. n.* the 31 pairs of nerves that leave the spinal cord and are distributed to the body, passing out from the vertebral canal through the spaces between the arches of the vertebrae.

spindle (spin-d'l) *n.* a collection of fibres seen in a cell when it is dividing. It plays an important part in chromosome movement in mitosis and meiosis and is also involved in division of the cytoplasm.

spine (spyn) *n.* 1. a sharp process on a bone. 2. the vertebral column (*see* backbone). —**spinal** *adj.*

spino- *prefix denoting* 1. the spine. 2. the spinal cord.

spiral bandage (spyr-ăl) *n.* a bandage wound round a part of the body, overlapping the previous section at each turn.

spiral organ *n. see* organ (of Corti).

Spirillum (spy-ril-ŭm) *n.* a genus of highly motile rigid spiral-shaped bacteria usually found in fresh and salt water containing organic matter. *S. minus* a species that causes rat-bite fever.

spiro- *prefix denoting* 1. spiral. 2. respiration.

spirochaetaemia (spy-roh-ki-tee-miă) *n.* the presence of spirochaetes in the bloodstream, occurring in the later stages of syphilis.

spirochaete (spy-roh-keet) *n.* any one of a group of spiral-shaped bacteria that lack a rigid cell wall and move by means of muscular flexions of the cell. The group includes the species *Borrelia*, *Leptospira*, and *Treponema*.

spirograph (spy-roh-grahf) *n.* an instrument for recording breathing movements. The record obtained is called a *spirogram*. —**spirography** *n.*

spirometer (spy-rom-it-er) *n.* an instrument for measuring the volume of air inhaled and exhaled. It is used in tests of ventilation. —**spirometry** *n.*

spironolactone (spy-rŏ-noh-lak-tohn) *n.* a synthetic corticosteroid that inhibits the activity of the hormone aldosterone and is administered by mouth to treat heart failure, high blood pressure, and fluid retention (oedema). Trade name: **Aldactone**.

Spitz-Holter valve (spits-hohl-ter) *n.* a valve used in the treatment of hydrocephalus to drain cerebrospinal fluid from the ventricles of the brain into the superior vena cava.

splanch- (splanchno-) *prefix denoting* the viscera.

splanchnic (splank-nik) *adj.* relating to the viscera. *Compare* somatic (def. 2). *s. nerves* the series of nerves in the sympathetic system that are distributed to the blood vessels and viscera.

splanchnology (splank-nol-ŏji) *n.* the study of the viscera.

spleen (spleen) *n.* a large dark-red ovoid organ situated on the left side of the body below and behind the stomach. The spongy interior (*pulp*) of the spleen consists of lymphoid tissue within a meshwork of reticular fibres. The spleen is a major component of the reticuloendothelial system, producing lymphocytes in the newborn and containing phagocytes, which remove worn-out red blood cells and other foreign bodies from the bloodstream.

Anatomical name: **lien**. —**splenic** (splen-ik) *adj.*

splen- (spleno-) *prefix denoting* the spleen.

splenectomy (spli-nek-tŏmi) *n.* surgical removal of the spleen. This is sometimes necessary in the emergency treatment of bleeding from a ruptured spleen.

splenic anaemia *n.* anaemia associated with portal hypertension and increased destruction of red blood cells by an overactive spleen.

splenitis (spli-ny-tis) *n.* inflammation of the spleen. *See also* perisplenitis.

splenomegaly (splee-noh-meg-ăli) *n.* enlargement of the spleen. It commonly occurs in malaria, blood disorders, leukaemia, and Hodgkin's disease. *See also* hypersplenism.

splenorenal anastomosis (splee-noh-ree-năl) *n.* a method of treating portal hypertension by joining the splenic vein to the left renal vein. *Compare* portacaval anastomosis.

splenovenography (splee-noh-vi-nog-răfi) *n.* X-ray examination of the spleen and veins associated with it following injection of a radio-opaque dye.

splint (splint) *n.* a rigid support to hold broken bones in position until healing has occurred.

spondyl- (spondylo-) *prefix denoting* a vertebra or the spine.

spondylitis (spon-di-ly-tis) *n.* inflammation of the synovial joints of the backbone. *ankylosing s.* a rheumatic disease in which there is pain and stiffness in the backbone and sacroiliac joints and sometimes also arthritis in the shoulder and hip. In severe cases the spine becomes completely rigid, through fusion of its joints, and kyphosis results. *See also* ankylosis.

spondylolisthesis (spon-di-loh-lis-thi-sis) *n.* a forward shift of one vertebra upon another, due to a defect of the joints that normally bind them together. This may be congenital or develop after injury.

spondylosis (spon-di-**loh**-sis) *n.* degeneration of the intervertebral discs in the cervical, thoracic, or lumbar regions of the backbone. Symptoms include pain and restriction of movement. Pain is relieved by wearing a collar (when the neck region is affected) or a surgical belt (for the lower spine), which prevents movement. Very severe cases sometimes require surgical fusion.

spondylosyndesis (spon-di-loh-sin-di-sis) *n.* surgical fusion of the intervertebral joints of the backbone.

spongioblastoma (spunji-oh-blas-toh-mǎ) *n. see* glioblastoma.

spontaneous (spon-**tay**-niǔs) *adj.* arising without apparent cause or outside aid. The term is applied in medicine to certain conditions, such as pathological fractures, that arise in the absence of outside injury.

sporadic (sper-**ad**-ik) *adj.* describing a disease that occurs only occasionally or in a few isolated places. *Compare* endemic, epidemic.

spore (spor) *n.* a small reproductive body produced by plants and microorganisms. Some kinds of spores function as dormant stages of the life cycle, enabling the organism to survive adverse conditions. Other spores are the means by which the organism can spread vegetatively. *See also* endospore.

sporicide (spor-i-syd) *n.* an agent that kills spores (e.g. bacterial spores). Most germicides are ineffective since spores are very resistant to chemical action. —**sporicidal** *adj.*

sporotrichosis (spor-oh-trik-**oh**-sis) *n.* a chronic infection of the skin and superficial lymph nodes that is caused by the fungus *Sporotrichum schenckii* and results in the formation of abscesses and ulcers.

Sporozoa (spor-ŏ-**zoh**-ǎ) *n.* a group of parasitic Protozoa that includes *Plasmodium*, the malaria parasite.

spotted fever (**spot**-id) *n. see* cerebrospinal fever, Rocky Mountain spotted fever, typhus.

sprain (sprayn) *n.* injury to a ligament, caused by sudden overstretching. Sprains should be treated by cold compresses (ice-packs) at the time of injury, and later by restriction of activity.

Sprengel's deformity (**spreng**-ělz) *n.* a congenital abnormality of the scapula, which is small and positioned high in the shoulder. [O. G. K. Sprengel (1852–1915), German surgeon]

sprue (**psilosis**) (sproo) *n.* deficient absorption of food due to disease of the small intestine. *tropical s.* sprue characterized by diarrhoea (usually steatorrhoea), glossitis, anaemia, and weight loss; the lining of the small intestine is inflamed and atrophied. Treatment with antibiotics and folic acid is usually effective. *See also* coeliac disease (nontropical sprue), malabsorption.

spud (spud) *n.* a blunt needle used for removing foreign bodies embedded in the cornea of the eye.

spur (sper) *n.* a sharp projection, especially one of bone.

sputum (spew-tŭm) *n.* saliva mixed with mucus coughed up from the respiratory tract. A sputum-productive cough occurs in many conditions in which examination of the sputum for microorganisms, cells, and other substances may help diagnosis.

squama (skway-mă) *n.* (*pl.* **squamae**) 1. a thin plate of bone. 2. a scale, such as any of the scales from the cornified layer of the epidermis. —**squamous** *adj.*

squamo- *prefix denoting* 1. the squamous portion of the temporal bone. 2. squamous epithelium.

squamous bone (skway-mŭs) *n. see* temporal (bone).

squamous epithelium *n. see* epithelium.

squint (skwint) *n. see* strabismus.

staccato speech (stă-**kah**-toh) *n.* abnormal speech in which there are pauses between words, sometimes associated with multiple sclerosis.

Stacke's operation (stak-ĕz) *n.* an operation in which the bone between the mastoid cells and the middle ear is removed to create a single cavity. It is performed when there is chronic infection of this area. [L. Stacke (1859–1918), German otologist]

stadium (stay-diŭm) *n.* a stage in the course of a disease. *s. invasioni* the period between exposure to infection and the onset of symptoms.

stagnant loop syndrome (stag-nănt) *n.* a condition in which a segment of the small intestine is out of continuity with the rest of the intestine or in which progress of contents through the small intes-

tine is delayed by an obstruction that allows an overgrowth of bacteria, causing malabsorption and steatorrhoea.

stain (stayn) 1. *n.* a dye used to colour tissues and other specimens for microscopical examination. 2. *vb.* to treat a specimen for microscopical study with a stain.

stammering (stuttering) (stam-er-ing) *n.* halting articulation with interruptions to the normal flow of speech and repetition of the initial consonants of words or syllables. The symptoms are most severe when the stammerer is under any psychological stress. Medical name: **dysphemia**. —**stammerer** *n.*

stanolone (stan-ŏ-lohn) *n.* a synthetic male sex hormone with anabolic activity, administered by mouth to treat wasting diseases, such as osteoporosis and anorexia, and breast cancer. Trade name: **Anabolex**.

St Anthony's fire (sănt **ant**-ŏ-niz fyr) *n.* a popular name for inflammation of the skin associated with ergot poisoning. *See* ergotism.

stapedectomy (stay-pi-**dek**-tŏmi) *n.* surgical removal of the stapes: part of the treatment for deafness due to otosclerosis.

stapediolysis (stă-pee-di-**ol**-i-sis) *n.* an operation to restore hearing in cases of otosclerosis, in which the stapes is freed from the fenestra ovalis.

stapes (stay-peez) *n.* a stirrup-shaped bone in the middle ear that articulates with the incus and is attached to the membrane of the fenestra ovalis. *See* ossicle.

staphylectomy (staf-i-**lek**-tŏmi) *n.* surgical removal of the uvula.

Staphylococcus (staf-i-loh-**kok**-ŭs) *n.* a genus of Gram-positive non-motile spherical bacteria occurring in grapelike clusters. Some species are saprophytes; others parasites. Many species produce exotoxins. *S. aureus* a species that causes boils and internal abscesses. *S. pyogenes* a species that is associated with most suppurative infections.

staphyloma (staf-i-**loh**-mă) *n.* abnormal bulging of the cornea or sclera (white) of the eye.

staphylorrhaphy (palatorrhaphy, uraniscorrhaphy) (staf-il-o-**răfi**) *n.* surgical suture of a cleft palate.

starch (starch) *n.* the form in which carbohydrates are stored in many plants and a major constituent of the diet. Starch consists of linked glucose units and occurs in two forms, *α-amylose* and *amylopectin*. Starch is digested by means of the enzyme amylase. *See also* dextrin.

starvation (star-**vay**-shŏn) *n. see* malnutrition.

stasis (**stay**-sis) *n.* stagnation or cessation of flow; for example, of blood or lymph whose flow is obstructed or of the intestinal contents when peristalsis is hindered.

-stasis *suffix denoting* stoppage of a flow of liquid; stagnation.

status asthmaticus (**stay**-tŭs ass-**mat**-ik-ŭs) *n.* an attack of asthma lasting for more than 24 hours. Treatment with corticosteroid drugs may be life-saving and artificial respiration may be needed.

status epilepticus (epi-**lep**-tik-ŭs) *n.* the occurrence of repeated epileptic fits without any recovery of consciousness between them. Prolonged status epilepticus causes a serious imbalance of the salts (electrolytes) in the body, which may lead to the patient's death.

status lymphaticus (lim-**fat**-ik-ŭs) *n.* enlargement of the thymus gland and other parts of the lymphatic system, formerly believed to be a predisposing cause to sudden death in infancy and childhood.

steapsin (sti-**ap**-sin) *n. see* lipase.

stearic acid (sti-**a**-rik) *n. see* fatty acid.

steat- (steato-) *prefix denoting* fat; fatty tissue.

steatoma (sti-ă-**toh**-mă) *n. see* sebaceous cyst. The term is also used for any tumour of a sebaceous gland.

steatopygia (sti-ă-toh-**pij**-iă) *n.* the accumulation of large quantities of fat in the buttocks.

steatorrhoea (sti-ă-tŏ-**ree**-ă) *n.* the passage of abnormally increased amounts of fat in the faeces due to reduced absorption of fat by the intestine (*see* malabsorption). The faeces are pale and may look greasy.

Stein-Leventhal syndrome (styn-lev-ĕn-thal) *n.* secondary amenorrhoea and sterility associated with multiple cysts in both ovaries. [I. F. Stein (1887–   ) and M. L. Leventhal (1901–71), US gynaecologists]

Steinmann's pin (styn-manz) *n.* a fine metal nail inserted through a fractured bone through which extension is applied to the distal bone fragment. [F. Steinmann (1872–1932), Swiss surgeon]

stellate (**stel**-ayt) *adj.* star-shaped. *s. fracture* a star-shaped fracture of the kneecap caused by a direct blow. *s. ganglion* a star-shaped collection of sympathetic nerve cell bodies in the root of the neck.

Stellwag's sign (stel-vagz) *n.* apparent widening of the distance between the upper and lower eyelids due to retraction of the upper lid and protrusion of the eyeball. It is a sign of exophthalmic goitre. [C. Stellwag von Carion (1823–1904), Austrian ophthalmologist]

steno- *prefix denoting* **1.** narrow. **2.** constricted.

stenosis (sti-**noh**-sis) *n.* the abnormal narrowing of a passage or opening, such as a blood vessel or heart valve. *See* aortic stenosis, mitral stenosis, pyloric stenosis.

stenostomia (stenostomy) (sten-ŏ-**stoh**-miă) *n.* the abnormal narrowing of an opening, such as the opening of the bile duct.

Stensen's duct (sten-sĕnz) *n.* the long secretory duct of the parotid salivary gland. [N. Stensen (1638–86), Danish physician]

sterco- *prefix denoting* faeces.

stercobilin (ster-koh-**by**-lin) *n.* a brownish-red pigment formed during the metabolism of the bile pigments biliverdin and bilirubin and subsequently excreted in the urine or faeces.

stercolith (**ster**-koh-lith) *n.* a stone formed of dried compressed faeces.

stercoraceous (ster-ker-**ay**-shŭs) *adj.* composed of or containing faeces.

stereognosis (ste-ri-og-**noh**-sis) *n.* the ability to recognize the three-dimensional shape of an object by touch alone. This is a function of the association areas of the parietal lobe of the brain. *See also* agnosia.

stereoscopic vision (ste-ri-ŏ-**skop**-ik) *n.* perception of the shape, depth, and distance of an object as a result of having binocular vision.

stereotaxy (ste-ri-ŏ-**taks**-i) *n.* a surgical procedure in which a deep-seated area in the brain is operated upon after its position has been accurately established by three-dimensional measurements. The operation may be performed using an electrical current or by heat, cold, or mechanical techniques. *See also* leucotomy.

stereotypy (ste-ri-ŏ-ty-pi) *n.* the constant repetition of a complex action, which is carried out in the same way each time. It is seen in catatonia and infantile autism; sometimes it is an isolated symptom in mental subnormality.

sterile (ste-ryl) *adj.* **1.** (of a living organism) barren; unable to reproduce its kind (*see* sterility). **2.** (of inanimate objects) completely free from microorganisms that could cause infection.

sterility (ster-il-iti) *n.* inability to have children, due either to infertility or (in someone who has been fertile) to a surgical operation (*see* sterilization).

sterilization (ste-ri-ly-**zay**-shŏn) *n.* **1.** a surgical operation or any other process that induces sterility in men or women; for example, by cutting the vasa deferentia in men (*see* vasectomy) and the Fallopian tubes in women (*see* salpingectomy). **2.** any means of rendering objects, wounds, etc., free of bacteria that would otherwise cause disease. Surgical instruments and dressings can be sterilized in an autoclave.

stern- (sterno-) *prefix denoting* the sternum.

sternocleidomastoid muscle (ster-noh-kly-doh-**mas**-toid) *n. see* sternomastoid muscle.

sternohyoid (ster-noh-**hy**-oid) *n.* a muscle in the neck, arising from the sternum and inserted into the hyoid bone. It depresses the hyoid bone.

sternomastoid muscle (ster-noh-**mas**-toid) (**sternocleidomastoid muscle**) *n.* a long muscle in the neck, extending from the mastoid process to the sternum and clavicle. It serves to rotate the neck and flex the head.

sternomastoid tumour *n.* a small painless nonmalignant swelling in the lower half of the sternomastoid muscle, appearing a few days after birth. It is most common after breech births. The tumour may cause a slight tilt of the head, which can be corrected by physiotherapy.

sternotomy (ster-**not**-ŏmi) *n.* surgical division of the sternum, performed to allow access to the heart and its major vessels.

sternum (ster-nŭm) *n.* (*pl.* **sterna**) the breastbone: a flat bone extending from the base of the neck to just below the diaphragm and forming the front part of the skeleton of the thorax. The sternum articulates with the collar bones (*see* clavicle) and the costal cartilages of the first seven pairs of ribs. —**sternal** *adj.*

sternutator (ster-new-tay-ter) *n.* an agent that produces sneezing.

steroid (**steer**-oid) *n.* one of a group of organic compounds that include the male and female sex hormones (androgens and oestrogens), the hormones of the adrenal cortex (*see* corticosteroid), progesterone, bile salts, and sterols. Synthetic steroids have been produced for therapeutic purposes.

sterol (**steer**-ol) *n.* one of a group of steroid alcohols. The most important sterols are cholesterol and ergosterol.

stertor (ster-ter) *n.* a snoring type of noisy breathing heard in deeply unconscious patients.

steth- (stetho-) *prefix denoting* the chest.

stethograph (steth-ŏ-grahf) *n.* an instrument for recording chest movements during breathing. —**stethography** (steth-**og**-răfi) *n.*

stethometer (steth-**om**-it-er) *n.* an instrument for measuring the expansion of the chest during breathing.

stethoscope (steth-ŏ-skohp) *n.* an instrument used for listening to sounds within the body (*see* auscultation). A simple stethoscope usually consists of a diaphragm or an open bell-shaped structure (which is applied to the body) connected by rubber or plastic tubes to shaped earpieces for the examiner.

Stevens-Johnson syndrome (stee-věnz jon-sŏn) *n.* an inflammatory condition characterized by fever, large blisters on the skin, and ulceration of the mucous membranes. It may be a severe allergic reaction to certain drugs or it may follow certain infections. [A. M. Stevens (1884–1945) and F. C. Johnson (1894–1934), US paediatricians]

sthenia (sthee-niă) *n.* a state of normal or greater than normal strength. *Compare* asthenia. —**sthenic** (sthen-ik) *adj.*

stibophen (stib-oh-fen) *n.* a sodium-containing salt of antimony administered by injection to treat schistosomiasis.

stigma (stig-mă) *n.* (*pl.* **stigmata**) **1.** a mark that characterizes a particular disease, such as the café-au-lait spots characteristic of neurofibromatosis. **2.** any spot or lesion on the skin.

stilboestrol (stil-bee-strŏl) *n.* a synthetic female sex hormone (*see* oestrogen) administered by mouth or injection to relieve menstrual disorders and symptoms of the menopause, to treat prostate and breast cancer, and to suppress lactation.

stilet (**stylet, stylus**) (sty-lit) *n.* **1.** a slender probe. **2.** a wire placed in the lumen of a catheter to give it rigidity while the instrument is passed along a body canal.

stillbirth (stil-berth) *n.* birth of a fetus that shows no evidence of life (heart beat, respiration, or independent movement) at any time later than 28 weeks after conception. A fetus born dead before this time is known as an abortion or miscarriage.

Still's disease (stilz) *n.* chronic arthritis developing in children before the age of 16. Some authorities confine the diagnosis of Still's disease to the following: a disease of childhood marked by arthritis (often involving several joints) with a swinging fever and a transitory red rash. The condition may be complicated by enlargement of the spleen and lymph nodes and inflammation of the pericardium and iris. [G. F. Still (1868–1941), British physician]

stimulant (stim-yoo-lănt) *n.* an agent that promotes the activity of a body system or function. Amphetamine and caffeine are stimulants of the central nervous system.

stimulus (stim-yoo-lŭs) *n.* (*pl.* **stimuli**) any agent that provokes a response, or particular form of activity, in a cell, tissue, or other structure.

stirrup (sti-rŭp) *n.* (in anatomy) *see* stapes.

stitch (stich) *n.* **1.** a sharp localized pain, commonly in the abdomen, associated with strenuous physical activity. It is a form of cramp. **2.** *see* suture.

stock culture (stok) *n. see* culture.

Stockholm technique (stok-hohm) *n.* a treatment for cervical cancer involving three successive applications of radium.

Stokes-Adams syndrome (stohks-ad-ămz) *n.* attacks of temporary loss of consciousness that occur when blood flow ceases due to ventricular fibrillation or asystole. This syndrome may complicate heart block. It is treated by means of a battery-operated pacemaker. [W. Stokes (1804–78) and R. Adams (1791–1875), Irish physicians]

stoma (stoh-mă) *n.* (*pl.* **stomata**) **1.** (in anatomy) the mouth or any mouthlike part. **2.** (in surgery) the artificial opening of a tube that has been brought to the abdominal surface (*see* colostomy, ileostomy). **s. therapist** a nurse specially trained in the care of these openings and the appliances used with them. **—stomal** *adj.*

stomach (stum-ăk) *n.* a distensible saclike organ that forms part of the alimentary canal between the oesophagus and the duodenum. The stomach lies just below the diaphragm, to the right of the spleen. Its function is to continue the process of digestion that begins in the mouth. Gastric juice, secreted by gastric glands

cardia

oesophagus

fundus

antrum

body

pylorus

greater omentum

Regions of the stomach seen from the front

in the mucosa, together with the churning action of the muscular layers of the stomach, reduces the food to a semiliquid partly digested mass.

stomachic (stŏ-**mak**-ik) *n.* an agent that stimulates the secretory activity of the stomach, used as a tonic to improve the appetite.

stomat- (stomato-) *prefix denoting* the mouth.

stomatitis (stoh-mǎ-**ty**-tis) *n.* inflammation of the mucous lining of the mouth.

stomatology (stoh-mǎ-**tol**-ŏji) *n.* the branch of medicine concerned with diseases of the mouth.

-stomy (-ostomy) *suffix denoting* a surgical opening into an organ or part.

stone (stohn) *n. see* calculus.

stool (stool) *n.* faeces discharged from the anus.

stop needle (stop) *n.* a surgical needle with a shank that has a protruding collar to stop it when the needle has been pushed a prescribed distance into the tissue.

strabismus (heterotropia) (strǎ-**biz**-mŭs) *n.* squint: any abnormal alignment of the two eyes. The strabismus is most commonly horizontal (*see* esotropia, exo-

tropia) but it may also be vertical (*see* hypertropia, hypotropia). Double vision is always experienced, but the image from the deviating eye usually becomes ignored. *See also* heterophoria.

strain (strayn) **1.** *n.* excessive stretching or working of a muscle, resulting in pain and swelling. *Compare* sprain. **2.** *n.* a group of organisms obtained from a particular source or having special properties distinguishing them from other members of the same species. **3.** *vb.* to damage a muscle by overstretching.

strangulated (strang-yoo-**layt**-id) *adj.* describing a part of the body whose blood supply has been interrupted by compression of a blood vessel. *s. hernia see* hernia.

strangulation (strang-yoo-**lay**-shŏn) *n.* the closure of a passage, such as the main airway to the lungs (resulting in the cessation of breathing), a blood vessel, or the gastrointestinal tract.

strangury (strang-yoor-i) *n.* severe pain in the urethra associated with an intense desire to pass urine, resulting from irritation of the base of the bladder. It may also occur in such conditions as cancer of the base of the bladder, cystitis, or prostatitis, when it is accompanied by the painful passage of a few drops of urine.

stratified (strat-i-fyd) *adj.* describing tissue consisting of several layers of cells. *See* epithelium.

stratum (strah-tŭm) *n.* a layer of tissue or cells, such as any of the layers of the epidermis. *s. corneum* the outermost layer of the epidermis.

streak (streek) *n.* (in anatomy) a line, furrow, or narrow band.

Streptobacillus (strep-toh-bă-sil-ŭs) *n.* a genus of Gram-negative aerobic nonmotile rodlike bacteria that tend to form filaments. *S. moniliformis* the cause of rat-bite fever in man.

Streptococcus (strep-toh-kok-ŭs) *n.* a genus of Gram-positive nonmotile spherical bacteria occurring in chains. Most species are saprophytes; some are pathogenic. Many pathogenic species are haemolytic. *S. pneumoniae see* pneumococcus. *S. pyogenes* a species containing different strains that produce infections such as scarlet fever and many exotoxins. *S. viridans* the species associated with bacterial endocarditis. *See also* Lancefield classification, streptokinase.

streptodornase (strep-toh-dor-nayz) *n.* an enzyme produced by some haemolytic bacteria of the genus *Streptococcus* that is capable of liquefying pus. *See also* streptokinase.

streptokinase (strep-toh-ky-nayz) *n.* an enzyme produced by some haemolytic bacteria of the genus *Streptococcus* that is capable of liquefying blood clots. It is injected to treat blockage of blood vessels and is also used in combination with streptodornase, ap-

plied topically or taken by mouth or injection, to liquefy pus and relieve inflammation.

streptolysin (strep-tol-i-sin) *n.* an exotoxin that is produced by *Streptococcus pyogenes* and destroys red blood cells.

Streptomyces (strep-toh-my-seez) *n.* a genus of aerobic mouldlike bacteria. They are important medically as a source of such antibiotics as streptomycin, actinomycin, chloramphenicol, and neomycin.

streptomycin (strep-toh-my-sin) *n.* an antibiotic, derived from the bacterium *Streptomyces griseus*, that is effective against a wide range of bacterial infections; it is administered by mouth or intramuscular injection. Streptomycin is an important drug in tuberculosis therapy but is usually given in conjunction with other drugs because bacteria soon become resistant to it.

stress (stres) *n.* any factor that threatens the health of the body or has an adverse effect on its functioning, such as injury, disease, or worry. Constant stress brings about changes in the balance of hormones in the body.

stretch reflex (myotatic reflex) (strech) *n.* the reflex contraction of a muscle in response to its being stretched.

stria (stry-ă) *n.* (*pl.* **striae**) (in anatomy) a streak, line, or thin band. *striae gravidarum* the lines that appear on the skin of the abdomen of pregnant women, due to stretching and rupture of the elastic fibres. Pinkish during pregnancy, they become white after delivery.

striated muscle (stry-ayt-id) *n.* a tissue comprising the bulk of the body's musculature. It is also known as *skeletal muscle*, because it is attached to the skeleton and is responsible for the movement of bones, and *voluntary muscle*, because it is under voluntary control.

stricture (**strik**-cher) *n.* a narrowing of any tubular structure in the body. A stricture may result from inflammation, muscular spasm, growth of a tumour within the affected part, or from pressure on it by neighbouring organs. *urethral s.* a fibrous narrowing of the urethra, usually resulting from injury or inflammation. The patient has increasing difficulty in passing urine and may develop retention.

stridor (**stry**-dor) *n.* the noise heard on breathing in when the trachea or larynx is obstructed. It tends to be louder and harsher than wheeze.

stroke (apoplexy) (strohk) *n.* a sudden attack of weakness affecting one side of the body, resulting from an interruption to the flow of blood to the brain. The primary disease is in the heart or blood vessels and the effect on the brain is secondary. The flow of blood may be prevented by thrombosis, embolus, or haemorrhage. A stroke can vary in severity from a passing weakness or tingling in a limb to a profound paralysis, coma, and death. *See also* cerebral haemorrhage.

stroma (**stroh**-mă) *n.* **1.** the supportive tissue of an organ, as opposed to the functional tissue (parenchyma). **2.** the spongy framework of protein strands within a red blood cell in which the blood pigment haemoglobin is packed.

strongyloidiasis (strongyloidosis) (stron-ji-loi-**dy**-ă-sis) *n.* an infestation of the small intestine with the parasitic nematode worm *Strongyloides stercoralis*. Larvae enter the body through the skin and migrate to the lungs, where they cause tissue destruction and bleeding. Adult worms burrow into the intestinal wall and may cause ulceration, diarrhoea, abdominal pain, nausea, anaemia, and weakness. Treatment involves use of the drugs thiabendazole and dithiazanine.

strontium (**stron**-tiŭm) *n.* a yellow metallic element, absorption of which causes bone damage when its atoms displace calcium in bone. Symbol: Sr. *strontium-90* a radioactive isotope used in radiotherapy for the contact therapy of skin and eye tumours.

struma (**stroo**-mă) *n.* (*pl.* **strumae**) a swelling of the thyroid gland (*see* goitre).

strychnine (**strik**-neen) *n.* a poisonous alkaloid produced in the seeds of the East Indian tree *Strychnos nux-vomica*. Poisoning causes painful muscular spasms similar to those of tetanus; death is likely to occur from spasm in the respiratory muscles.

stupe (stewp) *n.* any piece of material, such as a wad of cottonwool, soaked in hot water (with or without medication) and used to apply a poultice.

stupor (**stew**-per) *n.* a condition of near unconsciousness, with apparent mental inactivity and reduced ability to respond to stimulation.

Sturge-Weber syndrome (sterj-**web**-er) *n.* angioma associated with a purple birthmark on the face. [W. A. Sturge (1850–1919) and F. P. Weber (1863–1962), British physicians]

stuttering (**stut**-er-ing) *n. see* stammering.

St Vitus' dance (sănt vy-tŭs dahns) *n.* an archaic name for Sydenham's chorea.

stye (sty) *n.* acute inflammation of a gland at the base of an eyelash, caused by bacterial infection. The gland becomes hard and tender and a pus-filled cyst develops at its centre. Medical name: **hordeolum**.

stylet (**sty**-lit) *n. see* stilet.

stylo- *prefix denoting* the styloid process of the temporal bone.

styloid process (**sty**-loid) *n.* **1.** a long slender downward-pointing spine projecting from the lower surface of the temporal bone of the skull. It provides attachment for muscles and ligaments of the tongue and hyoid bone. **2.** any of various other spiny projections.

stylus (**sty**-lŭs) *n.* **1.** a pencil-shaped instrument, commonly used for applying external medication. **2.** *see* stilet.

styptic (**stip**-tik) *n. see* haemostatic.

sub- *prefix denoting* **1.** below; underlying. **2.** partial or slight.

subacute (sub-ă-**kewt**) *adj.* describing a disease that progresses more rapidly than a chronic condition but does not become acute.

subacute bacterial endocarditis *n.* a form of endocarditis characterized by a slow onset and protracted course. It is usually caused by species of *Streptococcus* or *Staphylococcus.*

subacute combined degeneration of the cord *n.* the neurological disorder complicating a deficiency of vitamin B_{12} and pernicious anaemia. There is selective damage to the motor and sensory nerve fibres in the spinal cord, resulting in spasticity of the limbs and a sensory ataxia.

subarachnoid haemorrhage (sub-ă-**rak**-noid) *n.* bleeding into the subarachnoid space, which causes severe headache with stiffness of the neck. The usual source of such a haemorrhage is a cerebral aneurysm that has burst.

subarachnoid space *n.* the space between the arachnoid and pia meninges of the brain and spinal cord, containing circulating cerebrospinal fluid and large blood vessels.

subclavian artery (sub-**klay**-vi-ăn) *n.* either of two arteries supplying blood to the neck and arms. The right subclavian artery branches from the innominate artery; the left subclavian arises directly from the aortic arch.

subclinical (sub-**klin**-ikăl) *adj.* describing a disease that is suspected but is not sufficiently developed to produce definite signs and symptoms in the patient.

subconscious (sub-**kon**-shŭs) *adj.* (in psychoanalysis) denoting the part of the mind that includes memories, motives, and intentions that are momentarily not present in consciousness but can more or less readily be recalled to awareness. *Compare* unconscious.

subcutaneous (sub-kew-**tay**-niŭs) *adj.* beneath the skin. *See also* injection. *s. tissue* loose connective tissue, often fatty, situated under the dermis.

subdural (sub-**dewr**-ăl) *adj.* below the dura mater; relating to the space between the dura mater and arachnoid. *s. haematoma see* haematoma.

subinvolution (sub-in-vŏ-**loo**-shŏn) *n.* failure of a part of the body to return to its normal size after being enlarged. *uterine s.* failure of the womb to revert to its normal size during the six weeks following childbirth. *Compare* hyperinvolution.

subjective (sub-**jek**-tiv) *adj.* apparent to the affected individual but not to others: applied particularly to symptoms.

sublimation (sub-li-**may**-shŏn) *n.* the replacement of socially undesirable means of gratifying motives or desires by means that are socially acceptable. *See also* defence mechanism, repression.

subliminal (sub-**lim**-inăl) *adj.* subconscious: beneath the threshold of conscious perception.

sublingual gland (sub-**ling**-wăl) *n.* one of a pair of salivary glands situated in the lower part of the mouth, one on either side of the tongue.

subluxation (sub-luks-**ay**-shŏn) *n.* partial dislocation of a joint, so that the bone ends are misaligned but still in contact.

submandibular gland (**submaxillary gland**) (sub-man-**dib**-yoo-ler) *n.* one of a pair of salivary glands situated below the parotid glands.

submaxillary gland (sub-maks-**il**-er-i) *n. see* submandibular gland.

submucosa (sub-mew-**koh**-sa) *n.* the layer of loose connective (areolar) tissue underlying a mucous membrane. —**submucosal** *adj.*

submucous (sub-**mew**-kŭs) *adj.* beneath a mucous membrane. *s. resection see* resection.

subnormality (sub-nor-**mal**-iti) *n.* a state of arrested or incomplete development of the mind. *intellectual s.* a scientific concept, denoting the state of those whose intellectual powers fall below some point on a standardized intelligence test. There are very many causes of intellectual subnormality, including Down's syndrome, inherited metabolic disorders, and brain injury. *mental s.* an administrative concept, describing the state of those whose intellectual powers have failed to develop to such an extent that they are in need of care and protection.

subphrenic abscess (sub-**fren**-ik) *n.* a collection of pus in the space below the diaphragm, usually on the right side, between the liver and diaphragm. Causes include postoperative infection and perforation of an organ.

substitution (sub-sti-**tew**-shŏn) *n.* (in psychoanalysis) the replacement of one idea by another: a form of defence mechanism.

substitution therapy *n.* treatment by providing a less harmful alternative to a drug or remedy that a patient has been receiving.

substrate (sub-**strayt**) *n.* the specific substance or substances on which a given enzyme acts.

subsultus (sub-**sul**-tus) *n.* abnormal twitching or tremor of muscles, such as may occur in feverish conditions.

subtertian fever (sub-**ter**-shăn) *n.* a form of malaria resulting from repeated infection by *Plasmodium falciparum* and characterized by continuous fever.

succus (**suk**-ŭs) *n.* any juice or secretion of animal or plant origin. *s. entericus* (*intestinal juice*) the clear alkaline fluid secreted by the glands of the small intestine. It contains mucus and digestive enzymes.

succussion (suk-**ush**-ŏn) *n*. a splashing noise heard when a patient who has a large quantity of fluid in a body cavity, such as the pleural cavity, moves suddenly or is deliberately shaken.

sucrose (**sewk**-rohz) *n*. a carbohydrate consisting of glucose and fructose. It is the principal constituent of cane sugar and sugar beet. The increasing consumption of sucrose in the last 50 years has coincided with an increase in the incidence of dental caries, diabetes, coronary heart disease, and obesity.

suction (**suk**-shŏn) *n*. the use of reduced pressure to remove unwanted fluids or other material through a tube for disposal. During surgery, suction tubes are used to remove blood from the area of operation.

sudamen (s'yoo-**day**-měn) *n*. (*pl*. **sudamina**) a white blister caused by sweat collecting in the sweat ducts or in the layers of the skin.

Sudeck's atrophy (**soo**-deks) *n*. rapid development of osteoporosis in a hand or foot, resulting from injury, infection, or malignancy. [P. H. M. Sudeck (1866–1938), German surgeon]

sudor (s'yoo-dor) *n*. *see* sweat.

sudorific (s'yoo-der-**if**-ik) *n*. *see* diaphoretic.

suffocation (suf-ŏ-**kay**-shŏn) *n*. cessation of breathing as a result of drowning, smothering, etc., leading to unconsciousness or death (*see* asphyxia).

suffusion (sŭ-**few**-*zh*ŏn) *n*. the spreading of a flush across the skin surface, caused by changes in the local blood supply.

sugar (**shuug**-er) *n*. any carbohydrate that dissolves in water, is usually crystalline, and has a sweet taste. Sugars are classified chemically as monosaccharides or disaccharides. Table sugar is virtually 100% pure sucrose. *See also* fructose, glucose, lactose.

suggestibility (sŭ-jes-ti-**bil**-iti) *n*. the state of readily accepting suggestions from others. —**suggestible** *adj*.

suggestion (sŭ-**jes**-chŏn) *n*. (in psychology) the process of changing a person's beliefs, attitudes, or emotions by telling him that they will change. It is sometimes used as a synonym for hypnosis. *See also* autosuggestion.

suicide (**soo**-i-syd) *n*. self-destruction as a deliberate act. **attempted s.** an attempt at self-destruction in which death is averted although the person concerned intended to kill himself (or herself). *Compare* parasuicide.

sulcus (**sul**-kŭs) *n*. (*pl*. **sulci**) one of the many clefts or infoldings of the surface of the brain.

sulphacetamide (sul-fǎ-**set**-ǎ-myd) *n*. a drug of the sulphonamide group that is used in eye drops to treat such infections as conjunctivitis. Trade names: **Albucid, Ocusol**.

sulphadimidine (sul-fǎ-**dy**-mi-deen) *n*. *see* sulphonamide.

sulphadoxine (sul-fǎ-**doks**-een) *n*. *see* sulphonamide.

sulpha drug (**sul**-fǎ) *n*. *see* sulphonamide.

sulphafurazole (sul-fǎ-**fewr**-ǎ-zohl) *n*. *see* sulphonamide.

sulphaguanidine (sul-fǎ-**gwan**-i-deen) *n*. *see* sulphonamide.

sulphamethizole (sul-fǎ-**meth**-i-zohl) *n*. *see* sulphonamide.

sulphamethoxazole (sul-fǎ-meth-**oks**-ǎ-zohl) *n*. a drug of the sulphonamide group. It is taken by mouth and is effective in the treatment of infections of the respiratory, urinary, and gastrointestinal tracts and the skin. The drug is frequently administered in a combined preparation with trimethoprim (*see* co-trimoxazole). Trade name: **Gantanol**.

sulphasalazine (sul-fă-sal-ă-zeen) *n.* a drug of the sulphonamide group, used in the treatment of ulcerative colitis. It is given by mouth or in the form of suppositories. Trade name: **Salazopyrin**.

sulphinpyrazone (sul-fin-py-răzohn) *n.* a uricosuric drug given by mouth for the treatment of chronic gout. It should not be taken by patients with impaired kidney function. Trade name: **Anturan**.

sulphonamide (sulpha drug) (sulfon-ă-myd) *n.* one of a group of drugs, derived from sulphanilamide (a red dye), that prevent the growth of bacteria. Sulphonamides are usually given by mouth and are effective against a variety of infections. Most of them are rapidly absorbed from the stomach and small intestine and should be taken at frequent intervals. Some, such as *sulphadoxine* (used for leprosy and malaria), are long-acting and need be taken only once a day. Others, including *sulphaguanidine*, are poorly absorbed and are therefore used to treat infections of the gastrointestinal tract. Many sulphonamides are rapidly excreted and very soluble in the urine and are used to treat infections of the urinary tract; examples are *sulphadimidine*, *sulphafurazole*, and *sulphamethizole*. Sulphonamides should be avoided in jaundice and kidney disease and in patients allergic to these drugs.

sulphone (sul-fohn) *n.* one of a group of drugs closely related to the sulphonamides. Sulphones possess powerful activity against the bacteria that cause leprosy and tuberculosis. The best known sulphone is dapsone.

sulphonylurea (sul-fŏ-nil-yoor-iă) *n.* one of a group of drugs, derived from a sulphonamide, that reduce the level of glucose in the blood. These drugs are given by mouth and are used in the treatment of diabetes mellitus. They include chlorpropamide, tolazamide, and tolbutamide.

sulphur (sul-fer) *n.* a nonmetallic element that is active against fungi and parasites. It is a constituent of ointments and other preparations used in the treatment of skin disorders and infections. Symbol: S.

sulphuric acid (sul-fewr-ik) *n.* a powerful corrosive acid, widely used in industry. Swallowing the acid causes severe burning of the mouth and throat. The patient should drink large quantities of milk or water or white of egg; gastric lavage should not be delayed. Formula: H_2SO_4.

sulthiame (sul-th'y-aym) *n.* an anticonvulsant drug administered by mouth in the treatment of severe forms of epilepsy. Trade name: **Ospolot**.

sunburn (sun-bern) *n.* damage to the skin by prolonged or unaccustomed exposure to the sun's rays. Sunburn may vary from reddening of the skin to the development of large painful fluid-filled blisters (*see* burn).

sunstroke (sun-strohk) *n. see* heatstroke.

super- *prefix denoting* **1.** above; overlying. **2.** extreme or excessive.

superciliary (soo-per-**sil**-i-er-i) *adj.* of or relating to the eyebrows (*supercilia*).

superego (soo-per-**ee**-goh) *n.* (in psychoanalysis) the part of the mind that functions as a moral conscience or judge. The superego is the result of the incorporation of parental injunctions into the child's mind.

superfecundation (soo-per-fee-kŭn-day-shŏn) *n.* the fertilization of two or more ova of the same age by spermatozoa from different males. *See* superfetation.

superfetation (soo-per-fee-**tay**-shŏn) *n.* the fertilization of a second ovum some time after the start of pregnancy, resulting in two fetuses of different maturity in the same womb.

superficial (soo-per-**fish**-ăl) *adj.* (in anatomy) situated at or close to a surface. Superficial blood vessels are those close to the surface of the skin.

superinfection (soo-per-in-**fek**-shŏn) *n.* an infection arising during the course of another infection and caused by a different microorganism, which is usually resistant to the drugs used to treat the primary infection.

superinvolution (soo-per-in-vŏ-loo-shŏn) *n. see* hyperinvolution.

superior (soo-**peer**-i-er) *adj.* (in anatomy) situated uppermost in the body in relation to another structure or surface.

supination (soo-pi-**nay**-shŏn) *n.* the act of turning the hand so that the palm is uppermost. *Compare* pronation.

supinator (**soo**-pi-nay-ter) *n.* a muscle of the forearm that extends from the elbow to the shaft of the radius. It supinates the forearm and hand.

supine (**soo**-pyn) *adj.* **1.** lying on the back or with the face upwards. **2.** (of the forearm) in the position in which the palm of the hand faces upwards. *Compare* prone.

suppository (sŭ-**poz**-it-er-i) *n.* a medicinal preparation in solid form suitable for insertion into a body cavity. *rectal s.* a suppository that is inserted into the rectum. It may contain drugs that act locally in the rectum or anus, drugs that are absorbed and act at other sites, or a simple lubricant. *vaginal s. see* pessary.

suppression (sŭ-**presh**-ŏn) *n.* **1.** the cessation or complete inhibition of any physiological activity. **2.** treatment that removes the outward signs of an illness or prevents its progress. **3.** (in psychology) a defence mechanism by which a person consciously and deliberately ignores an idea that is unpleasant to him.

suppuration (sup-yoor-**ay**-shŏn) *n.* the formation of pus.

supra- *prefix denoting* above; over.

supraorbital (soo-pră-**or**-bit'l) *adj.* of or relating to the area above the eye orbit. *s. reflex* the closing of the eyelids when the supraorbital nerve is struck, due to contraction of the muscle surrounding the orbit.

suprapubic (soo-pră-**pew**-bik) *adj.* above the pubic bone. *s. cystotomy see* cystotomy.

suprarenal glands (soo-pră-**ree**-năl) *pl. n. see* adrenal glands.

suramin (**s'yoor**-ă-min) *n.* a nonmetallic drug used in the treatment of trypanosomiasis. It is usually given by slow intravenous injection.

surfactant (ser-**fak**-tănt) *n*. a wetting agent: a substance that reduces surface tension. A surfactant is secreted by the cells (pneumocytes) lining the alveoli of the lungs to prevent the alveolar walls from sticking together.

blanket (skin)   continuous (skin)

surgeon (**serj**-ŏn) *n*. a qualified medical practitioner who specializes in surgery.

surgery (**serj**-er-i) *n*. the branch of medicine that treats injuries, deformities, or disease by operation or manipulation. *See also* cryosurgery, microsurgery. —**surgical** *adj*.

vertical mattress (skin)   interrupted (skin)

surgical neck (**serj**-ikǎl) *n*. the constriction of the shaft of the humerus, below the head. It is frequently the point at which fracture of the humerus occurs.

surgical spirit *n*. methylated spirit, usually with small amounts of castor oil and oil of wintergreen: used to sterilize the skin before surgery, injections, etc.

surrogate (**su**-rŏ-găt) *n*. (in psychology) a person or object in someone's life that functions as a substitute for another person.

purse string (intestine)

Types of surgical suture

susceptibility (sŭ-sep-ti-**bil**-iti) *n*. lack of immunity to disease. It is partly influenced by vaccination or other methods of increasing resistance to specific diseases.

suspensory bandage (su-**spen**-ser-i) *n*. a bandage arranged to support a hanging part of the body, such as the scrotum.

suspensory ligament *n*. a ligament that serves to support or suspend an organ, such as the lens of the eye, in position.

sustentaculum (sus-ten-**tak**-yoolŭm) *n*. any anatomical structure that supports another structure. —**sustentacular** *adj*.

suture (**soo**-cher) **1**. *n*. (in anatomy) a type of immovable joint, found particularly in the skull, characterized by a minimal amount of connective tissue between the two bones. **2**. *n*. (in surgery) the closure of a wound or incision with material such as silk or catgut, to facilitate the healing process. **3**. *n*. the material – silk, catgut, nylon, or wire – used to sew up a wound. **4**. *vb*. to close a wound by suture.

suxamethonium (suks-ă-měth-**oh**-niŭm) *n*. a drug that relaxes voluntary muscle (*see* muscle relaxant). It is administered by intravenous injection and is used mainly to produce muscle relaxation during surgery. Trade name: **Scoline**.

swab (swob) *n.* a pad of absorbent material (such as cotton), sometimes attached to a stick or wire, used for cleaning out or applying medication to wounds, operation sites, or body cavities.

swallowing (deglutition) (swol-oh-ing) *n.* the process by which food is transferred from the mouth to the oesophagus. Voluntary raising of the tongue forces food backwards towards the pharynx. This stimulates reflex actions in which the larynx and the nasal passages are closed so that food does not enter the trachea.

sweat (swet) *n.* the watery fluid secreted by the sweat glands. Its principal constituents in solution are sodium chloride and urea. The secretion of sweat is a means of excreting nitrogenous waste; it also has a cooling effect as the sweat evaporates from the surface of the skin. Anatomical name: **sudor**. *s. gland* a simple coiled tubular exocrine gland that lies in the dermis of the skin. Sweat glands occur over most of the surface of the body; they are particularly abundant in the armpits, on the soles of the feet and palms of the hands, and on the forehead.

sycosis (sy-koh-sis) *n.* inflammation of the hair follicles caused by bacterial infection. It commonly affects the beard area (*s. barbae*) and may cause intense itching.

Sydenham's chorea (sid-ĕn-ămz) *n.* see chorea. [T. Sydenham (1624–89), English physician]

symbiosis (sim-by-oh-sis) *n.* an intimate and obligatory association between two different species of organism (*symbionts*) in which there is mutual aid and benefit. *Compare* commensal, parasite.

symblepharon (sim-blef-er-on) *n.* a condition in which the eyelid adheres to the eyeball. It is usually the result of acid or alkali burns to the conjunctiva.

symbolism (sim-bŏl-izm) *n.* (in psychology) the process of representing an object or an idea by something else. Psychoanalytic theorists hold that conscious ideas frequently act as symbols for unconscious thoughts and that this is particularly evident in dreaming, in free association, and in the formation of psychological symptoms. —**symbolic** (sim-bol-ik) *adj.*

Syme's amputation (symz) *n.* amputation of the foot just above the ankle joint. [J. Syme (1799–1870), British surgeon]

symmetry (sim-it-ri) *n.* (in anatomy) the state of opposite parts of an organ or parts at opposite sides of the body corresponding to each other.

sympathectomy (sim-pă-thek-tŏmi) *n.* the surgical division of sympathetic nerve fibres. It is done to minimize the effects of normal or excessive sympathetic activity.

sympathetic nervous system (sim-pă-thet-ik) *n.* one of the two divisions of the autonomic nervous system, having fibres that leave the central nervous system in the thoracic and lumbar regions and are distributed to the blood vessels, sweat glands, salivary glands, heart, lungs, intestines, and other abdominal organs. The nerve endings release noradrenaline as a neutrotransmitter.

sympathin (sim-pă-thin) *n.* the name given by early physiologists to the substances released from sympathetic nerve endings, now known to be a mixture of adrenaline and noradrenaline.

sympatholytic (sim-pă-thoh-**lit**-ik) *n.* a drug that opposes the effects of the sympathetic nervous system. Sympatholytic drugs include guanethidine, phentolamine, and tolazoline.

sympathomimetic (sim-pă-thoh-mi-**met**-ik) *n.* a drug that has the effect of stimulating the sympathetic nervous system. The actions of sympathomimetic drugs are adrenergic (resembling those of noradrenaline). Sympathomimetic drugs include phenylephrine, salbutamol, ephedrine, and isoprenaline.

sympathy (**sim**-pă-thi) *n.* (in physiology) a reciprocal influence exercised by different parts of the body on one another.

symphysiectomy (sim-fizi-**ek**-tŏmi) *n.* removal of a part of the pubic symphysis in order to aid childbirth.

symphysiotomy (symphyseotomy) (sim-fizi-**ot**-ŏmi) *n.* incision into the pubic symphysis in order to enlarge the diameter of the birth passage and aid delivery.

symphysis (**sim**-fi-sis) *n.* **1.** a joint in which the bones are separated by fibrocartilage, which minimizes movement and makes the bony structure rigid. Examples are the pubic symphysis (*see* pubis) and the joints of the backbone, which are separated by intervertebral discs. **2.** the line that marks the fusion of two bones that were separate at an early stage of development.

symptom (**simp**-tŏm) *n.* an indication of a disease or disorder noticed by the patient himself. *Compare* sign.

symptomatology (semeiology) (simp-tŏm-ă-**tol**-ŏji) *n.* **1.** the branch of medicine concerned with the study of symptoms of disease. **2.** the symptoms of a disease, collectively.

syn- (sym-) *prefix denoting* union or fusion.

synalgia (sin-**al**-jiă) *n. see* referred pain.

synapse (**sy**-naps) *n.* the minute gap across which nerve impulses pass from one neurone to the next, at the end of a nerve fibre. Reaching a synapse, an impulse causes the release of a neurotransmitter, which diffuses across the gap and triggers an electrical impulse in the next neurone. *See also* neuromuscular junction.

synarthrosis (sin-arth-**roh**-sis) *n.* an immovable joint in which the bones are united by fibrous tissue. Examples are the cranial sutures. *See also* gomphosis, schindylesis.

synchondrosis (sin-kon-**droh**-sis) *n.* a slightly movable joint (*see* amphiarthrosis) in which the surfaces of the bones are separated by hyaline cartilage, as occurs between the ribs and sternum.

synchysis (**sink**-i-sis) *n.* softening of the vitreous humour of the eye.

syncope (fainting) (**sink**-ŏ-pi) *n.* loss of consciousness induced by a temporarily insufficient flow of blood to the brain. It commonly occurs in otherwise healthy people and may be caused by an emotional shock, by standing for prolonged periods, or by injury and profuse bleeding.

syncytium (sin-**sit**-iŭm) *n.* (*pl.* **syncytia**) a mass of protoplasm containing several nuclei. Muscle fibres are syncytia.

syndactyly (dactylion) (sin-**dak**-tili) *n.* congenital fusion of the fingers or toes. It varies in severity from no more than marked webbing of two or more fingers to virtually complete union of all the digits.

syndesm- (syndesmo-) *prefix denoting* connective tissue, particularly ligaments.

syndesmology (sin-des-**mol**-ŏji) *n.* the branch of anatomy dealing with joints and their components.

syndesmosis (sin-des-**moh**-sis) *n.* an immovable joint in which the bones are separated by connective tissue. An example is the articulation between the bases of the tibia and fibula.

syndrome (**sin**-drohm) *n.* a combination of signs and/or symptoms that forms a distinct clinical picture indicative of a particular disorder.

synechia (sin-**ek**-iă) *n.* an adhesion between the iris and another part of the eye. *anterior s.* synechia between the iris and the cornea. *posterior s.* synechia between the iris and the lens.

syneresis (sin-**eer**-i-sis) *n.* contraction of a blood clot to produce a firm mass that seals the damaged blood vessels.

synergist (**sin**-er-jist) *n.* **1.** a drug that interacts with another to produce increased activity, which is greater than the sum of the effects of the two drugs given separately. **2.** a muscle that acts with a prime mover (agonist) in making a particular movement. —**synergism** *n.*

syngraft (**sin**-grahft) *n. see* isograft.

synoptophore (sin-**op**-toh-for) *n. see* amblyoscope.

synostosis (sin-os-**toh**-sis) *n.* the joining by ossification of two adjacent bones. It occurs, for example, at the cranial sutures.

synovectomy (sy-noh-**vek**-tŏmi) *n.* surgical removal of the synovium of a joint. This is performed in cases of chronic synovitis, when other measures have been ineffective.

synovia (synovial fluid) (sy-**noh**-vi-ă) *n.* the thick colourless lubricating fluid that surrounds a joint or a bursa and fills a tendon sheath. It is secreted by the synovial membrane.

synovial joint (sy-**noh**-vi-ăl) *n. see* diarthrosis.

synovial membrane (synovium) *n.* the membrane that forms the sac enclosing a freely movable joint (*see* diarthrosis). It secretes the lubricating synovial fluid.

synovioma (sy-noh-vi-**oh**-mă) *n.* a benign or malignant tumour of the synovial membrane.

synovitis (sy-noh-**vy**-tis) *n.* inflammation of the synovial membrane, resulting in pain and swelling (arthritis). It is caused by injury, infection, or rheumatic disease.

synovium (sy-**noh**-vi-ŭm) *n. see* synovial membrane.

synthesis (**sin**-thi-sis) *n.* the formation of complex substances from simple constituents. —**synthetic** (sin-**thet**-ik) *adj.*

syphilide (syphilid) (**sif**-i-lyd) *n.* the skin rash that appears in the second stage of syphilis. Syphilides occur in crops that may last from a few days to several months. They denote a highly infectious stage of the disease.

syphilis (**sif**-i-lis) *n.* a chronic venereal disease caused by the bacterium *Treponema pallidum*. Bacteria usually enter the body during sexual intercourse; they may also pass from an infected pregnant woman across the placenta to the developing fetus, resulting in the disease being present at birth (*congenital s.*). The primary symptom is a hard ulcer (chancre) at the site of infection. Secondary stage symptoms include fever, malaise, general enlargement of lymph nodes, and a faint red rash on the chest. After months, or even years, the disease enters its tertiary stage with widespread formation of tumour-like masses (gummas). Tertiary syphilis may cause serious damage to the heart and blood vessels (*cardiovascular s.*) or to the brain and spinal cord (*neurosyphilis*), resulting in tabes dorsalis, blindness, and general paralysis of the insane. *See also* bejel. —**syphilitic** (sif-i-**lit**-ik) *adj.*

syring- (**syringo-**) *prefix denoting* a tube or long cavity, especially the central canal of the spinal cord.

syringe (si-**rinj**) *n.* an instrument consisting of a piston in a tight-fitting tube that is attached to a hollow needle or thin tube. A syringe is used to give injections, remove material from a part of the body, or to wash out a cavity.

syringobulbia (si-ring-oh-**bulb**-iă) *n.* see syringomyelia.

syringocystadenoma (syringoma) (si-ring-oh-sist-ad-i-**noh**-mă) *n.* a multiple benign tumour of the sweat glands, which shows as small hard swellings in the skin.

syringomyelia (si-ring-oh-my-**ee**-liă) *n.* a disease of the spinal cord in which longitudinal cavities form within the cord in the cervical (neck) region. Characteristically there is weakness and wasting of the muscles in the hands with a loss of awareness of pain and temperature. An extension of the cavitation into the lower brainstem is called *syringobulbia*. Cerebellar ataxia, a partial loss of pain sensation in the face, and weakness of the tongue and palate may occur.

syringomyelocele (si-ring-oh-my-**ĕl**-oh-seel) *n.* protrusion of the spinal cord through a defect in the spine together with a fluid-filled sac continuous with the central canal of the cord.

system (**sis**-tĕm) *n.* (in anatomy) a group of organs and tissues associated with a particular physiological function, such as the nervous system or respiratory system.

systemic (sis-**tem**-ik) *adj.* relating to or affecting the body as a whole, rather than individual parts and organs. *s. circulation see* circulation.

systole (**sis**-tŏ-li) *n.* the period of the cardiac cycle during which the heart contracts. —**systolic** (sis-**tol**-ik) *adj.*

systolic pressure *n. see* blood pressure.

T

tabes dorsalis (**locomotor ataxia**) (**tay**-beez dor-**sah**-lis) *n.* a form of neurosyphilis occurring 5–20 years after the original venereal infection. The infecting organisms progressively destroy the sensory nerves. Severe stabbing pains in the legs and trunk, an unsteady gait, and loss of bladder control are common. *See also* syphilis, general paralysis of the insane.

tablet (**tab**-lit) *n.* (in pharmacy) a small disc containing one or more drugs, made by compressing a powdered form of the drug(s). It is taken by mouth.

tabo-paresis (tay-boh-pă-**ree**-sis) *n.* a late effect of syphilitic infection of the nervous system in which the patient shows features of tabes dorsalis and general paralysis of the insane.

TAB vaccine *n.* a combined vaccine used to produce immunity against the diseases typhoid, paratyphoid A, and paratyphoid B.

tachy- *prefix denoting* fast; rapid.

tachycardia (tak-i-**kar**-diă) *n.* an increase in the heart rate above normal. *sinus t.* tachycardia that may occur normally with exercise or excitement. It may also be due to illness, such as fever.

tachyphrasia (tak-i-**fray**-ziă) *n.* rapid and voluble speech, such as that encountered in mania.

tachyphrenia (tak-i-**free**-niă) *n.* excessive rapidity of the mental processes, as in mania.

tachypnoea (tak-ip-**nee**-ă) *n.* rapid breathing.

tactile (**tak**-tyl) *adj.* relating to or affecting the sense of touch.

taenia (**tee**-niă) *n.* (*pl.* **taeniae**) a flat ribbon-like anatomical structure. *taeniae coli* the longitudinal ribbon-like muscles of the colon.

Taenia *n.* a genus of large tapeworms, some of which are parasites of the human intestine. *T. saginata* the beef tapeworm: the commonest tapeworm parasite of man. *See* taeniasis. *T. solium* the pork tapeworm. Its larval stage may develop in man, in whom it may cause cysticercosis.

taeniacide (**taenicide**) (**tee**-niă-syd) *n.* an agent that kills tapeworms.

taeniafuge (**tee**-niă-fewj) *n.* an agent, such as dichlorophen, that eliminates tapeworms from the body of their host.

taeniasis (tee-ny-ă-sis) *n.* an infestation with tapeworms of the genus *Taenia*, resulting from ingestion of raw or undercooked meat containing the larval stage of the parasite. Symptoms include increased appetite, hunger pains, weakness, and weight loss. *See also* cysticercosis.

Tagamet (**tag**-a-met) *n. see* cimetidine.

tal- (**talo-**) *prefix denoting* the ankle bone (talus).

talc (tal'k) *n.* a soft white powder consisting of magnesium silicate, used as a dusting powder.

talipes (**tal**-i-peez) *n.* club-foot: a deformity of one or both feet in which the patient cannot stand with the sole of the foot flat on the ground. *t. equinovarus* talipes in which the foot is twisted downwards and inwards so that the patient walks on the outer edge of the upper surface of his foot. *t. valgus* talipes in which the sole of the foot is twisted outwards. *t. varus* talipes in which the sole of the foot is turned inwards.

talus (**astragalus**) (**tay**-lŭs) *n.* the ankle bone. It forms part of the tarsus, articulating with the tibia above, the fibula to the side, and the calcaneus below.

tampon (**tam**-pon) *n.* a pack of gauze, cotton wool, or other absorbent material used to plug a cavity or canal in order to absorb blood or secretions.

tamponade (tam-pon-**ayd**) *n.* **1.** the insertion of a tampon. **2.** abnormal pressure on a part of the body; for example, as caused by the presence of excessive fluid between the pericardium and the heart.

taste

tantalum (tant-ă-lŭm) *n.* a rare heavy metal used in surgery. Tantalum sutures and plates are used for repair of defects in the bones of the skull. Symbol: Ta.

tapeworm (tayp-werm) *n.* any of a group of flatworms that have a long thin ribbon-like body and live as parasites in the intestines of man and other vertebrates. The body of a tapeworm consists of a head (*see* scolex), a short neck, and a chain of separate segments (*see* proglottis). Man is the primary host for some tapeworms (*see* Taenia). However, other genera are also medically important (*see* Echinococcus).

tapotement (ta-poht-**mahn**) *n.* a technique used in massage in which a part of the body is struck rapidly and repeatedly with the hands.

tapping (tap-ing) *n. see* paracentesis.

tar (tar) *n.* a blackish viscous liquid produced by the destructive distillation of pine wood (*pine t.*) or coal (*coal t.*), used in skin preparations to treat eczema and psoriasis. As a constituent of cigarettes, tar is known to have carcinogenic properties.

tars- (**tarso-**) *prefix denoting* 1. the ankle; tarsal bones. 2. the edge of the eyelid.

tarsal (tar-săl) 1. *adj.* relating to the bones of the ankle and foot (tarsus). 2. *adj.* relating to the eyelid, especially to its supporting tissue (tarsus). *t. glands see* meibomian glands. 3. *n.* any of the bones forming the tarsus.

tarsalgia (tar-sal-jiă) *n.* aching pain arising from the tarsus in the foot.

tarsectomy (tar-sek-tŏmi) *n.* 1. surgical excision of the tarsal bones

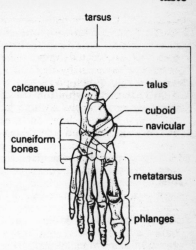

Bones of the right ankle and foot

of the foot. 2. surgical removal of a section of the tarsus of the eyelid.

tarsitis (tar-sy-tis) *n.* inflammation of the eyelid.

tarsorrhaphy (tars-o-răfi) *n.* an operation in which the upper and lower eyelids are joined together. It is performed to protect the cornea or to allow a corneal injury to heal.

tarsus (tar-sŭs) *n.* (*pl.* **tarsi**) 1. the seven bones of the ankle and proximal part of the foot (see illustration). The tarsus articulates with the metatarsals distally and with the tibia and fibula proximally. 2. the firm fibrous connective tissue that forms the basis of each eyelid.

tartar (tar-ter) *n.* an obsolete term for calculus, the hard deposit that forms on the teeth.

tartar emetic *n. see* antimony potassium tartrate.

taste (tayst) *n.* the sense for the appreciation of the flavour of substances in the mouth. There are four basic taste sensations – sweet, bitter, sour, and salt. *t. buds* the sensory receptors concerned with the sense of taste. They are located in the epithelium that covers the surface of the tongue and in the soft palate, the epiglottis, and parts of the pharynx. When a taste cell is stimulated by the presence of a dissolved substance impulses are sent via nerve fibres to the brain.

taurine (tor-een) *n.* an amino acid that is a constituent of the bile salt taurocholate and also functions as a neurotransmitter in the central nervous system.

taurocholic acid (tor-oh-**koh**-lik) *n.* see bile acids.

taxis (**tak**-sis) *n.* (in surgery) the returning to a normal position of displaced bones, organs, or other parts by manipulation only.

Tay-Sachs disease (amaurotic familial idiocy) (tay-**saks**) *n.* an inherited disorder of lipid metabolism (*see* lipidosis) in which abnormal accumulation of lipid in the brain leads to blindness, mental retardation, and death in infancy. [W. Tay (1843–1927), British physician; B. Sachs (1858–1944), US neurologist]

T bandage *n.* a T-shaped bandage used for the perineum and sometimes the head.

TCP *Trade name.* a solution of trichlorphenol: an effective antiseptic for minor skin injuries and irritations. It may also be used as a gargle for colds and sore throats.

tears (teerz) *pl. n.* the fluid secreted by the lacrimal glands to keep the front of the eyeballs moist and clean. Tears contain lysozyme, an enzyme that destroys bacteria.

technetium-131 (tek-**nee**-shi-ŭm) *n.* an isotope of the artificial radioactive element technetium. It emits gamma radiation and is used as a tracer in the technique of scintigraphy.

tectospinal tract (tek-toh-**spy**-năl) *n.* a tract that conveys nerve impulses from the midbrain to the spinal cord in the cervical (neck) region.

tectum (tek-tŭm) *n.* the roof of the midbrain, behind and above the cerebral aqueduct.

teeth (teeth) *pl. n. see* tooth.

tegmen (teg-měn) *n.* (*pl.* **tegmina**) a structure that covers an organ or part of an organ.

tegmentum (teg-men-tŭm) *n.* the region of the midbrain below and in front of the cerebral aqueduct.

tel- (tele-, telo-) *prefix denoting* **1.** end or ending. **2.** distance.

tela (**tee**-lă) *n.* any thin weblike tissue. *t. choroidea* a folded double layer of pia mater containing numerous small blood vessels that extends into several of the ventricles of the brain.

telangiectasis (til-an-ji-**ek**-tă-sis) *n.* (*pl.* **telangiectases**) a localized collection of distended blood capillary vessels. It is recognized as a red spot, sometimes spidery in appearance, that blanches on pressure. Telangiectases may be found in the skin or the lining of the mouth, gastrointestinal, respiratory, and urinary passages.

teleceptor (**tel**-i-sep-ter) *n.* a sensory receptor that is capable of responding to distant stimuli.

telecurietherapy (tel-i-kewr-i-**th'e**-ră-pi) *n.* a form of radiotherapy in which penetrating radiation is directed at a patient from a distance.

telencephalon (tel-en-**sef**-ă-lon) *n.* *see* cerebrum.

teleradiography (tel-i-ray-di-**og**-răfi) *n.* a form of radiography in which the X-ray source is situated about 2 metres from the patient, which produces X-ray pictures with less distortion.

temple (tem-pŭl) *n.* the region of the head in front of and above each ear.

temporal (temp-er-ăl) *adj.* of or relating to the temple. *t. arteritis* *see* arteritis. *t. artery* a branch of the external carotid artery that supplies blood mainly to the temple and scalp. *t. bone* either of a pair of bones of the cranium. The *squamous* portion forms part of the side of the cranium. The *petrous* part contributes to the base of the skull and contains the middle and inner ears. *See also* skull. *t. lobe* one of the main divisions of the cerebral cortex in each hemisphere of the brain, lying at the side within the temple. Areas of the cortex in this lobe are concerned with the appreciation of sound and spoken language. *t. lobe epilepsy see* epilepsy.

temporalis (tem-per-**ay**-lis) *n.* a fan-shaped muscle at the side of the head, extending from the temporal fossa to the mandible. This muscle lifts the lower jaw.

temporo- *prefix denoting* 1. the temple. 2. the temporal lobe of the brain.

temporomandibular joint (tem-per-oh-man-**dib**-yoo-ler) *n.* the articulation between the mandible and the temporal bone.

tenaculum (tin-ak-yoo-lŭm) *n.* 1. a sharp wire hook with a handle, used in surgical operations to

pick up pieces of tissue or the cut end of an artery. 2. a band of fibrous tissue that holds a part of the body in place.

tendinitis (ten-di-ny-tis) *n.* inflammation of a tendon. It occurs most commonly after excessive overuse but is sometimes due to bacterial infection (e.g. gonorrhoea) or a generalized rheumatic disease (e.g. rheumatoid arthritis, ankylosing spondylitis). *See also* tennis elbow. *Compare* tenosynovitis.

tendon (ten-dŏn) *n.* a tough whitish cord, consisting of numerous parallel bundles of collagen fibres, that serves to attach a muscle to a bone. Tendons assist in concentrating the pull of the muscle on a small area of bone. *t. sheath* a tubular sac, lined with synovial membrane and containing synovial fluid, that surrounds some tendons. *See also* aponeurosis. —**tendinous** (ten-din-ŭs) *adj.*

tendovaginitis (tenovaginitis) (ten-doh-vaj-i-ny-tis) *n.* inflammatory thickening of the fibrous sheath containing one or more tendons, usually caused by repeated minor injury. It usually occurs' at the back of the thumb (*de Quervain's t.*) and results in pain on wringing the wrists.

tenesmus (tin-ez-mŭs) *n.* a sensation of the desire to defecate, which is continuous or recurs frequently, without the production of significant amounts of faeces. It may be due to proctitis, prolapse of the rectum, rectal tumour, or irritable bowel syndrome.

tennis elbow (ten-iss) *n.* a painful inflammation of the tendon at the outer border of the elbow, caused by overuse of the forearm muscles. *See also* tendinitis.

teno- *prefix denoting* a tendon.

Tenon's capsule (tě-**nonz**) *n*. the fibrous tissue that lines the orbit and surrounds the eyeball. [J. R. Tenon (1724–1816), French surgeon]

tenoplasty (**ten**-oh-plasti) *n*. surgical repair of a ruptured or severed tendon.

tenorrhaphy (těn-o-**răfi**) *n*. the surgical operation of uniting the ends of divided tendons by suture.

tenosynovitis (peritendinitis) (ten-oh-sy-noh-**vy**-tis) *n*. inflammation of a tendon sheath, producing pain, swelling, and an audible creaking on movement. It may result from a bacterial infection or occur as part of a rheumatic disease.

tenotomy (tě-**not**-ŏmi) *n*. surgical division of a tendon. This may be necessary to correct a joint deformity caused by tendon shortening.

tenovaginitis (ten-oh-vaj-i-**ny**-tis) *n*. *see* tendovaginitis.

tensor (**ten**-ser) *n*. any muscle that causes stretching or tensing of a part of the body.

tent (tent) *n*. **1.** an enclosure of material (usually transparent plastic) around a patient in bed, into which a gas or vapour can be passed as part of treatment. *oxygen t.* a tent into which oxygen is passed. **2.** a piece of dried vegetable material, usually a seaweed stem, shaped to fit into an orifice, such as the cervical canal. As it absorbs moisture it expands, dilating the orifice.

tentorium (ten-tor-iŭm) *n*. a curved infolded sheet of dura mater that separates the cerebellum below from the occipital lobes of the cerebral hemispheres above.

terat- (terato-) *prefix denoting* a monster or congenital abnormality.

teratogen (te-ră-toh-jen) *n*. any substance, agent, or process that induces the formation of developmental abnormalities in a fetus. Known teratogens include the drug thalidomide, German measles, and irradiation with X-rays. *Compare* mutagen. —**teratogenic** *adj*.

teratogenesis (te-ră-toh-**jen**-i-sis) *n*. the process leading to developmental abnormalities in the fetus.

teratology (te-ră-**tol**-ŏji) *n*. the study of developmental abnormalities and their causes.

teratoma (te-ră-**toh**-mă) *n*. a tumour composed of a number of tissues not usually found at that site. Teratomas most frequently occur in the testis and ovary, possibly derived from remnants of embryological cells.

terbutaline (ter-**bew**-tă-leen) *n*. a bronchodilator drug administered by mouth, injection, or inhalation in the treatment of asthma, bronchitis, and other respiratory disorders. Trade name: **Bricanyl**.

teres (te-reez) *n*. either of two muscles of the shoulder, extending from the scapula to the humerus. *t. major* the muscle that rotates the arm inwards. *t. minor* the muscle that rotates the arm outwards.

Terramycin (te-ră-**my**-sin) *n*. *see* oxytetracycline.

tertian fever (ter-shăn) *n*. a type of malaria, caused by *Plasmodium ovale* or *P. vivax*, in which there is a two-day interval between fever attacks.

test (test) *n.* a laboratory examination or chemical analysis to determine the presence of a specific substance, microorganism, disease, etc. (See individual entries for named tests.)

testicle (test-ikŭl) *n.* either of the pair of male sex organs within the scrotum. It consists of the testis and its system of ducts (the vasa efferentia and epididymis).

testis (tes-tis) *n.* (*pl.* **testes**) either of the pair of male sex organs that produce spermatozoa and secrete the male sex hormone androgen under the control of gonadotrophins from the pituitary gland. The testes are contained within the scrotum (*see* reproductive system). *See also* spermatogenesis.

test meal *n.* a standard meal given to stimulate secretion of digestive juices, which can then be withdrawn by tube and measured as a test of digestive function. *fractional t. m.* a gruel preparation to stimulate gastric secretion. This test has been replaced by tests using histamine or pentagastrin as secretory stimulants.

testosterone (test-ost-er-ohn) *n.* the principal male sex hormone (*see* androgen).

test-tube baby (test-tewb) *n.* a baby born to a woman as a result of fertilization of one of her ova by her husband's sperm outside her body. Several ova are removed from the mother-to-be, mixed with sperm in a culture medium, and incubated until the blastocyst forms. The blastocyst is then implanted in the mother's womb and the pregnancy continues normally thereafter.

tetan- (**tetano-**) *prefix denoting* **1.** tetanus. **2.** tetany.

tetanus (**lockjaw**) (tet-ăn-ŭs) *n.* an acute infectious disease, affecting the nervous system, caused by the bacterium *Clostridium tetani.* Infection occurs by contamination of wounds by bacterial spores. Symptoms consist of muscle stiffness, spasm, and subsequent rigidity, first in the jaw and neck then in the back, chest, abdomen, and limbs; in severe cases the spasm may affect the whole body, which is arched backwards (*see* opisthotonos). Prompt treatment with penicillin and antitoxin is effective; immunization against tetanus is effective but temporary. —**tetanic** (tĕ-**tan**-ik) *adj.*

tetany (**tet**-ăn-i) *n.* spasm and twitching of the muscles, particularly those of the face, hands, and feet. Tetany is caused by a reduction in the blood calcium level, which may be due to underactive parathyroid glands, rickets, or alkalosis.

tetra- *prefix denoting* four.

tetrachloroethylene (tet-ră-klor-oh-eth-i-leen) *n.* an anthelmintic drug administered by mouth in the treatment of hookworm disease.

tetracycline (tet-ră-sy-kleen) *n.* **1.** one of a group of antibiotic compounds derived from cultures of *Streptomyces* bacteria. These drugs, including chlortetracycline, methacycline, and tetracycline, are effective against a wide range of bacterial infections, including respiratory-tract infections, syphilis, and acne. They are usually given by mouth. **2.** a particular antibiotic of the tetracycline group. Trade names: **Achromycin, Steclin.**

tetradactyly (tet-ră-**dak**-tili) *n.* a congenital abnormality in which there are only four digits on a hand or foot. —**tetradactylous** *adj.*

tetralogy of Fallot (te-**tral**-ŏji ŏv fa-**loh**) *n.* a form of congenital heart disease in which there is pulmonary stenosis, enlargement of the right ventricle, and a ventricular septal defect over which the origin of the aorta lies. The affected child is blue (cyanosed). [E. L. A. Fallot (1850–1911), French physician]

tetraplegia (tet-ră-**plee**-jiă) *n.* *see* quadriplegia.

thalam- (thalamo-) *prefix denoting* the thalamus.

thalamencephalon (thal-ăm-en-**sef**-ă-lon) *n.* the structures, collectively, at the anterior end of the brainstem, comprising the epithalamus, thalamus, hypothalamus, and subthalamus.

thalamic syndrome (thă-**lam**-ik) *n.* a raised threshold to pain stimuli combined with a highly unpleasant burning quality to any pain that is experienced once the threshold is exceeded. It is caused by disease affecting the thalamus.

thalamotomy (thal-ă-**mot**-ŏmi) *n.* an operation on the brain in which a lesion is made in a precise part of the thalamus. It has been used to control psychiatric symptoms of severe anxiety and distress. *See also* psychosurgery.

thalamus (**thal**-ă-mŭs) *n.* (*pl.* **thalami**) one of two egg-shaped masses of grey matter that lie deep in the cerebral hemispheres in each side of the forebrain. The thalami are relay stations for all the sensory messages that enter the brain, before they are transmitted to the cortex.

thalassaemia (Cooley's anaemia) (thal-ă-**see**-miă) *n.* a hereditary blood disease, widespread in the Mediterranean countries, Asia, and Africa, in which there is an abnormality in the protein part of the haemoglobin molecule. Symptoms include anaemia, enlargement of the spleen, and abnormalities of the bone marrow. Individuals inheriting the disease from both parents are severely affected (*t. major*), but those inheriting it from only one parent are usually symptom-free.

thalidomide (thă-**lid**-ŏ-myd) *n.* a drug that was formerly used as a sedative. If taken during the first three months of pregnancy, it was found to cause fetal abnormalities involving limb malformation.

thanat- (thanato-) *prefix denoting* death.

theca (**th'ee**-kă) *n.* a sheathlike surrounding tissue.

theine (**th'ee**-een) *n.* the active volatile principle found in tea (*see* caffeine).

thenar (**th'ee**-nar) *n.* 1. the palm of the hand. 2. the fleshy prominent part of the hand at the base of the thumb. *Compare* hypothenar. —**thenar** *adj.*

theobromine (thi-ŏ-**broh**-meen) *n.* an alkaloid, occurring in cocoa, that has a weak diuretic action and dilates coronary and other arteries.

theophylline (thi-**off**-i-leen) *n.* an alkaloid, occurring in the leaves of the tea plant, that has a diuretic effect and relaxes smooth muscles. Theophylline preparations, particularly aminophylline, are used mainly to control bronchial asthma.

therapeutics (th'e-ră-**pew**-tiks) *n.* the branch of medicine that deals with different methods of treatment and healing (*therapy*), particularly the use of drugs in the cure of disease.

therm (therm) *n.* a unit of heat equal to 100,000 British thermal units. 1 therm = 1.055×10^{8} joules.

therm- (**thermo-**) *prefix denoting* **1.** heat. **2.** temperature.

thermoanaesthesia (therm-oh-anis-**theez**-iă) *n.* absence of the ability to recognize the sensations of heat and coldness. It may indicate damage to the spinothalamic tract in the spinal cord.

thermocautery (therm-oh-**kaw**-ter-i) *n.* the destruction of unwanted tissues by heat (*see* cauterize).

thermocoagulation (therm-oh-koh-ag-yoo-**lay**-shŏn) *n.* the coagulation and destruction of tissues by cautery.

thermography (ther-**mog**-răfi) *n.* a technique for measuring and recording the heat produced by different parts of the body, by using photographic film sensitive to infrared radiation. The picture produced is called a *thermogram*. A tumour with an abnormally increased blood supply may be revealed on the thermogram as a 'hot spot'. *See also* mammothermography.

thermolysis (ther-**mol**-i-sis) *n.* (in physiology) the dissipation of body heat by such processes as the evaporation of sweat from the skin surface.

thermometer (ther-**mom**-i-ter) *n.* a device for registering temperature. *clinical t.* a sealed narrow-bore glass tube containing mercury, which expands when heated and rises up the tube. The tube is designed to register body temperatures between 35°C (95°F) and 43.5°C (110°F).

thermophilic (therm-oh-**fil**-ik) *adj.* describing organisms, especially bacteria, that grow best at temperatures of 48–85°C.

thermoreceptor (therm-oh-ri-sep-ter) *n.* a sensory nerve ending that responds to heat or to cold.

thermotaxis (therm-moh-**tak**-sis) *n.* the physiological process of regulating or adjusting body temperature.

thermotherapy (therm-oh-**th'e**-ră-pi) *n.* the use of heat to alleviate pain and stiffness in joints and muscles and to promote an increase in circulation.

thiacetazone (**thioparamizone**) (th'y-ă-**set**-ă-zohn) *n.* a drug administered by mouth in the treatment of leprosy and (in combination with isoniazid) tuberculosis.

thiamin (**vitamin B₁**) (th'y-ă-min) *n. see* vitamin B.

Thiersch's graft (**split-skin graft**) (teer-shĕz) *n.* a type of skin graft in which thin partial thicknesses of skin are cut in narrow strips and placed onto the wound area to be healed. [K. Thiersch (1822–95), German surgeon]

thigh (th'y) *n.* the upper part of the lower limb, between the hip and the knee. *t. bone see* femur.

thioguanine (th'y-oh-**gwah**-neen) *n.* a drug that prevents the growth of cancer cells and is administered by mouth in the treatment of leukaemia. Trade name: **Lanvis**.

thioparamizone (th'y-oh-pă-**ram**-i-zohn) *n. see* thiacetazone.

thiopentone (th'y-oh-**pen**-tohn) *n.* a short-acting barbiturate. It is given by intravenous injection to produce general anaesthesia or as a premedication prior to surgery. Trade name: **Pentothal**.

thiopropazate (th'y-oh-**proh**-pă-zayt) *n.* a major tranquillizer similar to chlorpromazine in its actions and effects. It is given by mouth to treat agitated psychotic patients with anxiety states and to control nausea and vomiting. Trade name: **Dartalan**.

thioridazine (th'y-oh-**rid**-ă-zeen) *n.* a major tranquillizer administered by mouth in the treatment of a wide range of mental and emotional disturbances, including schizophrenia and senile dementia. Trade name: **Melleril**.

thiotepa (th'y-oh-**tee**-pă) *n.* a cytotoxic drug given by injection to treat cancer of the breast or ovary, lymphoma, and sarcoma.

thiouracil (th'y-oh-**yoor**-ă-sil) *n.* a drug that is administered by mouth in the treatment of over-activity of the thyroid gland (thyrotoxicosis).

Thomas's splint (**tom**-ă-siz) *n.* a metal splint used for immobilizing a fractured lower limb, especially the femur. There is a ring at the hip, a cross-piece at the foot, and side-pieces for the attachment of material to support the leg. [H. O. Thomas (1834–1931), British orthopaedic surgeon]

thorac- (thoraco-) *prefix denoting* the thorax or chest.

thoracectomy (thor-ă-**sek**-tŏmi) *n.* an operation in which the chest cavity is opened (thoracotomy) and a rib or part of a rib is removed.

thoracentesis (thor-ă-sen-**tee**-sis) *n. see* pleurocentesis.

thoracic cavity (thor-**ass**-ik) *n.* the chest cavity. *See* thorax.

thoracic duct *n.* one of the two main trunks of the lymphatic system. It receives lymph from both legs, the lower abdomen, left thorax, left side of the head, and left arm and drains into the left innominate vein.

thoracic vertebrae *pl. n.* the 12 bones of the backbone to which the ribs are attached. *See also* vertebra.

thoracocentesis (thor-ă-koh-sen-**tee**-sis) *n. see* pleurocentesis.

thoracoplasty (**thor**-ă-koh-plasti) *n.* the surgical repair of abnormalities or defects of the thorax.

thoracoscopy (thor-ă-**kosk**-ŏpi) *n.* examination of the pleural cavity by means of an endoscope (*thorascope*).

thoracotomy (thor-ă-**kot**-ŏmi) *n.* surgical opening of the chest cavity to inspect or operate on the heart, lungs, or other structures within.

thorascope (**thor**-ă-skohp) *n.* an instrument used to inspect the pleural cavity.

thorax (**thor**-aks) *n.* the chest: the part of the body cavity between the neck and the diaphragm. The skeleton of the thorax is formed by the sternum, costal cartilages, ribs, and thoracic vertebrae. It encloses the lungs, heart, oesophagus, and associated structures. *Compare* abdomen. —**thoracic** *adj.*

thorium-X (**thor**-iŭm) *n.* the radio-active isotope radium-224, which emits alpha radiation and has several applications in radiotherapy. *See also* radium.

threadworm (**thred**-werm) *n. see* pinworm.

threonine (**three**-ŏ-neen) *n.* an essential amino acid. *See also* amino acid.

threshold (**thresh**-ohld) *n.* (in neurology) the point at which a stimulus begins to evoke a response, and therefore a measure of the sensitivity of a system under particular conditions.

thrill (thril) *n.* a vibration felt on placing the hand on the body.

-thrix *suffix denoting* a hair or hairlike structure.

thromb- (thrombo-) *prefix denoting* 1. a blood clot (thrombus). 2. thrombosis. 3. blood platelets.

thrombectomy (throm-**bek**-tŏmi) *n.* a surgical procedure in which a blood clot (thrombus) is removed from an artery or vein (*see* endarterectomy, phlebothrombosis).

thrombin (**throm**-bin) *n.* a substance (coagulation factor) that acts as an enzyme, converting the soluble protein fibrinogen to the insoluble protein fibrin in the final stage of blood coagulation. Thrombin is derived from the inactive substance prothrombin.

thromboangiitis obliterans (throm-boh-an-ji-**I**-tis ŏ-**blit**-er-anz) *n. see* Buerger's disease.

thromboarteritis (throm-boh-ar-ter-**I**-tis) *n.* inflammation of an artery (*see* arteritis) associated with thrombosis.

thrombocyte (**throm**-boh-syt) *n. see* platelet.

thrombocythaemia (throm-boh-si-**th'ee**-miă) *n.* a disease in which there is an abnormal proliferation of megakaryocytes, leading to an increased number of platelets in the blood.

thrombocytopenia (throm-boh-sy-toh-**pee**-niă) *n.* a reduction in the number of platelets in the blood. This results in bleeding into the skin (*see* purpura), spontaneous bruising, and prolonged bleeding after injury. —**thrombocytopenic** *adj.*

thrombocytosis (throm-boh-sy-**toh**-sis) *n.* an increase in the number of platelets in the blood. It may occur in a variety of diseases, including cancers and certain blood diseases, and is likely to cause an increased tendency to thrombosis.

thromboembolism (throm-boh-em-bŏ-lizm) *n.* the condition in which a blood clot (thrombus), formed at one point in the circulation, becomes detached and lodges at another point.

thromboendarterectomy (throm-boh-end-ar-ter-**ek**-tŏmi) *n. see* endarterectomy.

thromboendarteritis (throm-boh-end-ar-ter-**I**-tis) *n.* thrombosis complicating endarteritis, seen in temporal arteritis, polyarteritis nodosa, and syphilis.

thrombokinase (throm-boh-ky-nayz) *n. see* thromboplastin.

thrombolysis (throm-**bol**-i-sis) *n.* the dissolution of a blood clot (thrombus) by the infusion of an enzyme, such as streptokinase, into the blood.

thrombolytic (throm-boh-**lit**-ik) *adj.* describing an agent that breaks up blood clots (thrombi). *See* anticoagulant.

thrombophlebitis (throm-boh-fli-by-tis) *n.* a condition in which thrombosis is associated with inflammation of a vein wall (*see* phlebitis).

thromboplastin (thrombokinase) (throm-boh-**plast**-in) *n.* a substance formed during the earlier stages of blood coagulation. It acts as an enzyme, converting the inactive substance prothrombin to the enzyme thrombin.

thrombopoiesis (throm-boh-poi-ee-sis) *n.* the process of blood platelet production. Platelets are formed as fragments of cytoplasm shed from giant cells (megakaryocytes) in the bone marrow by a budding process.

thrombosis (throm-**boh**-sis) *n*. a condition in which the blood changes from a liquid to a solid state and produces a blood clot (*thrombus*). Thrombosis in an artery obstructs the blood flow to the tissue it supplies (*see* coronary thrombosis, stroke). Thrombosis can also occur in a vein, and it may be associated with inflammation (*see* phlebitis, phlebothrombosis).

thrombus (throm-**bŭs**) *n*. a blood clot (*see* thrombosis).

thrush (thrush) *n*. *see* candidiasis.

thym- (**thymo-**) *prefix denoting* the thymus.

thymectomy (th'y-**mek**-tŏmi) *n*. surgical removal of the thymus gland.

-thymia *suffix denoting* a condition of the mind.

thymine (th'y-meen) *n*. one of the nitrogen-containing bases (*see* pyrimidine) occurring in the nucleic acids DNA and RNA.

thymitis (th'y-my-tis) *n*. inflammation of the thymus gland.

thymocyte (th'y-moh-syt) *n*. a lymphocyte within the thymus.

thymol (th'y-mol) *n*. an antiseptic active against bacteria and fungi, used in mouthwashes, gargles, and skin preparations.

thymoma (th'y-**moh**-mă) *n*. a benign or malignant tumour of the thymus gland. It is sometimes associated with myasthenia gravis.

thymoxamine (th'y-**moks**-ă-meen) *n*. a drug that causes peripheral blood vessels to dilate (*see* vasodilator). It is administered by mouth in the treatment of Raynaud's disease and similar conditions. Trade name: **Opilon**.

thymus (th'y-mŭs) *n*. a bilobed or-

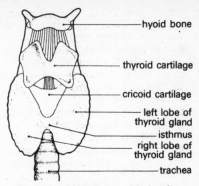

Position of the thyroid gland

gan in the root of the neck, above and in front of the heart. In relation to body size the thymus is largest at birth. It doubles in size by puberty, after which it gradually shrinks, its functional tissue being replaced by fatty tissue. In infancy the thymus controls the development of lymphoid tissue and immune response to microbes and foreign proteins. Its function in the adult is unclear. —**thymic** *adj*.

thyro- *prefix denoting* the thyroid gland.

thyrocalcitonin (calcitonin) (th'y-roh-kal-si-**toh**-nin) *n*. a hormone, produced in the thyroid gland, that lowers the levels of calcium and phosphate in the blood. Thyrocalcitonin is given by injection to treat hypercalcaemia and Paget's disease of the bone. *Compare* parathyroid hormone.

thyrocele (th'y-roh-seel) *n*. a swelling of the thyroid gland. *See* goitre.

thyroglobulin (th'y-roh-**glob**-yoo-lin) *n*. a protein in the thyroid gland from which the thyroid hormones are synthesized.

thyroglossal (th'y-roh-**glos**-ăl) *adj*. relating to the thyroid gland and the tongue. *t. duct* a duct in the embryo between the thyroid and the back of the tongue.

thyroid cartilage (th'y-roid) *n.* the main cartilage of the larynx, consisting of two broad plates that join at the front. *See also* Adam's apple.

thyroidectomy (th'y-roid-**ek**-tŏmi) *n.* surgical removal of the thyroid gland. *partial t.* thyroidectomy in which only the diseased part of the gland is removed. *subtotal t.* a method of treating thyrotoxicosis, in which the surgeon removes 90% of the gland.

thyroid gland *n.* a large endocrine gland situated in the base of the neck. It consists of two lobes, one on either side of the trachea, that are joined by an isthmus. The thyroid gland is concerned with regulation of the metabolic rate by the secretion of thyroid hormone. Thyroid extract is used in the treatment of thyroid deficiency diseases.

thyroid hormone *n.* an iodine-containing substance, synthesized and secreted by the thyroid gland, that is essential for normal metabolic processes and mental and physical development. There are two thyroid hormones, *triiodothyronine* and *thyroxine*. Lack of these hormones gives rise to cretinism in infants and myxoedema in adults. Excessive production of thyroid hormones gives rise to thyrotoxicosis.

thyroiditis (th'y-roid-**I**-tis) *n.* inflammation of the thyroid gland. *acute t.* thyroiditis due to bacterial infection. *chronic t.* thyroiditis that is commonly caused by an abnormal immune response (*see* autoimmunity) in which lymphocytes invade the tissues of the gland. *See* Hashimoto's disease.

thyroid-stimulating hormone (TSH, thyrotrophin) *n.* a hormone, synthesized and secreted by the anterior pituitary gland under the control of thyrotrophin-releasing hormone, that stimulates activity of the thyroid gland.

thyrotomy (th'y-**rot**-ŏmi) *n.* surgical incision of either the thyroid cartilage or the thyroid gland itself.

thyrotoxicosis (th'y-roh-toks-i-**koh**-sis) *n.* the syndrome due to excessive amounts of thyroid hormones in the bloodstream, causing a rapid heart beat, sweating, tremor, anxiety, increased appetite, loss of weight, and intolerance of heat. Causes include simple overactivity of the gland, a hormone-secreting tumour, and *Graves' disease* (*exophthalmic goitre*), in which there are additional symptoms including swelling of the neck (goitre) and protrusion of the eyes (exophthalmos). —**thyrotoxic** *adj.*

thyrotrophin (th'y-roh-**troh**-fin) *n.* *see* thyroid-stimulating hormone.

thyrotrophin-releasing hormone (TRH) *n.* a hormone-like substance from the hypothalamus (in the brain) that acts on the anterior pituitary gland to stimulate the release of thyroid-stimulating hormone.

thyroxine (th'y-**roks**-een) *n.* *see* thyroid hormone.

tibia (**tib**-iă) *n.* the shin bone: the inner and larger bone of the lower leg. It articulates with the femur above, with the talus below, and with the fibula to the side.

tibialis (tib-i-**ay**-lis) *n.* either of two muscles in the leg, extending from the tibia to the metatarsal bones of the foot. *t. anterior* the muscle that turns the foot inwards and flexes the toes backwards. *t. posterior* the muscle that extends the toes and inverts the foot.

tibio- *prefix denoting* the tibia.

tic (tik) *n.* a repeated and largely involuntary movement varying in complexity from the twitch of a muscle to elaborate well-coordinated actions. *t. douloureux see* neuralgia.

tick (tik) *n.* a bloodsucking parasite belonging to the order of arthropods (Acarina) that also includes the mites. Tick bites can cause serious skin lesions and occasionally paralysis, and certain tick species transmit typhus and relapsing fever. Dimethyl phthalate is used as a tick repellent. *t. fever* any infectious disease transmitted by ticks, especially Rocky Mountain spotted fever.

tincture (tink-cher) *n.* an alcoholic extract of a drug derived from a plant.

tinea (ringworm) (tin-iă) *n.* a ringlike intensely itching fungus infection of the skin, particularly the scalp and feet, and occasionally of the nails. It is caused by various species of the fungi *Microsporum, Trichophyton,* and *Epidermophyton* and is highly contagious, being spread by direct contact or via infected materials. The disease is treated with antifungal agents taken by mouth (such as griseofulvin) or applied locally. *t. barbis* ringworm of the skin under a beard. *t. capitis* ringworm of the scalp, of which favus is a severe form. *t. pedis see* athlete's foot.

tinnitus (ti-ny-tŭs) *n.* any noise (buzzing, ringing, etc.) in the ear.

The many causes include wax in the ear, damage to the eardrum, and diseases of the inner ear.

tintometer (tin-tom-it-er) *n.* an instrument for measuring the depth of colour in a liquid. The colour can then be compared with those on standard charts so that the concentration of a particular compound in solution can be estimated.

tissue (tis-yoo) *n.* a collection of cells specialized to perform a particular function. Aggregations of tissues constitute organs. *t. culture* the culture of living tissues, removed from the body, in a suitable medium supplied with nutrients and oxygen.

titration (ty-tray-shŏn) *n.* a method of determining the concentration of a substance in solution. A measured volume of a reagent of known concentration is added to a known volume of the test solution until the end point of the reaction has occurred.

titre (ty-ter) *n.* (in immunology) the extent to which a sample of blood serum containing antibody can be diluted before losing its ability to cause agglutination of the relevant antigen. It is used as a measure of the amount of antibody in the serum.

tobacco (tŏ-bak-oh) *n.* the dried leaves of the plant *Nicotiana tabacum* or related species, used in smoking and as snuff. Tobacco contains the stimulant but poisonous alkaloid nicotine, which enters the bloodstream during smoking.

toco- *prefix denoting* childbirth or labour.

tocography (tok-og-răfi) *n.* the measuring and recording of the force and frequency of uterine contractions during labour using an instrument called a *tocodynamometer*.

tocopherol (tok-off-er-ol) *n. see* vitamin E.

Todd's paralysis (Todd's palsy) (todz) *n.* transient paralysis of a part of the body that has previously been involved in a focal epileptic fit (*see* epilepsy). It is thought to be due to the exhaustion of the cells of the motor cortex of the brain. [R. B. Todd (1809–60), British physician]

tolazamide (tol-az-ă-myd) *n.* a drug administered by mouth in the treatment of maturity-onset diabetes. Trade name: **Tolanase**. *See also* sulphonylurea.

tolazoline (tol-az-oh-leen) *n.* a vasodilator drug, given by mouth for the treatment of peripheral vascular disorders, such as Raynaud's disease. Trade name: **Priscol**.

tolbutamide (tol-bew-tă-myd) *n.* a drug given by mouth in the treatment of diabetes mellitus. It is believed to act directly on the pancreas to stimulate insulin production and is particularly effective in elderly patients with mild diabetes. Trade names: **Pramidex, Rastinon**.

tolerance (tol-er-ăns) *n.* the reduction or loss of the normal response to a substance that usually provokes a reaction in the body. *drug t.* tolerance that may develop after taking a particular drug over a long period of time. In such cases increased doses are necessary to produce the desired effect. *See also* glucose tolerance test, immunological tolerance.

tolnaftate (tol-naf-tayt) *n.* an antiseptic applied topically as a cream, powder, or solution in the treatment of various fungal infections of the skin, including ringworm. Trade names: **Tinactin, Tinaderm**.

-tome *suffix denoting* a cutting instrument.

tomo- *prefix denoting* **1.** section or sections. **2.** surgical operation.

tomography (tŏ-mog-răfi) *n.* the technique of using X-rays or ultrasound waves to produce an image of structures at a particular depth within the body. The visual record of this technique is called a *tomogram*. *See also* CT scanner.

tomotocia (tom-oh-toh-siă) *n.* the delivery of a baby by cutting open the mother's abdomen and womb (*see* Caesarean section).

-tomy (-otomy) *suffix denoting* a surgical incision into an organ or part.

tone (tohn) *n. see* tonus.

tongue (tung) *n.* a muscular organ attached to the floor of the mouth. It is covered by mucous membrane and its surface is raised in minute projections (papillae), which give it a furred appearance. Taste buds are arranged in grooves around the papillae. The tongue helps in manipulating food during mastication and swallowing; it is the main organ of taste; and it plays an important role in the production of articulate speech. Anatomical name: **glossa**.

tonic (ton-ik) **1.** *adj.* **a.** relating to normal muscle tone. **b.** marked by continuous tension (contraction), e.g. a tonic muscle spasm. **2.** *n.* a medicinal substance taken to increase vigour and liveliness and produce a feeling of well-being.

tonicity (toh-nis-iti) *n.* **1.** the normal state of slight contraction, or readiness to contract, of

enamel

neck

gum (gingiva)

pulp cavity

nerves and blood vessels

dentine

periodontal membrane

root canal
alveolar bone

cementum

apical foramen

crown

root

Section of a molar tooth

healthy muscle fibres. **2.** the effective osmotic pressure of a solution. *See* hypertonic, hypotonic, osmosis.

tono- *prefix denoting* **1.** tone or tension. **2.** pressure.

tonography (toh-**nog**-răfi) *n.* measurement of the pressure within the eyeball in such a way as to record variations in pressure over periods of several minutes at a time.

tonometer (toh-**nom**-it-er) *n.* an instrument for measuring pressure in a part of the body, e.g. the eye (*see* ophthalmotonometer).

tonsil (**ton**-sil) *n.* a mass of lymphoid tissue on either side of the back of the mouth, between the anterior and posterior pillars of the fauces. The tonsils are concerned with protection against

infection. *See also* adenoids (pharyngeal tonsils).

tonsillectomy (ton-sil-**ek**-tŏmi) *n.* surgical removal of the tonsils.

tonsillitis (ton-sil-**I**-tis) *n.* inflammation of the tonsils due to bacterial or viral infection, causing a sore throat, fever, and difficulty in swallowing.

tonsillotome (ton-**sil**-ŏ-tohm) *n.* a surgical knife used for cutting into or removing a tonsil.

tonsillotomy (ton-sil-**ot**-ŏmi) *n.* surgical incision of a tonsil or removal of part of a tonsil.

tonus (**tone**) (**toh**-nŭs) *n.* the normal state of partial contraction of a resting muscle.

tooth (tooth) *n.* (*pl.* **teeth**) one of the hard structures in the mouth used for cutting and chewing food. Each tooth is embedded in a socket in the jawbone, to which it is attached by the periodontal membrane. The exposed part of the tooth (*crown*) is covered with enamel and the part within the bone (*root*) is coated with cementum; the bulk of the tooth consists of dentine enclosing the pulp. There are four different types of teeth (*see* canine, incisor, premolar, molar). *See also* dentition.

topagnosis (top-ag-**noh**-sis) *n*. inability to identify a part of the body that has been touched. It is a symptom of disease in the parietal lobes of the brain.

topectomy (toh-**pek**-tŏmi) *n*. an obsolete operation for the control of psychiatric symptoms by excising selected areas of the cerebral cortex. *See also* psychosurgery.

tophus (**toh**-fŭs) *n*. (*pl*. **tophi**) a hard deposit of crystalline uric acid and its salts in the skin, cartilage (especially of the ears), or joints: a feature of gout.

topical (**top**-ikăl) *adj*. local: used for the route of administration of a drug that is applied directly to the part being treated.

topo- *prefix denoting* place; position; location.

topography (tŏ-**pog**-răfi) *n*. the study of the different regions of the body, including the description of its. parts in relation to the surrounding structures. —**topographical** (top-ŏ-**graf**-ikăl) *adj*.

tormina (**tor**-min-ă) *n*. *see* colic.

torpor (**tor**-per) *n*. a state of sluggishness and diminished responsiveness: a characteristic of certain mental disorders and a symptom of certain forms of poisoning or metabolic disorder.

torsion (**tor**-shŏn) *n*. twisting.

torticollis (**wryneck**) (tor-ti-**kol**-iss) *n*. an irresistible turning movement of the head that becomes more persistent, so that eventually the head is held continually to one side. It may be caused by a birth injury to the sternomastoid muscle (*see* sternomastoid tumour).

tourniquet (**toor**-ni-kay) *n*. a device to press upon an artery and prevent flow of blood through it, usually a cord, rubber tube, or tight bandage. Tourniquets are no longer recommended as a first-aid measure to stop bleeding from a wound; direct pressure on the wound itself is considered less harmful.

tow (toh) *n*. the teased-out short fibres of flax, hemp, or jute, used in swabs, stupes, and for a variety of other purposes.

tox- (**toxi-**, **toxo-**, **toxic(o)-**) *prefix denoting* **1**. poisonous; toxic. **2**. toxins or poisoning.

toxaemia (toks-**eem**-iă) *n*. blood poisoning that is caused by toxins formed by bacteria growing in a local site of infection. *Compare* pyaemia, sapraemia, septicaemia. *t. of pregnancy* an illness of unknown cause affecting pregnant women. It includes the conditions of pre-eclampsia and eclampsia.

toxic (**toks**-ik) *adj*. having a poisonous effect; potentially lethal.

toxicity (toks-**iss**-iti) *n*. the degree to which a substance is poisonous.

toxicology (toks-i-**kol**-ŏji) *n*. the study of poisonous materials and their effects upon living organisms. —**toxicologist** *n*.

toxicosis (toks-i-**koh**-sis) *n*. the deleterious effects of a toxin; poisoning.

toxin (**toks**-in) *n.* a poison produced by a living organism, especially by a bacterium (*see* endotoxin, exotoxin). In the body toxins act as antigens (*see* antitoxin).

toxocariasis (**visceral larva migrans**) (toks-oh-kair-**I**-ă-sis) *n.* an infestation with the larvae of the dog and cat roundworms, *Toxocara canis* and *T. cati*. It is characterized by enlargement of the liver, pneumonitis, fever, joint and muscle pains, vomiting, an irritating rash, and convulsions.

toxoid (**toks**-oid) *n.* a preparation of a toxin that has been rendered harmless by chemical treatment while retaining its antigenic activity. Toxoids are used in vaccines.

toxoid-antitoxin *n.* a mixture of a toxoid and its antitoxin used as a vaccine to produce active immunity.

toxoplasmosis (toks-oh-plaz-**moh**-sis) *n.* a disease of mammals and birds due to the protozoan *Toxoplasma gondii*, which may be transmitted to man. Generally symptoms are mild but severe infection of lymph nodes can occur. *congenital t.* toxoplasmosis in which a woman infected during pregnancy transmits the organism to her fetus. It can produce blindness or mental retardation in the newborn.

trabecula (tră-**bek**-yoo-lă) *n.* (*pl.* **trabeculae**) **1.** any of the bands of tissue that pass from the outer part of an organ to its interior, dividing it into separate chambers. **2.** any of the thin bars of bony tissue in spongy bone. —**trabecular** *adj.*

trace element (trayss) *n.* an element required in minute amounts for the normal functioning of the body. Examples are copper, cobalt, and manganese.

tracer (**tray**-ser) *n.* a substance that is introduced into the body and whose progress can subsequently be followed so that information is gained about metabolic processes. Radioactive tracers are used for a variety of purposes, such as the investigation of thyroid disease or possible brain tumours.

trache- (**tracheo-**) *prefix denoting* the trachea.

trachea (**tray**-kiă) *n.* the windpipe: the part of the air passage between the larynx and the main bronchi. —**tracheal** (**tray**-ki-ăl) *adj.*

tracheal tugging *n.* a sign indicative of an aneurysm of the aortic arch: a downward tug is felt on the windpipe when the finger is placed in the midline at the root of the neck.

tracheitis (tray-ki-**I**-tis) *n.* inflammation of the trachea, usually secondary to bacterial or viral infection in the nose or throat. Tracheitis causes soreness in the chest and a painful cough and is often associated with bronchitis.

trachelorrhaphy (tray-kěl-o-**ră**fi) *n.* an operation for suturing tears in the cervix of the womb.

tracheobronchitis (tray-ki-oh-brong-**ky**-tis) *n.* inflammation of the trachea and bronchi.

tracheostomy (**tracheotomy**) (tray-ki-**ost**-ŏmi) *n.* a surgical operation in which a hole is made into the trachea through the neck to relieve obstruction to breathing, as in diphtheria. A curved metal, plastic, or rubber tube is usually inserted through the hole and held in position by tapes tied round the neck.

tracheotomy (tray-ki-**ot**-ŏmi) *n. see* tracheostomy.

trachoma (tră-**koh**-mă) *n.* a chronic contagious eye disease – a severe form of conjunctivitis – that is common in tropical regions. If untreated, the conjunctiva becomes scarred and shrinks, causing trichiasis; blindness usually follows. Treatment with tetracyclines is effective.

tract (trakt) *n.* **1.** a group of nerve fibres passing from one part of the brain or spinal cord to another, forming a distinct pathway. **2.** an organ or collection of organs providing for the passage of something, e.g. the digestive tract.

traction (trak-shŏn) *n.* the application of a pulling force as a means of counteracting the natural tension in the tissues surrounding a broken bone. Considerable force, exerted with weights, ropes, and pulleys, may be necessary to ensure that a broken femur is kept correctly positioned during the early stages of healing.

tractotomy (trak-**tot**-ŏmi) *n.* a neurosurgical operation for the relief of intractable pain, in which the nerve fibres that carry painful sensation to consciousness are severed within the medulla oblongata. *See also* cordotomy.

tragus (**tray**-gŭs) *n.* the projection of cartilage in the pinna of the outer ear that extends back over the opening of the external auditory meatus.

trance (trahns) *n.* a state in which reaction to the environment is diminished although awareness is

not impaired. It may be caused by hypnosis, meditation, catatonia, hysteria, or drugs.

tranquillizer (**trank**-wi-ly-zer) *n.* a drug that produces a calming effect, relieving anxiety and tension. *major t.* a drug, such as a phenothiazine or haloperidol, used to treat severe mental disorders. *minor t.* a drug, such as a benzodiazepine or meprobamate, used to treat neuroses and to relieve anxiety and tension.

trans- *prefix denoting* through or across.

transaminase (trans-**am**-in-ayz) *n.* an enzyme that is involved in the process of transamination. Examples are glutamic oxaloacetic transaminase (GOT) and glutamic pyruvic transaminase (GPT).

transamination (trans-am-i-**nay**-shŏn) *n.* a process involved in the metabolism of amino acids in which amino groups ($-NH_2$) are transferred from amino acids to certain α-keto acids, with the production of a second keto acid and amino acid. The reaction is catalysed by transaminases.

transcription (tran-**skrip**-shŏn) *n.* the process in which the information contained in the genetic code is transferred from DNA to RNA: the first step in the manufacture of proteins in cells. *See* messenger RNA, translation.

transection (tran-**sek**-shŏn) *n.* **1.** a cross section of a piece of tissue. **2.** cutting across the tissue of an organ (*see also* section).

transferase (**trans**-fer-ayz) *n.* an enzyme that catalyses the transfer of a group (other than hydrogen) between a pair of substrates.

transference (**trans**-fer-ĕns) *n.* (in psychoanalysis) the process by which a patient comes to feel and act towards the therapist as though he were somebody from the patient's past life, especially a powerful parent. The patient's transference feelings may be of love or of hatred.

transferrin (**siderophilin**) (**trans**-fer-in) *n.* a glycoprotein, found in the blood plasma, that acts as a carrier for iron in the bloodstream.

transfer RNA (**trans**-fer) *n.* a type of RNA whose function is to attach the correct amino acid to the protein chain being synthesized at a ribosome. *See also* translation.

transfusion (**trans**-few-*zh*ŏn) *n.* **1.** the injection of a volume of blood obtained from a healthy person into the circulation of a patient whose blood is deficient in quantity or quality, through accident or disease. The blood is allowed to drip, under gravity, through a needle inserted into one of the patient's veins. Blood transfusion is routine during major surgical operations in which much blood is likely to be lost. **2.** the administration of any fluid, such as plasma or saline solution, into a patient's vein by means of a drip.

transillumination (**tranz**-i-loo-mi-nay-shŏn) *n.* the technique of shining a bright light through part of the body to examine its structure. Transillumination of the paranasal sinuses is a means of detecting abnormalities.

translation (**tranz**-lay-shŏn) *n.* (in cell biology) the manufacture of proteins in a cell, which takes place at the ribosomes. *See* messenger RNA, transfer RNA.

translocation (**tranz**-loh-**kay**-shŏn) *n.* (in genetics) a type of chromosome mutation in which part of a chromosome is transferred to another part of the same chromosome or to a different chromosome. This can lead to serious genetic disorders, e.g. chronic myeloid leukaemia.

translumbar (**tranz**-**lum**-ber) *adj.* through the lumbar region: describing the route for injecting the aorta for aortography.

transmigration (**tranz**-my-gray-shŏn) *n.* the act of passing through or across, e.g. the passage of blood cells through the intact walls of capillaries and venules (*see* diapedesis).

transplacental (**trans**-plǎ-**sen**-t'l) *adj.* across the placenta: describing the transport of substances, etc., between mother and fetus.

transplantation (**trans**-plahn-tay-shŏn) *n.* the implantation of an organ or tissue from one part of the body to another, as in skin or bone grafting, or from one person to another, as in kidney or heart transplants. Transplanting organs or tissues between individuals is a difficult procedure because of the natural rejection processes in the recipient of the graft. Special treatment (e.g. with immunosuppressive drugs) is needed to prevent graft rejection.

transposition (**trans**-pŏ-**zish**-ŏn) *n.* the abnormal positioning of a part of the body such that it is on the opposite side to its normal site in the body. *t. of the great vessels* a congenital abnormality of the heart in which the aorta arises from the right ventricle and the pulmonary artery from the left ventricle.

transsexualism (tranz-**seks**-yoo-ăl-izm) *n.* the condition of one who firmly believes that he (or she) belongs to the sex opposite to his (or her) biological gender. In adults surgical sex reassignment is sometimes justifiable, to make the externals of the body conform to the individual's view of himself (or herself). —**transsexual** *adj.*, *n.*

transudation (trans-yoo-**day**-shŏn) *n.* the passage of a liquid through a membrane, especially of blood through the wall of a capillary vessel. The liquid is called the *transudate.*

transurethral (trans-yoor-**ee**-thrăl) *adj.* through the urethra. *t. resection see* resection.

transverse (tranz-**vers**) *adj.* (in anatomy) situated at right angles to the long axis of the body of an organ. *t. process* the long projection from the base of the neural arch of a vertebra.

transvestitism (tranz-**vest**-it-izm) *n.* the condition in which sexual pleasure is obtained by dressing in the clothes of the opposite sex. It may occur in both heterosexual and homosexual people. *See also* perversion. —**transvestite** *n.*

tranylcypromine (tran-il-sy-proh-meen) *n.* an antidepressant drug – one of the MAO inhibitors – given by mouth for the treatment of severe mental depressive states. Trade name: **Parnate.**

trapezium (tră-**pee**-ziŭm) *n.* a bone of the wrist (*see* carpus). It articulates with the scaphoid bone behind and with the first metacarpal in front.

trapezius (tră-**pee**-zi-ŭs) *n.* a flat triangular muscle covering the back of the neck and shoulder. It moves the scapula and draws the head backwards to either side.

trapezoid bone (tră-**pee**-zoid) *n.* a bone of the wrist (*see* carpus). It articulates with the second metatarsal bone in front, with the scaphoid bone behind, and with the trapezium and capitate bones on either side.

trauma (traw-mă) *n.* **1.** a physical wound or injury. **2.** (in psychology) an emotionally painful and harmful event, which may lead to neurosis. —**traumatic** (traw-**mat**-ik) *adj.*

traumatic fever *n.* a fever resulting from a serious injury.

traumatology (traw-mă-**tol**-ŏji) *n.* accident surgery: the branch of surgery that deals with wounds and disabilities arising from injuries.

travel sickness (motion sickness) (trav-ĕl) *n.* nausea, vomiting, and headache caused by motion during travel by sea, road, or air. The symptoms are due to overstimulation of the balance organs in the inner ear. Antihistamine drugs provide effective treatment.

trematode (trem-ă-tohd) *n. see* fluke.

tremor (trem-er) *n.* a rhythmical alternating movement that may affect any part of the body. Tremor is a prominent symptom of parkinsonism. *essential t.* a slow tremor that particularly affects the hands. *intention t.* tremor that occurs when a patient with disease of the cerebellum tries to touch an object. *physiological t.* a feature of the normal mechanism for maintaining posture. It may be more apparent in states of fatigue or anxiety.

trench foot (immersion foot) (trench) *n.* blackening of the toes and the skin of the foot due to death of the superficial tissues and caused by prolonged immersion in cold water.

Trendelenburg position (tren-del-ĕn-berg) *n.* a special operating-table posture for patients undergoing surgery of the pelvis or for patients suffering from shock. The patient is laid on his back with the pelvis higher than the head, inclined at an angle of about 45°. *See* position. [F. Trendelenburg (1844–1924), German surgeon]

Trendelenburg's operation *n.* ligation of the long saphenous vein at the groin: performed to remove weakened portions of varicose veins.

Trendelenburg's sign *n.* a sign indicating congenital dislocation of the hip: when the patient stands on the affected leg with the other leg flexed, the pelvis is lower on the side of the flexed leg.

trephine (trif-een) *n.* a surgical instrument used to remove a circular area of tissue, usually from the cornea of the eye or from bone.

Treponema (trep-ŏ-nee-mă) *n.* a genus of anaerobic spirochaete bacteria. All species are parasitic; some cause disease, such as *T. carateum* (pinta), *T. pallidum* (syphilis), and *T. pertenue* (yaws).

treponematosis (trep-ŏ-nee-mă-toh-sis) *n.* any infection caused by spirochaete bacteria of the genus *Treponema*.

triad (try-ad) *n.* (in medicine) a group of three united or closely associated structures or three symptoms or effects that occur together.

triamcinolone (try-am-sin-ŏ-lohn) *n.* a synthetic corticosteroid hormone with uses similar to cortisone; it reduces inflammation but does not cause salt and water retention. It is administered by mouth. Trade names: **Adcortyl, Ledercort**.

triamterene (try-am-ter-een) *n.* a diuretic that causes the loss of sodium and chloride from the kidneys and is administered by mouth in the treatment of various forms of fluid retention (oedema). Trade name: **Dytac**.

triangle (try-ang-ŭl) *n.* (in anatomy) a three-sided structure or area; for example, the femoral triangle.

triangular bandage (try-ang-yoo-ler) *n.* a piece of material cut or folded into a triangular shape and used for making an arm sling or holding dressings in position.

triaziquone (try-az-i-kwohn) *n.* a drug used in the treatment of various forms of cancer and administered by mouth, injection, or directly into the tumour. It has toxic actions on normal tissues, particularly the bone marrow. Trade name: **Trenimon**.

triceps (try-seps) *n.* a muscle with three heads of origin. *t. brachii* the muscle that is situated on the back of the upper arm and contracts to extend the forearm. It is the antagonist of the brachialis.

trich- (tricho-) *prefix denoting* hair or hairlike structures.

trichiasis (trik-I-ă-sis) *n.* a condition in which the eyelashes rub against the eyeball, producing discomfort and sometimes ulceration of the cornea. It accompanies all forms of entropion.

trichinosis (trichiniasis) (trik-i-noh-sis) *n.* a disease caused by larvae of the nematode worm *Trichinella spiralis*, contracted by eating imperfectly cooked infected meat. Symptoms include diarrhoea, nausea, fever, vertigo, delirium, and pains in the limbs. The larvae eventually settle within cysts in the muscles, which may result in pain and stiffness.

trichloracetic acid (try-klor-ă-**see**-tik) *n.* an astringent used in solution for a variety of skin conditions. It is also applied topically to produce sloughing, especially for the removal of warts.

trichobezoar (trik-oh-**bee**-zor) *n.* hairball; a mass of swallowed hair in the stomach. *See* bezoar.

Trichocephalus (trik-oh-**sef**-ă-lŭs) *n. see* whipworm.

trichology (trik-**ol**-ŏji) *n.* the study of hair.

Trichomonas (trik-oh-**moh**-năs) *n.* a genus of parasitic flagellate protozoans. *T. hominis* a species that lives in the large intestine. *T. vaginalis see* trichomoniasis.

trichomoniasis (trik-oh-mŏ-**ny**-ă-sis) *n.* **1.** an infection of the digestive system by the protozoan *Trichomonas hominis*, causing dysentery. **2.** an infection of the vagina due to the protozoan *Trichomonas vaginalis*, causing inflammation of genital tissues with vaginal discharge. It can be transmitted to males in whom it causes urethral discharge. Treatment with metronidazole is effective.

trichomycosis (trik-oh-my-**koh**-sis) *n.* any hair disease caused by infection with a fungus.

Trichophyton (trik-oh-**fy**-tŏn) *n.* a genus of fungi, parasitic to man, that frequently infect the skin,

nails, and hair and cause favus and ringworm.

trichophytosis (trik-oh-fy-**toh**-sis) *n.* a fungal infection caused by species of *Trichophyton*.

trichosis (trik-**oh**-sis) *n.* any abnormal growth or disease of the hair.

trichromatic (try-kroh-**mat**-ik) *adj.* describing or relating to the normal state of colour vision, in which a person is sensitive to all three of the primary colours. *Compare* dichromatic.

trichuriasis (trik-yoor-**I**-ă-sis) *n.* an infestation of the large intestine by the whipworm, *Trichuris trichiura*. Symptoms, including bloody diarrhoea, anaemia, weakness, and abdominal pain, are evident only in heavy infestations. Trichuriasis can be treated with various anthelmintics, including thiabendazole and piperazine salts.

Trichuris (trik-**yoor**-iss) *n. see* whipworm.

triclofos (**try**-kloh-fos) *n.* a sedative and hypnotic that is given by mouth, usually as a syrup, to induce sleep or as a daytime sedative, particularly in children. It is similar in its actions and effects to chloral hydrate. Trade name: **Tricloryl**.

tricuspid valve (try-**kusp**-id) *n.* the valve in the heart between the right atrium and right ventricle. It consists of three cusps that channel the flow of blood from the atrium to the ventricle and prevent any backflow.

tridactyly (try-**dak**-tili) *n.* a congenital abnormality in which there are only three digits on a hand or foot.

trifluoperazine (try-floo-oh-**pair**-ă-zeen) *n.* a major tranquillizer with uses and effects similar to those of chlorpromazine. Trade names: **Stelazine**, **Terfluzine**.

trigeminal nerve (try-**jem**-in-ăl) *n.* the fifth and largest cranial nerve (V), which is split into the ophthalmic, maxillary, and mandibular nerves. The motor fibres are responsible for controlling the muscles involved in chewing, while the sensory fibres relay information from the front of the head and from the meninges.

trigeminal neuralgia (tic douloureux) *n. see* neuralgia.

trigeminy (try-**jem**-in-i) *n.* a condition in which the heart beats can be subdivided into groups of three. The first beat is normal, but the second and third are premature beats (*see* ectopic beat).

trigger finger (**trig**-er) *n.* an impairment in the ability to extend a finger, resulting either from a nodular thickening in the flexor tendon or a narrowing of the flexor tendon sheath. On unclenching the fist, the affected finger at first remains bent then suddenly straightens.

triglyceride (try-**glis**-eryd) *n.* a lipid or neutral fat consisting of glycerol combined with three fatty-acid molecules. Triglycerides are the form in which fat is stored in the body.

trigone (**try**-gohn) *n.* a triangular region of tissue, such as the triangular region of the wall of the bladder that lies between the openings of the two ureters and the urethra.

trigonitis (try-goh-ny-tis) *n.* inflammation of the trigone (base) of the urinary bladder. This can occur as part of a generalized cystitis or it can be associated with inflammation in the urethra, prostate, or neck of the womb.

trigonocephaly (try-gŏ-noh-**sef**-ăli) *n.* a deformity of the skull in which the vault of the skull is sharply angled just in front of the ears, giving the skull a triangular shape. —**trigonocephalic** (try-gŏ-noh-si-**fal**-ik) *adj.*

triiodothyronine (try-I-oh-doh-th'y-rŏ-neen) *n. see* thyroid hormone.

trimeprazine (try-**mep**-ră-zeen) *n.* an antihistamine drug (a phenothiazine derivative) that also possesses sedative properties. Given by mouth, it is mainly used in the treatment of pruritus and as a preoperative medication, especially in children. Trade name: **Vallergan**.

trimester (try-**mest**-er) *n.* (in obstetrics) any one of the three successive three-monthly periods into which a pregnancy may be divided.

trimethoprim (try-**meth**-oh-prim) *n.* an antiseptic that is active against a range of microorganisms. It is used mainly in the treatment of chronic urinary-tract infections and malaria and is often administered, by mouth, in a combined preparation with sulphamethoxazole (*see* co-trimoxazole).

trimipramine (try-**mip**-ră-meen) *n.* a tricyclic antidepressant drug that also possesses sedative properties. It is given by mouth or by injection for the treatment of acute or chronic mental depression. Trade name: **Surmontil**.

trinitrophenol (try-ny-troh-**fee**-nol) *n. see* picric acid.

triploid (**trip**-loid) *adj.* describing cells, tissues, or individuals in which there are three complete chromosome sets. *Compare* haploid, diploid. —**triploid** *n.*

triquetrum (triquetral bone) (try-**kwee**-trŭm) *n.* a bone of the wrist (*see* carpus). It articulates with the ulna behind and with the pisiform, hamate, and lunate bones in the carpus.

trismus (triz-mŭs) *n.* spasm of the jaw muscles, keeping the jaws tightly closed. This is the characteristic symptom of tetanus but it also occurs with overuse of the phenothiazine drugs and in disorders of the basal ganglia.

trisomy (**try**-soh-mi) *n.* a condition in which there is one extra chromosome present in each cell in addition to the normal (diploid) chromosome set; the cause of such disorders as Down's syndrome. —**trisomic** (try-**soh**-mik) *adj.*

tritanopia (try-tă-**noh**-piă) *n.* a rare defect of colour vision in which affected persons are insensitive to blue light and confuse blues and greens. *Compare* deuteranopia, Daltonism.

tritium (**trit**-iŭm) *n.* an isotope of hydrogen that emits beta particles (electrons) during its decay. It has been used as a tracer in the investigation of diseases of the heart and the lungs. Symbol: T or ^{3}H.

trocar (**troh**-kar) *n.* an instrument used to draw off fluids from a body cavity. It comprises a metal tube containing a removable shaft with a sharp three-cornered point.

trochanter (troh-**kant**-er) *n.* either of the two protuberances that occur below the neck of the femur.

troche (trohsh) *n.* a medicinal lozenge, taken by mouth, used to treat conditions of the mouth, throat, or alimentary canal.

trochlea (**trok**-li-ă) *n.* an anatomical part having the structure or function of a pulley; for example the fibrocartilaginous ring in the frontal bone through which the tendon of the superior oblique eye muscle passes. —**trochlear** (**trok**-li-er) *adj.*

trochlear nerve *n.* the fourth cranial nerve (IV), which supplies the superior oblique eye muscle.

trochoid joint (pivot joint) (**troh**-koid) *n.* a form of diarthrosis (freely movable joint) in which a bone moves round a central axis, allowing rotational movement.

trometamol (troh-**met**-ă-mol) *n.* a diuretic that also reduces the acidity of body fluids. It is given by intravenous injection in conditions of acidosis to adjust the pH of the blood to normal levels. Trade name: **Tham-E**.

troph- (**tropho-**) *prefix denoting* nourishment or nutrition.

trophic (**trof**-ik) *adj.* relating to nutrition or to the supply of nutrients, etc., to a part of the body. *t. ulcer* an ulcer due to insufficient supply of blood or nutrients to the affected part.

trophoblast (**trof**-ŏ-blast) *n.* the tissue that forms the wall of the blastocyst.

-trophy *suffix denoting* nourishment, development, or growth.

-tropic *suffix denoting* **1.** turning towards. **2.** having an affinity for; influencing.

tropical medicine (**trop**-ikăl) *n.* the study of diseases more commonly found in tropical regions than elsewhere, such as malaria, trypanosomiasis, schistosomiasis, and leishmaniasis.

tropical ulcer (Naga sore) *n.* a skin disease prevalent in wet tropical regions. A large open sloughing sore usually develops at the site of a wound or abrasion. The ulcer is often infected with spirochaetes and bacteria and may extend deeply and cause destruction of muscles and bones.

Trousseau's sign (troo-**sohz**) *n.* a sign indicating low levels of calcium in the blood: a tourniquet placed around the upper arm stimulates spasm in the muscles of the hand. [A. Trousseau (1801–67), French physician]

troxidone (**troks**-i-dohn) *n.* an anticonvulsant drug given by mouth, alone or in conjunction with other drugs, in the treatment of epilepsy. It is highly toxic. Trade name: **Tridione**.

truncus (**trunk**-ŭs) *n.* a trunk: a main vessel or other tubular organ from which subsidiary branches arise. *t. arteriosus* the main arterial trunk arising from the fetal heart. It develops into the aorta and pulmonary artery.

trunk (trunk) *n.* **1.** *see* truncus. **2.** the body excluding the head and limbs.

truss (trus) *n.* a device for applying pressure to a hernia to prevent it from protruding. It usually consists of a pad attached to a belt worn under the clothing.

trypanocide (trip-**an**-ŏ-syd) *n.* an agent that kills trypanosomes. The main trypanocides are arsenic-containing compounds.

Trypanosoma (trip-ă-nŏ-**soh**-mă) *n. see* trypanosomiasis.

trypanosomiasis (trip-ă-nŏ-sŏ-**my**-ă-sis) *n.* any disease caused by the presence of parasitic protozoans of the genus *Trypanosoma*. The two most important diseases are Chagas' disease (*South American t.*), caused by *T. cruzi*, and sleeping sickness (*African t.*), caused

by *T. rhodesiense* or *T. gambiense*.

tryparsamide (trip-**ar**-să-myd) *n.* a drug used in the treatment of trypanosomiasis (sleeping sickness). Usually given by injection, it penetrates the cerebrospinal fluid and is highly active against the infective organism. Trade name: **Tryparsam**.

trypsin (**trip**-sin) *n.* an enzyme that continues the digestion of proteins by breaking down peptones into smaller peptide chains (*see* peptidase). It is secreted by the pancreas in an inactive form, *trypsinogen*, which is converted in the duodenum to trypsin by the action of the enzyme enteropeptidase.

trypsinogen (trip-**sin**-ŏ-jin) *n. see* trypsin.

tryptophan (**trip**-tŏ-fan) *n.* an essential amino acid. *See also* amino acid.

tsetse (**tet**-si) *n.* a large bloodsucking fly of tropical Africa belonging to the genus *Glossina*. Tsetse flies transmit the blood parasites that cause sleeping sickness, *Trypanosoma gambiense* and *T. rhodesiense*.

TSH *n. see* thyroid-stimulating hormone.

tsutsugamushi disease (tsoo-tsoo-gă-**moo**-shi) *n. see* scrub typhus.

tubal pregnancy (**oviducal pregnancy**) (**tew**-băl) *n. see* ectopic pregnancy.

tube (tewb) *n.* (in anatomy) a long hollow cylindrical structure, e.g. a Fallopian tube.

tuber (**tew**-ber) *n.* (in anatomy) a thickened or swollen part.

tubercle (**tew**-ber-kŭl) *n.* **1.** (in anatomy) a small rounded protuberance on a bone. **2.** the specific nodular lesion of tuberculosis.

tubercular (tew-**ber**-kew-ler) *adj.* having small rounded swellings or nodules, not necessarily caused by tuberculosis.

tuberculid (tew-**ber**-kew-lid) *n.* a papular lesion in the skin, probably due to an allergic reaction to tuberculosis infection.

tuberculin (tew-**ber**-kew-lin) *n.* a protein extract from cultures of tubercle bacilli, used to test whether a person has suffered from or been in contact with tuberculosis (*see* Mantoux test).

tuberculoma (tew-ber-kew-**loh**-mă) *n.* a mass of cheeselike material resembling a tumour, seen in some cases of tuberculosis. Tuberculomas are found in a variety of sites, including the lung or brain.

tuberculosis (tew-ber-kew-**loh**-sis) *n.* an infectious disease caused by the bacillus *Mycobacterium tuberculosis* and characterized by the formation of nodular lesions (tubercles) in the tissues. In the most common form of the disease (*pulmonary t.*) the bacillus is inhaled into the lungs where it sets up a primary tubercle and spreads to the nearest lymph nodes (the *primary complex*). Many people become infected but show no symptoms; they can, however, act as carriers. Symptoms of the active disease include fever, night sweats, weight loss, and the spitting of blood. In some cases the bacilli spread from the lungs to the bloodstream, setting up millions of tiny tubercles throughout the body (*miliary t.*). Bacilli entering by the mouth, usually in infected cows' milk, set up a primary complex in abdominal lymph nodes, leading to peritonitis, and sometimes spread to other or-

gans, joints, and bones (*see* Pott's disease).

Tuberculosis is curable by the antibiotics streptomycin, isoniazid (INH), and para-aminosalicylic acid (PAS). Preventive measures in the UK include the detection of carriers by X-ray screening of vulnerable populations and inoculation with BCG vaccine.

tuberculous (tew-**ber**-kew-lŭs) *adj.* relating to or affected with tuberculosis.

tuberose (tew-ber-ohz) *adj. see* tuberous.

tuberosity (tew-ber-**os**-iti) *n.* a large rounded protuberance on a bone.

tuberous (tuberose) (tew-ber-ŭs) *adj.* knobbed; having nodules or rounded swellings. *t. sclerosis* (*epiloia*) a congenital disorder in which the brain, skin, and other organs are studded with small plaques or tumours. Symptoms include epilepsy and mental retardation.

tubo- *prefix denoting* a tube, especially a Fallopian tube or auditory tube (meatus).

tuboabdominal (tew-boh-ab-**dom**-inăl) *adj.* relating to or occurring in a Fallopian tube and the abdomen.

tubocurarine (tew-boh-kewr-**ar**-een) *n.* a drug given by intravenous injection to produce relaxation of voluntary muscles before surgery and in such conditions as tetanus, encephalitis, and poliomyelitis (*see* muscle relaxant). Trade name: **Tubarine**.

tubo-ovarian (tew-boh-oh-**vair**-iăn) *adj.* relating to or occurring in a Fallopian tube and an ovary.

tubotympanal (tew-boh-**timp**-ăn-ăl) *adj.* relating to the tympanic cavity and the Eustachian tube.

tubule (tew-bewl) *n*. (in anatomy) a small cylindrical hollow structure. *See also* renal (tubule), seminiferous tubule.

tularaemia (rabbit fever) (tew-lă-ree-miă) *n*. a disease of rodents and rabbits, caused by the bacterium *Pasteurella tularense*, that may be transmitted to man. Symptoms include an ulcer at the site of infection, enlarged lymph nodes, headache, aching pains, loss of weight, and a fever lasting several weeks. Treatment with chloramphenicol, streptomycin, or tetracycline is effective.

tulle gras (tewl grah) *n*. a soft dressing consisting of open-woven silk (or other material) impregnated with a waterproof soft paraffin wax.

tumefaction (tew-mi-fak-shŏn) *n*. the process in which a tissue becomes swollen and tense by accumulation within it of fluid under pressure.

tumescence (tew-mes-ĕns) *n*. a swelling, or the process of becoming swollen, usually because of an accumulation of blood or other fluid within the tissues.

tumid (tew-mid) *adj*. swollen.

tumor (tew-mer) *n*. swelling: one of the four classical signs of inflammation in a tissue. *See also* calor, dolor, rubor.

tumour (tew-mer) *n*. any abnormal swelling in or on a part of the body. The term is usually applied to an abnormal growth of tissue, which may be benign or malignant. *Compare* cyst.

tunica (tew-nik-ă) *n*. a covering or layer of an organ or part; for example, a layer of the wall of a blood vessel (*see* adventitia, intima, media).

tunnel (tun-ĕl) *n*. (in anatomy) a canal or hollow groove.

TUR (transurethral resection) *n*. *see* resection.

turbinate bone (ter-bin-ayt) *n*. *see* nasal (concha).

turbinectomy (ter-bin-ek-tŏmi) *n*. the surgical removal of one of the turbinate bones.

turgescence (ter-jes-ĕns) *n*. a swelling, or the process by which a swelling arises in tissues, usually by the accumulation of blood or other fluid under pressure.

turgid (ter-jid) *adj*. swollen and congested, especially with blood.

turgor (ter-ger) *n*. a state of being swollen or distended.

Turner's syndrome (ter-nerz) *n*. a genetic defect in women in which there is only one X chromosome instead of the usual two. Affected women are infertile: they have female external genitalia but no ovaries. Characteristically they are short, mentally retarded, and have a webbed neck. [H. H. Turner (1892–), US endocrinologist]

turricephaly (tu-ri-sef-ăli) *n*. *see* oxycephaly.

tussis (tus-iss) *see* coughing.

twilight state (twy-lyt) *n*. a condition of disturbed consciousness in which the individual can still carry out some normal activities but is impaired in his awareness and has no memory of what he has done. It is encountered after epileptic attacks, in alcoholism, and in organic states of confusion.

twins (twinz) *n*. two individuals who are born at the same time and of the same parents. *fraternal* (or *dizygotic*) *t*. twins resulting from the simultaneous fertilization of two egg cells; they may be of different sexes and are no more alike than ordinary siblings. *identical* (or *monozygotic*) *t*.

twins resulting from the fertilization of a single egg cell that subsequently divides to give two separate fetuses. They are of the same sex and otherwise genetically identical. *See also* Siamese twins.

tylosis (ty-**loh**-sis) *n.* the development of a callus on the skin (*see* callosity).

tympan- (tympano-) *prefix denoting* **1.** the eardrum. **2.** the middle ear.

tympanic cavity (tim-**pan**-ik) *n. see* middle ear.

tympanic membrane (eardrum) *n.* the membrane at the inner end of the external auditory meatus, separating the outer and middle ears. When sound waves reach the ear the tympanum vibrates, transmitting these vibrations to the malleus.

tympanites (meteorism) (timp-ă-ny-teez) *n.* distension of the abdomen with air or gas: the abdomen is resonant on percussion. Causes include intestinal obstruction, irritable bowel syndrome, and aerophagy.

tympanitis (timp-ă-**ny**-tis) *n.* inflammation of the middle ear. *See* otitis.

tympanoplasty (**timp**-ă-noh-plasti) *n. see* myringoplasty.

tympanotomy (timp-ă-**not**-ŏmi) *n. see* myringotomy.

tympanum (**timp**-ă-nŭm) *n.* the middle ear (tympanic cavity) and/or the eardrum (tympanic membrane).

typhlitis (tif-**ly**-tis) *n.* inflammation of the caecum.

typho- *prefix denoting* **1.** typhoid fever. **2.** typhus.

typhoid fever (ty-foid) *n.* an infection of the digestive system by the bacterium *Salmonella typhi*, causing general weakness, high fever, a rash of red spots on the chest and abdomen, chills, sweating, and in serious cases inflammation of the spleen and bones, delirium, and erosion of the intestinal wall leading to haemorrhage. It is transmitted through contaminated food or drinking water. Treatment with ampicillin or chloramphenicol reduces the severity of symptoms. Vaccination with TAB provides temporary immunity. *Compare* paratyphoid fever.

typhus (spotted fever) (ty-fŭs) *n.* any one of a group of infections caused by rickettsiae and characterized by severe headache, a widespread rash, prolonged high fever, and delirium. They all respond to treatment with chloramphenicol or tetracyclines. The rickettsiae may be transmitted by lice (*epidemic, classical,* or *louse-borne t.*); rat fleas (*endemic, murine,* or *flea-borne t.*); ticks (*see* Rocky Mountain spotted fever); or mites (*see* rickettsial pox, scrub typhus).

tyramine (ty-ră-meen) *n.* an amine naturally occurring in cheese. It has a similar effect in the body to that of adrenaline. This effect can be dangerous in patients taking MAO inhibitors (antidepressants), in whom blood pressure may become very high.

tyrosine (ty-roh-seen) *n. see* amino acid.

tyrosinosis (ty-roh-si-**noh**-sis) *n.* an inborn defect of metabolism of the amino acid tyrosine causing excess excretion of parahydroxyphenylpyruvic acid in the urine.

tyrothricin (ty-roh-**thry**-sin) *n.* an antibiotic derived from the bacterium *Bacillus brevis*. It is used mainly in the treatment of infections of the mouth, throat, skin, wounds, and burns; it is applied topically as it is very toxic if taken into the body. Trade name: **Hydrotricine**.

U

ulcer (**ul**-ser) *n*. a break in the skin or in the mucous membrane lining the alimentary tract that fails to heal and is often accompanied by inflammation. *varicose u.* a complication of varicose veins, due to defective circulation. *See also* aphtha, bedsore, duodenal ulcer, gastric (ulcer), peptic (ulcer), rodent ulcer.

ulcerative colitis (**ul**-ser-ay-tiv) *n. see* colitis.

ulcerative gingivitis (**Vincent's angina**) *n*. acute painful inflammation and ulceration of the gums associated with infection by the microorganisms *Borrelia* and *Fusobacterium*.

ule- (ulo-) *prefix denoting* 1. scars; scar tissue. 2. the gums.

ulna (**ul**-nă) *n*. the inner and longer bone of the forearm. It articulates with the humerus and radius above and with the radius and indirectly with the wrist bones below. —**ulnar** (**ul**-ner) *adj*.

ulnar artery *n*. a branch of the brachial artery arising at the elbow and running deep within the muscles of the medial side of the forearm to the palm of the hand.

ulnar nerve *n*. one of the major nerves of the arm. It originates in the neck and runs down the inner side of the upper arm to behind the elbow. It supplies the muscles of the forearm and the skin of the palm and fourth and fifth fingers.

ultra- *prefix denoting* 1. beyond. 2. an extreme degree (e.g. of large or small size).

ultrafiltration (ultră-fil-**tray**-shŏn) *n*. filtration under pressure. In the kidney, blood is subjected to ultrafiltration to remove the waste material that goes to make up urine.

ultramicroscopic (ultra-my-krŏ-**skop**-ik) *adj*. too small to be seen by means of an ordinary light microscope.

ultrasonics (ultră-**sonn**-iks) *n*. the study of the uses and properties of ultrasound. —**ultrasonic** *adj*.

ultrasonography (ultră-sonn-**og**-răfi) *n*. the use of ultrasound to produce pictures of structures within the body.

ultrasonotomography (**echo-tomography**) (ultră-sonn-oh-tŏ-**mog**-răfi) *n*. the use of ultrasound to examine the internal structure of the body by producing images of the reflections from different depths.

ultrasound (**ultrasonic waves**) (**ul**-tră-sownd) *n*. sound waves of extremely high frequency (above 20,000 Hz), inaudible to the human ear. Ultrasound can be used to examine the structure of the inside of the body; the vibratory effect of the sound waves can also be used in the treatment of various disorders of deep tissues. *See also* echography.

ultraviolet rays (ultră-vy-ŏ-lit) *pl. n*. invisible short-wavelength radiation beyond the violet end of the visible spectrum. Sunlight contains ultraviolet rays, which are responsible for the production of both suntan and – on overexposure – sunburn.

umbilical cord (um-**bil**-ikăl) *n.* the strand of tissue connecting the fetus to the placenta. It contains two arteries that carry blood to the placenta and one vein that returns it to the fetus.

umbilicated (um-bil-i-kayt-id) *adj.* having a navel-like depression.

umbilicus (omphalus) (um-**bil**-ikŭs) *n.* the navel: a circular depression in the centre of the abdomen marking the site of attachment of the umbilical cord in the fetus. —**umbilical** *adj.*

umbo (**um**-boh) *n.* a projecting centre of a round surface, especially the projection of the inner surface of the eardrum to which the malleus is attached.

unciform bone (un-si-form) *n. see* hamate bone.

uncinate fits (un-sin-ayt) *pl. n.* a form of temporal lobe epilepsy in which hallucinations of taste and smell and inappropriate chewing movements are prominent features.

unconscious (un-kon-shŭs) *adj.* **1.** in a state of unconsciousness. **2.** (in psychoanalysis) denoting the part of the mind that includes memories, motives, and intentions that are not accessible to awareness and cannot be made conscious without overcoming resistances. *Compare* subconscious.

unconsciousness (un-**kon**-shŭs-nis) *n.* a condition of being unaware of one's surroundings, as in sleep, or of being unresponsive to stimulation. An unnatural state of unconsciousness may be caused by factors that produce reduced brain activity, such as lack of oxygen or a blow on the head, or it may be brought about deliberately during general anaesthesia. *See also* coma.

uncus (**unk**-ŭs) *n.* any hook-shaped structure, especially a projection of the lower surface of the cerebral hemisphere.

undecenoic acid (un-des-i-**noh**-ik) *n.* an antifungal agent, applied to the skin in the form of powder, ointment, lotion, or aerosol spray for the treatment of such infections as athlete's foot. Trade name: **Mycota**.

undine (**un**-deen) *n.* a small rounded container, usually made of glass, for solutions used to wash out the eye. It has a small neck for filling and a long tapering spout with a narrow outlet.

undulant fever (**un**-dew-länt) *n. see* brucellosis.

ungual (**ung**-wăl) *adj.* relating to the fingernails or toenails (ungues).

unguentum (ung-**wen**-tŭm) (in pharmacy) *n.* an ointment.

unguis (**ung**-wis) *n.* a fingernail or toenail. *See* nail.

uni- *prefix denoting* one.

unicellular (yoo-ni-**sel**-yoo-ler) *adj.* describing organisms or tissues that consist of a single cell.

unigravida (yoo-ni-**grav**-id-ă) *n. see* primigravida.

unilateral (yoo-ni-**lat**-erăl) *adj.* (in anatomy) relating to or affecting one side of the body or one side of an organ or other part.

union (**yoon**-yŏn) *n.* (in a fractured bone) the successful result of healing of a fracture, in which the bone ends have become firmly united by newly formed bone. *Compare* malunion.

uniovular (yoo-ni-**ov**-yoo-ler) *adj.* derived from a single ovum, as are identical twins. *Compare* binovular.

unipara (yoo-**nip**-er-ă) *n. see* primipara.

unipolar (yoo-ni-**poh**-ler) *adj.* (in neurology) describing a neurone that has one main process extending from the cell body. *Compare* bipolar.

Unna's paste (**oo**-năz) *n.* a dressing for varicose ulcers consisting of a mixture of zinc oxide, gelatin, and glycerine, applied between layers of a spiral bandage. [P. G. Unna (1850–1929), German dermatologist]

urachus (**yoor**-ă-kŭs) *n.* the remains of the cavity of the allantois. It usually disappears during embryonic development, leaving a solid fibrous cord connecting the bladder with the umbilicus. —**urachal** *adj.*

uracil (**yoor**-ă-sil) *n.* one of the nitrogen-containing bases (*see* pyrimidine) occurring in the nucleic acid RNA.

uraemia (yoor-**ee**-miă) *n.* the presence of excessive amounts of urea and other nitrogenous waste compounds in the blood. This occurs in kidney failure and results in nausea, vomiting, lethargy, drowsiness, and eventually (if untreated) death. Treatment may require haemodialysis on a kidney machine. —**uraemic** *adj.*

uramustine (yoor-ă-**must**-een) *n.* a cytotoxic drug administered by intravenous injection in the treatment of various forms of cancer, particularly chronic lymphatic leukaemia. Trade name: **Uracil Mustard**.

uran- (urano-) *prefix denoting* the palate.

uraniscorrhaphy (yoor-ăn-isk-o-răfi) *n. see* staphylorrhaphy.

uranism (**yoor**-ăn-izm) *n.* lead poisoning. *See* lead.

urataemia (yoor-ă-**tee**-miă) *n.* the presence in the blood of sodium urate and other urates, formed by the reaction of uric acid with bases. *See also* gout.

urate (**yoor**-ayt) *n.* a salt of uric acid, normally present in the urine. Excess amounts occur in the blood and joints in gout.

uraturia (yoor-ăt-**yoor**-iă) *n.* the presence in the urine of urates. Abnormally high concentrations of urates in urine occur in gout.

urea (yoor-**ee**-ă) *n.* the main breakdown product of protein metabolism. It is the chemical form in which unrequired nitrogen is excreted by the body in the urine. Urea is formed in the liver from ammonia and carbon dioxide.

urease (**yoor**-i-ayz) *n.* an enzyme that catalyses the hydrolysis of urea to ammonia and carbon dioxide.

urecchysis (yoor-**ek**-i-sis) *n.* the escape of uric acid from the blood into spaces in the connective tissue.

uresis (yoor-**ee**-sis) *n. see* urination.

ureter (yoor-**ee**-ter) *n.* either of a pair of tubes, 25–30 cm long, that conduct urine from the pelvis of kidneys to the bladder. —**ureteral**, **ureteric** (yoor-i-**te**-rik) *adj.*

ureter- (uretero-) *prefix denoting* the ureter(s).

ureterectomy (yoor-i-ter-ek-tŏmi) *n.* surgical removal of a ureter. This usually includes removal of the associated kidney as well (*see* nephroureterectomy).

ureteritis (yoor-i-ter-**I**-tis) *n.* inflammation of the ureter. This usually occurs in association with cystitis, particularly if caused by vesicoureteric reflux.

ureterocele (yoor-ee-ter-oh-seel) *n.* a cystic swelling of the wall of the ureter at the point where it passes into the bladder. It is associated with stenosis of the opening of the ureter and it may cause impaired drainage of the kidney with dilatation of the ureter and hydronephrosis.

ureteroenterostomy (yoor-ee-ter-oh-en-ter-**ost**-ŏmi) *n*. an artificial communication, surgically created, between the ureter and the bowel. *See also* ureterosigmoidostomy.

ureterolith (yoor-ee-ter-oh-lith) *n*. a stone in the ureter. *See* calculus, ureterolithotomy.

ureterolithotomy (yoor-ee-ter-oh-lith-**ot**-ŏmi) *n*. the surgical removal of a stone (calculus) from the ureter. If the stone occupies the lower portion of the ureter, it may be extracted by cystoscopy, thus avoiding open surgery.

ureteroneocystostomy (yoor-ee-ter-oh-nee-oh-sist-**ost**-ŏmi) *n*. the surgical reimplantation of a ureter into the bladder. This is most commonly performed to cure vesicoureteric reflux.

ureteronephrectomy (yoor-ee-ter-oh-ni-**frek**-tŏmi) *n*. *see* nephroureterectomy.

ureteroplasty (yoor-ee-ter-oh-plasti) *n*. surgical reconstruction of the ureter using a segment of bowel or a tube of bladder.

ureteropyelonephritis (yoor-ee-ter-oh-py-ĕ-loh-ni-**fry**-tis) *n*. inflammation involving both the ureter and the renal pelvis (*see* ureteritis, pyelitis).

ureterosigmoidostomy (yoor-ee-ter-oh-sig-moid-**ost**-ŏmi) *n*. the operation of implanting the ureters into the sigmoid colon. This method of permanent urinary diversion may be used after cystectomy or to bypass a diseased or damaged bladder. The urine is

passed together with the faeces, avoiding the need for an external opening and appliance to collect the urine.

ureterostomy (yoor-i-ter-**ost**-ŏmi) *n*. the surgical creation of an external opening into the ureter. This usually involves bringing the ureter to the skin surface so that the urine can drain into a suitable appliance (*cutaneous u.*).

ureterotomy (yoor-i-ter-**ot**-ŏmi) *n*. surgical incision into the ureter, most commonly performed in ureterolithotomy.

ureterovaginal (yoor-ee-ter-oh-vă-jy-năl) *adj*. relating to or between the ureter and vagina.

urethane (**yoor**-i-thayn) *n*. a drug administered by mouth to treat some forms of cancer.

urethr- (**urethro-**) *prefix denoting* the urethra.

urethra (yoor-ee-thră) *n*. the tube that conducts urine from the bladder to the exterior. The female urethra is quite short (about 3.5 cm) and opens just within the vulva, between the clitoris and vagina. The male urethra is longer (about 20 cm) and runs through the penis. It also serves as the ejaculatory duct. —**urethral** *adj*.

urethritis (yoor-i-**thry**-tis) *n*. inflammation of the urethra. This may be due to gonorrhoea (*specific u.*), a nonspecific venereal infection (*nonspecific u.*), or to the presence of a catheter in the urethra. The symptoms are those of urethral discharge with painful or difficult urination (dysuria).

urethrocele (yoor-ee-throh-seel) *n*. **1.** a pouch formed from a weakened portion of the wall of the urethra that encroaches on the vaginal canal. It may result from infection or from the pressure of the fetal head in prolonged labour. **2.** prolapse of the female urethra through its external opening.

urethrography (yoor-i-**throg**-răfi) *n.* X-ray examination of the urethra, after introduction of a radio-opaque fluid, so that its outline and any narrowing or other abnormalities may be observed in X-ray photographs (*urethrograms*).

urethroplasty (yoor-**ee**-throh-plasti) *n.* surgical repair of a urethral stricture. The operation entails the insertion of a flap or patch of skin from the scrotum or perineum into the urethra at the site of the stricture, which is laid widely open.

urethrorrhaphy (yoor-i-**thro**-răfi) *n.* surgical restoration of the continuity of the urethra. This may be required following laceration of the urethra.

urethrorrhoea (yoor-ee-thrŏ-**ree**-ă) *n.* a discharge from the urethra. This is a symptom of urethritis.

urethroscope (yoor-**ee**-thrŏ-skohp) *n.* an endoscope, consisting of a fine tube fitted with a light and lenses, for examination of the interior of the male urethra. —**urethroscopy** (yoor-i-**throsk**-ŏpi) *n.*

urethrostenosis (yoor-ee-throh-sti-**noh**-sis) *n.* a stricture of the urethra.

urethrostomy (yoor-i-**throst**-ŏmi) *n.* the operation of creating an opening of the urethra in the perineum in men. This can be permanent, to bypass a severe stricture of the urethra in the penis, or it can form the first stage of a urethroplasty.

urethrotomy (yoor-i-**throt**-ŏmi) *n.* the operation of cutting a stricture in the urethra. It is usually performed with a *urethrotome*: a type of endoscope that consists of a sheath down which is passed a fine knife.

-uria *suffix denoting* **1.** a condition of urine or urination. **2.** the presence of a specified substance in the urine.

uric acid (yoor-ik) *n.* a nitrogen-containing organic acid that is the end-product of nucleic acid metabolism and is a component of the urine. Crystals of uric acid are deposited in the joints of people suffering from gout.

uricosuric drug (yoor-i-koh-**sewr**-ik) *n.* a drug, such as probenecid or sulphinpyrazone, that increases the amount of uric acid excreted in the urine. Uricosuric drugs are used to treat gout and other conditions in which the levels of uric acid in the blood are increased.

uridrosis (yoor-i-**droh**-sis) *n.* the presence of excessive amounts of urea in the sweat; when the sweat dries, a white flaky deposit of urea may remain on the skin. The phenomenon occurs in uraemia.

urin- (urino-, uro-) *prefix denoting* urine or the urinary system.

urinalysis (yoor-in-**al**-i-sis) *n.* the analysis of urine, using physical, chemical and microscopical tests, to determine the proportions of its normal constituents and to detect alcohol, drugs, sugar, or other abnormal constituents.

urinary bladder (**yoor**-in-er-i) *n. see* bladder.

urinary tract *n.* the entire system of ducts and channels that conduct urine from the kidneys to the exterior. It includes the ureters, the bladder, and the urethra.

urination (micturition) (yoor-in-ay-shŏn) *n*. the periodic discharge of urine from the bladder through the urethra.

urine (yoor-in) *n*. the fluid excreted by the kidneys, which contains many of the body's waste products. It is the major route by which the end-products of nitrogen metabolism – urea, uric acid, and creatinine – are excreted. The other major constituent is sodium chloride. Biochemical analysis of urine is commonly used in the diagnosis of diseases and in pregnancy tests.

uriniferous tubule (yoor-in-**if**-er-ŭs) *n. see* renal (tubule).

urinogenital (urogenital) (yoor-in-oh-**jen**-it'l) *adj*. of or relating to the organs and tissues concerned with excretion and reproduction.

urinometer (yoor-in-om-it-er) *n*. a hydrometer for measuring the specific gravity of urine.

urobilin (yoor-oh-**by**-lin) *n. see* urobilinogen.

urobilinogen (yoor-oh-by-**lin**-ŏ-jin) *n*. a colourless product of the reduction of the bile pigment bilirubin. Urobilinogen is formed from bilirubin in the intestine by bacterial action. Part of it is reabsorbed and returned to the liver; part of it is excreted. When exposed to air, urobilinogen is oxidized to a brown pigment, *urobilin*.

urocele (yoor-oh-seel) *n*. a cystic swelling in the scrotum, containing urine that has escaped from the urethra. This may arise following urethral injury.

urochesia (yoor-oh-**kee**-ziă) *n*. the passage of urine through the rectum. This may follow a penetrating injury involving both the lower urinary tract and the bowel.

urochrome (yoor-oh-krohm) *n*. the pigment responsible for the colour of urine.

urogenital (yoor-oh-**jen**-it'l) *adj. see* urinogenital.

urography (yoor-**og**-răfi) *n*. X-ray examination of any part of the urinary tract. *See* pyelography.

urokinase (yoor-oh-ky-nayz) *n*. an enzyme, produced by the kidney, that activates the system involved in dissolving blood clots. It has been used for treating pulmonary embolism.

urolith (yoor-oh-lith) *n*. a stone in the urinary tract. *See* calculus.

urology (yoor-**ol**-ŏji) *n*. the branch of medicine concerned with the study and treatment of diseases of the urinary tract. —**urological** (yoor-ŏ-**loj**-ikăl) *adj*. —**urologist** *n*.

urticaria (hives, nettle rash) (er-ti-**kair**-iă) *n*. an acute or chronic allergic reaction in which red round wheals develop on the skin, ranging in size from small spots to several inches across. These itch intensely and may last for hours or days; the cause is sensitivity to certain foods, such as shellfish or strawberries. *See also* angioneurotic oedema.

uter- (utero-) *prefix denoting* the womb (uterus).

uterine (yoo-teryn) *adj*. of or relating to the womb (uterus).

uterocele (yoo-ter-oh-seel) *n. see* hysterocele.

uterogestation (yoo-ter-oh-jes-tay-shŏn) *n*. the development of a fetus in the womb, i.e. a normal pregnancy. *Compare* ectopic pregnancy.

uterography (yoo-ter-og-răfi) *n*. radiography of the womb.

utero-ovarian (yoo-ter-oh-oh-vair-iăn) *adj*. relating to or occurring in the womb and an ovary.

uterosalpingography (hysterosalpingography) (yoo-ter-oh-sal-ping-**og**-răfi) *n*. radiography of the interior of the womb and the Fallopian tubes following injection of a radio-opaque fluid.

uterovesical (yoo-ter-oh-**ves**-ikăl) *adj*. relating to the womb and bladder.

uterus (womb) (**yoo**-ter-ŭs) *n*. the part of the female reproductive tract that is specialized to allow the embryo to become implanted in its inner wall and to nourish the growing fetus from the maternal blood. The nonpregnant uterus is a pear-shaped organ, about 7.5 cm long, suspended in the pelvic cavity. The upper part is connected to the two Fallopian tubes and the lower part joins the vagina at the cervix.

utricle (utriculus) (**yoo**-trik-ŭl) *n*. **1.** the larger of the two membranous sacs within the vestibule of the ear. It contains a macula, which responds to gravity and relays information to the brain about the position of the head. **2.** a small sac (the *prostatic u.*) extending out of the urethra of the male into the substance of the prostate gland.

uvea (uveal tract) (**yoo**-vi-ă) *n*. the vascular pigmented layer of the eye, which lies beneath the outer layer (sclera). It consists of the choroid, ciliary body, and iris. —**uveal** *adj*.

uveitis (yoo-vi-**I**-tis) *n*. inflammation of any part of the uveal tract of the eye, either the iris (*iritis*), ciliary body (*cyclitis*), or choroid (*choroiditis*). All types may lead to visual impairment, and uveitis is an important cause of blindness.

uveoparotitis (uveoparotid fever) (yoo-vi-oh-pa-rŏ-**ty**-tis) *n*. inflammation of the uvea and swelling of the parotid salivary gland: one of the more common varieties of the chronic disease sarcoidosis.

uvula (**yoov**-yoo-lă) *n*. a small soft extension of the soft palate that hangs from the roof of the mouth above the root of the tongue. It is composed of muscle, connective tissue, and mucous membrane.

uvulectomy (yoov-yoo-**lek**-tŏmi) *n*. surgical removal of the uvula.

uvulitis (yoov-yoo-**ly**-tis) *n*. inflammation of the uvula.

V

vaccination (vak-si-**nay**-shŏn) *n*. a means of producing immunity to a disease by using a vaccine. The name was applied originally only to treatment with vaccinia (cowpox) virus, which gives protection against cowpox and smallpox. However, it is now used synonymously with inoculation as a method of immunization against any disease. A vaccine is usually given by injection but may be introduced into the skin through light scratches; for some diseases, oral vaccines are available.

vaccine (**vak**-seen) *n*. a special preparation of antigenic material that can be used to stimulate the development of antibodies and thus confer active immunity against a specific disease or number of diseases. Many vaccines are produced by culturing bacteria or viruses under conditions that lead to a loss of their virulence but not of their antigenic nature. Other vaccines consist of specially treated toxins (toxoids) or of dead bacteria that are still antigenic. *See* immunization.

vaccinia (vak-sin-iă) *n. see* cowpox.

vaccinotherapy (vak-sin-oh-th'e-răpi) *n.* the treatment of disease by the use of vaccines.

vacuole (vak-yoo-ohl) *n.* a space within the cytoplasm of a cell, formed by infolding of the cell membrane, that contains material taken in by the cell.

vacuum extractor (vak-yoo-ŭm) *n.* a suction cup that can be attached to the head of a fetus in order to aid delivery.

vagal (vay-găl) *adj.* relating to the vagus nerve.

vagin- (vagino-) *prefix denoting* the vagina.

vagina (vă-jy-nă) *n.* the lower part of the female reproductive tract: a muscular tube, lined with mucous membrane, connecting the cervix of the uterus to the exterior. It receives the erect penis during coitus. —**vaginal** *adj.*

vaginismus (vaj-i-niz-mŭs) *n.* sudden and painful contraction of the muscles surrounding the vagina, usually in response to the vulva or vagina being touched. The condition may be associated with fear of or aversion to coitus; other causative factors include vaginal injury and dryness of the lining membrane of the vagina. *See also* dyspareunia.

vaginitis (vaj-i-ny-tis) *n.* inflammation of the vagina, which may be caused by infection (commonly with *Trichomonas vaginalis*), ill-fitting contraceptive devices, dietary deficiency, or poor hygiene. There is often irritation, increased vaginal discharge, and

pain on passing urine. *postmenopausal v.* vaginitis caused by a deficiency of female sex hormones.

vaginoplasty (colpoplasty) (vă-jy-noh-plasti) *n.* a tissue-grafting operation on the vagina.

vaginoscope (vaj-in-oh-skohp) *n. see* colposcope.

vago- *prefix denoting* the vagus nerve.

vagotomy (vag-ot-ŏmi) *n.* the surgical cutting of any of the branches of the vagus nerve. This is usually performed to reduce secretion of acid and pepsin by the stomach in order to cure a peptic ulcer.

vagus nerve (vay-gŭs) *n.* the tenth cranial nerve (X), which supplies motor nerve fibres to the muscles of swallowing and parasympathetic fibres to the heart and organs of the chest cavity and abdomen. Sensory branches carry impulses from the viscera and the sensation of taste from the mouth.

valgus (val-gŭs) *adj.* describing any deformity that displaces the hand or foot away from the midline. *See* knock-knee (genu valgum), talipes.

valine (vay-leen) *n.* an essential amino acid. *See also* amino acid.

Valium (val-iŭm) *n. see* diazepam.

valve (valv) *n.* a structure found in some tubular organs or parts that restricts the flow of fluid within them to one direction only (*see* cusp). Valves are important structures in the heart, veins, and lymphatic vessels. *See also* mitral valve, tricuspid valve, semilunar valve.

valvotomy (valvulotomy) (val-vot-ŏmi) *n.* surgical cutting through a valve. The term is usually used to describe the op-

(A) cut vein showing the two cusps
of a valve; (B) action of
a venous valve

eration to relieve obstruction
caused by stenosed valves in the
heart.

valvula (val-vew-lă) *n.* (*pl.* **valvulae**)
a small valve. *valvulae con-
niventes* circular folds of mucous
membrane in the small intestine.

valvulitis (val-vew-ly-tis) *n.* inflammation of one or more valves,
particularly the heart valves. This
is most often due to rheumatic
fever (*see* endocarditis).

vancomycin (vank-oh-my-sin) *n.* an
antibiotic, derived from the bacterium *Streptomyces orientalis*,
that is effective against most
Gram-positive organisms. It is
given by intravenous infusion for
infections due to strains that are
resistant to other antibiotics.
Trade name: **Vancocin**.

van den Bergh's test (van-den-
bergz) *n.* a test to determine
whether jaundice in a patient is
due to haemolysis or to disease
of the liver or bile duct. [A. A.
H. van den Bergh (1869–1943),
Dutch physician]

vaporizer (vay-per-I-zer) *n.* a piece
of equipment for producing an
extremely fine mist of liquid
droplets by forcing a jet of liquid through a narrow nozzle
with a jet of air. *See also* aerosol.

Vaquez-Osler disease (vak-ay
ohs-ler) *n. see* polycythaemia
(vera). [L. H. Vaquez (1860–
1936), French physician; Sir W.
Osler (1849–1919), Canadian
physician]

varicectomy (va-ri-sek-tŏmi) *n. see*
phlebectomy.

varicella (va-ri-sel-ă) *n. see*
chickenpox.

varices (va-ri-seez) *pl. n. see* varix.

varicocele (va-ri-koh-seel) *n.* a collection of dilated veins in the
spermatic cord. It usually produces no symptoms apart from
occasional aching discomfort. In
some cases varicocele is associated with oligospermia, which
can be improved by surgical correction of the varicocele (*var-
icocelectomy*).

varicose veins (va-ri-kohs) *pl. n.*
veins that are distended, length-
ened, and tortuous. The superficial veins of the legs are most
commonly affected; other sites
include the rectum (*see* haemorrhoids) and testes (*see* varicocele). There is an inherited ten-

dency to varicose veins but obstruction to blood flow is responsible in some cases. Treatment includes elastic support and sclerotherapy, but stripping or excision is required in some cases.

varicotomy (va-ri-**kot**-ŏmi) *n.* incision into a varicose vein (*see* phlebectomy).

variola (vă-**ry**-ŏ-lă) *n. see* smallpox.

varioloid (**vair**-i-ŏ-loid) **1.** *n.* a mild form of smallpox in people who have previously had smallpox or have been vaccinated against it. **2.** *adj.* resembling smallpox.

varix (**vair**-iks) *n.* (*pl.* **varices**) a single varicose vein.

varus (**vair**-ŭs) *adj.* describing any deformity that displaces the hand or foot towards the midline. *See* bow-legs (genu varum), talipes.

vas- (vaso-) *prefix denoting* **1.** vessels, especially blood vessels. **2.** the vas deferens.

vasa efferentia (**vay**-să ef-er-en-shiă) *pl. n.* (*sing.* **vas efferens**) the many small tubes that conduct spermatozoa from the testis to the epididymis.

vasa vasorum (vas-or-ŭm) *pl. n.* the tiny arteries and veins that supply the walls of blood vessels.

vascular (**vas**-kew-ler) *adj.* relating to or supplied with blood vessels. *v. system see* cardiovascular system.

vascularization (vas-kew-ler-I-zay-shŏn) *n.* the development of blood vessels (usually capillaries) within a tissue.

vasculitis (vas-kew-**ly**-tis) *n. see* angiitis.

vas deferens (vas **def**-er-ĕnz) *n.* (*pl.* **vasa deferentia**) either of a pair of ducts that conduct spermato-

zoa from the epididymis to the urethra on ejaculation.

vasectomy (vă-**sek**-tŏmi) *n.* the surgical operation of cutting the vas deferens. Bilateral vasectomy causes sterility and is an increasingly popular means of birth control.

vaso- *prefix. see* vas-.

vasoactive (vay-zoh-**ak**-tiv) *adj.* affecting the diameter of blood vessels, especially arteries. Examples of vasoactive agents are emotion, pressure, carbon dioxide, and temperature.

vasoconstriction (vay-zoh-kŏn-strik-shŏn) *n.* a decrease in the diameter of blood vessels, especially arteries.

vasoconstrictor (vay-zoh-kŏn-strik-ter) *n.* an agent that causes narrowing of the blood vessels and therefore a decrease in blood flow. Examples are cyclopentamine, methoxamine, and phenylephrine. Vasoconstrictors are used to raise the blood pressure in disorders of the circulation, shock, or severe bleeding and to maintain blood pressure during surgery.

vasodilatation (vay-zoh-dy-lă-tay-shŏn) *n.* an increase in the diameter of blood vessels, especially arteries.

vasodilator (vay-zoh-dy-**lay**-ter) *n.* a drug that causes widening of the blood vessels and therefore an increase in blood flow. Vasodilators are used to lower blood pressure in cases of hypertension. *coronary v.* a drug, such as glyceryl trinitrate or pentaerythritol, that increases the blood flow through the heart and is used to relieve and prevent angina. *peripheral v.* a drug, such as cyclandelate, phenoxybenzamine, or tolazoline, that affects the blood vessels of the limbs and is used to treat conditions of poor circulation.

vasoligation (vay-zoh-ly-**gay**-shŏn) *n.* the surgical tying of the vas deferens. This is performed to prevent infection spreading from the urinary tract causing recurrent epididymitis.

vasomotion (vay-zoh-**moh**-shŏn) *n.* an increase or decrease in the diameter of blood vessels, particularly the arteries. *See* vasoconstriction, vasodilatation.

vasomotor (vay-zoh-**moh**-ter) *adj.* controlling the muscular walls of blood vessels, especially arteries, and therefore their diameter. *v. centre* a collection of nerve cells in the medulla oblongata that brings about reflex changes in the rate of the heart beat and in the diameter of blood vessels, so that the blood pressure can be adjusted. *v. nerve* any nerve, usually belonging to the autonomic nervous system, that controls the circulation of blood through blood vessels by its action on the muscle fibres within their walls or its action on the heart beat.

vasopressin (antidiuretic hormone, ADH) (vay-zoh-**pres**-in) *n.* a hormone, released by the pituitary gland, that increases the reabsorption of water by the kidney and causes constriction of blood vessels. It is administered either nasally or by injection to treat diabetes insipidus.

vasopressor (vay-zoh-**pres**-er) *adj.* stimulating the contraction of blood vessels and therefore bringing about an increase in blood pressure.

vasospasm (**vay**-zoh-spazm) *n. see* Raynaud's disease.

vasovagal (vay-zoh-**vay**-găl) *adj.* relating to the action of impulses in the vagus nerve on the circulation. The vagus reduces the rate at which the heart beats, and so lowers its output. *v. attack* excessive activity of the vagus nerve, causing slowing of the heart and a fall in blood pressure, which leads to fainting. *See* syncope.

vasovesiculitis (vay-zoh-ve-sik-yoo-ly-tis) *n.* inflammation of the seminal vesicles and vas deferens. This usually occurs in association with prostatitis and causes pain in the perineum, groin, and scrotum and a high temperature.

vectis (**vek**-tis) *n.* a curved instrument used to assist the delivery of an infant.

vector (**vek**-ter) *n.* an animal, usually an insect or a tick, that transmits parasitic microorganisms – and therefore the diseases they cause – from person to person or from infected animals to human beings.

vectorcardiography (vek-ter-kar-di-**og**-răfi) *n. see* electrocardiography.

vegetation (vej-i-**tay**-shŏn) *n.* (in pathology) an abnormal outgrowth from a membrane. In ulcerative endocarditis, such outgrowths, consisting of fibrin with enmeshed blood cells, are found on the membrane lining the heart valves.

vegetative (**vej**-i-tă-tiv) *adj.* **1.** relating to growth and nutrition rather than to reproduction. **2.** functioning unconsciously; autonomic.

vehicle (**vee**-ikŭl) *n.* (in pharmacy) any substance, such as sterile water or dextrose solution, that acts as the medium in which a drug is administered.

The principal veins of the body

vein (vayn) *n.* a blood vessel conveying blood towards the heart. All veins except the pulmonary vein carry deoxygenated blood from the tissues to the vena cava. Veins contain valves that assist the flow of blood back to the heart. Anatomical name: **vena.** —**venous** (vee-nŭs) *adj.*

vena cava (vee-nă kay-vă) *n.* either of the two main veins, conveying blood from the other veins to the right atrium of the heart. *inferior v. c.* the vein that receives blood from parts of the body below the diaphragm. *superior v. c.* the vein that drains blood from the head, neck, thorax, and arms.

vene- (**veno-**) *prefix denoting* veins.

venene (ven-een) *n.* a mixture of two or more venoms: used to produce antiserum against venoms (antivenene).

venepuncture (venipuncture) (ven-i-punk-cher) *n.* the puncture of a vein for any therapeutic purpose; for example, to extract blood for laboratory tests. *See also* phlebotomy.

venereal disease (VD) (vin-eer-iăl) *n.* any infectious disease transmitted by sexual intercourse. Examples are gonorrhoea, genital herpes, and syphilis.

venereology (vin-eer-i-ol-ŏji) *n.* the study of venereal diseases.

venesection (ven-i-sek-shŏn) *n. see* phlebotomy.

veno- *prefix. see* vene-.

venoclysis (vi-nok-li-sis) *n.* the continuous infusion into a vein of saline or other solution.

venography (phlebography) (vi-nog-răfi) *n.* X-ray examination to show up the course of veins in a particular region of the body. A radio-opaque contrast medium is injected slowly into a vein and X-ray photographs (*venograms*) taken as the compound is carried towards the heart. *See also* angiography.

venom (ven-ŏm) *n.* the poisonous material produced by snakes, scorpions, etc. Some venoms produce no more than local pain and swelling; others can prove lethal.

ventilation (ven-ti-lay-shŏn) *n.* the passage of air into and out of the respiratory tract. In the alveoli of the lungs gas exchange is most efficient when matched by an adequate blood flow (perfusion). Ventilation/perfusion imbalance is an important cause of anoxia and cyanosis.

ventilator (ven-ti-lay-ter) *n.* **1.** a device to ensure a supply of fresh air. **2.** equipment that is manually or mechanically operated to maintain a flow of air into and out of the lungs of a patient who is unable to breathe normally. *See also* respirator.

ventral (ven-trăl) *adj.* relating to or situated at or close to the front of the body or to the anterior part of an organ.

ventricle (ven-trik-ŭl) *n.* **1.** either of the two lower chambers of the heart. The left ventricle receives blood from the pulmonary vein and pumps it into the aorta. The right ventricle pumps blood from the venae cavae into the pulmonary artery. **2.** one of the four fluid-filled cavities within the brain. The paired first and second ventricles (lateral ventricles) communicate with the third ventricle. This leads to the fourth ventricle in the hindbrain, which is continuous with the spinal canal. Cerebrospinal fluid circulates through all the cavities. —**ventricular** (ven-trik-yoo-ler) *adj.*

ventricul- (ventriculo-) *prefix denoting* a ventricle (of the brain or heart).

ventricular folds *pl. n. see* vocal cords.

ventriculitis (ven-trik-yoo-ly-tis) *n.* inflammation in the ventricles of the brain, usually caused by infection.

ventriculoatriostomy (ven-trik-yoo-loh-ay-tri-**ost**-ŏmi) *n.* an operation for the relief of raised pressure due to the build-up of cerebrospinal fluid that occurs in hydrocephalus.

ventriculography (ven-trik-yoo-**log**-răfi) *n.* X-ray examination of the ventricles of the brain after the introduction of a contrast medium.

ventriculoscopy (ven-trik-yoo-**losk**-ŏpi) *n.* observation of the ventricles of the brain through a fibre-optic instrument. *See* endoscope, fibre optics.

ventriculostomy (ven-trik-yoo-**lost**-ŏmi) *n.* an operation to introduce a hollow needle (cannula) into one of the lateral ventricles of the brain. This may be done to relieve raised intracranial pressure, to obtain cerebrospinal fluid for examination, or to introduce antibiotics or contrast material for X-ray examination.

ventro- *prefix denoting* **1.** ventral. **2.** the abdomen.

ventrofixation (ven-troh-fiks-ay-shŏn) *n.* an operation to secure a retroverted womb to the wall of the abdomen.

ventrosuspension (ven-troh-sus-pen-shŏn) *n.* the stitching of the round ligaments of a displaced womb to the abdominal wall.

venule (ven-yool) *n.* a minute vessel that drains blood from the capillaries.

verbigeration (ver-bij-er-ay-shŏn) *n.* repetitive utterances of the same words over and over again. It is most common in institutionalized schizophrenics.

vermicide (verm-i-syd) *n.* a chemical agent used to destroy parasitic worms living in the intestine. *Compare* vermifuge.

vermiform appendix (verm-i-form) *n. see* appendix.

vermifuge (verm-i-fewj) *n.* any drug or chemical agent used to expel worms from the intestine. *See also* anthelmintic.

vermix (ver-miks) *n.* the vermiform appendix.

vernix caseosa (ver-niks kay-si-oh-să) *n.* the layer of greasy material that covers the skin of a fetus or newborn baby. It is produced by the sebaceous glands and contains skin scales and fine hairs.

verruca (ver-oo-kă) *n. see* wart.

A typical thoracic vertebra
(from above)

version (ver-shŏn) *n.* the changing of the position of a fetus in the womb. This may be done to facilitate delivery by applying manual pressure to the outside of the abdomen or by inserting the hand into the womb. *spontaneous v.* a change in the position of the fetus caused by the natural contractions of the womb muscles. *See also* cephalic version, podalic version.

vertebra (ver-tib-ră) *n.* (*pl.* **vertebrae**) one of the 33 bones of which the backbone is composed. Each vertebra typically consists of a *body*, from the back of which arises an arch of bone (the *neural arch*) enclosing a cavity through which the spinal cord passes. Individual vertebrae are bound together by ligaments and intervertebral discs. —**vertebral** *adj.*

vertebral column (ver-tib-răl) *n.* *see* backbone.

vertex (ver-teks) *n.* the crown of the head.

vertigo (vert-i-goh) *n.* a disabling sensation in which the affected individual feels that either he himself or his surroundings are in a state of constant movement. It is a symptom of disease either in the labyrinth of the inner ear or in the vestibular nerve or its nuclei in the brainstem.

vesical (ves-ikăl) *adj.* relating to or affecting a bladder, especially the urinary bladder.

vesicant (epispastic) (ves-i-kănt) *n.* an agent that causes blistering of the skin.

vesicle (ves-ikŭl) *n.* **1.** a very small blister in the skin that contains serum. Vesicles occur in a variety of skin disorders, including eczema and herpes. **2.** (in anatomy) any small bladder, especially one filled with fluid. —**vesicular** (ves-ik-yoo-ler) *adj.*

vesico- *prefix denoting* the urinary bladder.

vesicofixation (ves-i-koh-fiks-ay-shŏn) *n.* *see* cystopexy.

vesicoureteric reflux (ves-i-koh-yoor-i-te-rik) *n.* the backflow of urine from the bladder into the ureters, due to defective valves. Infection is conveyed to the kidneys, causing recurrent attacks of acute pyelonephritis and scarring of the kidneys in childhood.

vesicovaginal (ves-i-koh-vă-jy-năl) *adj.* relating to the bladder and vagina.

vesicular breath sounds *pl. n.* normal breath sounds, which may be increased or decreased in disease states.

vesicular mole *n.* *see* hydatidiform mole.

vesiculitis (ve-sik-yoo-ly-tis) *n.* inflammation of the seminal vesicles. *See* vasovesiculitis.

vesiculography (ve-sik-yoo-log-răfi) *n.* X-ray examination of the seminal vesicles. This is usually performed by injecting radio-opaque contrast material into the exposed vasa deferentia.

vesiculopapular (ve-sik-yoo-loh-pap-yoo-ler) *adj.* describing a skin condition typified by having both vesicles and papules.

vesiculopustular (ve-sik-yoo-loh-pus-tew-ler) *adj.* describing a skin condition that has both vesicles and pustules.

vessel (ves-ĕl) *n.* a tube conveying a body fluid, especially a blood vessel or a lymphatic vessel.

vestibular glands (ves-tib-yoo-ler) *pl. n.* the two pairs of glands that open at the junction of the vagina and vulva. Their function is to lubricate the entrance to the vagina during coitus.

vestibular nerve *n.* the division of the vestibulocochlear nerve that carries impulses from the semicircular canals, utricle, and saccule of the inner ear, conveying information about posture, movement, and balance.

vestibule (vest-i-bewl) *n.* (in anatomy) a cavity situated at the entrance to a hollow part. The vestibule of the ear is the cavity of the bony labyrinth that contains the saccule and utricle.

vestibulocochlear nerve (acoustic nerve, auditory nerve) (ves-tib-yoo-loh-**kok**-li-er) *n.* the eighth cranial nerve (VIII), responsible for carrying sensory impulses from the inner ear to the brain. It has two branches (*see* cochlear nerve, vestibular nerve).

vestigial (ves-**tij**-iăl) *adj.* existing only in a rudimentary form. The term is applied to organs whose structure and function have diminished during the course of evolution.

viable (vy-ăbŭl) *adj.* capable of surviving. The term is applied to a fetus from about the 28th week of gestation.

Vibramycin (vy-bră-**my**-sin) *n. see* doxycycline.

Vibrio (**vib**-ri-oh) *n.* a genus of Gram-negative motile commashaped bacteria widely distributed in soil and water. *V. cholerae* the species that causes cholera.

vicarious (vik-**air**-iŭs) *adj.* describing an action or function performed by an organ not normally involved in the function. *v. menstruation* a rare disorder in which monthly bleeding occurs from places other than the vagina, such as the sweat glands, breasts, nose, or eyes.

villus (**vil**-ŭs) *n.* (*pl.* **villi**) one of many short finger-like processes that project from some membranous surfaces. *arachnoid v. see* arachnoid. *chorionic v.* a fold of the chorion. They are particularly numerous in the placenta, where they provide an extensive area for the exchange of oxygen, food, etc., between maternal and fetal blood. *intestinal v.* any of numerous projections that line the small intestine. Each contains a network of blood capillaries and a lacteal. Their function is to absorb the products of digestion and they greatly increase the surface area over which this can take place.

vinblastine (vin-**blas**-teen) *n.* a cytotoxic drug that is given by intravascular injection mainly in the treatment of cancers of the lymphatic system, such as Hodgkin's disease. It is highly toxic. Trade names: **Velban, Velbe**.

Vincent's angina (vin-sěnts) *n. see* ulcerative gingivitis. [H. Vincent (1862–1950), French physician]

vincristine (vin-**kris**-teen) *n.* a cytotoxic drug with uses and side-effects similar to those of vinblastine. Trade name: **Oncovin**.

vinyl ether (vy-nil) *n.* a general anaesthetic, used mainly for inducing anaesthesia and for minor surgery under short anaesthesia. It is sometimes given in combination with nitrous oxide or ether. Trade name: **Vinethene**.

viomycin (vy-oh-**my**-sin) *n.* an antibiotic derived from bacteria of the genus *Streptomyces*. It is given by intramuscular injection in the treatment of tuberculosis, particularly against strains that are resistant to other antibiotics. Trade name: **Viocin**.

viprynium (vi-**pry**-niŭm) *n.* a drug administered by mouth for the treatment of threadworm infestation. It stains the stools a red colour. Trade name: **Vanquin**.

viraemia (vyr-**ee**-miă) *n.* the presence in the blood of virus particles.

virilism (vi-**ril**-izm) *n.* the development in a female of increased body hair, muscle bulk, deepening of the voice, and male psychological characteristics.

virilization (vi-ri-ly-**zay**-shŏn) *n.* the induction in a female of male characteristics (*see* virilism) as a result of hormone imbalance or hormone therapy.

virology (vyr-**ol**-ŏji) *n.* the science of viruses. *See also* microbiology.

virulence (vi-**rew**-lĕns) *n.* the disease-producing (pathogenic) ability of a microorganism. *See also* attenuation.

virus (**vy**-rŭs) *n.* a minute particle that is capable of replication but only within living cells. Viruses are too small to be visible with a light microscope or to be trapped by filters. They infect animals, plants, and microorganisms. Viruses cause many diseases, including herpes, influenza, mumps, polio, and rabies. Antibiotics are ineffective against them, but many viral diseases are controlled by means of vaccines. —**viral** *adj.*

viscera (**vis**-er-ă) *pl. n.* (*sing.* **viscus**) the organs within the body cavities, especially the organs of the abdominal cavities. —**visceral** (**vis**-er-ăl) *adj.*

visceral pouch *see* pharyngeal pouch.

viscero- *prefix denoting* the viscera.

visceroptosis (vis-er-op-**toh**-sis) *n.* downward displacement of the abdominal organs.

viscid (**vis**-id) *adj.* glutinous and sticky.

viscus (**vis**-kŭs) *n. see* viscera.

visual acuity (**vizh**-yoo-ăl) *n.* sharpness of vision. The commonest way of assessing visual acuity is the Snellen chart.

visual field *n.* the area in front of the eye in any part of which an object can be seen without moving the eye.

visual purple *n. see* rhodopsin.

vital capacity (vy-**t'l**) *n.* the maximum volume of air that a person can exhale after maximum inhalation.

vital centre *n.* any of the collections of nerve cells in the brain that act as governing centres for different vital body functions, such as breathing, blood pressure, etc.

Vitallium (vy-**tal**-iŭm) *n. Trademark.* an alloy of chromium and cobalt that is used in instruments, prostheses, surgical appliances, and dentures.

vital statistics *pl. n.* statistics relating to the births, marriages, deaths, and incidence of disease within a population.

vitamin (**vit**-ă-min) *n.* any of a group of substances that are required, in very small amounts, for healthy growth and development: they cannot be synthesized in the body and are therefore essential constituents of the diet. Vitamins are divided into two groups, according to whether they are soluble in water or fat.

vitamin A (retinol) *n.* a fat-soluble vitamin that occurs preformed in foods of animal origin (especially milk products, egg yolk, and liver) and is formed in the body from the pigment β-carotene, present in some vegetable foods (for example cabbage, lettuce, and carrots). Retinol is essential for growth, vision in dim light, and the maintenance of soft mucous tissue. A deficiency causes stunted growth, night blindness, xerophthalmia, keratomalacia, and eventual blindness. Recommended daily intake: 750 µg retinol equivalents.

vitamin B *n.* any one of a group of water-soluble vitamins that are often found together in the same kinds of food, such as liver, yeast, and eggs, and all function as coenzymes. B_1 *(thiamin, aneurin)* a vitamin deficiency of which leads to beriberi. Recommended daily intake: 1 mg. B_2 *(riboflavin)* a vitamin important in tissue respiration. A deficiency causes ariboflavinosis. Recommended daily intake: 1.7 mg. B_6 *(pyridoxine)* a vitamin from which the coenzyme pyridoxal phosphate is formed. Deficiency is very rare. B_{12} *(cyanocobalamin)* a vitamin that can be absorbed only in the presence of intrinsic factor, secreted in the stomach. A deficiency can lead to pernicious anaemia and degeneration of the nervous system. Recommended daily intake: 3–4 µg. *See also* biotin, folic acid, nicotinic acid, pantothenic acid.

vitamin C (ascorbic acid) *n.* a water-soluble vitamin that is essential in maintaining healthy connective tissues. A deficiency of vitamin C leads to scurvy. Recommended daily intake: 30 mg; rich sources are citrus fruits and vegetables.

vitamin D *n.* a fat-soluble vitamin that enhances the absorption of calcium and phosphorus from the intestine and promotes their deposition in the bone. D_2 *(ergocalciferol, calciferol)* a form obtained from the diet; good sources are fatty fish, eggs, and margarine. D_3 *(cholecalciferol)* a form manufactured in the skin in the presence of sunlight. A deficiency of vitamin D leads to rickets and osteomalacia. Recommended daily intake: 10 µg (for a child up to five years); 2.5 µg (thereafter).

vitamin E *n.* any of a group of chemically related compounds *(tocopherols* and *tocotrienols)* that are thought to stabilize cell membranes. Good sources of the vitamin are vegetable oils, eggs, butter, and wholemeal cereals. It is fairly widely distributed in the diet and a deficiency is therefore unlikely.

vitamin K *n.* a fat-soluble vitamin occurring in two main forms – *phytomenadione* and *menaquinone* – essential for the normal clotting of blood. A dietary deficiency does not often occur as the vitamin is synthesized by bacteria in the large intestine and is widely distributed in green leafy vegetables and meat.

vitellus (vi-**tel**-ŭs) *n.* the yolk of an ovum.

vitiligo (leucoderma) (vit-i-**ly**-goh) *n.* a condition in which areas of skin lose their pigment and become white. The cause is unknown and treatment is unsatisfactory in Europeans.

vitreous humour (vitreous body) (**vit**-ri-ŭs) *n.* the transparent jelly-like material that fills the chamber behind the lens of the eye.

vivisection (viv-i-**sek**-shŏn) *n.* a surgical operation on a living animal for experimental purposes.

vocal cords (vocal folds) (**voh**-kăl) *pl. n.* the two folds of tissue protruding from the sides of the lar-root of the tongue

epiglottis

vocal fold (true vocal cord)

ventricular fold (false vocal cord)

glottis

larynx

The vocal cords

ynx to form a narrow slit (glottis) across the air passage (see illustration). Their controlled interference with the expiratory air flow produces audible vibrations that make up speech, song, and all other vocal noises.

vocal fremitus *n. see* fremitus.

vocal resonance *n.* the sounds heard through the stethoscope when the patient speaks. These are normally just audible but they become much louder (*bronchophony*) if the lung under the stethoscope is consolidated. Vocal resonance is lost over pleural fluid except at its upper surface, when it has a bleating quality (*aegophony*). *See also* pectoriloquy.

volar (**voh**-ler) *adj.* relating to the palm of the hand or the sole of the foot (the *vola*).

volatile (**vol**-ă-tyl) *adj.* describing a liquid that evaporates at room temperature.

volition (vŏl-**ish**-ŏn) *n.* the act of or capacity for exercizing the will. ·

Volkmann's contracture (**fohlk**-mahnz) *n.* shrinkage and shortening of the muscles of the forearm and hand due to inadequate blood supply, caused by injury or pressure (e.g. from a tight bandage) in the elbow re-

gion. [R. von Volkmann (1830–89), German surgeon]

volsella (**vulsella**) (vol-**sel**-ă) *n.* surgical forceps with clawlike hooks at the ends of both blades.

volt (vohlt) *n.* the SI unit of electric potential. Symbol: V.

voluntary admission (vol-ŭn-ter-i) *n.* entry of a patient into a psychiatric hospital with his (or her) agreement. *Compare* compulsory admission.

voluntary muscle *n. see* striated muscle.

volvulus (vol-**vew**-lŭs) *n.* twisting of part of the digestive tract, usually leading to partial or complete obstruction and sometimes reducing the blood supply, causing gangrene.

vomer (**voh**-mer) *n.* a thin plate of bone that forms part of the nasal septum.

vomica (**vom**-ik-ă) *n.* **1.** an abnormal cavity in an organ, usually a lung, sometimes containing pus. **2.** the abrupt expulsion from the mouth of a large quantity of pus or decaying matter originating in the throat or lungs.

vomit (**vom**-it) **1.** *vb.* to eject the contents of the stomach through the mouth (*see* vomiting). **2.** *n.* the contents of the stomach ejected during vomiting. Medical name: **vomitus**.

vomiting (**vom**-it-ing) *n.* the reflex action of ejecting the contents of the stomach through the mouth. Vomiting is controlled by a special centre in the brain that may be stimulated by drugs acting directly on it or by impulses transmitted from the stomach (e.g. after ingesting irritating substances), the intestine (e.g. in intestinal obstruction), or from the inner ear (in travel sickness). Medical name: **emesis**.

wart

von Recklinghausen's disease (von rek-ling-how-zĕnz) *n.* 1. a syndrome due to hyperparathyroidism, characterized by loss of mineral from bones, which become weakened and fracture easily, and formation of kidney stones. Medical name: **osteitis fibrosa. 2.** *see* neurofibromatosis. [F. D. von Recklinghausen (1833–1910), German pathologist]

von Willebrand's disease (von wil-i-brandz) *n.* an inherited disorder of the blood vessels characterized by spontaneous bleeding from mucous membrane. It may or may not be associated with deficiency of coagulation factor VIII (*see* haemophilia). [A. von Willebrand (1870–1949), Swedish physician]

vulsella (vul-sel-ă) *n. see* volsella.

vulv- (**vulvo-**) *prefix denoting* the vulva.

vulva (vul-vă) *n.* the female external genitalia. Two pairs of fleshy folds (*see* labium) surround the openings of the vagina and urethra and extend forward to the clitoris. *See also* vestibular glands.

vulvectomy (vul-vek-tŏmi) *n.* surgical removal of the vulva.

vulvitis (vul-vy-tis) *n.* inflammation of the vulva, which is often accompanied by intense itching and burning pain. It may be caused by fungal or bacterial infection or by ill-fitting underwear.

vulvovaginitis (vul-voh-vaj-i-ny-tis) *n.* 1. inflammation of the vulva and vagina (*see* vaginitis, vulvitis). 2. *see* bartholinitis.

W

wafer (way-fer) *n.* a thin sheet made from moistened flour, formerly used to enclose a powdered medicine that is taken by mouth.

waiting list (wayt-ing) *n.* a list of the names of patients who are awaiting admission to hospital after having been assessed either as an out-patient or on a domiciliary consultation involving a specialist. In general the patients are offered places in the order in which their names were placed on the list.

Waldeyer's ring (vahl-dy-erz) *n.* the ring of lymphoid tissue formed by the tonsils. [H. W. G. von Waldeyer (1836–1921), German anatomist]

Wangensteen tube (wang-ĕn-steen) *n.* a tube with a suction apparatus that is passed into the stomach through the nose and is used to drain the contents of the stomach and duodenum to relieve abdominal distention. [O. H. Wangensteen (1898–1980), US surgeon]

warfarin (wor-fer-in) *n.* an anticoagulant used mainly in the treatment of coronary or venous thrombosis to reduce the risk of embolism. It is given by mouth or injection. Trade names: **Coumadin, Marevan.**

wart (**verruca**) (wort) *n.* a small (often hard) benign growth in the skin. Caused by a virus, warts usually occur on the face, fingers, hands, elbows, and knees. They usually disappear spontaneously but there is a wide range of treatments, including local application of chemicals and electrocautery. *common w.* a large rough wart occurring on the hand. *plantar w.* a painful wart occurring on the sole of the foot. *venereal w.* a wart found on the genitals or around the anus.

Wassermann reaction (wass-er-măn) *n.* the most commonly used test for the diagnosis of syphilis. A sample of the patient's blood is examined for the presence of antibodies to the organism *Treponema pallidum.* [A. P. von Wassermann (1866–1925), German bacteriologist]

water bed (waw-ter) *n.* a bed with a flexible water-containing mattress. The surface of the bed adapts itself to the patient's posture, which leads to greater comfort and fewer bedsores.

waterbrash (waw-ter-brash) *n.* a sudden filling of the mouth with dilute saliva. This often accompanies dyspepsia, particularly if there is nausea.

water-hammer pulse *n. see* Corrigan's pulse.

Waterhouse-Friderichsen syndrome (waw-ter-howss frid-er-ik-sĕn) *n.* fever, cyanosis, and bleeding into the skin resulting from haemorrhage of both adrenal glands, caused by septicaemia resulting from bacterial meningitis. [R. Waterhouse (1873–1958), British physician; C. Friderichsen (1886–), Danish physician]

Waterston's operation (waw-ter-stŏnz) *n.* the operation of joining the right pulmonary artery to the ascending aorta, performed to relieve tetralogy of Fallot. [D. Waterston (1910–), British surgeon]

watt (wot) *n.* the SI unit of power, equal to 1 joule per second. Symbol: W.

weal (weel) *n. see* wheal.

Weber-Christian disease (web-er-
kris-chăn) *n.* a form of panniculitis in which there is fever and enlargement of the liver and spleen. [F. P. Weber (1863–1962), British physician; H. A. Christian (1876–1951), US physician]

Weber's test (vay-berz) *n.* a hearing test in which a vibrating tuning fork is placed at the midpoint of the forehead. If one ear is affected by conductive deafness the sound appears louder in the affected ear. [F. E. Weber (1832–91), German otologist]

Weil-Felix reaction (vyl fay-liks) *n.* a diagnostic test for typhus. A sample of the patient's serum is tested for the presence of antibodies against the organism *Proteus vulgaris.* [E. Weil (1880–1922), German physician; A. Felix (1887–1956), Czech bacteriologist]

Weil's disease (vylz) *n. see* leptospirosis. [A. Weil (1848–1916), German physician]

Welch's bacillus (welch-ŭz) *n. see* Clostridium. [W. H. Welch (1850–1934), US pathologist]

wen (wen) *n. see* sebaceous cyst.

Wernicke's encephalopathy (ver-nik-ĕz) *n.* mental confusion or delirium occurring in combination with paralysis of the eye muscles, nystagmus, and an unsteady gait. It is caused by a deficiency of vitamin B_1 and is most commonly seen in alcoholics and in patients with persistent vomiting. [K. Wernicke (1848–1905), German neurologist]

Wertheim's operation (ver-tymz) *n.* surgery for cervical cancer involving removal of the entire womb, the connective tissue and lymph nodes close to it, and the upper part of the vagina. [E. Wertheim (1864–1920), Austrian gynaecologist]

Wharton's duct (wor-t'nz) *n.* the secretory duct of the submandibular salivary gland. [T. Wharton (1614–73), English physician]

Wharton's jelly *n.* the mesoderm tissue of the umbilical cord, which becomes converted to a loose jelly-like mesenchyme surrounding the umbilical blood vessels.

wheal (weal) (weel) *n.* a temporary red or pale raised area of the skin, often accompanied by severe itching. Wheals are sometimes the sign of a local or general allergy (*see* urticaria). *See also* dermographia.

Wheelhouse's operation (weel-howss-ŭz) *n.* an operation to relieve urethral stricture in which the incision is made through the perineum. [G. Wheelhouse (1826–1909), British surgeon]

wheeze (weez) *n.* low-pitched breathing sounds associated with bronchospasm, such as occurs in asthma and byssinosis. *Compare* stridor.

whiplash injury (wip-lash) *n.* damage to the ligaments, vertebrae, spinal cord, or nerve roots in the neck region, caused by sudden jerking back of the head and neck.

Whipple's disease (wip-ŭlz) *n.* a rare disease, occurring only in males, in which there is malabsorption, usually accompanied by skin pigmentation and arthritis. [G. H. Whipple (1878–1976), US pathologist]

Whipple's operation *n.* *see* pancreatectomy. [A. O. Whipple (1881–1963), US surgeon]

whipworm (wip-werm) *n.* a small parasitic whiplike nematode worm, *Trichuris trichiura* (*Trichocephalus dispar*), that lives in the large intestine. Human infection (*see* trichuriasis) results from the consumption of water or food contaminated with faecal material.

white blood cell (wyt) *n.* *see* leucocyte.

white leg (milk leg) *n.* a condition that may affect women after childbirth in which there is clotting and inflammation in a vein in the leg. The leg becomes pale, swollen, tense, and painful. Medical name: **phlegmasia alba dolens**.

white matter *n.* nerve tissue of the central nervous system that is paler in colour than the associated grey matter because it contains more nerve fibres and thus larger amounts of myelin.

whites (wyts) *n.* *see* leucorrhoea.

Whitfield's ointment (wit-feeldz) *n.* an ointment containing benzoic and salicylic acids, used to treat fungal infections of the skin. [A. Whitfield (1868–1947), British dermatologist]

whitlow (felon) (wit-loh) *n.* an abscess affecting the pulp of the fingertip. *See also* paronychia.

whoop (hoop) *n.* *see* whooping cough.

whooping cough (hoop-ing) *n.* an acute contagious disease, primarily affecting children, due to infection of the mucous membranes lining the air passages by the bacterium *Haemophilus pertussis*. It is characterized by a paroxysmal cough: series of short coughs are followed by a noisy involuntary drawing in of the breath (*whoop*). Bleeding from the nose and mouth and vomiting often occur after a paroxysm. Immunization reduces the incidence and severity of the disease; an attack usually also confers immunity. Medical name: **pertussis**.

Widal reaction (vi-**dahl**) *n.* an agglutination test for the presence of antibodies against the *Salmonella* organisms that cause typhoid fever. [G. F. I. Widal (1862–1929), French physician]

Wilms' tumour (vilmz) *n. see* nephroblastoma. [M. Wilms (1867–1918), German surgeon]

Wilson's disease (wil-sŏnz) *n.* an inborn defect of copper metabolism in which there is a deficiency of caeruloplasmin (which normally forms a nontoxic complex with copper). The free copper may be deposited in the liver, causing jaundice and cirrhosis, or in the brain, causing mental retardation and symptoms resembling parkinsonism. Medical name: **hepatolenticular degeneration**. [S. A. K. Wilson (1878–1936), British neurologist]

windpipe (**wind**-pyp) *n. see* trachea.

wisdom tooth (wiz-dŏm) *n.* the third molar tooth on each side of either jaw, which erupts normally around the age of 20.

witch hazel (**hamamelis**) (wich hay-zĕl) *n.* a preparation made from the leaves and bark of the tree *Hamamelis virginiana*, used as an astringent, especially for the treatment of sprains and bruises.

withdrawal (wi*th*-**draw**-ăl) *n.* **1.** (in psychology) the removal of one's interest from one's surroundings. **2.** *see* coitus (interruptus).

withdrawal symptoms *pl. n. see* dependence.

Wolffian body (vol-fi-ăn) *n. see* mesonephros. [K. F. Wolff (1733–94), German anatomist]

Wolffian duct *n.* the mesonephric duct (*see* mesonephros).

womb (woom) *n. see* uterus.

Wood's glass (wuudz) *n.* a nickel-oxide filter that holds back all but a few rays projected from an ultraviolet light source. These rays (*W. light*) cause fluorescence in hair and skin affected by some fungal and bacterial infections and are therefore useful in diagnosis. [R. W. Wood (1868–1955), US physician]

woolsorter's disease (**wuul**-sor-terz) *n. see* anthrax.

word blindness (werd) *n. see* alexia.

worm (werm) *n.* any of various soft-bodied legless animals, including flatworms, nematode worms, earthworms, and leeches.

wound (woond) *n.* a break in the structure of an organ or tissue caused by an external agent; for example, a bruise, cut, or burn.

wrist (rist) *n.* **1.** the joint between the forearm and hand. It consists of the proximal bones of the carpus, which articulate with the radius and ulna. **2.** the whole region of the wrist joint, including the carpus and lower parts of the radius and ulna.

wrist drop *n.* paralysis of the muscles that raise the wrist, which is caused by damage to the radial nerve.

wryneck (ry-nek) *n. see* torticollis.

Wuchereria (voo-ker-**eer**-iă) *n.* a genus of white threadlike parasitic worms (*see* filaria) that live in the lymphatic vessels. *W. bancrofti* the species that causes elephantiasis.

X

xanthaemia (carotenaemia) (zanth-ee-mia) *n.* the presence in the blood of the yellow pigment carotene, from excessive intake of carrots, tomatoes, or other vegetables containing the pigment.

xanthelasma (zanth-ĕ-laz-mă) *n.* one or more yellow deposits of fatty material in the skin around the eyes.

xanthine (zanth-een) *n.* a nitrogenous breakdown product of the purines adenosine and guanine. Xanthine is an intermediate product of the breakdown of nucleic acids to uric acid.

xantho- *prefix denoting* yellow colour.

xanthochromia (zanth-oh-kroh-miă) *n.* yellow discoloration, such as may affect the skin in jaundice or the cerebrospinal fluid when it contains the breakdown products of haemoglobin from red blood cells that have entered it.

xanthoma (zanth-oh-mă) *n.* (*pl.* **xanthomata**) a yellowish swelling, nodule, or plaque in the skin resulting from deposits of fat and usually accompanied by a raised blood cholesterol level. *xanthomata palpebrarum* the yellowish plaques that may appear on the eyelids in the elderly (*see* xanthelasma).

xanthomatosis (zanth-oh-mă-toh-sis) *n.* the presence of multiple small fatty tumours in the skin, the eyes, and the internal organs due to an excess of fats in the blood (hyperlipidaemia).

xanthopsia (zanth-op-siă) *n.* yellow vision: the condition in which all objects appear to have a yellowish tinge. It is sometimes experienced in digitalis poisoning.

X chromosome *n.* the sex chromosome present in both sexes. Women have two X chromosomes and men one. Genes for some important genetic disorders, including haemophilia, are carried on the X chromosomes. *Compare* Y chromosome.

xeno- *prefix denoting* different; foreign; alien.

xenograft (zen-oh-grahft) *n. see* heterograft.

Xenopsylla (zen-op-sil-ă) *n.* a genus of tropical and subtropical fleas. *X. cheopis* the rat flea, which occasionally attacks man and can transmit plague; it also transmits murine typhus and two tapeworms.

xero- *prefix denoting* a dry condition.

xeroderma (zeer-oh-der-mă) *n.* a mild form of the hereditary disorder ichthyosis, in which the skin develops slight dryness and forms branlike scales.

xerophthalmia (zeer-off-thal-miă) *n.* a progressive disease of the eye due to deficiency of vitamin A. The cornea and conjunctiva become dry, thickened, and wrinkled. This may progress to keratomalacia and eventual blindness.

xerosis (zeer-oh-sis) *n.* abnormal dryness of the conjunctiva, the skin, or the mucous membranes. In xerosis of the conjunctiva, the membrane becomes thickened and grey in the area exposed when the eyelids are open.

xerostomia (zeer-oh-stoh-miă) *n.* dryness of the mouth resulting from diminished secretion of saliva. The phenomenon may be caused by drugs or poisons or be associated with disease. *Compare* ptyalism.

xiphi- (xipho-) *prefix denoting* the xiphoid process of the sternum.

xiphisternum (zif-i-ster-nŭm) *n. see* xiphoid process.

xiphoid process (xiphoid cartilage) (zif-oid) *n.* the lowermost section of the breastbone (*see* sternum): a flat pointed cartilage that gradually ossifies until it is completely replaced by bone, a process not completed until after middle age. It does not articulate with any ribs. Also called: **ensiform process** *or* **cartilage, xiphisternum**.

X-rays *pl. n.* electromagnetic radiation of extremely short wavelength (beyond the ultraviolet), with great penetrating powers in matter opaque to light. X-rays are used in diagnosis in the techniques of radiography and also in certain forms of radiotherapy. Great care is needed to avoid unnecessary exposure, because the radiation is harmful in large quantities. *See* radiation (sickness).

xylene (dimethylbenzene) (zy-leen) *n.* a liquid used for increasing the transparency of tissues prepared for microscopic examination after they have been dehydrated.

xylometazoline (zy-loh-mi-taz-ohleen) *n.* a drug that constricts blood vessels (*see* vasoconstrictor). It is applied topically as a nasal decongestant in the relief of the common cold and sinusitis. Trade name: **Otrivine**.

xylose (zy-lohz) *n.* a pentose sugar that is involved in carbohydrate interconversions within cells.

Y

yawning (yawn-ing) *n.* a reflex action in which the mouth is opened wide and air is drawn into the lungs then slowly released. It is a result of drowsiness, fatigue, or boredom.

yaws (pian, framboesia) (yawz) *n.* a tropical infectious disease caused by the presence of the spirochaete *Treponema pertenue* in the skin and its underlying tissues. Yaws occurs chiefly in conditions of poor hygiene. It is characterized by small tumours, each covered by a yellow crust of dried serum, on the hands, face, legs, and feet. These tumours may deteriorate into deep ulcers. The disease responds well to treatment with penicillin and other antibiotics.

Y chromosome *n.* a sex chromosome that is present in men but not in women; it is believed to carry the genes for maleness. *Compare* X chromosome.

yeast (yeest) *n.* any unicellular fungus of the genus *Saccharomyces*. Yeasts ferment carbohydrates, producing alcohol and carbon dioxide, and are important in brewing and breadmaking. They are also a commercial source of proteins and of vitamins of the B complex.

yellow fever (yel-oh) *n.* an infectious disease, caused by an arborvirus, occurring in tropical Africa and South America. It is transmitted by mosquitoes, principally *Aëdes aegypti*. The virus causes degeneration of the tissues of the liver and kidneys. Symptoms include chill, headache, pains in the back and limbs, fever, vomiting, constipation, a reduced flow of urine (which contains high levels of albumin), and jaundice. Yellow fever often proves fatal.

yellow spot *n*. *see* macula (lutea).

yolk sac (vitelline sac) (yohk) *n*. the membranous sac that lies ventral to the embryo. It probably assists in transporting nutrients to the early embryo and is one of the first sites where blood cells are formed.

yttrium-90 (it-riŭm) *n*. an artificial radioactive isotope of the element yttrium, used in radiotherapy. It can be used in the form of 1 mm spheres scattered around a tumour or injected directly into a tumour in the form of a solution.

Z

zein (zee-in) *n*. a protein found in maize.

zinc chloride (zink) *n*. a caustic substance having strong astringent properties. It is used as a solution for cleansing wounds and ulcers and also as a mouth wash and deodorant.

zinc oxide *n*. a mild astringent used in various skin conditions, usually mixed with other substances. It is applied as a cream, ointment, dusting powder, or as a paste.

zinc sulphate *n*. an astringent applied in a lotion for the treatment of ulcers of the skin and mouth. It is also used in eye drops and, occasionally, as an emetic.

zinc undecenoate (zinc undecylenate) *n*. an antifungal agent with uses similar to those of undecenoic acid.

Zollinger-Ellison syndrome (zol-inj-er el-i-sŏn) *n*. a rare disorder in which there is excessive secretion of gastric juice due to high levels of circulating gastrin, which is produced by a pancreatic tumour or an enlarged pancreas. The high levels of stomach acid cause peptic ulcers. [R. M. Zollinger (1903–) and E. H. Ellison (1918–70), US physicians]

zona pellucida (zoh-nă pel-oo-sid-a) *n*. the thick membrane that develops around the mammalian oocyte within the ovarian follicle. *See* ovum.

zonula (zon-yoo-lă) *n*. *see* zonule.

zonule (zonula) (zon-yool) *n*. (in anatomy) a small band or zone. *z. of Zinn* (*zonula ciliaris*) the suspensory ligament of the lens of the eye. —**zonular** *adj*.

zonulolysis (zon-yoo-lol-i-sis) *n*. dissolution of the zonule of Zinn, which facilitates removal of the lens in cases of cataract.

zoo- *prefix denoting* animals.

zoonosis (zoh-ŏ-noh-sis) *n*. any infectious disease of animals that can be transmitted to man, such as anthrax or rabies.

zygoma (zy-goh-mă) *n*. *see* zygomatic arch, zygomatic bone.

zygomatic arch (zygoma) (zy-goh-mat-ik) *n*. the horizontal arch of bone on either side of the face, just below the eyes, formed by connected processes of the zygomatic and temporal bones. *See* skull.

zygomatic bone (zygoma, malar bone) *n*. either of a pair of bones that form the prominent part of the cheeks and contribute to the orbits. *See* skull.

zygote (zy-goht) *n*. the fertilized ovum before cleavage begins.

zym- (zymo-) *prefix denoting* **1.** an enzyme. **2.** fermentation.

zymogen (zy-moh-jen) *n. see* proenzyme.

zymosis (zy-moh-sis) *n.* **1.** the process of fermentation, brought about by yeast organisms. **2.** the changes in the body that occur in certain infectious diseases, once thought to be the result of a process similar to fermentation. —**zymotic** (zy-mot-ik) *adj.*

zymotic disease *n.* an old name for a contagious disease.

Appendix 1 Normal values for biochemical data

(B = whole blood; P = plasma; S = serum; U = urine)

Table 1.1 Everyday tests

Determination	Sample	Normal range
alcohol	B or P	legal limit (UK) < 17.4 mmol/l
α-amylase	P	0–180 somogyi units/dl
albumin	P	35–50 g/l
albumin – pregnancy	P	25–38 g/l
anion gap ($Na^+ + K^+$)–($HCO_3^- + Cl^-$)	P	12–17 mmol/l
barbiturate	B	possibly fatal if:
short acting		> 35 μmol/l
medium acting		> 105 μmol/l
long acting		> 215 μmol/l
bilirubin	P	3–17 μmol/l
bromide	P	0 mmol/l
bromsulphthalein retention	P	< 5% dye remains
bicarbonate	P	24–30 mmol/l
bicarbonate – pregnancy	P	20–25 mmol/l
calcium (ionized)	P	1.0–1.25 mmol/l
calcium (total)	P	2.12–2.65 mmol/l
calcium (total) – pregnancy	P	1.95–2.35 mmol/l
chloride	P	95–105 mmol/l
copper	P	12–26 μmol/l
creatinine	P	70–150 μmol/l
creatinine – pregnancy	P	24–68 μmol/l
cholesterol	P	3.9–7.8 mmol/l
glucose (fasting)	P	4.0–6.0 mmol/l
iron	S	(male) 14–31 μmol/l
		(female) 11–30 μmol/l
total iron-binding capacity (TIBC)	S	54–75 μmol/l

Table 1.1 *(cont.)*

Determination	Sample	Normal range
lead	B	0.3 – 1.8 μmol/l
lithium	P	(therapeutic) 0.5 – 1.5 mmol/l
		(toxic)> 2.0 mmol/l
magnesium	P	0.75 – 1.05 mmol/l
osmolality	P	278 – 305 mosm/kg
phenylalanine	P	(infants) 42 – 73 μmol/l
phosphate (inorganic)	P	0.8 – 1.45 mmol/l
potassium	P	3.5 – 5.0 mmol/l
protein (total)	P	60 – 80 g/l
sodium	P	135 – 145 mmol/l
urea	P	2.5 – 6.7 mmol/l
urea – pregnancy	P	2.0 – 4.2 mmol/l
uric acid	P	(male) 210 – 480 μmol/l
		(female) 150 – 390 μmol/l
uric acid – pregnancy	P	100 – 270 μmol/l

Table 1.2 Blood gases

Measurement	Normal range
arterial carbon dioxide (P_{aCO_2})	4.7 – 6.0 kPa
venous P_{CO_2}	> 10.6 kPa
arterial oxygen (P_{aO_2})	> 10.6 kPa
newborn P_{aO_2}	5.33 – 8.0 kPa
for every year over 60 add	0.13 kPa
arterial pH	7.35 – 7.45
base excess	$\pm$ 2 mmol/l
carbon monoxide	toxic at > 20%
	coma at > 50%

Table 1.3 Diagnostic enzymes

Enzyme	Sample	Normal range
acid phosphatase		
total	S	1 – 5 iu/l
prostatic	S	0 – 1 iu/l
alkaline phosphatase	P	adult 30 – 300 iu/l
alanine-amino transferase (ALT)	P	5 – 35 iu/l
aspartate-amino transferase (AST)	P	5 – 35 iu/l
α-amylase	P	0 – 180 somogyi units/dl
creatine kinase (CPK)	P	(female) 25 – 170 iu/l (male) 25 – 195 iu/l
gamma-glutamyl transpeptidase (γGT)	P	(female) 7 – 33 iu/l (male) 11 – 51 iu/l
aldolase	P	0.5 – 7.6 u/l
α-hydroxybutyric dehydrogenase	P	53 – 144 iu/l
lactate dehydrogenase	P	240 – 525 iu/l
glutathione reductase	B	7.8 $\pm$ 1.09/g Hb at 37°C
5′-nucleotidase	P	3 – 17 iu/l
cholinesterase	P	2.25 – 7.0 iu/l

Table 1.4   Proteins

Protein	Sample	Normal range
total protein	P	69–85 g/l
	S	60–80 g/l
albumin	P	35–50 g/l
globulin fractions		
α₁-globulin	S	2–4 g/l
α₂-globulin	S	5–9 g/l
β-globulin	S	6–11 g/l
γ-globulin	S	7–17 g/l
α₁-antitrypsin	S	1.3–3.28 g/l
α₂-haptoglobin	S	0.3–2.0 g/l
α₂-caeruloplasmin	S	0.3–0.6 g/l
β₁-transferrin	S	1.2–2.0 g/l
immunoglobulins		
IgG		7.2–19 g/l
IgA		0.8–5.0 g/l
IgM		0.5–2.0 g/l
complement C₃		0.69–1.3 g/l
complement C₄		0.12–0.27 g/l
caeruloplasmin	P	100–400 mg/l
β₂-microglobulin	S	1.1–2.4 mg/l
	U	4–370 µg/l or 30–370 µg/24 h
fibrinogen	P	2–4 g/l
fibrinogen degradation products	S	less than 0.8 µg/l

Table 1.5 Lipids and lipoproteins

Lipid	Sample	Normal range
cholesterol	P	3.9–7.8 mmol/l
triglyceride	P	0.55–1.90 mmol/l
phospholipid	S	2.9–5.2 mmol/l
non-esterified fatty acids	S	(male) 0.19–0.78 mmol/l
		(female) 0.06–0.9 mmol/l
lipoproteins (as cholesterol)		
very low density	S	0.128–0.645 mmol/l
low density	S	1.55–4.4 mmol/l
high density	S	0.9–1.93 mmol/l

Table 1.6 Vitamins

Vitamin	Sample	Normal range
β-carotene	S	0.9–5.6 μmol/l
vitamin A	S	0.7–1.7 μmol/l
thiamin (B_1)	P	> 40 nmol/l
riboflavine (B_2)	P	free < 21.3 nmol/l
	P	total < 85.0 nmol/l
pyridoxine (B_6)	S	> 178 nmol/l
folate	S	5–63 nmol/l (2.1–2.8 μg/l)
vitamin B_{12}	S	0.13–0.68 nmol/l (> 150 ng/l)
ascorbate	B	34–68 μmol/l
vitamin D	S	23.8–111 nmol/l
vitamin D metabolites		
25–OHD		12.5–125 nmol/l
24,25 $(OH)_2$ D_3		1.25–7.5 nmol/l
1,25 $(OH)_2$ D_3		50–100 pmol/l
red cell transketolase	B	40–90 iu/l
red cell folate	B	0.36–1.44 μmol/l (160–640 μg/l)

Table 1.7 Urine

Determination	*Normal range*
calcium	2.5 – 7.5 mmol/24 h
copper	0.2 – 1.0 μmol/24 h
iron	< 1.0 mg/24 h
lead	< 0.39 μmol/24 h
magnesium	3.3 – 4.9 mmol/24 h
phosphate (inorganic)	15 – 50 mmol/24 h
potassium	40 – 120 mmol/24 h
sodium	100 – 250 mmol/24 h
creatinine	9 – 17 mmol/24 h
amylase	8000 – 30 000 Wohlegmuth U/24 h
	35 – 260 somogyi units/dl
ascorbic acid	34 – 68 μmol/l
glucose	0.06 – 0.84 mmol/l
hydroxyindole acetic acid (5 HIAA)	16 – 73 μmol/24 h
oxalate	< 450 μmol/24 h
urate	2 – 6 mmol/24 h
urea	250 – 500 mmol/24 h
urobilinogen	up to 6.7 μmol/24 h
zinc	2.1 – 11.0 μmol/24 h
δ-amino laevulinic acid	up to 15.3 μmol/24 h
coproporphyrin	0.09 – 0.43 μmol/24 h
porphobilinogen	0.9 – 8.8 μmol/24 h
uroporphyrin	5 – 30 μg/24 h
β_2-microglobulin	4 – 370 μg/l
	30 – 370 μg/24 h
osmolality	350 – 1000 mosm/kg
cortisol	< 280 nmol/24 h
hydroxymethylmandelic acid	16 – 48 μmol/24 h

Table 1.7 (*cont.*)

Determination	Normal range
24-hour urinary excretion	
protein	up to 150 mg
pregnancy	up to 300 mg
albumin	up to 25 mg
creatinine	
male	9.0 – 17.0 mmol
female	7.5 – 12.5 mmol
pregnancy	8.0 – 13.5 mmol
uric acid	up to 5.0 mmol
pregnancy (except late)	up to 7.0 mmol
cystine	0.04 – 0.42 mmol

Table 1.8   Faeces

Determination	Normal range
fat (on normal diet)	11 – 18 mmol/l
	(3 – 5 g/24 h)
nitrogen	70 – 140 mmol/24 h
	(1 – 2 g/24 h)
urobilinogen	50 – 500 μmol/24 h
	(30 – 300 mg/24 h)
coproporphyrin	0.018 – 1.20 μmol/24 h
	(0.012 – 0.832 mg/24 h)
protoporphyrin	0 – 4 μmol/24 h
	(0 – 2.09 mg/24 h)

Appendix 2 Normal haematological values in adults

Measurement	Value
haemoglobin	(male) 13.5–18.0 g/dl
	(female) 11.5–16.0 g/dl
packed red cell volume of haematocrit (PCV)	(male) 0.40–0.54 l/l
	(female) 0.37–0.47 l/l
red cell count	(male) 4.5–6.5 × 10^{12}/l
	(female) 3.9–5.6 × 10^{12}/l
mean cell volume (MCV)	81–100 fl
mean cell haemoglobin (MCH)	27–32 pg
mean cell haemoglobin concentration (MCHC)	32–36 g/dl
reticulocyte count	0.8–2.0 per cent
absolute count	25–100 × 10^9/l
total blood volume	70 ± 10 ml/kg
plasma volume	45 ± 5 ml/kg
red cell volume	(male) 30 ± 5 ml/kg
	(female) 25 ± 5 ml/kg
white cell count	4.0–11.0 × 10^9/l
neutrophils	2.0–7.5 × 10^9/l
lymphocytes	1.3–3.5 × 10^9/l
eosinophils	0–0.44 × 10^9/l
basophils	0–0.10 × 10^9/l
monocytes	0.2–0.8 × 10^9/l
platelet count	150–400 × 10^9/l
bleeding time	1–9 min
coagulation time	5–11 min
thrombin time	10–15 s
prothrombin time	10–14 s
activated partial thromboplastin time	35–45 s
fibrinogen concentration	1.6–4.2 g/l
fibrinogen titre	normal – up to 1/128
erythrocyte sedimentation rate	(male) 0–10 mm
	(female) 0–15 mm
cold agglutinin titre at 4 °C	less than 64

Appendix 3 Standard values for body weight

Table 3.1 Appropriate body weight and lower limits for defining overweight and obesity in adults

Men

Height (cm)	Average (kg)	Acceptable range (kg)	Overweight (kg)	Obese (kg)
158	55.8	44–64	70	77
160	57.6	44–65	72	78
162	58.6	46–66	73	79
164	59.6	47–67	74	80
166	60.6	48–69	76	83
168	61.7	49–71	78	85
170	63.5	51–73	80	88
172	65.0	52–74	81	89
174	66.5	53–75	83	90
176	68.0	54–77	85	92
178	69.4	55–79	87	95
180	71.0	58–80	88	96
182	72.6	59–82	90	98
184	74.2	60–84	92	101
186	75.8	62–86	95	103
188	77.6	64–88	97	106
190	79.3	66–90	99	108
192	81.0	68–93	102	112

Women

Height (cm)	Average (kg)	Acceptable range (kg)	Overweight (kg)	Obese (kg)
146	46.0	37–53	58	64
148	46.5	37–54	59	65
150	47.0	38–55	61	66
152	48.5	39–57	63	68
156	49.5	39–58	64	70
158	50.4	40–58	64	70
160	51.3	41–59	65	71
162	52.6	42–61	67	73
164	54.0	43–62	68	74
166	55.4	44–64	70	77
168	56.8	45–65	72	78
170	58.1	45–66	73	79
172	60.0	46–67	74	80
174	61.3	48–69	76	83
176	62.6	49–70	77	84
178	64.0	51–72	79	86
180	65.3	52–74	81	89

Table 3.2 Median and range of standard values for weight for height of children

Boys

Height (cm)	Weight (kg) Median	Range	Height (cm)	Weight (kg) Median	Range
50	3.3	2.5 – 4.4	102	16.3	13.4 – 19.6
52	3.7	2.8 – 4.8	104	16.8	13.9 – 20.2
54	4.1	3.1 – 5.3	106	17.4	14.4 – 20.8
56	4.6	3.4 – 5.9	108	18.1	14.9 – 21.5
58	5.1	3.9 – 6.4	110	18.7	15.5 – 22.2
60	5.7	4.4 – 7.1	112	19.4	16.1 – 23.0
62	6.2	4.9 – 7.7	114	20.0	16.7 – 23.9
64	6.8	5.4 – 8.7	116	20.7	17.3 – 24.8
66	7.4	6.0 – 9.0	118	21.5	17.9 – 25.8
68	8.0	6.5 – 9.6	120	22.2	18.6 – 26.9
70	8.5	7.0 – 10.2	122	23.0	19.3 – 28.2
72	9.1	7.5 – 10.8	124	23.9	20.0 – 29.5
74	9.6	8.0 – 11.4	126	24.8	20.7 – 30.9
76	10.0	8.4 – 11.9	128	25.7	21.5 – 32.3
78	10.5	8.8 – 12.4	130	26.7	22.3 – 33.9
80	10.9	9.2 – 12.9	132	27.8	23.1 – 35.6
82	11.3	9.6 – 13.3	134	29.0	23.9 – 37.4
84	11.7	9.9 – 13.8	136	30.2	24.8 – 39.3
86	12.1	10.3 – 14.2	138	31.5	25.7 – 41.3
88	12.5	10.6 – 14.7	140	33.0	26.6 – 43.4
90	13.0	11.0 – 15.1	142	34.5	27.5 – 45.5
92	13.4	11.4 – 15.6	144	36.1	28.4 – 47.8
94	13.9	11.9 – 16.1			
96	14.4	12.3 – 16.6			
98	14.9	12.8 – 17.1			
100	15.5	13.3 – 17.7			

Girls

Height (cm)	Weight (kg) Median	Range	Height (cm)	Weight (kg) Median	Range
50	3.4	2.6 – 4.2	100	15.4	12.7 – 18.8
52	3.7	2.8 – 4.7	102	15.9	13.1 – 19.4
54	4.1	3.1 – 5.2	104	16.5	13.6 – 20.0
56	4.5	3.5 – 5.7	106	17.0	14.0 – 20.6
58	5.0	3.9 – 6.3	108	17.6	14.5 – 21.3
60	5.5	4.3 – 6.9	110	18.2	15.0 – 22.0
62	6.1	4.8 – 7.5	112	18.9	15.6 – 22.8
64	6.7	5.3 – 8.1	114	19.6	16.2 – 23.7
66	7.3	5.8 – 8.7	116	20.3	16.8 – 24.7
68	7.8	6.3 – 9.3	118	21.0	17.4 – 25.8
70	8.4	6.8 – 9.9	120	21.8	18.1 – 27.0
72	8.9	7.2 – 10.5	122	22.7	18.8 – 28.3
74	9.4	7.7 – 11.0	124	23.6	19.5 – 29.8
76	9.8	8.1 – 11.4	126	24.6	20.3 – 31.4
78	10.2	8.5 – 11.9	128	25.7	21.0 – 33.2
80	10.6	8.8 – 12.3	130	26.8	21.9 – 35.1
82	11.1	9.3 – 12.9	132	28.0	22.7 – 37.3
84	11.4	9.6 – 13.2	134	29.4	23.6 – 39.6
86	11.8	9.9 – 13.6	136	30.8	24.5 – 42.2
88	12.2	10.3 – 14.1			
90	12.6	10.7 – 14.5			
92	13.0	11.1 – 15.0			
94	13.5	11.5 – 15.6			
96	14.0	12.0 – 16.1			
98	14.6	12.5 – 16.8			
100	15.2	13.1 – 17.4			

Appendix 4 Nutrition and energy

Table 4.1 The approximate normal composition of a 70 kg man

	kg
water	42
intracellular	28
extracellular	14
solids	
fat	12.6
protein	11.2
intracellular (muscle)	8.4
extracellular (collagen)	2.8
minerals	3.8
carbohydrate	0.4

Table 4.2 Daily requirements for energy at different ages

	Age	Energy kcal/kg	Energy kJ/kg
infant	3 months	120	500
child	4–6 years	90	380
adolescent			
male	13–15 years	57	240
female	13–15 years	50	210
adult			
male		46	190
female		40	170

Table 4.3 Estimate of energy expenditure of a normal adult

	Time	kcal	kJ	Total range kcal (kJ)
male				
bed	8 h	500	2100	
non-occupational activities	8 h	700– 1500	3000– 6300	
work				
light	8 h	1100	4600	2300–3100 (9660–13 000)
very heavy		2400	10 100	3600–4400 (15 100–18 500)
female				
bed	8 h	420	1760	
non-occupational activities	8 h	580– 980	2430– 4120	
work				
light	8 h	800	3360	1800–2200 (7560–9240)
heavy		1400	5880	2400–2700 (10 100–11 340)

Appendix 5   Hospital episodes

Table 5.1   Annual number of hospital episodes (discharges from and deaths in hospital) and beds occupied daily: England, 1977. (Figures in thousands of patients and thousands of beds)

Specialty	Hospital episodes		Hospital beds occupied daily	
	No.	*%*	*No.*	*%*
acute medical	1350.7	25.3	42.1	13.8
acute surgical	2595.1	48.6	58.3	19.0
maternity	694.7	13.0	12.9	4.2
geriatrics	226.0	4.2	51.8	16.9
mental illness	177.8	3.3	80.8	26.4
mental handicap	19.6	0.4	47.9	15.6
other	281.1	5.2	12.6	4.1
total	5345.0	100.0	306.4	100.0

Table 5.2 Some common reasons for hospital admission: number of episodes, England and Wales, 1977. (Percentage of all admissions for each sex in parentheses)

Disease	Number of episodes Males		Females	
malignant neoplasm of lung	38 310	(1.8)	10 370	(0.4)
malignant neoplasm of breast	560	(<0.1)	36 510	(1.6)
other malignant neoplasms	113 560	(5.5)	105 660	(4.6)
diabetes mellitus	22 940	(1.1)	25 960	(1.1)
cataract	16 090	(0.8)	24 210	(1.0)
acute myocardial infarction	61 020	(2.0)	29 070	(1.3)
other ischaemic heart disease	31 360	(1.5)	19 990	(0.9)
cerebrovascular disease	46 940	(2.3)	58 280	(2.5)
pneumonia	31 390	(1.5)	28 130	(1.2)
bronchitis and emphysema	29 410	(1.4)	13 420	(0.6)
hypertrophy of tonsils and adenoids	40 240	(1.9)	43 640	(1.9)
appendicitis	36 090	(1.7)	36 830	(1.6)
hernia	80 220	(3.9)	21 750	(0.9)
cholelithiasis, cholecystitis	18 380	(0.9)	43 510	(1.9)
hyperplasia of prostate	32 840	(1.6)		
disorders of menstruation			94 770	(4.1)
abortion			102 400	(4.4)
arthritis	23 780	(1.1)	47 980	(2.1)
fractures, dislocations, sprains	102 300	(4.9)	88 480	(3.8)
intracranial injury	75 940	(3.7)	43 030	(1.9)
adverse effects of drugs	39 640	(1.9)	67 070	(2.9)
all causes	2 071 500	(100.0)	2 315 560	(100.0)

Appendix 6 Range of incidence rates of common cancers (men, unless specified otherwise)

Site of origin of cancer	High incidence area	Cumulative incidence (%) in high incidence area	Low incidence area	Ratio of rates in high and low incidence areas
skin	Australia (Queensland)	> 20	India (Bombay)	> 200
oesophagus	Iran, N. E.	20	Nigeria	300
lung	England	11	Nigeria	35
stomach	Japan	11	Uganda	25
*cervix of uterus	Columbia	10	Israel (Jewish)	15
prostate	USA (blacks)	9	Japan	40
liver	Mozambique	8	England	100
*breast	Canada (British Columbia)	7	Israel (non-Jewish)	7
colon	USA (Connecticut)	3	Nigeria	10
*uterus	USA (California)	3	Japan	30
buccal cavity	India (Bombay)	2	Denmark	25
rectum	Denmark	2	Nigeria	20
bladder	USA (Connecticut)	2	Japan	6
*ovary	Denmark	2	Japan	6
nasopharynx	Singapore (Chinese)	2	England	40
pancreas	New Zealand (Maori)	2	India (Bombay)	8
larynx	Brazil (Sao Paulo)	2	Japan	10
pharynx	India (Bombay)	2	Denmark	20
penis	Parts of Uganda	1	Israel (Jewish)	300

* women

Appendix 7 The Knoll scale of liability to pressure sores

Parameters	0	1	2	3	Score
general state of health	good	fair	poor	moribund	......
mental status	alert	lethargic	semi-comatose	comatose	......
activity	ambulatory	needs help	*chairfast	*bedfast	......
mobility	full	limited	*very limited	*immobile	......
incontinence	none	occasional	*usually of urine	*total of urine and faeces	......
oral nutrition intake	good	fair	poor	none	......
oral fluid intake	good	fair	poor	none	......
predisposing disease (diabetes, neuropathies, vascular disease, anaemias)	absent	slight	moderate	severe	......

* Count these conditions as double

The higher the score, the greater is the potential to develop bedsores.
Patients with scores above 12 should be considered at risk.

Appendix 8   Poison Information Centres

United Kingdom

London	National Poisons Information Service	01-407 7600
	New Cross Hospital	Ext. 4001
	Avonley Road	
	London SE14 5ER	
Edinburgh	Scottish Poisons Information Bureau	031-229 2477
	The Royal Infirmary	Ext. 2233
	Lauriston Place	
	Edinburgh 3	
Cardiff	Poisons Information Service	0222-492233
	Cardiff Royal Infirmary	Ext. 200
	Cardiff CF2 1SZ	
Belfast	Poisons Information Service	0232-40503
	Royal Victoria Hospital	Ext. 2140
	Grosvenor Road	
	Belfast BT12 6BB	

Republic of Ireland

Dublin	Poisons Information Service	0001-72 3355
	Jervis Street Hospital	
	Dublin 1	

Appendix 9   SI units

Table 9.1   Base and supplementary SI units

Physical quantity	Name	Symbol
length	metre	m
mass	kilogram	kg
time	second	s
electric current	ampere	A
thermodynamic temperature	kelvin	K
luminous intensity	candela	cd
amount of substance	mole	mol
*plane angle	radian	rad
*solid angle	steradian	sr

*supplementary units

Table 9.2   Derived SI units with special names

Physical quantity	Name of SI unit	Symbol for SI unit
frequency	hertz	Hz
energy	joule	J
force	newton	N
power	watt	W
pressure	pascal	Pa
electric charge	coulomb	C
electric potential difference	volt	V
electric resistance	ohm	Ω
electric conductance	siemens	S
electric capacitance	farad	F
magnetic flux	weber	Wb
inductance	henry	H
magnetic flux density (magnetic induction)	tesla	T
luminous flux	lumen	lm
illuminance (illumination)	lux	lx
absorbed dose	gray	Gy
activity	becquerel	Bq
dose equivalent	sievert	Sv

Table 9.3 Decimal multiples and submultiples to be used with SI units

Submultiple	Prefix	Symbol	Multiple	Prefix	Symbol
10^{-1}	deci	d	10^1	deca	da
10^{-2}	centi	c	10^2	hecto	h
10^{-3}	milli	m	10^3	kilo	k
10^{-6}	micro	μ	10^6	mega	M
10^{-9}	nano	n	10^9	giga	G
10^{-12}	pico	p	10^{12}	tera	T
10^{-15}	femto	f	10^{15}	peta	P
10^{-18}	atto	a	10^{18}	exa	E

Table 9.4 Conversion of units to and from SI units

From	To	Multiply by
in	m	0.0254
ft	m	0.3048
sq in	m^2	0.00064516
sq ft	m^2	0.092903
cu in	m^3	0.0000164
cu ft	m^3	0.0283168
l(itre)	m^3	0.001
gal(lon)	m^3	0.0045609
gal(lon)	litres	4.5609
lb	kg	0.453592
g cm^{-3}	kg m^{-3}	1000
lb/in^3	kg m^{-3}	27679.9
mmHg	Pa	133.322
cal	J	4.1868
m	in	39.3701
cm	in	0.393701
cm^2	sq in	0.155
m^2	sq in	1550
m^2	sq ft	10.7639
m^3	cu in	61023.6
m^3	cu ft	35.3146
m^3	l(itre)	1000
m^3	gal(lon)	219.969
kg	lb	2.20462
kg m^{-3}	g cm^{-3}	0.001
kg m^{-3}	lb/in^3	0.0000363
Pa	mmHg	0.0075006
J	cal	0.238846

Sources

Appendix 1
Tables 1.1 to 1.8: from A. M. Giles and B. D. Ross (1983), Normal or reference values for biochemical data, *Oxford Textbook of Medicine* (edited by D. J. Weatherall, J. G. G. Ledingham, and D. A. Warrell).

Appendix 2
Adapted from D. J. Weatherall (1983), Introduction [to disease of the blood], *Oxford Textbook of Medicine*.

Appendix 3
Table 3.1: from W. P. T. James (1983), Obesity, *Oxford Textbook of Medicine*. Table 3.2: from World Health Organization (1979) Monograph (WHO/FAP/79.1), reproduced in W. P. T. James (1983), Obesity, *Oxford Textbook of Medicine*.

Appendix 4
Table 4.1: from R. Smith and D. H. Williamson (1983), Biochemical background [to nutrition], *Oxford Textbook of Medicine*. Tables 4.2, 4.3: from R. Smith and W. P. T. James (1983), Introduction [to nutrition], *Oxford Textbook of Medicine*.

Appendix 5
Tables 5.1, 5.2: from M. J. Goldacre and M. P. Vessey (1983), Health and Sickness in the Community, *Oxford Textbook of Medicine* (Table 5.2 derived from *Hospital Inpatient Enquiry*).

Appendix 6
From R. Doll and R. Peto (1983), Epidemiology of cancer, *Oxford Textbook of Medicine*.

Appendix 7
By courtesy of Knoll Pharmaceutical Co., New Jersey.